Fundamentals SUCCESS

NCLEX®-Style Q&A Review

FIFTH EDITION

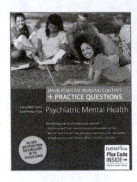 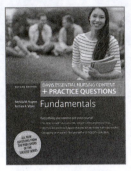 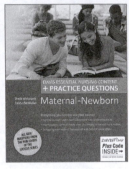 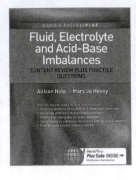 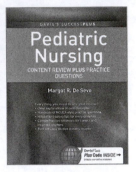

Fundamentals **SUCCESS**

NCLEX®-Style Q&A Review

FIFTH EDITION

Patricia M. Nugent, RN, MA, MS, EdD
Professor Emeritus
Adjunct Professor
Nassau Community College
Garden City, New York
Private Practice—President of Nugent Books, Inc.

Barbara A. Vitale, RN, MA
Professor Emeritus
Nassau Community College
Garden City, New York
Private Practice—Professional Resources for Nursing

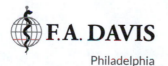

F.A. DAVIS

Philadelphia

F. A. Davis Company
1915 Arch Street
Philadelphia, PA 19103
www.fadavis.com

Copyright © 2019 by F. A. Davis Company

Printed in the United States of America

Last digit indicates print number: 10 9 8 7 6 5 4 3 2 1

Acquisitions Editor: Jacalyn Sharp
Senior Content Project Manager: Julia L. Curcio
Electronic Project Editor: Sandra A. Glennie
Design and Illustrations Manager: Carolyn O'Brien

ISBN: 978-0-8036-7745-6

Dedicated to

Joseph Vitale
and
Neil Nugent

For their love, support, sense of humor, enthusiasm for life,
and attempts to keep our compulsive natures under control.

Acknowledgments

Many people at F. A. Davis were essential to the production of this book. We want to thank Jacalyn Sharp, Acquisitions Editor, whose expertise in publishing was instrumental to the production of this edition. We especially thank Julia Curcio, Senior Content Project Manager, who always was available, answered every question, and supported and encouraged us throughout this project. We salute Mauri Loemker, Senior Project Manager, who managed every detail proficiently, kept us on track, and was never ruffled. Trumpets for Carolyn O'Brien, Design and Illustrations Manager, who skillfully implemented our line drawings and managed our illustrations with finesse. We would like to acknowledge the efforts of Will Welsh, Development Manager, for his expert review of the diversity and spirituality content, and to Linda Conheady, copy editor, who was phenomenal with the details of grammar and content. In addition, we want to thank Bob Butler, Production Manager, who ensured that this project progressed from a manuscript to a book and Sandra A. Glennie, Electronic Project Editor, for her efforts on our behalf.

We want to express our appreciation to Lera Salmon, Marketing Coordinator, and the F. A. Davis sales consultants, who have done a spectacular job of highlighting the strengths of our texts to nursing faculty. Special recognition goes to all the nursing students and faculty who participated in field-testing sessions and focus groups for their commitment to excellence and generosity in sharing their time, energy, and intellect. This input helped us to fine-tune the content and its presentation.

Finally, and most importantly, we thank our husbands, Joseph and Neil, for their love and support, which were essential to the revision of this book. They are loved and appreciated by us.

A Message to Nursing Educators

Nurses are required to use critical thinking in every domain of nursing practice.

- Accrediting bodies of educational programs have increased the emphasis on maximizing the cognitive abilities of learners.
- Licensing examinations are designed to evaluate the test taker's ability to engage in clinical reasoning.
- Agency accrediting bodies have developed standards that require creative, evidence-based practice.
- Health care, health-care environments, and technology have increased in complexity, requiring sophisticated health-care practitioners.

The premise of this book is based on the beliefs that:

- People use critical thinking all the time in their daily lives.
- People can enhance their critical-thinking skills.
- Students can use critical-thinking skills when taking a nursing examination.
- Nurses continue to use critical thinking in their professional lives.

How can nursing educators help students think critically?

- Help students develop their critical-thinking abilities through the information contained in Chapter 1.
- Help students identify and develop their cognitive and personal competencies by exploring the Helix of Critical Thinking.
- Support students who are maximizing their critical-thinking abilities by their being positive, reflective, inquisitive, and creative.
- Help students use the RACE Model, a formula for applying critical thinking, when answering nursing questions.
- Encourage students to practice test taking by answering the questions and reviewing the answers and their rationales in Chapters 2 through 5 to:
  - Reinforce what they know.
  - Learn new information.
  - Identify what still needs to be learned.
  - Set priorities for future learning.
- Have students practice answering alternate-format questions (e.g., exhibit, multiple-response, drag and drop [ordered response], hot-spot, fill-in-the-blank, and items using a chart, table, or graphic image) presented in Chapter 6. This practice allows test takers to develop critical-thinking skills in relation to questions that authentically evaluate unique nursing interventions (e.g., calculations, setting priorities, and analyzing data from multiple sources).
- Have students practice taking a comprehensive examination with integrated fundamental content gleaned from subunits of nursing information. Chapter 7, Comprehensive Final Book Exam, has a 100-item integrated examination. The RACE Model is applied to every question on this 100-item examination. This approach role-models the clinical reasoning that can be employed when one is answering a nursing test question.

- Encourage students to review the keywords at the beginning of each clinical subunit in Chapters 2 through 5. Knowing the definition of these words and understanding concepts and principles associated with them will build a theoretical base for answering the questions in the content area.
- Encourage students, particularly those who speak English as a second language, to learn the words in the Glossary of English Words Commonly Encountered on Nursing Examinations. This will allow students taking a test to concentrate on nursing content rather than being distracted by a lack of comprehension of English words.
- Encourage students to practice answering nursing questions on the computer. Students who purchase this book will have a free 30-day access to a comprehensive review question platform, *Davis Edge for NCLEX-RN®*. This platform includes thousands of NCLEX-style questions.

A Message to Nursing Students

If you are similar to the average nursing student, you study assigned chapters in your textbook, read articles in nursing journals and on the Internet, review your classroom notes, complete computer instruction programs related to nursing content, practice nursing skills in a simulated laboratory, and apply in the clinical area what you have learned. All these activities are excellent ways for you to expand and strengthen your theoretical base and become a safe practitioner of nursing. However, these activities may not be enough for you to be successful when taking a nursing examination. You must practice test taking as early as possible in your program of study with questions appropriate for your level of nursing education. In addition, you must be aware of, strengthen, and expand your cognitive competencies (intellectual reasoning skills) and personal competencies (individual attitudes or qualities) reflected in the **Helix of Critical Thinking** and then utilize these components of critical thinking when answering nursing questions.

Nursing students keep making the same statements:

- I need more examples of nursing test questions, especially alternate-format items.
- I need to practice taking nursing examinations on the computer.
- I need to learn how to answer a nursing test question.
- **I need to pass my nursing examinations!**

This book addresses these needs.

WHY YOU SHOULD READ THIS TEXTBOOK

FEATURES

BENEFITS

FEATURES	BENEFITS
This book contains more than 1,200 fundamentals of nursing questions. The emphasis is on the thinking process levels of application and analysis.	Reviewing the rationales for every question will: • Reinforce what you know—this increases trust in your ability and promotes a sense of security. • Teach you new information—this increases your knowledge and builds self-confidence. • Identify what you still need to learn—this focuses and prioritizes your study activities so that the return on your effort is maximized.
Every question has the rationales for the correct and the incorrect answers.	Practicing answering questions will enhance your critical-thinking skills, promote your self-confidence, build your stamina when taking tests, and reduce your test anxiety—and it should increase your test performance.
Chapter 1 • A discussion of maximizing your critical-thinking abilities is presented, including the attitudes and qualities of successful critical thinkers and strategies to overcome barriers to critical thinking.	• An exploration of your critical-thinking abilities should motivate you to maintain a positive mental attitude and be reflective, inquisitive, and creative when thinking.

Continued

Continued

• The levels of thinking processes (e.g., knowledge, comprehension, application, and analysis) are explored. Several questions addressing similar nursing content are carried across these levels to demonstrate the progression from a simple, concrete level of thinking (e.g., remembering or understanding information) to a complex, abstract level of thinking (e.g., using or scrutinizing information). • The **RACE Model** is introduced and applied to a variety of increasingly complex sample questions.	• Your understanding of the levels of thinking processes will enable you to identify what level of thinking is required to answer a question. This will influence which strategies to use to answer the question. • When you use the RACE Model to critically analyze a question and answer it correctly, you will feel empowered, your test anxiety will decrease, and your test performance should improve.
Chapters 2 through 5 • Questions are grouped into content areas common to fundamentals of nursing courses. • A keyword list is provided at the beginning of each unit of nursing content. These lists include vocabulary and nursing/medical terminology essential to the content of nursing.	• Practicing answering questions that are grouped by nursing content permits a focused study of related information when preparing for a unit examination in your nursing curriculum. • Focusing on critical words expands your theoretical base and provides a strong foundation for more advanced concepts.
Chapter 6 Each type of alternate-format item is introduced, followed by several examples. Thirty-six percent of the questions (446) in the book are alternate-format items. 33—Exhibit items 25—Hot-spot items 37—Illustration/graphic items 56—Drag and drop items 36—Fill-in-the-blank items 259—Multiple-response items	• Practicing answering these questions will help to reduce anxiety concerning alternate-format questions encountered on examinations and increase your ability to identify the correct answer.
Chapter 7 • This chapter contains a 100-item Comprehensive Final Book Exam. • The RACE Model and rationales for the correct and incorrect answers are included with each question.	• Taking this test provides an opportunity to experience an examination with information presented from a variety of units of study within a nursing curriculum. • Reviewing the application of the RACE Model to every question should encourage you to develop similar critical-thinking skills when answering test questions.
Glossary A glossary is included that identifies and defines ordinary English words that appear frequently in nursing examinations.	Familiarity with these words reduces the challenge of a test question because you can center your attention on the theoretical content presented in the question.

Continued

Davis Edge	
Davis Edge Students can access on the Internet a comprehensive review platform that contains thousands of nursing questions. *Davis Edge's* offerings include:	
• Test-taking strategies and tips	• Test-taking strategies and tips will expand your cognitive and personal competencies, which should increase your critical-thinking abilities.
• Progressive quizzing	• Progressive quizzing allows you to customize quizzes to your level of knowledge. You can progressively receive more difficult questions or different content areas to challenge you to reach higher levels of understanding.
• Test builder	• The test builder lets you design comprehensive tests that reflect content and alternate-format items from client needs categories in the same proportions as NCLEX® examinations. Practicing test taking increases knowledge, stamina, and self-confidence.
• Rationales for correct and incorrect answers	• Rationales help you to analyze options critically and understand why an option is correct or incorrect. A review of rationales helps you attain and reinforce a comprehensive body of fundamental nursing information.
• Self-grading	• This provides immediate feedback, which is motivating and identifies areas of content that requires additional study.

To increase your knowledge of fundamentals of nursing theory and be successful on nursing examinations, it is important for you to use this book—*Fundamentals Success: NCLEX® Style Q & A Review, Fifth Edition.* Although this book is valuable for all nursing students regardless of their level of nursing education, it is essential for beginning nursing students. The related knowledge, attitudes, and skills that you develop early in your fundamental nursing courses influence your present and future educational performance. A house will stand and survive only when it is built on a strong foundation. The same concept can be applied to your nursing education. The components of a strong foundation in nursing are a comprehensive understanding of the fundamentals of nursing theory, well-developed critical-thinking abilities, and an inventory of strategies for successful test taking.

Another textbook you may find helpful toward maximizing your success when preparing for and taking examinations in nursing is *Test Success: Test-Taking Techniques for Beginning Nursing Students* (Nugent & Vitale, F. A. Davis Company). This book focuses on empowerment, critical thinking, study techniques, the multiple-choice question, the nursing process, test-taking techniques, testing formats other than multiple-choice questions (including alternate formats on NCLEX® examinations), and computer applications in education and evaluation. It also contains hundreds of fundamentals of nursing questions, of which 44% are alternate-format items. Every question has the rationales for correct and incorrect answers and test-taking techniques when appropriate. It includes a 100-item Comprehensive Final Book Exam.

We are firm believers in the old sayings, "You get out of it what you put into it!" and "Practice makes perfect!" The extent of your learning, the attitudes you develop, and the skills you acquire depend on the energy you are willing to expend. It is our belief that if you give this book your best effort, you will strengthen and expand your theoretical foundation of fundamentals of nursing and your critical-thinking abilities in testing situations. We expect your efforts to be rewarded with success on your nursing examinations!

Table of Contents

Fundamentals of Critical Thinking Related to Test Taking

INTRODUCTION

To prepare for writing this chapter, we did what all writers should do. We performed a detailed search of the literature about critical thinking, we reviewed all the significant materials that related to test taking or nursing practice, and we wrote an outline for a comprehensive discussion of critical thinking in relation to nursing examinations. The introductory section of the chapter was to be titled "The Historical Perspective of Critical Thinking." When we typed the chapter heading and reread it, we had written "Hysterical" instead of "Historical." Because we have a relatively good sense of humor and the ability to laugh at ourselves, our response was peals of laughter. We realized that this was a Freudian slip! Loosely defined, a *Freudian slip* occurs when unconscious mental processes result in a verbal statement that reflects more accurately the true feelings of the speaker than does the originally intended statement. Being true believers in the statement that *all behavior has meaning*, we could not continue until we explored why we wrote what we wrote.

When we looked up the word *hysterical* in the dictionary, its definitions were *an uncontrollable outburst of emotion* or *out of control* and *extremely comical* or *hilarious*. Associating the word "hysterical" with the concept of critical thinking raised two thoughts. Are we overwhelmed, frantic, and out of control when considering the relationship between critical thinking and nursing, or do we find this relationship funny, comical, and hilarious? If you feel overwhelmed, frenzied, or out of control when considering critical thinking, carefully read the section in this chapter titled *Be Positive: You Can Do It!* When we personalized the word "hysterical" to our own experiences, we recalled that when we believe that something is funny, our internal communication is, "Isn't that hysterically funny?" So, now we were faced with the task of exploring why we thought reviewing the historical perspective of critical thinking was so funny or why it could be overwhelming. We actually spent several hours pursuing this goal. At the completion of this process, we arrived at three conclusions:

- The words "critical thinking" are just buzzwords. *Critical thinking* is a skill that we all possess uniquely, and we use this skill routinely in all the activities of our daily living. It is funny to profess that critical thinking is something new and different.
- Who cares about the historical perspectives of critical thinking! Information about the abstract topic of critical thinking must be presented in a manner in which the information learned today can be implemented tomorrow.
- Feelings of being overwhelmed can be conquered because critical-thinking abilities can be enhanced.

Definition of Critical Thinking

As we sat back and reflected on our morning's work in relation to Alfaro-LeFevre's (1995) definition of critical thinking, we recognized and appreciated that we had been thoroughly involved with critical thinking. We had:

- Engaged in purposeful, goal-directed thinking.
- Aimed to make judgments based on evidence (fact) rather than conjecture (guesswork).

- Employed a process based on principles of science (e.g., problem solving, decision making).
- Used strategies (e.g., metacognition, reflection, Socratic questioning) that maximized our human potential and compensated for problems caused by human nature.

Critical thinking is a cognitive strategy by which you reflect on and analyze your thoughts, actions, and decisions. Critical thinking often is integrated into traditional linear processes. Linear processes usually follow a straight line, with a beginning and a product at the end. Some linear-like processes, such as the nursing process, are considered cyclical because they repeat themselves. Some formal reasoning processes include the following:

- **Problem Solving** involves identifying a problem, exploring alternative interventions, implementing selected interventions, and arriving at the end product, which is a solution to the problem.
- **Decision Making** involves carefully reviewing significant information, using methodical reasoning, and arriving at the end product, which is a decision.
- **Diagnostic Reasoning** involves collecting information, correlating the collected information to standards, identifying the significance of the collected information, and arriving at the end product, which is a conclusion or nursing diagnosis.
- **The Scientific Method** involves identifying a problem to be investigated, collecting data, formulating a hypothesis, testing the hypothesis through experimentation, evaluating the hypothesis, and arriving at the end product, which is acceptance or rejection of the hypothesis.
- **The Nursing Process** involves collecting information (Assessment); determining significance of information (Analysis); identifying priorities, goals, expected outcomes, and nursing interventions (Planning); carrying out nursing interventions (Implementation/Intervention); and assessing the client's response to interventions and comparing the actual outcomes with expected outcomes (Evaluation), ultimately to arrive at the end product of meeting a person's needs.

Each of these methods of manipulating and processing information incorporates critical thinking. They all are influenced by intellectual standards, such as being focused, methodical, deliberate, logical, relevant, accurate, precise, clear, comprehensive, creative, and reflective. It is helpful to incorporate critical thinking into whatever framework or structure that works for you.

The purpose of this discussion is to impress on you that you:

- Use critical thinking in your personal life.
- Will continue to use critical thinking in your professional life.
- Should enhance your critical-thinking abilities when studying.
- Can use critical-thinking skills when taking a nursing examination.

In an attempt to make the abstract aspects of critical thinking more concrete, we have schematically represented our concept of critical thinking by the **Helix of Critical Thinking.** In Figure 1-1, the Helix of Critical Thinking has been unwound and enlarged so that the components of the cognitive competencies and personal competencies can be viewed easily. The *cognitive competencies* are the intellectual or reasoning processes employed when thinking. The *personal competencies* are the characteristics or attitudes of the individual thinker. These lists of competencies represent the cognitive abilities or personal qualities commonly associated with critical thinkers. No one possesses all of these competencies, and you may identify competencies that you possess that are not on these lists. The lists are not all-inclusive. Make lists of your own cognitive and personal competencies. Your lists represent your repertoire or inventory of thinking skills. As you gain knowledge and experience, your lists will expand. The more cognitive and personal competencies you possess, the greater your potential to think critically.

The Helix of Critical Thinking, when wound (Fig. 1-2), demonstrates the integration of cognitive competencies and personal competencies essential to thinking critically. Not all of these competencies are used in every thinking situation. You can pick or choose from them

Cognitive Competencies	Personal Competencies
Dissect	Thinking independently
Modify	Tolerant of ambiguity
Analyze	Self-confident
Interpret	Open-minded
Examine	Accountable
Correlate	Courageous
Synthesize	Persevering
Investigate	Imaginative
Recall facts	Disciplined
Categorize	Risk taking
Summarize	Committed
Understand	Inquisitive
Demonstrate	Motivated
Self-examine	Confident
Translate data	Reflective
Query evidence	Objective
Make inferences	Authentic
Manipulate facts	Assertive
Present arguments	Intuitive
Establish priorities	Rational
Make generalizations	Creative
Compare and contrast	Humble
Determine significance	Curious
Determine implications	Honest
Determine consequences	Moral

Figure 1–1. The Helix of Critical Thinking is schematically elongated to demonstrate the components of cognitive competencies and personal competencies. The more cognitive competencies and personal competencies a person possesses, the greater the potential the person has to think critically.

as from a smorgasbord when you are confronted with situations that require critical thinking. Initially, you may have to stop and consciously consider what cognitive competencies (i.e., intellectual skills) or personal competencies (i.e., abilities, attitudes) to use. As you gain knowledge and experience and move toward becoming an expert critical thinker, the use of these competencies will become second nature. The Helix will contract or expand depending on the competencies you use in a particular circumstance. In addition, there is constant interaction among cognitive competencies, among personal competencies, and between cognitive competencies and personal competencies.

The interactive nature of the Helix of Critical Thinking and the Nursing Process is demonstrated in Figure 1-3. **The Nursing Process is a critical thinking framework that involves assessing and analyzing human responses to plan and implement nursing care that meets client needs as evidenced by the evaluation of client outcomes.** The

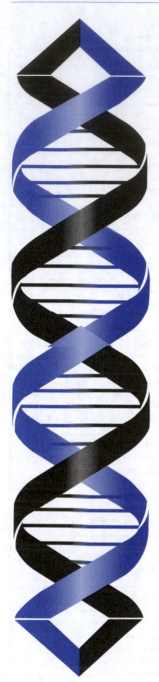

Figure 1–2. The Helix of Critical Thinking demonstrates the interwoven relationship between cognitive competencies and personal competencies essential to thinking critically. Throughout the thinking process, there is constant interaction among cognitive competencies, among personal competencies, and between cognitive and personal competencies.

Nursing Process provides a precise framework in which purposeful thinking occurs. Critical thinking is an essential component within, between, and among the phases of the Nursing Process. Different combinations of cognitive and personal competencies may be used during different phases of the Nursing Process.

The interactive nature of the Helix of Critical Thinking and the Problem-Solving Process is demonstrated in Figure 1-4. **The Problem-Solving Process is a dynamic, linear process that has a beginning and an end, with a resolution of the identified problem.** It provides a progressive step-by-step method in which goal-directed thinking occurs. Critical thinking is an essential component within and between the steps of the Problem-Solving Process, and different combinations of cognitive and personal competencies may be used during the various steps involved.

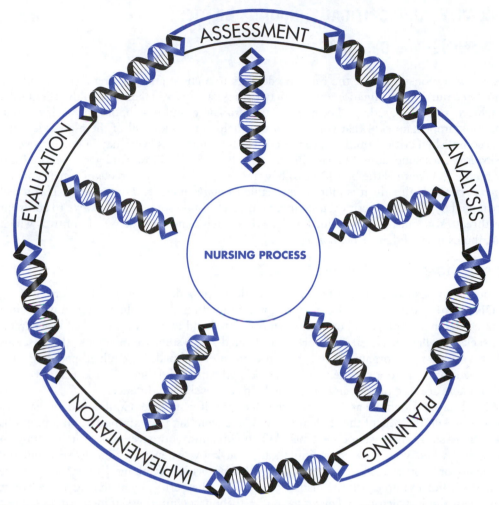

Figure 1–3. The interactive nature of the Helix of Critical Thinking within the Nursing Process. The Nursing Process is a dynamic, cyclical process in which each phase interacts with and is influenced by the other phases of the process. Critical thinking is an essential component within, between, and among phases of the Nursing Process. Different combinations of cognitive and personal competencies may be used during the different phases of the Nursing Process.

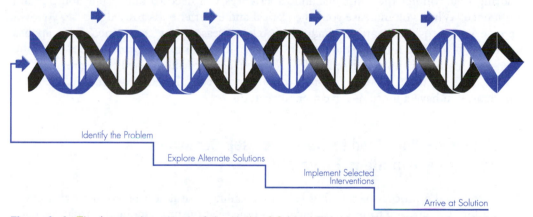

Figure 1–4. The interactive nature of the Helix of Critical Thinking within the Problem-Solving Process. The Problem-Solving Process is a dynamic, linear process that has a beginning and an end, with the resolution of the identified problem. Different combinations of cognitive and personal competencies may be used during the different steps of the Problem-Solving Process.

MAXIMIZE YOUR CRITICAL-THINKING ABILITIES

Be Positive: You Can Do It!

Assuming responsibility for the care one delivers to a client and desiring a commendable grade on a nursing examination raise anxiety because a lot is at stake: to keep the client safe; to achieve a passing grade; to become a nurse ultimately; and to support one's self-esteem. The most important skill that you can learn to help you achieve all of these goals is to be an accomplished critical thinker. We use critical-thinking skills every day in our lives when we explore these questions: "What will I have for breakfast?" "How can I get to school from my home?" "Where is the best place to buy my clothes?" Once you recognize that you are *thinking critically* already, it is more manageable to *think* about *thinking critically*. If you feel threatened by the idea of critical thinking, then you must do something positive to confront the threat. You must be disciplined and work at increasing your sense of control, which contributes to confidence! *You can do it!*

OVERCOME BARRIERS TO A POSITIVE MENTAL ATTITUDE

Supporting a positive mental attitude requires developing discipline and confidence.

Discipline is defined as self-command or self-direction. A disciplined person works in a planned manner, explores all options in an organized and logical way, checks for accuracy, and seeks excellence. When you work in a planned and systematic manner with conscious effort, you are more organized and therefore more disciplined. Disciplined people generally have more control over the variables associated with an intellectual task. Effective critical thinkers are disciplined, and discipline helps to develop confidence.

Confidence is defined as poise, self-reliance, or self-assurance. Confidence increases as one matures in the role of the student nurse. Understanding your strengths and limitations is the first step to increasing confidence. When you know your strengths, you can draw on them, and when you know your limitations, you know when it is time to seek out the instructor or another resource to help you with your critical thinking. Either way, you are in control! For example, ask the instructor for help when critically analyzing a case study, share with the instructor any concerns you have about a clinical assignment, and seek out the instructor in the clinical area when you feel the need for support. Failing to use your instructor is like putting your head in the sand. Learning needs must be addressed, not avoided. Although your instructor is responsible for your clinical practice and for stimulating your intellectual growth as a nursing student, you are the consumer of your nursing education. As the consumer, you must be an active participant in your own learning by ensuring that you get the assistance and experiences you need to build your abilities and confidence. When you increase your theoretical and experiential knowledge base, you will increase your sense of control, which ultimately increases your confidence. This applies not just to beginning nursing students but to every level of nursing practice because of the explosion in information and technology. When you are disciplined, you are more in control; when you are more in control, you are more confident; and when you are more confident, you have a more positive mental attitude.

Be Reflective: You Need to Take One Step Backward Before Taking Two Steps Forward!

Reflection is the process of thinking back or recalling a situation or event to rediscover its meaning. It helps you to seek and understand the relationships among information, concepts, and principles and to apply them in future clinical or testing situations. Reflection can be conducted internally as quiet, thoughtful consideration, in a one-on-one discussion with an instructor or another student, or in a group.

As a beginning nursing student, you are just starting to develop an experiential background from the perspective of a provider of nursing care. However, you have a wealth of experiences, personal and educational, that influence your development as a licensed nurse.

Your personal experiences include activities using verbal and written communication, such as delegating tasks to family members or coworkers, setting priorities for daily activities, using mathematics when shopping or balancing a checkbook, and so on. A nursing program of study incorporates courses from a variety of other disciplines, such as anatomy and physiology, chemistry, physics, psychology, sociology, reading, writing, mathematics, and informatics. Every experience is a potential valuable resource for future learning. Recognize the value of the "you" you bring to your nursing education and incorporate it into your reflective processes.

Engaging in reflection is a highly individualized mental process. One form of reflection is writing a journal. A **journal** is an objective and subjective diary of your experiences. It is a chronicle that includes cognitive learning, feelings, and attitudes, and it requires you actively to develop skills related to assessing, exploring the meaning of critical incidents, documenting, developing insights into thoughts and actions that comprise clinical practice, and evaluating. Journal writing is a rich resource that provides a written record of where you have been, where you are, and where you are going. It helps you to incorporate experiences into the development of your professional being. After an examination, explore your feelings and attitudes regarding the experience. Be honest with yourself. Did you prepare adequately for the test? Did you find the content harder or easier than content on another test? Were you anxious before, during, or after the test and, if so, was your anxiety low, medium, or high? What would a low score or a high score on the test mean to you? When you were confronted with a question that you perceived as difficult, how did you feel and how did you cope with the feeling? You do not necessarily have to ask yourself all of these questions. You should ask yourself those questions that have meaning for you.

Another form of reflection is making mental pictures. **Mental pictures** are visual images that can be recalled in the future. For example, when caring for a client who has Parkinson's disease, compare the client's signs and symptoms with the classic clinical manifestations associated with the disease. Then make a visual picture in your mind. Visualize the pill-rolling tremors, masklike face, drooling, muscle rigidity, and so on, so that in the future you can recall the visual picture rather than having to remember a memorized list of symptoms.

Retrospective (after the event) reflection involves seeking an understanding of relationships between previously learned information and the application of this information in client-care situations or testing experiences. This type of reflection helps you to judge your personal performance against standards of practice. A self-assessment requires the willingness to be open to identifying one's successful and unsuccessful interventions, strengths and weaknesses, and knowledge and lack of knowledge. The purpose of retrospective reflection is not to be judgmental or to second-guess decisions but rather to learn from the situation. The worth of the reflection depends on the abilities that result from it. When similar situations arise in subsequent clinical practice, previous actions that were reinforced or modified can be accessed to have a present successful outcome.

A *clinical postconference* is an example of retrospective reflection. Students often meet in a group (formally or informally) after a clinical experience to review the day's events. During the discussion, students have an opportunity to explore feelings and attitudes, consider interventions and alternative interventions, assess decision-making and problem-solving skills, identify how they and other students think through a situation, and so on. You also can review your own thinking when reviewing an experience with a client by speaking aloud what you were thinking. For example:

"When I went into the room to take my postoperative client's vital signs, I realized that the client had an IV in the right arm. I knew that if I took a blood pressure reading in the arm that had an IV, the reading could interfere with the IV, so I knew I had to take the blood pressure reading in the left arm. When I looked at my client, he looked very pale and sweaty. I got a little nervous, but I continued to get the other vital signs. I put the thermometer in the client's mouth and started to take his pulse. It was very fast, and I knew that this was abnormal, so I paid special attention to its rhythm and volume. It was very thready, but it was regular. The temperature and respirations were within the high side of the expected range."

A beginning nursing student may immediately respond by saying, "I don't know what is going on here, so I better take this information to my instructor." A more advanced student could say, "What could be happening? Maybe the client is bleeding or has an infection. I think I should inform my instructor, but I'll inspect the incision first."

When you review an experience such as this example, you can identify your thinking skills. Taking the blood pressure in the left arm and assessing the rate, rhythm, and volume of the pulse were habits because you did not have to figure out a new method when responding to the situation. Remembering the expected range for the various vital signs used the thinking skill of total recall because you memorized and internalized these values. Determining further assessments after obtaining the vital signs required inquiry. You collected and analyzed information and did not take the vital sign results at face value. You recognized abnormalities and gaps in information, collected additional data, considered alternative conclusions, and identified alternative interventions.

Another example of retrospective reflection is reviewing an examination. When reviewing each question, determine why you got a question wrong. For example, several statements you could make are:

- "I did not understand what the question was asking because of the English or medical vocabulary used in the question."
- "I did not know or understand the content being tested."
- "I knew the content being tested, but I did not apply it correctly in the question."

When a limited English or medical vocabulary prevents you from answering a question correctly, you must spend time expanding this foundation. A list of English words that appear repeatedly in nursing examinations is included in the glossary at the end of this textbook. In addition, nursing/medical keyword lists have been included in each content area in this textbook. You can use these word lists to review key terminology used in nursing-related topics. To expand your vocabulary, look up new words when studying, write flash cards for words you need to learn, and explore unfamiliar words with which you are confronted on tests.

When you answered a question incorrectly because you did not understand the content, make a list so that you can design a study session devoted to reviewing this information. This study session should begin with a brief review of what you do know about the topic (5 minutes or less). Then your efforts should be devoted to studying what you identified as what you need to know. You should do this after reviewing every test. This exercise is based on the axiom *Strike while the iron is hot*. The test is over, so your anxiety level is reduced, and how nursing-related content is used in a test question is fresh in your mind. Study sessions that are goal directed tend to be more focused and productive.

When you know the content being tested but have applied the information incorrectly, it is an extremely frustrating experience. However, do not become discouraged. It is motivating to recognize that you actually know the content! Your next task is to explore how to tap into your knowledge successfully. Sometimes restating or summarizing what the question is asking places it into your own perspective, which helps to clarify the content in relation to the test question. Also, you can view the question in relation to specific past experiences or review the information in two different textbooks to obtain different perspectives on the same content. Another strategy to reinforce your learning is to use the left page of your notebook for taking class notes and leave the facing page blank. After an examination, use the blank page to make comments to yourself about how the content was addressed in test questions or add information from your textbook to clarify class notes. How to review thinking strategies in relation to cognitive levels of nursing questions is explored later in this chapter.

Examine your test-taking behaviors. For example, if you consistently changed your initial answers on a test, it is wise to explore what factors influenced you to change your answers. In addition, determine how many questions were converted to either right or wrong answers. The information you collect from this assessment should influence your future behaviors. If you consistently changed correct answers to incorrect answers, you should examine the factors that caused you to change your answers. If you identify a thinking process that consistently led you to change a correct answer to an incorrect answer, you may want to consider abandoning this type of thinking. If you are unable to identify the thinking process that consistently led you to change a correct answer to an incorrect answer, you may decide to not change any answers until you determine what thinking process made you question your initial answer. If you changed incorrect answers to correct answers, you should identify what thinking process was used to arrive at your second choice so that you can use it the first time you look at a question.

Reflection is an essential component of all learning. How can you know where you are going without knowing where you have been? Therefore, to enhance your critical-thinking abilities, you must *take one step backward before taking two steps forward!*

OVERCOME BARRIERS TO EFFECTIVE REFLECTION

Reflecting on your knowledge, strengths, and successes is easy, but reflecting on your lack of knowledge, weaknesses, and mistakes takes courage and humility. **Courage** is the attitude of confronting anything recognized as dangerous or difficult without avoiding or withdrawing from the situation. Courage is necessary because when people look at their shortcomings, they tend to be judgmental and are their own worst critics. This type of negativity must be avoided because it promotes defensive thinking, interferes with the reception of new information, and limits self-confidence.

Humility is having a modest opinion of one's own abilities. Humility is necessary because it is important to admit your limitations. Only when you identify what you do and do not know can you make a plan to acquire the knowledge necessary to be successful on nursing examinations and practice safe nursing care. Arrogance or a "know-it-all" attitude can interfere with maximizing your potential. For example, when reviewing examinations with students, the students who benefit the most are the ones who are willing to listen to their peers or instructor as to why the correct answer is correct. The students who benefit the least are the ones who consistently and vehemently defend their wrong answers. A healthy amount of inquiry, thoughtful questioning, and not accepting statements at their face value are important critical-thinking competencies; however, self-righteous or obstructionist attitudes more often than not impede, rather than promote, learning.

Be Inquisitive: If You Don't Go There, You'll Never Get Anywhere!

To **inquire** means to question or investigate. The favorite words of inquisitive people are *what, where, when,* and, more importantly, *how, why, if … then,* and *it depends.* When studying, ask yourself these words to delve further into a topic under consideration. The following are examples:

- You raise the head of the bed when a client is short of breath. You recognize that this intervention will facilitate respirations. Ask yourself the question, "*How* does this intervention facilitate respirations?" The answer could be, "Raising the head of the bed allows the abdominal organs to drop by gravity, which reduces pressure against the diaphragm, which, in turn, permits maximal thoracic expansion."
- You insert an indwelling urinary catheter and are confronted with the decision as to where to place the drainage bag. Ask yourself *what* questions. "*What* will happen if I place the drainage bag on the bed frame?" The answer could be, "Urine will flow into the drainage bag by gravity." "*What* will happen if I place the drainage bag on an IV pole?" The answer could be, "Urine will remain in the bladder because the IV pole is above the level of the bladder and fluid does not flow uphill, and if there is urine in the bag, it will flow back into the bladder."
- When palpating a pulse, you should use gentle compression. Ask yourself the question, "*Why* should I use gentle compression?" The answer could be, "Gentle compression allows you to feel the pulsation of the artery and prevents excessive pressure on the artery that will cut off circulation and thus obliterate the pulse."

- The textbook says that in emergencies nurses should always assess the airway first. Immediately ask, "*Why* should I assess the airway first?" There may be a variety of answers. "In an emergency, follow the ABCs (Airway, Breathing, and Circulation) of assessment, which always begin with the airway. Maslow's Hierarchy of Needs identifies that physiological needs should be met first. Because an airway is essential for the passage of life-sustaining gases in and out of the lungs, this is the priority." Although all of these responses answer the question *why*, only the last answer really provides an in-depth answer to the *why* question. If your response to the original *why* question raises another *why* question, you need to delve deeper. "*Why* do the ABCs of assessment begin with the airway?" "*Why* should physiological needs be met first?"

- When talking with a client about an emotionally charged topic, the client begins to cry. You are confronted with a variety of potential responses. Use the method of *if … then* statements. *If … then* thinking links an action to a consequence. For example, *if* I remain silent, *then* the client may refocus on what was said. *If* I say, "You seem very sad," *then* the client may discuss the feelings being felt at the time. *If* I respond with an open-ended statement, *then* the client may pursue the topic in relation to individualized concerns. After you explore a variety of courses of action with the *if … then* method, you should be in a better position to choose the most appropriate intervention for the situation.

- You will recognize that you have arrived at a more advanced level of critical thinking when determining that your next course of action is based on the concept of *it depends*. For example, a client suddenly becomes extremely short of breath, and you decide to administer oxygen during this emergency. When considering the amount and route of delivery of the oxygen, you recognize that *it depends*. You need to collect more data. You need to ask more questions, such as, "Is the client already receiving oxygen? Does the client have chronic obstructive pulmonary disease? Is the client a mouth breather? What other signs and symptoms are identified?" The answers to these questions will influence your choice of interventions.

When exploring the *what, where, when, how, why, if … then*, and *it depends* methods of inquiry, you are more likely to arrive at appropriate inferences, assumptions, and conclusions that will ensure effective nursing care.

These same techniques of inquiry can be used when practicing test taking. Reviewing questions that have rationales is an excellent way to explore the reasons for correct and incorrect answers. When answering a question, state why you think your choice is the correct answer and why you think each of the other options is an incorrect answer. This method encourages you to focus on the reasons why you responded in a certain way in a particular situation. It prevents you from making quick judgments before exploring the rationales for your actions. After you have done this, compare your rationales with the rationales for the correct and incorrect answers that are provided. Are your rationales focused, methodical, deliberate, logical, relevant, accurate, precise, clear, comprehensive, creative, and reflective? This method of studying not only reviews nursing content but also fosters critical thinking and applies critical thinking to test taking.

During or after the review of an examination, these techniques of inquiry also can be employed, particularly with those questions you got wrong. Although you can conduct this review independently, it is more valuable to review test questions in a group. Your peers and the instructor are valuable resources you should use to facilitate your learning. Different perspectives, experiential backgrounds, and levels of expertise can enhance your inquiry. Be inquisitive. *If you don't go there, you'll never get anywhere.*

OVERCOME BARRIERS TO BEING INQUISITIVE

Effective inquiry requires more than just a simplistic, cursory review of a topic. Therefore, critical thinkers must have curiosity, perseverance, and motivation. **Curiosity** is the desire to learn or know and is a requirement to delve deeper into a topic. If you are uninterested in or apathetic about a topic, you are not going to go that extra mile. Sometimes you may have to "psych yourself up" to study a particular topic. Students frequently say they are overwhelmed by topics such as fluids and electrolytes, blood gases, or chest tubes. As a result, they develop a minimal understanding of these topics and are willing to learn by trial and error in the clinical area or surrender several questions on an examination. Never be willing to let a lack of knowledge be the norm, because this results in incompetence and an unsafe nursing care provider. Overcome this attitude by maximizing your perseverance.

Perseverance means willingness to continue in some effort or course of action despite difficulty or opposition. Critical thinkers never give up until they obtain the information that satisfies their curiosity. To perform a comprehensive inquiry when studying requires time. Make a schedule for studying at the beginning of the week and adhere to it. This prevents procrastination later in the week when you may prefer to rationalize doing something else and postpone studying. In addition, studying 1 hour a day is more effective than studying 7 hours in 1 day. Breaks between study periods allow for the processing of information, and they provide time to rest and regain focus and concentration. The greatest barrier to perseverance is a deadline. When working under a time limit, you may not have enough time to process and understand information. The length of time to study for a test depends on the amount and type of content to be tested and how much previous studying has been done. If you study 2 hours every day for 2 weeks during a unit of instruction, a 1-hour review may be adequate for an examination addressing this content. If you are preparing for a comprehensive examination for a course at the end of the semester, you may decide to study 3 hours a night for 1 to 2 weeks. If you are studying for a National Council Licensure Examination (NCLEX), you may decide to study 2 hours a day for 3 months. Only you can determine how much time you need to study or prepare for a test. Perseverance can be enhanced by the use of motivation strategies.

Motivation strategies inspire, prompt, encourage, or instigate you to act. For example, divide the information to be learned into segments and set multiple short-term goals for studying. Cross a segment off the list after you reach a goal. Also, this is the time to use incentives. Reward yourself after an hour of studying. Think about how proud you will be when you earn an excellent grade on the examination. Visualize yourself walking down the aisle at graduation or working as a nurse during your career. Incentives can be more tangible (e.g., eating a snack, reading a book for 10 minutes, playing with a child, or doing anything that strikes your fancy). You should identify the best pattern of studying that satisfies your needs; use motivation techniques to increase your enthusiasm, and then draw on your determination to explore in depth the *what, where, when, how, why, if … then*, and *it depends* of nursing practice.

Be Creative: You Must Think Outside the Box!

Creative people are imaginative, inventive, innovative, resourceful, original, and visionary. To find solutions beyond common and standardized procedures or practices, you must be creative. Creativity is what allows you to be yourself and individualize the nursing care you provide to each client. With the explosion of information and technology, the importance of thinking creatively will increase in the future because the "old" ways of doing things will be inadequate. No two situations or two people are ever alike. Therefore, *you must think outside the box!*

OVERCOME BARRIERS TO CREATIVITY

It is difficult to think outside the box when you are not willing to color outside the lines! To be creative, you must be open-minded, have independence of thought, and be a risk taker. Being **open-minded** requires you to consider a wide range of ideas, concepts, and opinions before framing an opinion or making judgments. You must identify your opinions, beliefs, biases, stereotypes, and prejudices. We all have them to one extent or another, so do not deny them. However, they must be recognized, compartmentalized, and not imposed on clients. Unless these attitudes are placed in perspective, they will interfere with critical thinking. In every situation, you must remain open to all perspectives, not just your own. When you think that your opinion is the only right opinion, you are engaging in egocentric thinking. *Egocentric thinking* is based on the belief that the world exists or can be known only in relation to the individual's mind. This rigid thinking creates a barrier around your brain that obstructs the inflow of information, imaginative thinking, and the outflow of innovative ideas. An example of an instance in which you have been open-minded is one in which you have changed your mind after having had a discussion with someone else. The new information persuaded you to think outside of your original thoughts and opinions.

Independence of thought means the ability to consider all the possibilities and then arrive at an autonomous conclusion. To do this, you need to feel comfortable with ambiguity. *Ambiguous* means having two or more meanings and is therefore being uncertain, unclear, indefinite, and vague. For example, a nursing student may be taught by an instructor to establish a sterile field for a sterile dressing change by using the inside of the package of the sterile gloves. When following a sterile dressing change procedure in a clinical skills book, the directions may state to use a separate sterile cloth for the sterile field. When practicing this procedure with another student, the other student may open several 4 × 4 gauze packages and leave them open as their sterile fields. As a beginning nursing student, this concept is difficult to understand because of a limited relevant knowledge base and experiential background. Frequently, thinking is concrete and follows rules and procedures, is black and white, or is correct or incorrect. It takes knowledge and experience to recognize that you have many options and may still follow the principles of sterile technique. Remember, "There is more than one road to Rome!"

To travel a different path requires taking risks. *Risk* in the dictionary means the chance of injury, damage, or loss. However, **risk taking** in relation to nursing refers to considering all the options, eliminating potential danger to a client, and acting in a reasoned, logical, and safe manner when implementing unique interventions. Being creative requires intellectual stamina and a willingness to go where no one has been before. Risk takers tend to be leaders, not followers. The greatest personal risk of creativity is the blow to the ego when confronted with failure. However, you must recognize that throughout your nursing career you will be faced with outcomes that are successful as well as those that are unsuccessful. How you manage your feelings with regard to each, particularly those that are unsuccessful, will influence your willingness to take future creative risks. Successful outcomes build confidence. Unsuccessful outcomes should not be defeating or prevent future creativity when appropriately examined. The whole purpose of evaluation in the nursing process is to compare and contrast client outcomes with expected outcomes. If expected outcomes are not attained, the entire process must be reexamined and then reperformed. You must recognize that:

- Unsuccessful outcomes do occur.
- Unsuccessful outcomes may not be a reflection of your competence.
- The number of successful outcomes far outnumbers the number of unsuccessful outcomes.

When you accept these facts, then you may feel more confident to take risks with your creativity.

CRITICAL THINKING APPLIED TO TEST TAKING

Educational Domains

Nursing as a discipline includes three domains of learning—affective, psychomotor, and cognitive. The **affective domain** is concerned with attitudes, values, and the development of appreciations. An example of nursing care in the affective domain is the nurse quietly accepting a client's statement that there is no God without the nurse imposing personal beliefs on the client. The **psychomotor domain** is concerned with manipulative or motor skills related to procedures or physical interventions. An example of nursing care in the psychomotor domain is the nurse administering an intramuscular injection to a client. The **cognitive domain** is concerned with recall, recognition of knowledge, comprehension, and the development and application of intellectual skills and abilities. An example of nursing care in the cognitive domain is the nurse clustering collected information and determining its significance.

Components of a Multiple-Choice Question

A multiple-choice question is called an **item.** Each item has two parts. The **stem** is the part that contains the information that identifies the topic and its parameters and then asks a question. The second part consists of one or more possible responses, which are called **options.** One of the options is the **correct answer,** and the others are wrong answers (also called **distractors**).

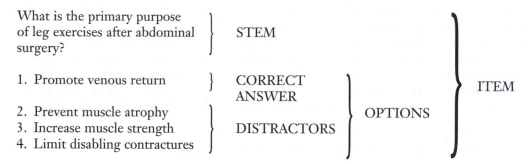

Cognitive Levels of Nursing Questions

Questions on nursing examinations reflect a variety of thinking processes that nurses use when caring for clients. These thinking processes are part of the cognitive domain, and they progress from the simple to the complex, from the concrete to the abstract, and from the tangible to the intangible. Four major types of thinking processes are represented by nursing questions:

- **Knowledge-Level Questions,** in which the emphasis is on recalling remembered information.
- **Comprehension-Level Questions,** in which the emphasis is on understanding the meaning and intent of remembered information.
- **Application-Level Questions,** in which the emphasis is on remembering understood information and utilizing the information in new situations.
- **Analysis-Level Questions,** in which the emphasis is on comparing and contrasting a variety of elements of information.

CRITICAL-THINKING STRATEGY TO ANSWER NURSING QUESTIONS: THE RACE MODEL

Answering a test question is like participating in a race. Of course, you want to come in first and be the winner. However, the thing to remember about a race is that success is based not just on speed but also on strategy and tactics. The same is true about success on nursing examinations. Although speed may be a variable that must be considered when taking a timed test so that the amount of time spent on each question is factored into the test strategy, the emphasis should be on the use of critical-thinking strategies to answer test questions. The RACE model presented here is a critical-thinking strategy to use when answering nursing questions. If you follow the RACE model every time you examine a test question, its use will become second nature. This methodical approach will improve your abilities to analyze a test question critically and will improve your chances of selecting the correct answer.

The RACE model has four steps to answering a test question:

R - *Recognize keywords.*

A - *Ask what the question is asking.*

C - *Critically analyze every option in relation to the question and the other options.*
  - Critically scrutinize *every* option in relation to the information in the stem.

- Critically identify a rationale for *every* option.
- Critically compare and contrast *every* option in relation to the information in the stem and its significance in relation to the other options.

E - **Eliminate incorrect options.**
- *Eliminate* one option at a time.
- *Eliminate* as many incorrect options as possible.

The following discussion explores this critical-thinking strategy in relation to the thinking processes represented in nursing test questions. Thoughtfully read the *Cognitive Requirements* under each type of question (e.g., Knowledge, Comprehension, Application, and Analysis). It is important to understand this content to apply the critical-thinking strategies inherent in each type of cognitive-level question. In addition, three sets of sample test questions are presented to demonstrate the increasing complexity of thinking reflected in the various cognitive levels focusing on specific fundamentals of nursing content. Also, each cognitive level includes the RACE model applied to an alternate-type item.

Knowledge-Level Questions: Remember Information!

Knowledge is information that is filed or stored in the brain. It represents the elements essential to the core of a discipline. In nursing, this information consists of contents such as terminology, steps of procedures, expected laboratory values, classifications of medications, expected ranges of vital signs, and common human responses. A knowledge-level question does not require complex understanding, comparative analysis, or application skills; it requires only recall of information. The information is recalled or recognized in the form in which it was originally learned and requires no alteration from one use or application to another because it is concrete. This information is the foundation of critical thinking. You must have adequate, accurate, relevant information on which to base your more theoretical, abstract thinking.

Beginning nursing students find knowledge-level questions the easiest because they require the recall or regurgitation of information. Information may be memorized, which involves repeatedly reviewing information to place it and keep it in the brain. Information also can be committed to memory through repeated experiences with the information. Repetition is necessary because information is forgotten quickly unless reinforced. When answering knowledge-level questions, you either know the information or you don't. The challenge of answering knowledge-level questions is defining what the question is asking and tapping your knowledge. See our textbook *Test Success: Test-Taking Techniques for Beginning Nursing Students* (F.A. Davis) for specific study techniques related to knowledge-level questions.

USE THE RACE MODEL TO ANSWER KNOWLEDGE-LEVEL QUESTIONS

1. Which is the classification of the medication docusate sodium?
    1. Stool softener
    2. Cardiac glycoside
    3. Histamine-2 antagonist
    4. Calcium channel blocker

IMPLEMENT THE RACE MODEL: A CRITICAL-THINKING STRATEGY

Recognize keywords.	Which is the **classification** of the medication **docusate sodium**?
Ask what the question is asking.	What category of medication is docusate sodium?
Critically analyze each option in relation to the question and the other options.	The words in the stem that indicate that this is a knowledge-level question are *which* and *classification*. Recall the classification of each drug listed in the question. Identify which one is the stool softener and which ones are not. **Rationales:** 1. **Docusate sodium is a stool softener. Stool softeners are medications that promote the elimination of fecal material. Water is pulled into the intestinal lumen, resulting in a softer fecal mass.** 2. Docusate sodium is not a cardiac glycoside. Cardiac glycosides increase cardiac output by decreasing the heart rate and strengthening cardiac contractions. 3. Docusate sodium is not a histamine-2 antagonist. Histamine-2 antagonists are medications that inhibit histamine at histamine-2 receptor sites in the parietal cells in the stomach, which reduces gastric acid secretion. 4. Docusate sodium is not a calcium channel blocker. Calcium channel blockers are medications that inhibit calcium ion influx across cell membranes during cardiac depolarization. They dilate coronary and peripheral arteries, relax coronary vascular smooth muscles, and slow sinoatrial/atrioventricular node conduction time.
Eliminate incorrect options.	If you know the classification or physiological action of one or more of the incorrect options, you can reduce the number of options from which to identify the correct answer. Because options 2, 3, and 4 are not the names of the classification of docusate sodium, they can be eliminated.

2. Which is the description of the interviewing technique of paraphrasing?
  1. Condensing a discussion into an organized review
  2. Asking the client to elaborate on a previous comment
  3. Restating what the client has said by using similar words
  4. Asking goal-directed questions concentrating on key concerns

IMPLEMENT THE RACE MODEL: A CRITICAL-THINKING STRATEGY

Recognize keywords.	Which is the **description** of the interviewing technique of **paraphrasing**?
Ask what the question is asking.	How is the interviewing technique of paraphrasing implemented?
Critically analyze each option in relation to the question and the other options.	The words in the stem that indicate that this is a knowledge-level question are *which* and *description*. Recall and compare the characteristics of paraphrasing and the other interviewing techniques to the statements in the options. **Rationales:** 1. Reviewing a discussion is known as summarizing, not paraphrasing. 2. Asking a client to elaborate on a previous comment or unclear message is known as clarifying, not paraphrasing. **3. Paraphrasing, or restating a client's message, is an interviewing skill in which the nurse listens for a client's basic message and then repeats the content in similar words. This validates information from the client without changing the meaning of the statement and provides an opportunity for the client to hear what was said.** 4. Asking goal-directed questions that concentrate on key concerns is known as focusing, not paraphrasing.
Eliminate incorrect options.	Recalling the characteristics of other interviewing techniques can help eliminate incorrect options. Options 1, 2, and 4 are not examples of paraphrasing and can be eliminated.

3. What is another name for a decubitus ulcer?
   1. Skin tear
   2. Pressure ulcer
   3. Surface abrasion
   4. Penetrating wound

IMPLEMENT THE RACE MODEL: A CRITICAL-THINKING STRATEGY

Recognize keywords.	What is **another name** for a **decubitus ulcer**?
Ask what the question is asking.	What is an alternate name for a decubitus ulcer?
Critically analyze each option in relation to the question and the other options.	The words in the stem that indicate that this is a knowledge-level question are *what* and *another name*. Recall the description of or visualize a decubitus ulcer. Now recall the description of or visualize the wound in each option. The description or visualization of the wound in the correct option should match that of a decubitus ulcer. **Rationales:** 1. A skin tear is not a decubitus ulcer. A skin tear is a break in the continuity of thin, fragile skin caused by friction or shearing force. 2. **Pressure ulcer is another name for decubitus ulcer. A pressure ulcer is impaired skin (reddened area, sore, or lesion characterized by sloughing of tissue) over a bony prominence that is caused by pressure that interferes with the delivery of oxygen to body cells.** 3. An abrasion is not a decubitus ulcer. An abrasion is the scraping or rubbing away of the superficial layers of the skin. 4. A penetrating wound is not a decubitus ulcer. A penetrating wound occurs when a sharp object pierces the skin and injures underlying tissues.
Eliminate incorrect options.	Knowing the descriptions of various types of wounds will help to eliminate incorrect options. Options 1, 3, and 4 are not other names for a decubitus ulcer and can be eliminated.

4. Which is the name of this type of syringe?
1. Piston
2. Insulin
3. Intradermal
4. Subcutaneous

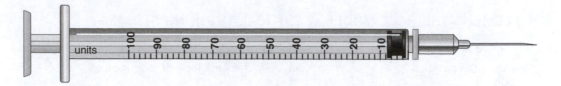

IMPLEMENT THE RACE MODEL: A CRITICAL-THINKING STRATEGY

Recognize keywords.	Which is the **name** of **this** type of **syringe**?
Ask what the question is asking.	Identify the name of the type of syringe that is marked in units and depicted in the illustration?
Critically analyze each option in relation to the question and the other options.	The words in the stem that indicate that this is a knowledge-level question are *which* and *name*. To answer this question, you must identify that the syringe in the illustration is an insulin syringe. This question does not require complex understanding, comparative analysis, or application skills; it requires only recall of the name of this type of syringe. **Rationales:** 1. This is not an illustration of a syringe used for irrigating a wound. Generally, a piston syringe that can contain up to 50 mL of solution is used to irrigate a wound; it has a tip to which a catheter can be attached. **2. This is an illustration of an insulin syringe. It is a U-100 syringe marked in units, of which there are 100 units per mL.** 3. This is not an illustration of a syringe used to administer a medication via the intradermal route. Generally, a 1-mL tuberculin syringe marked in 0.01 mL (1/100th of a milliliter) and minims (16 minims is equal to 1 mL) is used to administer a medication via the intradermal route. 4. This is not an illustration of a syringe that is used to administer a medication via the subcutaneous route. Generally, a 3-mL standard syringe marked in whole milliliters and 0.1 mL (1/10th of a milliliter) with a ⅝-, ½-, or 1-inch length needle is used to administer a medication into subcutaneous tissue.
Eliminate incorrect options.	Because options 1, 3, and 4 are not the names of the type of syringe depicted in the illustration, they can be eliminated.

Comprehension-Level Questions: Understand Information!

Comprehension is the ability to understand that which is known. To be safe practitioners, nurses must understand information such as reasons for nursing interventions, physiology and pathophysiology, consequences of actions, and responses to medications. To reach an understanding of information in nursing, you must be able to translate information into your own words to personalize its meaning. Once information is rearranged in your own mind, you must interpret the essential components for their intent, corollaries, significance, implications, consequences, and conclusions in accordance with the conditions described in the original communication. The information is manipulated within its own context without being used in a different or new situation.

Beginning nursing students generally consider comprehension-level questions slightly more difficult than knowledge-level questions but less complicated than application-level and analysis-level questions. Students often try to deal with comprehension-level information by memorizing the content. For example, when studying local signs and symptoms of an infection, students may memorize the following list: heat, erythema, pain, edema, and exudate. Although this can be done, it is far better to understand why these adaptations occur. Erythema and heat occur because of increased circulation to the area. Edema occurs because of increased permeability of the capillaries. Pain occurs because the accumulating fluid in the tissue presses on nerve endings. Exudate occurs because of the accumulation of fluid, cells, and other substances at the site of infection. The mind is a wonderful machine, but unless you have a photographic memory, lists of information without understanding often become overwhelming and confusing. The challenge of answering comprehension-level questions is to understand the information. See our textbook *Test Success: Test-Taking Techniques for Beginning Nursing Students* for specific study techniques related to comprehension-level questions.

USE THE RACE MODEL TO ANSWER COMPREHENSION-LEVEL QUESTIONS

5. How does the medication docusate sodium facilitate defecation?
  1. Softens stool
  2. Forms a bulk residue
  3. Irritates the intestinal wall
  4. Dilates the intestinal lumen

IMPLEMENT THE RACE MODEL: A CRITICAL-THINKING STRATEGY

Recognize keywords.	**How** does the medication **docusate sodium facilitate defecation**?
Ask what the question is asking.	How does docusate sodium work in the body to promote the passage of stool?
Critically analyze each option in relation to the question and to the other options.	The words in the stem that indicate this is a comprehension-level question are *how* and *facilitate*. You should scrutinize each option to identify whether the description in the option correctly explains *how* or *why* docusate sodium works to facilitate defecation. **Rationales:** **1. Docusate sodium softens and delays the drying of feces by lowering the surface tension of water, permitting water and fat to penetrate the feces.** 2. Bulk-forming laxatives, such as psyllium hydrophilic mucilloid, increase the fluid, gaseous, or solid bulk in the intestines. 3. Irritants or stimulants, such as bisacodyl, irritate the intestinal mucosa or stimulate intestinal wall nerve endings, which precipitates peristalsis. 4. Large-volume enemas, not medications, enlarge the lumen of the intestine, which precipitates peristalsis.
Eliminate incorrect options.	Options 2, 3, and 4 do not accurately describe the therapeutic action of docusate sodium and can be eliminated. Knowing the therapeutic action of the other medications may help you eliminate incorrect options.

6. How does the interviewing technique of paraphrasing promote communication?
   1. Requires clients to defend their points of view
   2. Limits clients from continuing a rambling conversation
   3. Allows clients to take their conversations in any desired direction
   4. Offers clients an opportunity to develop a clearer idea of what they said

IMPLEMENT THE RACE MODEL: A CRITICAL-THINKING STRATEGY

Recognize keywords.	**How** does the interviewing technique of **paraphrasing promote communication**?
Ask what the question is asking.	How does paraphrasing encourage communication?
Critically analyze each option in relation to the question and to the other options.	The words in the stem that indicate that this is a comprehension-level question are *how* and *promote*. You should scrutinize each option to identify whether the description in the option correctly explains the consequence of using paraphrasing as a communication technique. **Rationales:** 1. Requiring clients to defend their points of view describes the results of challenging statements that usually are barriers to communication. 2. Limiting clients from continuing a rambling conversation describes one purpose of the interviewing skill of focusing, which is the use of questions or statements to center on one concern mentioned within a wordy, confusing conversation. 3. Allowing clients to take their conversations in any desired direction is the purpose of open-ended questions or statements. **4. Paraphrasing involves actively listening for the client's concerns, which are then restated by the nurse in similar words. This intervention conveys that the nurse has heard and understood the message and gives the client an opportunity to review what was said.**
Eliminate incorrect options.	Options 1, 2, and 3 do not accurately describe how paraphrasing works to promote communication and can be eliminated. You do not have to know how other interviewing skills work to facilitate communication to answer the question correctly. However, this information may help you eliminate incorrect options.

7. Why does turning clients every 2 hours prevent pressure ulcers from developing?
   1. Promotes muscle contractions, increasing the basal metabolic rate of the body
   2. Relieves weight on capillaries, allowing oxygen to reach peripheral body cells
   3. Keeps the extremities dependent, permitting blood to flow to distal cells by gravity
   4. Drops the organs in the abdominal cavity by gravity, relieving pressure against the diaphragm

IMPLEMENT THE RACE MODEL: A CRITICAL-THINKING STRATEGY

Recognize keywords.	**Why** does **turning** clients every 2 hours **prevent pressure ulcers** from developing?
Ask what the question is asking.	What are the physiological responses of the body to relieving pressure on body tissues?
Critically analyze each option in relation to the question and to the other options.	The words in the stem that indicate that this is a comprehension-level question are *why* and *prevent*. You should scrutinize each option to identify whether the description in the option correctly explains why turning a client relieves pressure and prevents a pressure ulcer. You also can use the strategy "If … then." If you change a client's position every 2 hours, then it will…! Recall your understanding about this issue and compare your "If … then" response to the options presented. **Rationales:** 1. Muscle contraction expends energy that raises the basal metabolic rate; however, this is unrelated to the development of pressure ulcers. **2. Capillary beds are compressed and blood flow is obliterated with excessive external pressure (12 to 32 mm Hg). Changing position removes the weight of the body off dependent areas, permitting blood to flow through the capillaries, thus supporting gaseous exchange at the cellular level.** 3. Blood flow to the extremities increases when the extremities are kept below the level of the heart; however, this is unrelated to the development of pressure ulcers. 4. Relieving pressure against the diaphragm by abdominal organs allows for greater thoracic expansion; however, this is unrelated to the development of pressure ulcers.
Eliminate incorrect options.	Options 1, 3, and 4 do not accurately explain why turning relieves pressure, thereby preventing a pressure ulcer, and can be eliminated. Understanding the concept of gravity in relation to options 1, 3, and 4 may help you eliminate these options because they are unrelated to pressure ulcer development in body tissues.

8. What is the purpose of administering a medication using a 45° angle and 1½-inch needle length as indicated in the illustration?
   1. Injects medication into a muscle
   2. Injects medication into intradermal tissue
   3. Injects medication into subcutaneous tissue
   4. Injects medication into the intravascular compartment

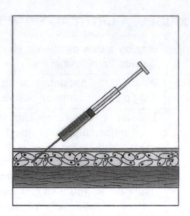

IMPLEMENT THE RACE MODEL: A CRITICAL-THINKING STRATEGY

Recognize keywords.	Which is the **purpose of administering** a medication using a 45° angle and 1½-inch needle length **as indicated in the illustration**?
Ask what the question is asking.	What tissue will be accessed when administering an injection using a 1½-needle at a 45° angle?
Critically analyze each option in relation to the question and to the other options.	The words in the stem that indicate that this is a comprehension-level question are *what* and *purpose*. To answer this question, you must know that when using a 1½-inch length needle at a 45° angle medication is injected into subcutaneous tissue. **Rationales:** 1. A muscle is not accessed via a 45° angle using a 1½-inch needle. A 90° angle of insertion is standard for administering medication via the intramuscular route. A muscle is below the level of subcutaneous tissue. A needle length of 1½ inches is necessary to reach muscle tissue in most adults, a 2-inch length needle is used to administer an intramuscular injection to an obese adult, and a 1-inch needle length is used when administering an intramuscular injection in the deltoid muscle. 2. The area below the epidermis is not accessed via a 45° angle using a 1½-inch needle. A 15° angle of insertion is used to administer medication via the intradermal route. **3. This is an illustration of a medication injected via the subcutaneous route. A syringe with a 1½-inch needle inserted at a 45° angle ensures that medication is injected into subcutaneous tissue and not into a muscle or intradermal tissue.**

Continued

	4. A vein is not accessed via a 45° angle using a 1½-inch needle. The intravascular route requires administration of a medication directly into a vein. This can be accomplished by adding medication to a large-volume bag of intravenous fluid, a single dose of medication mixed with a small volume of fluid in its own intravenous bag via secondary tubing attached to a current primary intravenous line (Piggyback) or via a Bolus (push) single dose of medication inserted directly into a primary line or venous access device.
Eliminate incorrect options.	Options 1, 2, and 4 can be eliminated because these routes inject medication into areas of the body other than subcutaneous tissue that is depicted in the illustration. If you know the names of the routes that require other than a 45° angle of insertion, such as option 1 (intramuscular—90° angle) or option 2 (intradermal—15° angle), you can eliminate these two options from consideration, thereby increasing your chances of selecting the correct answer.

Application-Level Questions: Use Information!

Application is the ability to use known and understood information in new situations. It requires more than just understanding information because you must demonstrate, solve, change, modify, or manipulate information in other than its originally learned form or context. With application-level questions, you are confronted with a new situation that requires you to recall information and manipulate the information from within a familiar context to arrive at abstractions, generalizations, or consequences regarding the information that can be used in the new situation to answer the question. Application-level questions require you to make rational, logical judgments.

Beginning nursing students frequently find application-level questions challenging because they require a restructuring of understood information into abstractions, commonalities, and generalizations, which are then applied to new situations. You do this all the time. Although there are parts of your day that are routine, every day you are exposed to new, challenging experiences. The same concept holds true for application-level questions. With application-level questions, you will be confronted by situations that you learned about in a book, experienced personally, relived through other students' experiences, or never heard about or experienced before. This will happen throughout your entire nursing career. The challenge of answering application-level questions is going beyond rules and regulations and using information in a unique, creative way. See our textbook *Test Success: Test-Taking Techniques for Beginning Nursing Students* for specific study techniques related to application-level questions.

USE THE RACE MODEL TO ANSWER APPLICATION-LEVEL QUESTIONS

9. A client reports not having had a bowel movement in 3 days. Which classification of drugs is helpful in relieving this problem?
1. Stool softener
2. Cardiac glycoside
3. Histamine-2 antagonist
4. Calcium channel blocker

IMPLEMENT THE RACE MODEL: A CRITICAL-THINKING STRATEGY

Recognize keywords.	A client reports **not having had a bowel movement** in 3 days. Which **classification** of **drugs** is **helpful** in **relieving** this problem?
Ask what the question is asking.	Which classification of drugs is most helpful in facilitating defecation, thus relieving constipation?
Critically analyze each option in relation to the question and to the other options.	The words in the stem that indicate that this is an application-level question are *helpful in relieving*. To choose which classification of drugs will be most helpful in relieving this client's problem, you must know that a client who has not had a bowel movement in 3 days may be constipated, the therapeutic action and outcome of various classifications of drugs, and which classification of drugs would be helpful in relieving constipation. **Rationales:** 1. **Docusate sodium is a stool softener. It increases water and fat penetration of feces, which softens the stool.** 2. Cardiac glycosides increase the force of cardiac contractions, which increases the cardiac output (positive inotropic effect), and decreases electrical conduction in the heart, which decreases the heart rate (negative chronotropic effect). Docusate sodium is not a cardiac glycoside. 3. Histamine-2 antagonists inhibit histamine at histamine-2 receptor sites in parietal cells, and this inhibits gastric acid secretion. Docusate sodium is not a histamine-2 antagonist. 4. Calcium channel blockers inhibit calcium ion influx across cell membranes during cardiac depolarization. They relax coronary vascular smooth muscles, dilate coronary and peripheral arteries, and slow sinoatrial/atrioventricular node conduction times. Docusate sodium is not a calcium channel blocker.
Eliminate incorrect options.	Because options 2, 3, and 4 are unrelated to facilitating the passage of stool, they can be eliminated. You do not have to know the expected outcome of the drug classifications in the incorrect options to answer the question correctly. However, if you know this information, it may help you eliminate these options.

10. A client scheduled for major surgery, who is perspiring and nervously picking at the bed linen, says, "I don't know if I can go through with this surgery." The nurse responds, "You'd rather not have surgery now?" Which interviewing technique was used by the nurse?
1. Focusing
2. Reflection
3. Clarification
4. Paraphrasing

IMPLEMENT THE RACE MODEL: A CRITICAL-THINKING STRATEGY

Recognize keywords.	A client scheduled for major surgery, who is perspiring and nervously picking at the bed linen, says, "I don't know if I can go through with this surgery." The nurse responds, **"You'd rather not have surgery now?" Which** interviewing **technique was used** by the nurse?
Ask what the question is asking.	What interviewing technique is being used by the nurse when the nurse says in response to the client, "You'd rather not have surgery now?"
Critically analyze each option in relation to the question and to the other options.	The words in the stem that indicate that this is an application-level question are *which interviewing technique was used*. To identify which technique was used by the nurse, you have to understand the elements of a paraphrasing statement, and you must recognize a paraphrasing statement when it is used. **Rationales:** 1. The example in the stem is not using focusing because the client's statement was short and contained one message that was reiterated by the nurse. Focusing is used to explore one concern among many statements made by the client. 2. The example in the stem is not using reflection because the nurse's statement is concerned with the content, not the underlying feeling, of the client's statement. An example of reflection is, "You seem anxious about having major surgery." 3. The example in the stem is not using clarification. When clarification is used, the nurse is asking the client to further explain what is meant by the client's statement. An example of clarification is, "I am not quite sure that I know what you mean when you say you would rather not have surgery now." **4. The nurse used paraphrasing because the client's and nurse's statements contain the same message but are expressed with different words.**
Eliminate incorrect options.	Options 1, 2, and 3 can be eliminated because these techniques are different from the technique portrayed in the nurse's response in the stem. It is helpful to understand the elements of the other interviewing techniques because it will help you eliminate incorrect options.

11. A nurse identifies that a client on prolonged bedrest may be developing a pressure ulcer. Which color of the skin over a bony prominence supports this conclusion?
1. Red
2. Blue
3. Black
4. Yellow

IMPLEMENT THE RACE MODEL: A CRITICAL-THINKING STRATEGY

Recognize keywords.	A nurse identifies that a client on prolonged bedrest may be **developing a pressure ulcer. Which color of** the **skin** over a **bony prominence** supports this conclusion?
Ask what the question is asking.	Which skin color is a sign of a beginning pressure ulcer?
Critically analyze each option in relation to the question and to the other options.	The words in the stem that indicate that this is an application-level question are *identifies* and *developing a pressure ulcer*. To answer this question, you have to understand how and why pressure can cause an ulcer and know a common early sign that indicates the beginning of a pressure ulcer. **Rationales:** 1. **Erythema is a red discoloration generally caused by local vasodilation in an attempt to bring more oxygen to the area. Red skin is a sign of a developing pressure ulcer.** 2. Cyanosis is a bluish color caused by an increased amount of deoxygenated hemoglobin associated with hypoxia, not pressure. 3. Eschar generally appears black and is the scab or dry crust that results from death of tissue. This is a late, not early, sign of a pressure ulcer. 4. Jaundice is a yellow-orange color caused by increased deposits of bilirubin in tissue, not a response to pressure.
Eliminate incorrect options.	Options 2, 3, and 4 are not signs of a pressure ulcer and are incorrect answers. It is helpful to know what is happening when the skin reflects each of the colors indicated in the options so that you can eliminate incorrect answers.

12. A client has a prescription for regular insulin coverage before meals. The prescription states to administer regular insulin based on blood glucose results.

150 to 175 mg/dL: 2 units
176 to 225 mg/dL: 4 units
226 to 275 mg/dL: 6 units
276 mg/dL or more: notify primary health-care provider

The client's blood glucose level before breakfast is 177 mg/dL. How many units of regular insulin should the nurse administer? **Record your answer using a whole number.**

Answer: _____ units

IMPLEMENT THE RACE MODEL: A CRITICAL-THINKING STRATEGY

Recognize keywords.	A client has a prescription for regular insulin coverage before meals. The prescription states to administer regular insulin based on blood glucose results. **150 to 175 mg/dL: 2 units** **176 to 225 mg/dL: 4 units** **226 to 275 mg/dL: 6 units** **276 mg/dL or more: notify primary health-care provider** The client's **blood glucose level** before breakfast is **177 mg/dL. How many units of regular insulin should the nurse administer?** Record your answer using a **whole number.** Answer: _____units
Ask what the question is asking.	How many units of regular insulin should the nurse administer when the client's blood glucose level is 177 mg/dL?
Critically analyze each option in relation to the question and to the other options.	The words in the stem that indicate that this is an application-level question are *how many units* and *should administer*. A fill-in-the-blank question does not have several options within the question. Generally, you have to insert the information contained in the question into a mathematical formula to manipulate the information to arrive at an answer. However, this fill-in-the-blank item does not require a formula to answer the question. You have to compare the client's glucose level of 177 mg/dL with the regular insulin prescription to arrive at the correct answer. **Rationale: Answer: 4 units. The client's glucose level is 177 mg/dL. The prescription for regular insulin indicates that if the client's glucose level is 176 to 225 mg/dL, the client should receive 4 units of regular insulin.**
Eliminate incorrect options.	Because the client's glucose level is 177 mg/dL, the other parameters for glucose levels and their accompanying regular insulin doses can be eliminated.

Analysis-Level Questions: Scrutinize Information!

Analysis is the separation of an entity into its constituent parts and examination of their essential features in relation to each other. Analysis-level questions assume that you know, understand, and can apply information. They ask you to engage in higher-level critical-thinking strategies. To answer analysis-level questions, you first must examine each element of information as a separate entity. Second, you need to investigate the differences among the various elements of information. In other words, you must compare and contrast information. Third, you must analyze the structure and organization of the compared and contrasted information to arrive at a conclusion or answer. Analysis-level questions often ask you to set priorities and in the stem frequently use words such as *first, initially, best, priority,* and *most important.*

Beginning nursing students find analysis-level questions the most difficult to answer. Analysis-level questions demand scrutiny of individual elements of information as well as require identification of differences among elements of information. Sometimes students cannot identify the structural or organizational relationship of elements of information. The challenge of answering analysis-level questions is performing a complete scrutiny of all the various elements of information and their interrelationships without overanalyzing or "reading into" the questions. See our textbook *Test Success: Test-Taking Techniques for Beginning Nursing Students* for specific study techniques related to analysis-level questions.

USE THE RACE MODEL TO ANSWER ANALYSIS-LEVEL QUESTIONS

13. A frail, malnourished older adult has been experiencing constipation. Which medication does the nurse anticipate that the primary health-care provider will **most** likely prescribe?
    1. Bisacodyl
    2. Mineral oil
    3. Docusate sodium
    4. Magnesium hydroxide

IMPLEMENT THE RACE MODEL: A CRITICAL-THINKING STRATEGY

Recognize keywords.	A **frail, malnourished older adult** has been experiencing **constipation.** Which **medication** does the nurse anticipate that the primary health-care provider will **most likely prescribe?**
Ask what the question is asking.	Which medication that promotes defecation is most appropriate for a debilitated older adult?
Critically analyze each option in relation to the question and the other options.	Analysis-level questions often ask you to set priorities, as indicated by the words *most likely prescribe* in the stem of this question. This question requires you to understand that frail, malnourished older adults have minimal compensatory reserve in various body systems to manage responses to cathartics and laxatives; know the physiological action, outcome, side effects, and toxic effects of all four medications presented in the item; and contrast and compare the drugs and the risks they pose in the older adult to arrive at which drug would be the most appropriate for this client. **Rationales:** 1. Bisacodyl irritates the intestinal mucosa, stimulates nerve endings in the wall of the intestines, and causes rapid propulsion of waste from the body. Bisacodyl is not the best choice of a laxative for an older adult because it can cause intestinal cramps, fluid and electrolyte imbalances, and irritation of the intestinal mucosa. 2. Mineral oil lubricates feces in the colon; however, it can inhibit the absorption of fat-soluble vitamins and is not the best medication to promote defecation in a malnourished older adult. **3. Docusate sodium permits fat and water to penetrate feces, which soften stool. Of all the options, docusate sodium has the fewest side effects in malnourished older adults.**

Continued

	4. Magnesium hydroxide draws water into the intestine by osmosis, which stimulates peristalsis. It is contraindicated for a malnourished older adult because it can cause fluid and electrolyte imbalances and inhibit absorption of fat-soluble vitamins.
Eliminate incorrect options.	Options 1, 2, and 4 are more potent than the correct answer and therefore are least likely to be prescribed to relieve constipation in a debilitated older adult. Because you must compare and contrast the drugs in the options presented, the more you know about these medications, the more options you may be able to eliminate, increasing your chances of selecting the correct answer.

14. The mother of a terminally ill child says, "I never thought that I would have such a sick child." Which is the **best** initial response by the nurse?
    1. "How do you feel right now?"
    2. "What do you mean by sick child?"
    3. "Life is not fair to do this to a child."
    4. "A sick child is something you never expected."

IMPLEMENT THE RACE MODEL: A CRITICAL-THINKING STRATEGY

Recognize keywords.	The mother of a terminally ill child says, "I never thought that I would have such a sick child." What is the **best initial response** by the nurse?
Ask what the question is asking.	Which is an example of the best interviewing technique to use when initially responding to a statement made by the mother of a terminally ill child?
Critically analyze each option in relation to the question and the other options.	Analysis-level questions often ask you to set priorities, as indicated by the words *best initial response* in the stem of this question. To answer this question, you need to identify which interviewing techniques are portrayed in the statements in each option; understand how and why each interviewing skill works; compare and contrast the pros and cons of each technique if used in this situation; and identify which technique is the most supportive, appropriate, and best initial response by the nurse. **Rationales:** 1. Direct questions cut off communication and should be avoided. 2. This response focuses on the seriousness of the child's illness, which is not the issue raised in the mother's statement. 3. This statement reflects the beliefs and values of the nurse, which should be avoided. **4. This is a declarative statement that paraphrases the mother's comment. It communicates to the mother that the nurse is listening attentively and invites the mother to expand on her thoughts if she feels ready.**
Eliminate incorrect options.	Options 1, 2, and 3 can be eliminated because they do not focus on the content of the mother's statement.

15. Which client has the highest risk for developing a pressure ulcer?
  1. An older adult on bedrest
  2. A toddler learning to walk
  3. A thin young woman in a coma
  4. An emotionally unstable middle-age man

IMPLEMENT THE RACE MODEL: A CRITICAL-THINKING STRATEGY

Recognize keywords.	Which client has the **highest risk** for **developing** a **pressure ulcer**?
Ask what the question is asking.	Which client with an associated age and health issue is at the greatest risk for a pressure ulcer?
Critically analyze each option in relation to the question and to the other options.	Analysis-level questions often ask you to set priorities, as indicated by the words *highest risk* in the stem of this question. To answer this question, you need to know what major risk factors contribute to the development of a pressure ulcer, such as what age group is most vulnerable and what situations are associated with pressure ulcer development. Compare and contrast the four options and assign a level of risk to each of the individuals identified in the options. Once you complete this intellectual analysis, you will identify the individual at the highest risk. **Rationales:** 1. Although the skin of older adults is vulnerable to the development of pressure ulcers because of decreased subcutaneous fat, reduced thickness and vascularity of the dermis, and decreased sebaceous gland activity, older adults are still capable of changing position and moving around in bed, which relieves pressure on integumentary tissue. 2. A toddler learning to walk is not immobile. In addition, the skin of toddlers is supple and usually has adequate circulation, subcutaneous tissue, and hydration. A toddler may fall and develop bruises (contusions) or scrapes (abrasions), not pressure ulcers. **3. Of the options presented, a thin young woman in a coma is the most vulnerable for developing a pressure ulcer. A thin person has little protective subcutaneous fat over bony prominences, and a person in a coma is immobile and unable to move or turn purposefully. Immobility results in prolonged pressure, which interferes with the oxygen supply to peripheral body cells.** 4. Middle-age men usually do not exhibit the effects of aging on the integumentary system. In addition, emotionally unstable people are able to move and change positions, which permits circulation to the cells of the skin.
Eliminate incorrect options.	Individuals presented in options 1, 2, and 4 are at less of a risk for the development of pressure ulcers than a thin person who is immobile.

16. A client has a prescription for 20 units of NPH insulin and 6 units of regular insulin to be administered subcutaneously at 0800. Insert an arrow at the line on the barrel of the syringe to where the total insulin solution will fill the syringe.

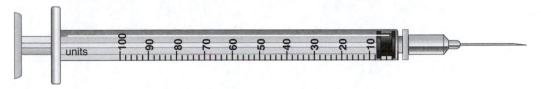

IMPLEMENT THE RACE MODEL: A CRITICAL-THINKING STRATEGY

Recognize keywords.	A client has a prescription for **20 units** of NPH insulin and **6 units** of regular insulin to be administered subcutaneously at 0800. **Insert an arrow** at the line on the **barrel of the syringe** where the **total insulin solution will fill the syringe**.
Ask what the question is asking.	What is the total amount of units of insulin to be administered, and where is this amount of solution on an insulin syringe?
Critically analyze each option in relation to the question and to the other options.	The words in the stem that indicate that this is an analysis-level, hot-spot question are *insert an arrow*. There are no options to consider in a hot-spot item. To answer this question, you must add the two doses of insulin (20 units + 6 units = 26 units) and then identify where the resulting single dose will be on the insulin syringe.
	Rationale: The prescription is for 20 units of NPH insulin and 6 units of regular insulin. These medications can be combined into one syringe. The total dose is 26 units (20 units of NPH insulin and 6 units of regular insulin). Each line on this insulin syringe represents 2 units of insulin. Therefore, the answer should indicate that the total solution of insulin will reach line 26 on the insulin syringe.
Eliminate incorrect options.	There are no incorrect options presented.

SUMMARY

Thinking about thinking is more strenuous than physical labor. A physical task is always easier if you use the right tool. This concept also is true for mental labor. A critical-thinking strategy, such as the RACE model, provides a methodical, analytical approach to answering questions in nursing. As with any strategy, it takes practice and experience to perfect its use. Therefore, you are encouraged to use this critical-thinking strategy when practicing test taking or reviewing examinations.

Nursing Within the Context of Contemporary Health Care

2

Theory-Based Nursing Care

KEYWORDS

The following words include nursing/medical terminology, concepts, principles, and information relevant to content specifically addressed in the chapter, or information associated with topics presented in it. English dictionaries, nursing textbooks, and medical dictionaries, such as *Taber's Cyclopedic Medical Dictionary,* are resources that can be used to expand your knowledge and understanding of these words and related information.

Actualization

Adaptive capacity

Beliefs

Critical time

Defense mechanism

Developmental task

Erikson, Erik—Personality Development

Freud, Sigmund—Psychoanalytic Theory

Gordon, Marjorie—Functional Health Patterns

Health

Health belief

Health-illness continuum

Homeostasis

Human behavior

Jung, Carl—Personality Theory

Kübler-Ross, Elisabeth—Stages of Grieving

Libido

Maslow, Abraham—Hierarchy of Basic Human Needs

Model

Moral development

Multiplicity of stressors

Philosophy of nursing

Piaget, Jean—Theory of Cognitive Development

Stress

Stressor (primary, secondary)

Theory

Values

Wellness

THEORY-BASED NURSING CARE: QUESTIONS

1. A nurse is considering the Faith Development Theory by James Fowler while assessing several clients. Which clients does the nurse expect to assume responsibility for their own beliefs about faith?
   1. Older adolescents
   2. Young adolescents
   3. Older school-age children
   4. Young school-age children

2. A nurse is caring for a group of clients. A client experiencing which of the following situations does the nurse anticipate will have the hardest time coping?
   1. Scheduled for a biopsy
   2. Unable to control the course of illness
   3. Challenged by a multiplicity of stressors
   4. Having to relocate to an assisted-living facility

3. A nurse inadvertently commits a medication error without the knowledge of other nursing team members. According to Freud, which part of the personality guides the nurse to initiate an Incident Report?
   1. Superego
   2. Libido
   3. Ego
   4. Id

4. Which statement does the nurse understand is **most** related to adaptations associated with the General Adaptation Syndrome?
   1. Adaptations depend on the nature of the stressor.
   2. Adaptations can be conscious or unconscious.
   3. Adaptations become secondary stressors.
   4. Adaptations are maladaptive responses.

5. A client with terminal cancer is willing to try new therapies. Which stage of Kübler-Ross Stages of Grieving does the nurse identify that the client is experiencing?
   1. Denial
   2. Depression
   3. Bargaining
   4. Acceptance

6. A nurse gives a client in a nursing home a choice about which color shirt to wear. Which level need, according to Maslow's Hierarchy of Needs, has the nurse just met?
   1. Self-esteem
   2. Physiological
   3. Safety and Security
   4. Love and Belonging

7. A nurse is assessing a child in relation to the stages of Jean Piaget's Theory of Cognitive Development. Which behavior indicates that the child has reached the Formal Operations stage of cognitive development according to Piaget?
   1. Utilizes deductive reasoning when examining alternatives
   2. Uses logical thought to organize collected information
   3. Investigates objects by placing them in the mouth
   4. Employs language to communicate with others

8. Which statement **best** reflects a principle common to all theories of health, wellness, and illness?
   1. A sense of well-being is synonymous with health.
   2. People are able to control factors that affect health.
   3. Many variables influence a person's perception of health.
   4. A person who is able to meet the demands of one's role is necessary for health.

9. According to Maslow, which characteristic is **least** associated with a person who is self-actualized?
   1. Is autonomous
   2. Is able to see the good in others
   3. Has the ability to problem-solve
   4. Has an external locus of control

10. Which concept identified by the nurse is basic to the health-illness continuum model?
    1. People can be both healthy and ill at the same time on the continuum.
    2. Actualization must be achieved to be on the healthy end of the continuum.
    3. When variables are balanced, people are in the exact center of the continuum.
    4. There is no distinct boundary between health and illness along the continuum.

11. A prospective nurse is being interviewed for a job by the nurse manager in an urgent care center. The nurse manager states that the facility adheres to a clinical model of health/illness. Which should the nurse anticipate will be expected of the nurses within this facility?
    1. Consider clients as holistic human beings.
    2. Make assessment of clients in the physiological domain.
    3. Identify the relationship between clients' beliefs and actions.
    4. Recognize if clients are able to perform their role within the family.

12. Which person is considered healthy when referring to the Role-Performance Model of Health?
    1. Coal miner who retires after acquiring black lung disease
    2. Coach who continues to coach after becoming a paraplegic
    3. Brick layer who takes a leave of absence while recovering from hernia surgery
    4. Police officer who sells alarm systems after leaving the force because of being shot while on duty

13. Freedom from which situation demonstrates a safety and security need in Maslow's Hierarchy of Human Needs?
    1. Pain
    2. Hunger
    3. Ridicule
    4. Loneliness

14. A nurse is caring for a client who was exposed to a stressful event. Which statement about the General Adaptation Syndrome should the nurse consider when caring for this client?
    1. A stressful event is an iatrogenic stress.
    2. An individual exposed to a stressful event will adapt in a unique way.
    3. A stressful event will precipitate an autonomic nervous system response.
    4. An individual exposed to a stressful event eventually will achieve homeostasis.

15. A nurse is facilitating a support group for people who are coping with the death of a significant other. Which client behavior reflects complicated grieving?
    1. Remarrying within 6 months after the death of a wife
    2. Being continuously angry 3 months after the death of a parent
    3. Exhibiting indicators of depression 9 months after the death of a husband
    4. Keeping a child's room unchanged for 4 years after the death of the child

16. A nurse identifies that love and belonging needs associated with Maslow's Hierarchy of Needs are related to which of Gordon's Functional Health Patterns?
    1. Values-belief pattern
    2. Role-relationship pattern
    3. Cognitive-perceptual pattern
    4. Sexuality-reproductive pattern

17. Which statement identifies a basic principle associated with Sigmund Freud and his work?
    1. The reality principle reflects a person's essential need for immediate gratification.
    2. Defense mechanisms are a common means of mainly conscious coping.
    3. The id controls the personality.
    4. No behavior is accidental.

18. Which concept about health do nurses need to appreciate?
1. Perceptions of health vary among cultures.
2. To be considered healthy, a person needs to be productive.
3. There must be an absence of illness for a person to be considered healthy.
4. Underlying consensus exists among theorists about the definition of health.

19. A nurse is caring for an immobilized client who was admitted to the hospital with a pressure ulcer. Which type of stressor precipitated the pressure ulcer?
1. Microbiological
2. Physiological
3. Chemical
4. Physical

20. The Health Belief Model attempts to explain and predict health behaviors and focuses on which of the following?
1. One's ability to fulfill one's assigned roles
2. Constructs associated with perceived threat and net benefit
3. Locus of control being important in one making choices about health behaviors
4. People moving along a continuum from health on one end to illness on the other end

21. A nurse is assessing a client who is experiencing prolonged stress. For which **most** serious complication should the nurse monitor the client?
1. Altered sleeping
2. Impaired immunity
3. Increased muscle tension
4. Decreased intestinal peristalsis

22. A nurse is analyzing information about a client. Which of the following does Maslow's Hierarchy of Needs theory help the nurse to identify?
1. Client's problem that has top priority
2. Developmental level of the client
3. Coping patterns of the client
4. Client's health beliefs

23. A nurse is teaching a course about death and dying to a community group. Which is **most** important for the nurse to teach parents about preparing a child for the death of a grandparent?
1. Wait until the child asks a question about the situation.
2. Have the child participate in mourning rituals.
3. Begin at the child's level of understanding.
4. Praise the child for being strong.

24. A nurse is assessing a client who experienced an emotional stress. Which **most** common response should the nurse anticipate the client will exhibit?
1. Anger
2. Denial
3. Anxiety
4. Depression

25. A nurse is assessing clients in the postanesthesia care unit. For which response to stress should the nurse monitor clients? **Select all that apply.**
1. _____ Dilated pupils
2. _____ Fast, bounding pulse
3. _____ Shorter response time
4. _____ Rapid, shallow breathing
5. _____ Increased muscle tension

26. Which nursing intervention **supports** a client with a problem in the Role-Relationship Pattern category of Gordon's Functional Health Patterns? **Select all that apply.**
    1. _____ Seeking the assistance of a spiritual advisor
    2. _____ Teaching the client self-care in preparation for going home
    3. _____ Referring a client to a self-help group to learn colostomy care
    4. _____ Assessing a family member's readiness to provide care in the home
    5. _____ Protecting a client from family members who disagree with the client's medical choices

27. A nurse is differentiating between primary and secondary stressors. Which stressor is an example of a secondary stressor? **Select all that apply.**
    1. _____ Pain
    2. _____ Tachycardia
    3. _____ Death of a spouse
    4. _____ Shortness of breath
    5. _____ Ingested microorganisms
    6. _____ Increased blood pressure

28. Of the clients presented, which client's level of wellness does the nurse determine **best** represents the placement of the X on Dunn's Health Grid?
    1. A healthy, active older adult who has an apartment in an independent living facility that provides daily meals, weekly housekeeping, and services such as activities, medical and dental care on-site, and banking available 2 days a week
    2. A person with a diagnosis of diabetes with a stable blood glucose who receives weekly visits from a public health nurse and has a home health aide who visits three mornings a week
    3. A person with a diagnosis of stage II-A lung cancer who lives in a men's shelter and who consistently misses clinic appointments
    4. A relatively healthy homeless person with a diagnosis of pneumonia and who is responding to medication

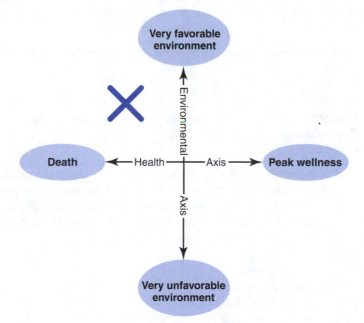

29. Which is an example of a health belief? **Select all that apply.**
1. _____ Eating foods that are low in fat
2. _____ Accepting grim results of diagnostic tests
3. _____ Engaging in physical exercise twice a week
4. _____ Recognizing that smoking can cause lung cancer
5. _____ Respecting a client's decision regarding therapeutic treatment

30. Which is an example of a response to a physiological stressor? **Select all that apply.**
1. _____ A sunburn after being outside all day
2. _____ Diarrhea after eating contaminated food
3. _____ Shortness of breath when walking up a hill
4. _____ A rapid heart rate during a final examination
5. _____ Excess fluid volume as a result of renal disease

31. The Kübler-Ross Stages of Grieving theory reflects a process that progresses through several stages to final acceptance. List these client statements in order according to the Kübler-Ross Stages of Grieving.
1. "I am going to get a second opinion."
2. "I find it so hard to think about the fact that I don't have long to live."
3. "I've never smoked in my life. I shouldn't be the one with lung cancer."
4. "I'll have the chemotherapy because I want to see my children grow up."
5. "I don't want a big funeral because I want people to remember me and be happy."

Answer: _____

32. A nurse is caring for a client recently diagnosed with advanced cancer. Which client statement reflects the Kübler-Ross stage of denial in the grief process? **Select all that apply.**
1. _____ "Why did this have to happen to me now?"
2. _____ "How could this happen when I quit smoking cigarettes?"
3. _____ "Maybe they mixed up my records with someone else's records."
4. _____ "I probably will not live long enough to see my children married."
5. _____ "What's the point in doing anything? They tell me I am going to die soon anyway."

33. Which word describes the concept of adaptive capacity? **Select all that apply.**
1. _____ Adjust
2. _____ Modify
3. _____ Change
4. _____ Etiology
5. _____ Remission
6. _____ Compliance

34. A nurse educator is conducting a class about child development for nurses. The nurse reviews the Stages of Moral Development Theory by Lawrence Kohlberg, emphasizing the reason an individual makes a moral decision in each of six stages. Place the following client statements in the order that reflects the motives for moral decisions as an individual progresses from stage one to stage six.
1. "I was following the rules."
2. "I did not want to get punished."
3. "I expected to receive a reward."
4. "I thought it was the right thing to do."
5. "I wanted others to see me as a good person."
6. "I was doing what is acceptable in our community."

Answer: _____

35. A nurse is caring for a newly admitted client. The nurse collects data and reviews the client's clinical record. Which level need is the **priority** for this client according to Maslow's Hierarchy of Needs?
1. Physiologic
2. Self-esteem
3. Safety and security
4. Love and belonging

CLIENT'S CLINICAL RECORD

Vital Signs
Temperature: 99.8°F, temporal
Pulse: 110 beats per minute
Respirations: 24 breaths per minute

Pain Assessment
Reports a pain level of 9 on a scale of 0 to 10
"Sharp, piercing pain"
Located in lower left abdomen
Pain started 3 days ago and became progressively worse

Social History
65-year-old female
Smokes one pack of cigarettes daily for 45 years
Drinks alcohol socially on weekends
Husband of 45 years died of colon cancer 1 year ago
States that she "misses him a lot"
Daughter wants her to move in with her, but client states she wants to remain independent
    because she is able to take care of herself
Participates in a sewing group at her church, making pillowcases for hospitalized
    children

1. 1. **Older adolescents and young adults assume responsibility for their own commitments, beliefs, and attitudes about faith. This reflects the individuative-reflective stage of faith development.**
   2. Young adolescents begin to examine life-guiding beliefs, values, and attitudes about faith. This reflects the synthetic-conventional stage of faith development.
   3. Older school-age children may accept the concept of God and appreciate the perceptions of others. This reflects the mythic-literal stage of faith development.
   4. Children between 3 and 7 years of age imitate parental behaviors without thorough understanding. This reflects the intuitive-projective stage of faith development.

2. 1. Although waiting for the results of a biopsy is stressful, it is not as stressful as one of the other options presented.
   2. Although being unable to control the course of illness is stressful, it is not as stressful as one of the other options presented.
   3. **As the multiplicity of stressors increases, it becomes harder for a person to cope. As each stress is added, the accumulated impact is greater than just the sum of each individual stressor.**
   4. Relocation is stressful whether it is voluntary or involuntary. However, it is not as stressful as one of the other options presented.

3. 1. **The superego monitors the ego. The superego is concerned with social standards, ethics, self-criticism, moral standards, and conscience. If the nurse initiates an Incident Report, it is the superego that directs the achievement of ego-ideal behavior. If the nurse does not initiate an Incident Report, it is the superego that criticizes, punishes, and causes a sense of guilt.**
   2. Libido refers to the psychic energy derived from basic biological urges, not the center of the conscience.
   3. The ego seeks compromise between the id and superego and represents the psychological aspect of the personality, not the center of the conscience.
   4. The id will not guide a nurse to initiate an incident report because the id is the source of instinctive and unconscious urges, not the center of the conscience.

4. 1. The General and Local Adaptation Syndromes involve automatic nonspecific responses that are not dependent on specific stressors. The body automatically responds in the same way physiologically regardless of the nature of the stressor.
   2. **Reactions to stress are both conscious and unconscious. In the General and Local Adaptation Syndromes, automatic physiological responses are not under conscious control. Adaptations, such as behavioral responses, are often under conscious control.**
   3. Although an adaptation may become a secondary stressor, many do not.
   4. Adaptations can be maladaptive and fail to help a person achieve or maintain balance, or they can be positive and help a person achieve or maintain balance.

5. 1. A client in the denial stage of grieving refuses to believe that the event is happening and is unable to deal with practical problems, such as trying new therapies.
   2. A client in the depression stage of grieving usually will acknowledge the reality and inevitability of the impending loss, will grieve the loss of present relationships and future experiences, and may stop all but palliative therapy.
   3. **A client in the bargaining stage of grieving seeks to avoid the loss and will try new therapies to gain more time.**
   4. A client in the acceptance stage of grieving comes to terms with the loss. The client begins to detach from surroundings and supportive people and generally no longer has the emotional or physical energy to try new therapies.

6. 1. **Choosing which color shirt to wear provides a person with the opportunity to make a choice and supports feelings of independence, competence, and self-respect, which all contribute to a positive self-esteem.**
   2. Providing choices does not meet needs on the physiological level of Maslow's Hierarchy of Needs. Physiological needs are related to having adequate air, food, water, rest, shelter, and the ability to eliminate and regulate body temperature.
   3. Providing choices does not meet needs on the safety and security level of Maslow's Hierarchy of Needs. Safety and security needs are related to being and feeling protected in the physiological and interpersonal realms.

4. Providing choices does not meet needs on the love and belonging level of Maslow's Hierarchy of Needs. Love and belonging needs are related to giving and receiving affection, attempting to avoid loneliness and isolation, and wanting to feel as though one belongs.

7. 1. **Utilizing deductive reasoning to examine alternatives reflects the Formal Operations stage of cognitive development. These individuals use symbols related to abstract concepts and are capable of hypothetical and deductive reasoning.**

2. Using logical thought to organize information reflects the Concrete Operations stage of cognitive development. These individuals use logical thought to organize information and solve concrete problems. Also, they are less egocentric than when in previous stages.

3. Investigating objects by placing them in the mouth reflects the Sensorimotor stage of cognitive development. These individuals process information on the physical or emotional level primarily through the senses.

4. Employing language to communicate with others reflects the Preoperational stage of cognitive development. These individuals demonstrate an increasing ability to connect cognitively through language and actions.

8. 1. Not all models of health agree with this view of health. For example, the Clinical Model has a narrow interpretation that views health as the absence of signs and symptoms of disease or injury. Well-being is a subjective perception of energy and vigor. A person able to carry out daily tasks, interact successfully with others, manage stress and emotions, and strive for continued growth and who has meaning or purpose in life has a sense of well-being, regardless of the severity of disease or infirmity.

2. Not all definitions of health identify that a person is able to control factors that affect health. The Adaptive Model is one of the few that addresses a person's ability to use purposeful adaptive responses and processes in response to internal and external stimuli to achieve health.

3. **There is little consensus about any one definition of health, wellness, and illness. However, all definitions of health, wellness, and illness address the fact that there are a number of factors that influence health.**

4. Not all definitions of health define health in terms of an individual's ability to fulfill societal roles. For example, the Clinical Model views people from the perspective of a physiological system with related functions with health being the absence of disease or injury.

9. 1. Self-actualized people are autonomous, independent, self-directed, and governed from within.

2. Self-actualized people are friendly and loving. They respect themselves and others and seek out the good in others.

3. Self-actualized people are accurate in predicting future events, highly creative, and open to new ideas and have superior perception. All these qualities contribute to problem-solving abilities.

4. **An external locus of control least describes self-actualized people. People with an external locus of control respond to a reward or recognition that comes from outside the self. People who are self-actualized strive to develop their maximum potential based on motivation from within.**

10. 1. Where people place themselves on the health-illness continuum is a self-perception of their status in relation to health and illness. From their perspectives, they cannot be healthy and ill at the same time.

2. Only the Eudaemonistic Model of Health incorporates the concept of actualization, or realization of a person's potential, as the major component of a definition of health.

3. Variables, such as genetic makeup, race, gender, age, lifestyle, risk factors, culture, environment, standard of living, support system, spiritual beliefs, and emotional factors, may be in balance and individuals may view themselves at the extremes of the continuum, or they may be out of balance and people may view themselves in the center of the continuum.

4. **Health and illness are on opposite ends of the health-illness continuum, and there is no distinct boundary between health and illness. Only a person can place herself or himself somewhere along the health-illness continuum based on his or her own perceptions about what constitutes health and illness.**

11. 1. Holistic health care involves viewing all dimensions of the person, including emotional, mental, spiritual, and physical. This is a broad approach when compared with the clinical model.

2. **The clinical model, also known as the medical model, is concerned with the**

presence or absence of signs and symptoms of illness, disease, or injury. It is a narrow interpretation of health/illness because the focus is on the identification and treatment of a defect or dysfunction. Urgent care centers are concerned with meeting acute health-care needs.

3. Identifying the relationship between clients' beliefs and actions is a component of the Health Belief Model of Health Behavior. It is unrelated to the clinical model of health/illness.

4. Performing societal roles (e.g., parent, spouse, friend, and employee) is related to the Role Performance Model of Health. It is a narrow interpretation of health and is unrelated to the clinical model of health/illness.

12. 1. If a person retires because of illness, the person has not met society's expectation in terms of role performance and, therefore, is considered unhealthy in light of the Role-Performance Model of Health.

2. According to the Role-Performance Model of Health, as long as a person can perform work associated with societal roles, even if a person is limited physically, the person is considered healthy. A coach who continues coaching even though ill or disabled is considered healthy in light of the Role-Performance Model of Health.

3. According to the Role-Performance Model of Health, a person who cannot fulfill responsibilities associated with one's job is considered sick. Therefore, a person who takes a leave of absence from work to recover is someone who is considered unhealthy in this model.

4. A strict interpretation of the Role-Performance Model of Health will most likely describe a police officer who changes jobs because of a physical or emotional inability to continue the first job as unhealthy. Even though the former police officer is still a wage earner, it is not in the same job.

13. **1. According to Maslow's Hierarchy of Needs, freedom from pain is considered a safety and security need. Confusion sometimes occurs because other theorists, such as R. A. Kalish, believe that pain should be categorized along with adequate air, food, water, rest/sleep, shelter, elimination, and temperature regulation as a first-level physiological need.**

2. According to Maslow's Hierarchy of Needs, freedom from hunger is considered a first-level physiological need, not a safety and security need.

3. According to Maslow's Hierarchy of Needs, freedom from ridicule is associated with self-esteem needs, not safety and security needs.

4. According to Maslow's Hierarchy of Needs, freedom from loneliness is associated with the need to feel loved and to belong, not to feel safe and secure.

14. 1. Not all stressful events are iatrogenic stresses. An iatrogenic stress is a stimulus caused by a treatment or diagnostic procedure.

2. The General Adaptation Syndrome is a common physiological response to stress that follows a uniform, not unique, pattern in everyone.

3. Stressors precipitate the General Adaptation Syndrome, which is a neuroendocrine response and part of the autonomic nervous system.

4. Not everyone achieves homeostasis. Some individuals reach the stage of exhaustion.

15. 1. Moving on with one's life is a sign of successful grieving. Mourning periods may be abbreviated if the loss is replaced immediately by another equally respected person or if the person experienced anticipatory grieving, which is grieving experienced before the death.

2. Being continuously angry 3 months after the death of a parent is within the realm of expected grieving behavior and is not complicated grieving. If a person is continuously angry after 1 year, it is considered complicated grieving.

3. Depression of this length is not uncommon, particularly if the relationship was meaningful or intense or no one was able to fill the role of the deceased. If depression does not resolve within a year after the death, it is considered complicated grieving.

4. Keeping a deceased child's room unchanged for years is outside the usual limits of grieving. Often, a person can get stuck in a stage of grieving and is unable to progress to the next stage. Keeping a room unchanged for years reflects an inability to face the reality of the loss or to deal with the feelings associated with the loss.

16. 1. Love and belonging needs identified in Maslow's Hierarchy of Needs are not

associated with Gordon's Value-Belief Pattern category. Gordon's Value-Belief Pattern category addresses topics such as spiritual distress and well-being, not love and belonging needs.

2. **Love and belonging needs identified in Maslow's Hierarchy of Needs are associated with Gordon's Role-Relationship Pattern category. Gordon's Role-Relationship Pattern category addresses topics such as social issues, loneliness, and relationships among family members and others.**

3. Love and belonging needs identified in Maslow's Hierarchy of Needs are not associated with Gordon's Cognitive-Perceptual Pattern category. Gordon's Cognitive-Perceptual Pattern category addresses topics such as comfort, confusion, conflict, knowledge deficit, disturbed thought processes, and sensory perception, not love and belonging needs.

4. Love and belonging needs identified in Maslow's Hierarchy of Needs are not associated with Gordon's Sexuality-Reproduction Pattern category. Gordon's Sexuality-Reproduction Pattern category addresses topics such as altered sexuality patterns and dysfunction, not love and belonging needs.

17. 1. The reality principle, according to Freud, is a learned ego function whereby a person is able to delay the need for pleasure rather than seek immediate gratification.

2. Defense mechanisms are mainly unconscious, not conscious, coping patterns that deny, distort, or reduce awareness of a stressful event in an attempt to protect the personality from anxiety. Suppression is the only defense mechanism under conscious control. It is when a person chooses to force unwanted information out of conscious awareness.

3. The ego, not the id, controls the personality. The ego mediates the urges of the id and the conscience of the superego and is therefore the part of the psyche that controls the personality.

4. **Freud believed that all behavior has meaning and called this theory psychic determinism. He believed that every psychic event is determined by prior events. Behavior, mental phenomena, and even dreams are not accidental but rather an expression of thoughts, feelings, or needs that have a relationship to the rest of a person's life.**

18. 1. **Every individual is influenced by family, ethnic, and cultural beliefs and values. These beliefs and values influence a person's lifestyle through how one perceives, experiences, and copes with health, illness, and disability. The nurse must assess the impact of these influences on the client's health and health practices.**

2. Only in the Role-Performance Model of Health is productivity or performance of one's role a necessary component to be considered healthy. Although it is important to understand, it is a narrow definition of health and fails to include the multitude of other factors that impact on a definition of health.

3. Absence of disease or injury is the foundation of the Clinical Model of Health and fails to include the multitude of other factors that have an impact on a definition of health.

4. Health cannot be easily measured or defined in common terms. There is no consensus on a definition of health, because health is unique to each individual and is based on personal expectations and values.

19. 1. Pressure is not a microbiological stressor. Microbiological stressors precipitate infection.

2. Pressure is not a physiological stressor. Physiological stressors are disturbances in structure or function of any tissue, organ, system, or body part.

3. Pressure is not a chemical stressor. Chemical stressors are drugs, poisons, and toxins.

4. **The force of pressure is a physical stressor. Pressure is the continuous force of a body part on a surface as a result of gravity; compression of tissue occurs between a bony prominence and the surface on which the body part is resting. This force is external to the body. The pressure ulcer, which is the response, becomes a secondary stressor that is then physiological in nature.**

20. 1. Fulfilling one's roles is the focus of the Role-Performance Model of Health and Wellness. This model states that health is defined in terms of a person's ability to fulfill societal roles; if roles are met, people perceive themselves as healthy even if they have an illness.

2. **The Health Belief Model focuses on perceived threats, severity, benefits, barriers, cues to action, and self-efficacy, which all influence a person's "readiness to act" in response to a health threat;**

Rosenstock first proposed this model during the 1950s.

3. Locus of control is the focus of the Health Locus of Control Model. If the nurse knows that a client is motivated by either internal or external forces, then the nurse can plan internal or external reinforcement to motivate a client toward better health.

4. This is the focus of the Health-Illness Continuum Model of health and wellness. This model focuses on health being on one end of the continuum and illness being on the other end. People move back and forth along the continuum based on their own perceptions, with no distinct boundary between health and illness.

21. 1. Difficulty sleeping is a common response to stress, but it is not life-threatening. Although it can contribute to fatigue, it is not as serious a concern as one of the other options presented.

2. Impaired immunity is a serious threat caused by prolonged periods of stress. Stressors elevate blood cortisone levels, which decrease anti-inflammatory responses, deplete energy stores, lead to a state of exhaustion, and decrease resistance to disease.

3. Increased muscle tension is a physiological indicator of stress. However, it is not as serious a concern as one of the other options presented.

4. When stressed, the client's parasympathetic nervous system precipitates a decrease in intestinal peristalsis. Constipation is a concern, but it is not as serious as one of the other options presented.

22. **1. Client problems/needs can be ranked in order of ascending importance according to how essential they are for survival using Maslow's Hierarchy of Needs as a framework. Maslow identifies five levels of human needs. A person must meet lower-level needs before addressing higher-level needs. Physiological needs are first-level needs: air, food, water, sleep, shelter, etc.; safety and security needs are second; love and belonging needs are third; self-esteem needs are fourth; and self-actualization is the fifth-level need.**

2. Erikson's Developmental Theory is designed to identify a client's developmental level, not Maslow's Hierarchy of Needs.

3. Maslow's Hierarchy of Needs is not designed to identify a person's coping patterns in response to stress.

4. Rosenstock's and Becker's Health Belief Models, not Maslow's Hierarchy of Needs, identify the relationship between health beliefs and the use of preventive actions to promote health.

23. 1. Waiting until the child asks a question is not an effective way to deal with childhood grieving. Children are perceptive and capable of recognizing that something is wrong but may not know what questions to ask. Avoiding discussing the loss with the child may make the child feel afraid, lonely, or even abandoned.

2. The child's age, level of understanding, feelings, and fears will determine how much the child should engage in mourning rituals. Children should not be forced to attend mourning rituals, nor should they be pushed aside in an attempt to protect them from pain, because this can lead to feelings of abandonment, fear, or loneliness.

3. Beginning at the child's level of understanding is essential when preparing a child for the death of a grandparent. Because there is such a difference regarding how children of different ages view the concept of death, it is important first to assess the child's level of understanding.

4. No one should be told how to feel or behave when it comes to reacting to loss. Expression of diverse feelings is essential if a child is to cope with the loss of the grandparent or develop positive coping strategies to deal with loss later as an adult.

24. 1. Although anger may be identified as a reaction to stress, it is not the most common response to stress. Anger is more classically seen in the Kübler-Ross second stage of dying/grieving.

2. Denial is more commonly seen in the Kübler-Ross first stage of dying/grieving, not as the most common response to stress.

3. Anxiety is the most common response to all new experiences that serve as an emotional threat.

4. Depression is an extreme response to prolonged stress and is not the most common human response to stress.

25. 1. Dilated pupils increase visual perception in reaction to a perceived threat.
    2. A fast, bounding pulse is a physiological response to the body's neurohormonal reaction to stress. During the alarm phase of the General Adaptation Syndrome, the autonomic nervous system initiates the fight-or-flight response and releases large amounts of epinephrine and cortisone into the body that contribute to a rapid, bounding pulse.
    3. The response time is shorter when a person is exposed to a stressor as a result of an increase in alertness and energy associated with the alarm phase of the General Adaptation Syndrome.
    4. Rapid, shallow breathing is a physiological response associated with the fight-or-flight response of the autonomic nervous system when large amounts of cortisone and epinephrine are released into the body as a person perceives a threat.
    5. Increased muscle tension prepares the body for fight or flight.

26. 1. This action supports the achievement of a goal in the Value-Belief category, not the Role-Relationship category.
    2. This action supports achievement of a goal in the Cognitive-Perceptual category, not the Role-Relationship category.
    3. This action supports the achievement of a goal in the Health Perception/Health Management category, not the Role-Relationship category.
    4. This action supports achievement of a goal in the Role-Relationship category.
    5. This action supports achievement of a goal in the Role-Relationship category. Clients have a right to make medical decisions for themselves.

27. 1. Pain initially is a response to some previous primary stressor, threat, or stimulus. However, when pain stimulates additional responses in an effort to manage the pain, the pain becomes a secondary stressor.
    2. Tachycardia is a response to a primary stressor, such as trauma or a cardiac

problem. Tachycardia then becomes a secondary stressor precipitating further adaptations in the individual.
    3. Death of a spouse is a primary psychosocial stressor, not a response to some previous stressor.
    4. Shortness of breath is a response to a primary stressor, such as cancer of the lung or a respiratory tract infection. Shortness of breath then becomes a secondary stressor precipitating further adaptations in the individual.
    5. Ingested microorganisms are a primary microbiological stressor, not a response to some previous stressor.
    6. An increase in blood pressure. It is a response to a primary stressor, such as a systemic infection or fear of the unknown. Then the increased blood pressure may become a secondary stressor.

28. 1. This person is healthy, active, and lives in a favorable, supportive environment. This person reflects high-level wellness and should be plotted on the upper right side of Dunn's Health Grid.
    2. This person is in poor health but receives routine care from health team members. This person reflects protected poor health and should be plotted on the upper left side of Dunn's Health Grid.

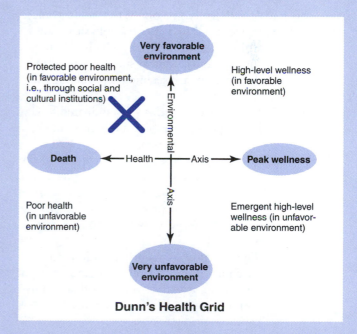

Dunn's Health Grid

3. This person has a chronic health problem, is not receiving consistent heath care, and lives in a men's shelter. This person reflects poor health, lives in an unfavorable environment, and should be plotted on the lower left side of Dunn's Health Grid.

4. This person is relatively healthy and is recovering from pneumonia but is homeless, which is an environment that is unfavorable. This person reflects emergent high-level wellness and should be plotted on the lower right side of Dunn's Health Grid.

29. 1. Eating foods low in fat is a behavior, not a health belief.
2. Accepting grim results of diagnostic tests reflects a behavior in response to bad news, rather than a behavior reflecting a health belief.
3. Engaging in physical exercise twice a week is a behavior, not a health belief.
4. **This is an example of a health belief. If a person believes that smoking cigarettes can cause lung cancer, then the person may refrain from smoking.**
5. Respecting a client's decision is not an example of a health belief. It reflects the nurse's acceptance of a client as a unique individual and recognizes the client's right to make personal choices about health care.

30. 1. A sunburn is a response to the ultraviolet rays of the sun, which is a physical, not a physiological, stressor. The body's responses to a sunburn, such as pain or inflammation, are secondary physiological stressors.
2. Diarrhea after eating contaminated food is a response to a microbiological, not a physiological, stressor.
3. **Shortness of breath is a response to the physiological stress of walking up a hill. The body is reacting via physiological mechanisms to take in more oxygen to meet the oxygen demand of cells when walking.**
4. The threat of a final examination is a psychological, not a physiological, stressor. The rapid heart rate during a final examination is a physiological response to a psychological stressor.
5. **Excess fluid volume is a response to the physiological stress of kidney impairment. Because of impaired kidney function, the body is unable**

to secrete urine, and excess fluid volume occurs.

31. 1. **This statement reflects "doctor shopping," which is a form of denial, the first stage of the Kübler-Ross Stages of Grieving theory. The client is experiencing shock and disbelief.**
3. **This statement reflects the anger stage, the second stage of the Kübler-Ross Stages of Grieving theory. The client is aware of the reality of the situation and is resentful and angry.**
4. **This statement characterizes the bargaining stage, the third stage of the Kübler-Ross Stages of Grieving theory. The client is negotiating for more time.**
2. **This statement reflects depression, the fourth stage of the Kübler-Ross Stages of Grieving theory. The client is grieving over what is happening and what will never be.**
5. **This statement characterizes acceptance, the fifth stage of the Kübler-Ross Stages of Grieving theory. The client has accepted the inevitable and is looking toward the future.**

32. 1. This statement characterizes the anger, not denial, stage in the grieving process. During the anger stage, the person may vent hostile feelings or displace these feelings on others through acting-out behaviors.
2. This statement characterizes the anger, not denial, stage of the grieving process. During the anger stage, the person may question, "Why me, when I did everything right?"
3. **This statement characterizes the denial stage of the grieving process. When in denial, a client may identify reasons why the diagnosis is not possible.**
4. This statement characterizes the depression stage of the grieving process. During the depression stage, the client realizes the full impact of the situation and grieves future losses.
5. This statement characterizes the depression stage of the grieving process. During the depression stage, the client realizes the full impact of the situation and grieves future losses.

33. 1. **Adaptive capacity refers to the quality and quantity of resources one can**

draw on to regain balance after one is threatened. This process requires an individual to adjust consciously or unconsciously in the physical, emotional, mental, or spiritual dimension in an effort to achieve balance, or homeostasis.

2. Adaptive capacity refers to the quality and quantity of resources one can draw on to regain balance after one is threatened. This process requires an individual to modify consciously or unconsciously in the physical, emotional, mental, or spiritual dimension in an effort to achieve balance, or homeostasis.

3. Adaptive capacity refers to the quality and quantity of resources one can draw on to regain balance after one is threatened. This process requires an individual to change consciously or unconsciously in the physical, emotional, mental, or spiritual dimension in an effort to achieve balance, or homeostasis.

4. Etiology refers to the stressor or threat to homeostasis that stimulates a person to draw on personal resources within the physical, emotional, mental, or spiritual dimension.

5. Remission refers to the abatement or lessened intensity of the symptoms of a disease or illness, not adaptive capacity.

6. Compliance refers to adherence to an established therapeutic action plan, not adaptive capacity.

34. 2. The first stage of moral development is Obedience and Punishment. The motivation for behavior is fear of negative consequences (e.g., punishment, disapproval).

3. The second stage of moral development is Individualism and Exchange.

The motivation for behavior is the desire for a positive consequence (e.g., reward, good result).

5. The third stage of moral development is Interpersonal Relationships. The motivation for behavior is based on pleasing others because it is what others expect.

1. The fourth stage of moral development is Maintaining Social Order. The motivation for behavior is based on following the rules to uphold the law.

6. The fifth stage of moral development is Social Contract and Individual Rights. The motivation for behavior is based on differing beliefs and values but adheres to standards agreed upon by society.

4. The sixth stage of moral development is Universal Principles. Motivation for behavior is based on abstract reasoning, universal ethical principles, and principles of justice.

35. 1. A need in the *physiologic* level is not the priority. Although the pulse and respiratory rates are slightly higher than the expected (normal) ranges, they most likely are a response to the pain experienced by the client.

2. There are no data to support the conclusion that a need in the *self-esteem* level exists. The client reports that she wants to remain independent and is able to care for herself.

3. Pain is a *safety and security* level need based on Maslow's Hierarchy of Needs. Pain relief is the client's priority need.

4. A need in the *love and belonging* level is not the priority. The client's daughter appears to be concerned about the client's well-being. However, the client disagrees with moving in with her daughter.

Legal and Ethical Issues

The following words include nursing/medical terminology, concepts, principles, and information relevant to content specifically addressed in the chapter, or information associated with topics presented in it. English dictionaries, nursing textbooks, and medical dictionaries, such as *Taber's Cyclopedic Medical Dictionary,* are resources that can be used to expand your knowledge and understanding of these words and related information.

Accountability

Accreditation

Act of commission/omission

Advance directives:
   Do Not Resuscitate
   Health-care proxy
   Power of attorney

American Nurses Association Standards of Nursing Practice

Assault

Battery

Beneficence

Breach of duty

Certification

Civil law

Code of Ethics

Common law

Confidentiality

Contract

Controlled substances

Crime

Criterion, Criteria

Defamation

Defendant

Defense

Ethics

Euthanasia

False imprisonment

Fraud

Functions of the nurse:
   Dependent
   Independent
   Interdependent

Good Samaritan law

Health-Care Quality Improvement Act

Incident Report

Informed consent

Invasion of privacy

Liability

Libel

Licensure

Litigation

Malpractice

National Council Licensing Examinations (NCLEX)

Accreditation Commission for Education in Nursing

Negligence

Nonmaleficence

Nurse Practice Act

Occupational Safety and Health Acts (OSHA)

Patient Care Partnership (formerly called Patients' Bill of Rights)

Plaintiff

Professional liability insurance

Quality of life

Reciprocity

Res ipsa loquitur

Respondeat superior

Risk management

Sigma Theta Tau International, Honor Society of Nursing

Slander

Standards of care

State Board of Nursing

The Joint Commission (formerly the Joint Commission on Accreditation of Healthcare Organizations)

Tort

Veracity

LEGAL AND ETHICAL ISSUES: QUESTIONS

1. When a nurse is administering a medication to a confused client, the client says, "This pill looks different from the one I had before." Which should the nurse do?
   1. Explain the purpose of the medication.
   2. Ask what the other medication looked like.
   3. Check the original medication prescription.
   4. Encourage the client to take the medication.

2. A nurse administers an incorrect dose of a medication to a client. Which is the **primary** purpose of documenting this event in an Incident Report?
   1. Record the event for future litigation.
   2. Provide a basis for designing new policies.
   3. Prevent similar situations from happening again.
   4. Ensure accountability for the cause of the accident.

3. When preparing to administer a medication, the nurse identifies that the dose is larger than the standard dose recommended by the manufacturer. Which should the nurse do?
   1. Inform the supervisor.
   2. Give the drug as prescribed.
   3. Give the average dose of the medication.
   4. Discuss the prescription with the primary health-care provider.

4. When a nurse attempts to administer a medication to a client, the client refuses to take the medication because it causes diarrhea. The nurse provides teaching about the medication, but the client continues adamantly to refuse the medication. Which should the nurse do **first**?
   1. Discuss with a family member the need for the client to take the medication.
   2. Explain again to the client the consequences of refusing to take the medication.
   3. Document in the client's clinical record the client's refusal to take the medication.
   4. Notify the primary health-care provider of the client's refusal to take the medication.

5. When caring for a terminally ill client, a family member says, "I need your help to hasten my mother's death so that she is no longer suffering." Which should the nurse do based on the position of the American Nurses Association in relation to assisted suicide?
   1. Not participate in active euthanasia
   2. Participate based on personal values and beliefs
   3. Participate when the client is experiencing severe pain
   4. Not participate unless two primary health-care providers are consulted and the client has had counseling

6. Which of the following is responsible for ensuring that Registered Nurses are minimally qualified to practice nursing?
   1. American Nurses Association
   2. Sigma Theta Tau International
   3. National Council of State Boards of Nursing
   4. Constituent Leagues of the National League for Nursing

7. For which **primary** reason is an expert nurse called to testify in a lawsuit regarding professional nursing malpractice?
   1. Strengthen the defense.
   2. Support the prosecution.
   3. Present standards of nursing care as they apply to the facts in the case.
   4. Make judgments associated with laws governing the practice of nursing.

8. A nurse initiates a visit from a member of the clergy for a client. How is the nurse functioning when initiating this visit?
   1. Interdependently
   2. Independently
   3. Dependently
   4. Collegially

9. A client is asked to participate in a medical research study. Which document should the nurse explain to the client because it protects the client's rights?
   1. Code of Ethics
   2. Informed Consent
   3. Nurse Practice Act
   4. Constitution of the United States

10. A client with a prolonged history of smoking cigarettes is being considered for a lung transplant. Which element of ethical practice is associated with fair policies and procedures guiding allocation of organs for transplantation?
    1. Justice
    2. Fidelity
    3. Veracity
    4. Nonmaleficence

11. A primary health-care provider prescribes out of bed to a chair as the activity level for a client. How is the nurse functioning when moving this client out of bed to a chair?
    1. Interdependently
    2. Collaboratively
    3. Independently
    4. Dependently

12. A Registered Nurse witnesses an accident and assists the victim, who has a life-threatening injury. Which should the nurse do to meet an important standard of care when acting as a Good Samaritan at the scene of an accident?
    1. Seek consent from the injured party before rendering assistance.
    2. Implement every critical-care intervention necessary to sustain life.
    3. Stay at the scene until another qualified person takes over responsibility.
    4. Insist on helping because a nurse is the best-qualified person to provide care.

13. A faculty member of a nursing program is conducting an informational session for potential nursing students. Which information about licensure to practice nursing upon completion of a nursing program should the faculty member include in the session?
    1. "It is a responsibility of the American Nurses Association."
    2. "It is granted on graduation from a nursing program."
    3. "It is approved by the National League for Nursing."
    4. "It is required by law in each individual state."

14. When considering legal issues, the word *contract* is to *liable* as *standard* is to which word?
    1. Rights
    2. Negligence
    3. Malpractice
    4. Accountability

15. An anxious client repeatedly uses the call bell to get the nurse to come to the room. Finally, the nurse says to the client, "If you keep ringing, there will come a time I won't answer your bell." Which legal term is related to this statement?
    1. Slander
    2. Battery
    3. Assault
    4. Libel

16. A nurse is informed that a credentialing team has arrived and is in the process of assessing the quality of care delivered at the hospital. Which organization is associated with the credentialing of hospitals?
    1. The Joint Commission
    2. National League for Nursing
    3. American Nurses Association
    4. National Council Licensure Examination

17. A nurse changes a client's dry sterile dressing. How is the nurse functioning when performing this task?
    1. Interdependently
    2. Collaboratively
    3. Independently
    4. Dependently

18. A nurse must administer a medication. Which should the nurse do **first**?
    1. Verify the prescription for accuracy.
    2. Check the client's identification armband.
    3. Ensure the medication is in the medication cart.
    4. Determine the appropriateness of the prescribed medication.

19. When choosing a nursing school in the United States that awards an associate degree, a future student nurse should consider schools that have met the standards of nursing education established by which organization?
    1. Accreditation Commission for Education in Nursing
    2. North American Nursing Diagnosis Association
    3. Sigma Theta Tau International
    4. American Nurses Association

20. A client's diet prescription is "clear liquids to regular as tolerated." How is the nurse functioning when progressing the client's diet to full liquid?
    1. Dependently
    2. Independently
    3. Collaboratively
    4. Interdependently

21. The licensure of Registered Professional Nurses protects which of the following?
    1. Nurses
    2. Clients
    3. Common law
    4. Health-care agencies

22. Which factor is unique to malpractice when comparing negligence and malpractice?
    1. The action did not meet standards of care.
    2. The inappropriate care is an act of commission.
    3. There is harm to the client as a result of the care.
    4. There is a contractual relationship between the nurse and client.

23. A nurse completes an Incident Report after a client falls while getting out of bed unassisted. Which is the purpose of this report?
    1. Ensure that all parties have an opportunity to document what happened.
    2. Help establish who is responsible for the situation.
    3. Make data available for quality-control analysis.
    4. Document the situation on the client's chart.

24. How is the nurse functioning when administering a drug that has prn as part of the prescription?
    1. Collegially
    2. Dependently
    3. Independently
    4. Interdependently

25. Which is the main role of the American Nurses Association?
　1. Establish standards of nursing practice.
　2. Recognize academic achievement in nursing.
　3. Monitor educational institutions granting degrees in nursing.
　4. Prepare nurses to become members of the nursing profession.

26. A nurse says, "If you do not let me do this dressing change, I will not let you eat dinner with the other clients in the dining room." Which legal term is related to this statement?
　1. Battery
　2. Assault
　3. Negligence
　4. Malpractice

27. For which are state legislatures responsible?
　1. Standardized care plans
　2. Enactment of Nurse Practice Acts
　3. Accreditation of educational nursing programs
　4. Certification in specialty areas of nursing practice

28. Nursing practice is influenced by the doctrine of *respondeat superior*. Which is the basic concept related to this theory of liability?
　1. Nurses must respond to the Supreme Court when they commit acts of malpractice.
　2. Health-care facilities are responsible for the negligent actions of the nurses whom they employ.
　3. Nurses are responsible for their actions when they have contractual relationships with clients.
　4. The law absolves nurses from being sued for negligence if they provide inappropriate care at the scene of an accident.

29. When attempting to administer a 10 p.m. sleeping medication, the nurse assesses that the client appears to be asleep. Which should the nurse do?
　1. Withhold the drug.
　2. Notify the primary health-care provider.
　3. Awaken the client to administer the drug.
　4. Administer it later if the client awakens during the night.

30. Which is the **primary** purpose of the American Nurses Association (ANA) Standards of Clinical Nursing Practice?
　1. Define the philosophy of nursing practice.
　2. Establish criteria for quality nursing practice.
　3. Identify the legal definition of nursing practice.
　4. Determine educational standards for nursing practice.

31. Which person requires a co-signature for a valid consent for surgery?
　1. 15-year-old mother whose infant requires exploratory surgery
　2. 40-year-old client in a home for developmentally disabled adults
　3. 90-year-old adult who wants more information about the risks of surgery
　4. 50-year-old unconscious trauma victim who needs insertion of a chest tube

32. A client living in Oregon has been receiving hospice care in the home. One day, the client tells the nurse, "Dying takes forever. I hate it that I am a burden to my family. I can't stand this anymore. Can you help me end my life?" The nurse's personal ethical values do not include complying with this client's request. Which is the nurse's **best** response?
　1. "I will inform your primary health-care provider of your desire to die."
　2. "Your family members probably do not consider you a burden."
　3. "Let's talk a little more about your wanting to die."
　4. "Nurses cannot participate in assisted suicide."

33. A nurse working in a hospital administers a medication to the wrong client and is sued by the client. Under contract law, which liability occurs when the hospital is additionally identified as a defendant in the legal action? **Select all that apply.**
    1. _____ Vicarious liability
    2. _____ *Borrowed servant*
    3. _____ *Captain of the ship*
    4. _____ *Respondeat superior*
    5. _____ Quasi-intentional tort

34. A student nurse about to graduate is actively developing a personal ethical foundation for nursing practice. Place the following actions in the order in which they should progress.
    1. Clarify personal values and beliefs.
    2. Identify ethical issues when working.
    3. Identify a personal ethical foundation.
    4. Work continuously to improve ethical decision-making abilities.
    5. Integrate one's personal ethical foundation within the ethics of the profession.

    Answer: _____

35. A client sustained a serious injury as a result of malpractice by a nurse. Several legal elements must be met to prove the nurse committed malpractice in a civil suit. Which statement is associated with the element of causation? **Select all that apply.**
    1. _____ A nurse-client relationship existed between the nurse and the client.
    2. _____ A nurse's omission or commission of an act failed to meet standards of care.
    3. _____ A nurse's action or inaction was the immediate reason for the plaintiff's injury.
    4. _____ A nurse should have known that the action or inaction could result in harm or injury to the client.
    5. _____ A nurse's action or inaction that did not meet a standard of care resulted in a client experiencing pain, suffering, and disability.

36. A client is scheduled to have surgery, and informed consent is to be obtained. Place the following steps in the order in which they should be performed.
    1. The client is willing to sign the consent voluntarily.
    2. The client signs the consent in the presence of the nurse.
    3. The nurse determines that the client is alert and competent to give consent.
    4. The primary health-care provider informs the client of the risks and benefits of the procedure.

    Answer: _____

37. Identify the action that is an example of slander. **Select all that apply.**
    1. _____ Volunteer telling another volunteer a client's age
    2. _____ Discussing confidential information on an elevator used by visitors
    3. _____ Personal care assistant sharing information about a client with another client
    4. _____ Unit manager documenting a nurse's medication error in a performance appraisal
    5. _____ Housekeeper who is angry at a nurse falsely telling another staff member that the nurse uses cocaine

38. An older adult male is admitted to the hospital after sustaining a brain attack (cerebrovascular accident, stroke). Intravenous fluids, resuscitative medications, and mechanical ventilation are instituted in the emergency department. Eventually, testing indicates absence of brain functions. A nurse interviews the client's son and daughter and reviews the client's advance directives. Legally, which is the **most** likely outcome in this scenario?
    1. The son will request that life-sustaining interventions be stopped.
    2. The daughter will legally be able to prevent the withdrawal of medical interventions.
    3. The nurse should refer this situation to the agency's ethics committee for consideration.
    4. The primary health-care provider should concur with another health-care provider to arrive at a course of action.

CLIENT'S CLINICAL RECORD

Interview With Client's Daughter
Client's daughter stated, "I love my dad, and I don't want him to die." Daughter indicated that she has been the person caring for her father when he is ill and stated that she will do everything she can to keep her dad alive.

Interview With Client's Son
Client's son stated, "I love my dad, too, but if there is no hope for recovery, why are we doing all these things? What is the point?" Son indicated that he knows that he and his sister disagree on what should be done.

Client's Advance Directives
The client's Health Care Proxy identifies the son as his representative.

39. A student nurse is about to graduate from an accredited nursing program. Which does the student nurse understand is an action **unrelated** to a state Nurse Practice Act? **Select all that apply.**
    1. _____ Setting guidelines for nurses' salaries in the state
    2. _____ Establishing reciprocity for licensure between states
    3. _____ Determining minimum requirements to be licensed as a nurse
    4. _____ Maintaining a list of nurses who can legally practice in the state
    5. _____ Providing legal counsel for a nurse who is being sued for malpractice

40. A primary health-care provider asks a nurse to witness informed consents by several clients. Which client identified by the nurse is **unable** to give an informed consent for surgery? **Select all that apply.**
    1. _____ 16-year-old boy who is married
    2. _____ 50-year-old woman who is confused
    3. _____ 35-year-old woman who is depressed
    4. _____ 50-year-old woman who does not speak English
    5. _____ 94-year-old man who recently suffered the death of his spouse

1. 1. This intervention ignores the client's concern. Although this ultimately may be done, it is not the priority action.
2. This action by itself is unsafe because the client is confused and the information obtained may be inaccurate.
3. **This is the safest intervention because it goes to the original source of the prescription.**
4. This action ignores the client's statement and is unsafe without first obtaining additional information.

2. 1. Although documentation of an incident may be used in a court of law, it is not the primary reason for an Incident Report.
2. Providing a basis for designing new policies is not the primary reason for Incident Reports. New policies may or may not have to be written and implemented.
3. **Risk-management committees use statistical data about accidents and incidents to identify patterns of risk and prevent future accidents and incidents.**
4. Although nurses are always accountable for their actions, accountability for the cause of an incidence is the role of the courts.

3. 1. It is unnecessary to call the supervisor in this situation.
2. Giving the drug as prescribed may be unsafe for the client and may result in malpractice.
3. Changing a medication prescription is not within the scope of nursing practice.
4. **Nurses have a professional responsibility to know or investigate the standard dose for prescribed medications being administered. In addition, nurses are responsible for their own actions regardless of whether there is a written prescription. The nurse has a responsibility to question and/or refuse to administer a prescription that appears unreasonable.**

4. 1. Discussing the situation with a family member without the client's consent is a violation of confidentiality.
2. The client has been taught about the medication and adamantly refuses the medication. Further teaching at this time may be viewed by the client as badgering.
3. **Withholding the medication and documenting the client's refusal are the appropriate interventions. Clients have a right to refuse care.**
4. Notifying the primary health-care provider eventually should be done, but it is not the priority at this time.

5. 1. **Nursing actions must comply with the law, and the law states that euthanasia is legally wrong. Euthanasia can lead to criminal charges of homicide or civil lawsuits for providing an unacceptable standard of care.**
2. A nurse's beliefs, values, or moral convictions should not be imposed on clients. In addition, nurses cannot participate in euthanasia.
3. Compassion and good intentions are not an acceptable basis for actions beyond the scope of nursing practice.
4. Nurses cannot legally be involved with euthanasia. In some states in the U.S., a primary health-care provider can prescribe a medication that can be taken by a client to cause death (e.g., Oregon, Washington, Vermont, Colorado, California, and the District of Columbia). The ANA, according to its Code for Nurses with Interpretive Statements, indicates that nurses should not participate in active euthanasia or assistive suicide.

6. 1. The American Nurses Association (ANA) is the national professional organization for nursing in the United States. It fosters high standards of nursing.
2. Sigma Theta Tau International, Honor Society of Nursing, recognizes academic achievement and leadership qualities, encourages high professional standards, fosters creative endeavors, and supports excellence in the profession of nursing.
3. **The National Council of State Boards of Nursing is responsible for the NCLEX examinations. Passing the NCLEX examination establishes competencies required to perform safely and effectively as a newly licensed nurse. Passing an NCLEX examination assists State Boards of Nursing in making licensure decisions.**
4. The National League for Nursing (NLN) is committed to promoting and improving nursing service and nursing.

7. 1. A nurse expert can testify for either the defense or the prosecution.
2. A nurse expert can testify for either the prosecution or the defense.
3. **The American Nurses Association Standards of Clinical Nursing Practice are authoritative statements by which the national organization for nursing describes the responsibilities for which nurses are accountable. An expert nurse**

is capable of explaining these standards as they apply to the situation under litigation. These professional standards are criteria that help a judge or jury determine if a nurse committed malpractice or negligence.

4. An expert nurse is not an authority in the law. The expert nurse's role is not to make judgments about the laws as they apply to the practice of nursing.

8. 1. A nurse does not need a primary health-care provider's prescription to make a referral to a member of the clergy. An interdependent intervention requires a primary health-care provider's prescription associated with a parameter.

  2. When a nurse initiates a referral to a member of the clergy, the nurse is working independently. Nurses legally are permitted to diagnose and treat human responses to actual or potential health problems.

  3. A nurse can make a referral to a member of the clergy. This action is within the scope of nursing practice.

  4. The nurse can make a referral to a member of the clergy without collaborating with another professional health-care team member.

9. 1. A code of ethics is the official statement of a group's ideals and values. It includes broad statements that provide a basis for professional actions.

  2. Informed consent is an agreement by a person to accept a course of treatment or a procedure after receiving complete information necessary to make a knowledgeable decision.

  3. Nurse Practice Acts define the scope of nursing practice; they are unrelated to participation in research studies.

  4. The Constitution of the United States addresses broad individual rights and responsibilities. The rights related to nursing practice and clients include the rights of privacy, freedom of speech, and due process.

10. 1. **The ethical principle of *Justice* refers to fairness and that all clients should be treated equally, impartially, and without prejudice regardless of individual factors.**

  2. The scenario in the stem does not reflect fidelity. *Fidelity* refers to making only promises or commitments that can be kept.

3. The scenario in the stem does not reflect veracity. *Veracity* refers to being truthful, which is essential to a trusting nurse-client relationship.

4. The scenario in the stem does not reflect nonmaleficence. *Nonmaleficence* refers to preventing harm, avoiding actions that can cause harm, or removing a client from harm.

11. 1. The nurse is following the primary health-care provider's prescription to get the client out of bed. There are no restrictions or parameters in relation to the prescription. However, the nurse must use judgment before, during, and after a transfer if a client's condition changes.

  2. A nurse does not work collaboratively when moving this client out of bed.

  3. The responsibility to determine a client's activity level is not within the legal scope of nursing practice.

  4. Determining the extent of activity desirable for a client is within the primary health-care provider's, not a nurse's, scope of practice. Following activity prescriptions is a dependent function of the nurse.

12. 1. Depending on the injured person's physical and emotional status, the person may or may not be able to provide consent for care.

  2. When a nurse helps in an emergency, the nurse is required to render care that is consistent with care that any reasonably prudent nurse would provide under similar circumstances. The nurse should not attempt interventions that are beyond the scope of nursing practice.

  3. When a nurse renders emergency care, the nurse has an ethical responsibility not to abandon the injured person. The nurse should not leave the scene until the injured person leaves or another qualified person assumes responsibility.

  4. A nurse should offer assistance, not insist on assisting, at the scene of an emergency.

13. 1. The American Nurses Association (ANA) Standards of Clinical Nursing Practice do not address licensure.

  2. When a person graduates from a school of nursing, the individual receives a diploma that indicates completion of a course of study; the diploma is not a license to practice nursing.

3. The National League for Nursing (NLN) promotes nursing service and nursing education; it is not involved with licensure.

4. The Nurse Practice Act in a state stipulates the requirements for licensure within the state.

14. 1. Although clients have a right to receive care that meets appropriate standards, the word *right* does not have the same relationship to the word *standard* as the relationship between the words *contract* and *liable*.

2. The words *standard* and *negligence* do not have the same relationship as the words *contract* and *liable*. Negligence involves an act of commission or omission that a reasonably prudent person would not do.

3. The words *standard* and *malpractice* do not have the same relationship as the words *contract* and *liable*. Malpractice is negligence by a professional person.

4. Liable means a person is accountable for fulfilling a contract that is enforceable by law. Accountable means a person is responsible (liable) for meeting standards, which are expectations established for making judgments or comparisons.

15. 1. This is not an example of slander, which is a false spoken statement resulting in damage to a person's character or reputation.

2. This is not an example of battery, which is the unlawful touching of a person's body without consent.

3. This is an example of assault. Assault is a verbal attack or unlawful threat causing a fear of harm. No actual contact is necessary for a threat to be an assault.

4. This is not an example of libel, which is a false printed statement resulting in damage to a person's character or reputation.

16. **1. The Joint Commission (formerly the Joint Commission on Accreditation of Healthcare Organizations) evaluates health-care organizations' compliance with standards stipulated by The Joint Commission. Accreditation indicates that the organization has the capabilities to provide quality care. In addition, federal and state regulatory agencies and insurance companies require accreditation by The Joint Commission.**

2. The National League for Nursing (NLN) fosters the development and improvement of nursing education and nursing service.

3. The American Nurses Association (ANA) is the national professional organization for nursing in the United States. Its purposes are to promote high standards of nursing practice and to support the educational and professional advancement of nurses.

4. In the United States, graduates of educational programs that prepare students to become Licensed Practical Nurses or Registered Professional Nurses must successfully complete the National Council Licensure Examination-PN (NCLEX-PN®) and the National Council Licensure Examination-RN (NCLEX-RN®), respectively, as part of the criteria for licensure.

17. 1. The changing of a dry sterile dressing is an interdependent action by the nurse when the primary health-care provider's prescription for wound care includes a parameter such as "change the sterile dressing whenever necessary."

2. In this situation, the nurse is not working with other health-care professionals to implement a primary health-care provider's prescription.

3. This intervention is not within the scope of nursing practice without a primary health-care provider's prescription.

4. A nurse is not permitted legally to prescribe wound care. The nurse needs a prescription from a primary health-care provider to implement wound care.

18. **1. The administration of medications is a dependent function of the nurse. The primary health-care provider's prescription should be verified for accuracy. The prescription must include the name of the client, the name of the drug, the size of the dose, the route of administration, the number of times per day to be administered, and any related parameters.**

2. Although checking the client's identification armband is essential for the safe administration of a medication, it is not the first step when preparing to administer a medication to a client.

3. Although ensuring that the medication is available may be done as a time-management practice, it is not the first step when preparing to administer a medication to a client.

4. A nurse is legally responsible for the safe administration of medications; therefore,

the nurse should assess if a medication prescription is reasonable. However, this is not the first step when preparing to administer a medication to a client.

19. 1. **Accreditation Commission for Education in Nursing (ACEN) is an organization that appraises and grants accreditation status to nursing programs that meet predetermined structure, process, and outcome criteria.**
2. The North American Nursing Diagnosis Association (NANDA) developed a constantly evolving taxonomy of nursing diagnoses to provide a standardized language that focuses on clients and related nursing care.
3. Sigma Theta Tau International, Honor Society of Nursing, recognizes academic achievement. It does not accredit schools of nursing.
4. The American Nurses Association (ANA) is the national professional organization for nursing in the United States. It does not accredit schools of nursing.

20. 1. This dietary prescription has parameters that exceed a simple dependent function of the nurse.
2. Prescribing a diet for a client is outside the scope of nursing practice.
3. Collaborative or collegial interventions are actions the nurse carries out in conjunction with other health-care team members.
4. **The primary health-care provider's prescription implies a progression in the diet as tolerated. The nurse uses judgment to determine the time of this progression, which is an interdependent action.**

21. 1. Licensure does not protect nurses. Licensure only ensures that the individual has met the requirements to practice nursing. Earning a license to practice as a Licensed Practical Nurse or Registered Nurse is granted to an individual who passes the NCLEX-PN® or NCLEX-RN® examination, respectively, according to the licensure requirements for the state in which the license is issued.
2. **Licensure indicates that a person has met minimal standards of competency, thus protecting the public's safety.**
3. Licensure does not protect common law. Common law comprises standards and rules based on the principles established in prior judicial decisions.

4. Licensure does not protect health-care agencies. The Joint Commission determines if agencies meet minimal standards of health-care delivery, thus protecting the public.

22. 1. There is a violation of standards of care with both negligence and malpractice.
2. Negligence and malpractice both involve acts of either commission or omission.
3. The client must have sustained injury, damage, or harm with both negligence and malpractice.
4. **Only malpractice is misconduct performed in professional practice, where there is a contractual relationship between the client and nurse that results in harm to the client.**

23. 1. The nurse who identified or created the potential or actual harm completes the Incident Report. The report identifies the people involved in the incident, describes the incident, and records the date, time, location, actions taken, and other relevant information.
2. Documentation should be as factual as possible and avoid accusations. Questions of liability are the responsibility of the courts.
3. **Incident Reports help to identify patterns of risk so that corrective action plans can take place.**
4. An Incident Report is not part of the client's clinical record, and reference to the report should not be made in the client's clinical record.

24. 1. Collegial or collaborative interventions are actions the nurse performs in conjunction with other health-care team members.
2. Dependent interventions are those activities performed under a primary health-care provider's direction and supervision.
3. Independent interventions are those activities the nurse is licensed to initiate based on knowledge and expertise.
4. **An interdependent intervention requires a primary health-care provider's prescription associated with a set parameter. The parameter, prn (whenever necessary), requires that the nurse use judgment when implementing the prescription.**

25. 1. **The American Nurses Association has established Standards of Care and Standards of Professional Performance.**

These standards reflect the values of the nursing profession, provide expectations for nursing practice, facilitate the evaluation of nursing practice, and define the profession's accountability to the public.

2. Sigma Theta Tau International, Honor Society of Nursing, recognizes academic achievement and scholarship in nursing.
3. The National League for Nursing Accrediting Commission, the Commission on Collegiate Nursing Education, and state education departments monitor educational institutions granting degrees in nursing.
4. Schools of nursing award a diploma, associate degree, or baccalaureate degree in nursing after successful completion of the program. These graduates are eligible to take the licensing examination for entry into the practice of nursing.

26. 1. This statement is not an example of battery. Battery is the actual willful touching of another person that may or may not cause harm.
    2. **This statement is an unjust threat. Assault is the threat to harm another person without cause.**
    3. This statement is not an example of negligence. Negligence occurs when harm or injury is caused by an act of either commission or omission.
    4. This statement is not an example of malpractice. Malpractice is negligence by a professional person as compared with the actions of another professional person in a similar circumstance when a contract exists between the client and nurse.

27. 1. Nursing team members or an interdisciplinary team of health-care providers write standardized care plans.
    2. **Every state has its own Nurse Practice Act that describes and defines the legal boundaries of nursing practice within the state.**
    3. The National League for Nursing Accrediting Commission, the Commission on Collegiate Nursing Education, and state education departments are the major organizations accrediting nursing education programs in the United States.
    4. The American Nurses Association and other specialty organizations offer certification in specialty areas in nursing practice.

28. 1. This is unrelated to *respondeat superior*. Negligence and malpractice, which are unintentional torts, are litigated in local courts by civil actions between individuals.
    2. **The ancient legal doctrine *respondeat superior* means "let the master answer." By virtue of the employer-employee relationship, the employer is responsible for the conduct of its employees.**
    3. Individual responsibility is unrelated to *respondeat superior*. A nurse can have an independent contractual relationship with a client. When a nurse works for an agency, the contract between the nurse and client is implied. In both instances, the nurse is responsible for the care provided.
    4. This is unrelated to *respondeat superior*. Good Samaritan laws do not provide absolute immunity. Nurses must function as a reasonable prudent nurse would function in a similar situation. Nurses can be held responsible if there is gross departure from the normal standard of care or if there is willful wrongdoing on the nurse's part.

29. 1. This is a violation of the primary healthcare provider's prescription. Drug administration is a dependent nursing function.
    2. Notifying the primary health-care provider is unnecessary.
    3. **Administering a medication is a dependent function of the nurse. The prescription should be followed as written if the prescription is reasonable and prudent. This medication was not a prn medication but rather a standing prescription.**
    4. The drug should be administered as prescribed, not at a later time.

30. 1. A philosophy incorporates the values and beliefs about the phenomena of concern to a discipline. The ANA Standards of Clinical Nursing Practice reflect, not define, a philosophy of nursing. Each nurse and nursing organization should define its own philosophy of nursing.
    2. **The ANA Standards of Clinical Nursing Practice describe the nature and scope of nursing practice and the responsibilities for which nurses are accountable.**
    3. The laws of each state define the practice of nursing within the state.
    4. Educational standards are established by accrediting bodies, such as the National

League for Nursing Accrediting Commission, the Commission on Collegiate Nursing Education, and state education departments.

31. 1. A mother may legally make medical decisions for her children, even if the mother is younger than 18 years of age.

  2. **A person living in a protected environment, such as a home for developmentally disabled adults, may not have the mental capacity to make medical decisions and requires the signature of a court-appointed legal representative. This person can be a parent, sibling, relative, or unrelated individual.**

  3. Older adults can make decisions for themselves as long as they understand the risks and benefits of the surgery and are not receiving medication that may interfere with cognitive ability.

  4. The insertion of a chest tube to inflate a lung is an emergency intervention to facilitate respiration and oxygenation. This emergency procedure is implemented to sustain life and does not require a signed consent if the client is incapacitated.

32. 1. This statement eventually may be made, but at this time it is not the priority. By this response, the nurse is functioning as a client advocate without violating personal values against assisted suicide. In states such as Oregon, Washington, and Vermont, Colorado, and California and in the District of Columbia, primary health-care providers can prescribe medications that may be used by clients to cause their own deaths; this is called assisted suicide. Certain criteria must be met, depending on the state, such as being 18 years of age or older, having a terminal illness with fewer than 6 months to live, being capable of self-administering the medication, and meeting specific psychiatric criteria (e.g., counseling, no psychiatric diagnosis, exploration of palliative options). Nurses do not have the legal or ethical right or obligation to help clients die. The American Nurses Association Code of Ethics states that nurses should not participate in assisted suicide or euthanasia.

  2. This minimizes the client's concerns. Also, the nurse may or may not know if this is a true statement; the family members may believe that caring for a dying family member is a burden.

  3. **This statement is an open-ended question that encourages the client to discuss feelings and explore future options, including assisted suicide.**

  4. Although this may be a true statement, it does not meet the client's physical or emotional needs. This statement focuses on the nurse rather than the client.

33. 1. **Vicarious liability applies in this situation. Vicarious liability applies when accountability for a wrong is assigned to a person or entity that did not directly cause an injury but has a contractual relationship with the person who did cause the wrong. The nurse is still liable for his or her own actions.**

  2. A *borrowed servant* does not apply to this situation. A *borrowed servant* applies when an employer directs a nurse to work for a second employer (e.g., agency nurse); the second employer is held accountable for the nurse's actions.

  3. **The liability of *Captain of the ship* applies in this situation. The liability of *Captain of the ship* occurs when a health-care provider is held liable for a nurse who is working under the direction of the health-care provider. The nurse is still liable for his or her own actions.**

  4. *Respondeat superior* refers to "Let the master answer" and applies in this situation. When an agency hires a nurse, the nurse functions as a representative of the institution and must perform within its policies and procedures; the hospital is responsible for the actions of the nurse. The nurse is still liable for his or her own actions.

  5. A quasi-intentional tort is not related to this situation. An example of a quasi-intentional tort is making false statements, verbally (slander) or in writing (libel), about another person that harm the person's reputation (defamation of character) or holds the person up to ridicule or contempt.

34. 1. **A nurse must know oneself before helping others. The first step is to identify and explore personal values and beliefs.**

3. Once values and beliefs are explored, then a basis for an ethical foundation of nursing practice can be identified for oneself.

5. After a nurse identifies a personal ethical foundation, it should be compared to the ethics of the nursing profession (American Nurses Association Code of Ethics). This ensures that the nurse works within the standards of the nursing profession.

2. Identifying ethical issues when working in the nursing profession facilitates nursing actions that preserve personal integrity while meeting the needs of clients without imposing personal values or beliefs onto clients or their family members.

4. A nurse's ethical decision-making abilities should never remain static. These abilities grow as one matures within the profession and as a variety of factors (e.g., new technology, evolving social policy) influence one's ethical foundation.

35. 1. This statement reflects the element of *duty*, not *causation*. The element of duty is met when a nurse has a legal obligation to provide nursing care to the client.
    2. This statement reflects the element of *breach of duty*, not *causation*. The element of breach of duty is met when a nurse's action or inaction fails to meet standards of care established by a job description, agency policy or procedures, the state nurse practice act, and standards established by professional organizations.
    3. *Causation* relates to malpractice when a client's injury is directly the result of a nurse's action or inaction (proximate cause).
    4. *Causation* relates to malpractice when a nurse should have known that an action or inaction that is a breach of a nursing standard could result in harm or injury to a client (foreseeability).
    5. This statement reflects the element of *damages*, not *causation*. The element of damages is met when the plaintiff proves that physical, emotional, or financial harm or injury was the result of a standard of care not being met.

36. 4. It is the responsibility of the primary health-care provider to include all the information necessary to make a knowledgeable decision. Clients have a legal right to have adequate and accurate information to make informed decisions.
    3. Clients must be competent to sign a consent form. The client must be alert, competent, and in touch with reality. Confused, sedated, unconscious, or minor clients may not give consent. Minor clients who are married, parents, emancipated, or serving in the United States military can provide a legal consent.
    1. Clients must give their consent voluntarily and without coercion.
    2. The health-care provider witnessing the signing of the consent must ensure that the signature is genuine.

37. 1. This is a violation of the client's right to confidentiality, not slander.
    2. This is a violation of a client's right to confidentiality, not slander.
    3. This is a violation of the client's right to confidentiality, not slander.
    4. This is not slander because it is a written, not spoken, statement and it documents true, not false, information.
    5. This is an example of slander. It is a malicious, false statement that may damage the nurse's reputation.

38. 1. The son, by law, as a result of the client's Health Care Proxy, can make health-care decisions for his father, including withdrawing all life-sustaining interventions.
    2. The daughter lacks legal authority to act on behalf of her father.
    3. This is unnecessary. Legally, this situation is not an ethical dilemma.
    4. This is unnecessary. There are legal documents that will dictate the future course of action.

39. 1. The salary of nurses is determined through negotiations between nurses or their representatives, such as a union or a professional nursing organization, and the representatives of the agency for which they work.
    2. A state's Nurse Practice Act determines the criteria for reciprocity for licensure.
    3. A state's Nurse Practice Act stipulates minimum requirements required for a person to be licensed as a Registered Professional Nurse or Licensed Practical Nurse within the state.

4. A state's Nurse Practice Act defines the criteria for licensure within the state. However, actual functions, such as maintaining a list of nurses who can legally practice in the state, usually are delegated to another official body, such as a State Board of Nursing or State Education Department.

5. State Nurse Practice Acts do not provide legal counsel for a nurse who is sued for malpractice. A nurse should purchase malpractice insurance upon graduation from a nursing program or may be provided legal counsel by an employer.

40. 1. Legally, individuals younger than 18 years old can provide informed consent if they are married, pregnant, parents, members of the military, or emancipated.

2. A person who is confused is unable to understand the risks and benefits associated with making an informed decision. In this situation, a person designated as a health-care proxy or legal guardian has to make decisions for the confused individual.

3. A depressed person is capable of making health-care decisions until proven to be mentally incompetent.

4. This person can provide informed consent after interventions ensure that the person understands the facts and risks concerning the treatment.

5. This person is considered functionally competent and able to make decisions for himself. There is no indication that the client is impaired because of grieving.

Leadership and Management

The following words include nursing/medical terminology, concepts, principles, and information relevant to content specifically addressed in the chapter, or information associated with topics presented in it. English dictionaries, nursing textbooks, and medical dictionaries, such as *Taber's Cyclopedic Medical Dictionary,* are resources that can be used to expand your knowledge and understanding of these words and related information.

Accountable, accountability
Case management
Change theory
Consensus
Controlling
Cooperation
Creative
Delegate
Directing
Documentation
Efficiency
Empower
Feedback
Five Rights of Delegation:
  Right Task
  Right Person
  Right Communication
  Right Time
  Right Supervision
Flexible
Human resource management
Incentives
Job description
Leadership
Leadership styles—classic:
  Autocratic—directive
  Democratic—participative, consultative
  Laissez-faire—nondirective, permissive
Leadership styles—contemporary:
  Charismatic leadership

Connective leadership
Transactional leadership
Transformational leadership
Shared leadership
Managers:
  First-line managers
  Unit managers
  Middle managers
  Nurse executives
Motivation
Network
Organization
Performance evaluation
Power types:
  Expert
  Influence
  Legitimate
  Referent
  Reward
Preceptor
Primary nursing
Problem solving
Productivity
Resistance to change
Resource management
Role model
Subordinate
Systems theory
Table of organization
Time management

LEADERSHIP AND MANAGEMENT: QUESTIONS

1. An accurate assessment drives the rest of the steps of the nursing process. Which management function drives effective management?
   1. Planning
   2. Directing
   3. Organizing
   4. Controlling

2. Which is **most** basic for a nurse to have when working in a management position?
   1. Strong interpersonal communication skills
   2. Awareness of when to be confrontational
   3. Knowledge of the role of a change agent
   4. Recognition by peers as a leader

3. A unit manager mentors a new unit manager as part of orientation to the position. Which type of power is being used by the unit manager mentor?
   1. Influence
   2. Coercive
   3. Referent
   4. Expert

4. A nurse manager considers that there are "Five Rights of Delegation." Which is a right of delegation in addition to *right task*, *right person*, *right communication*, and *right time*?
   1. Place
   2. Route
   3. Feedback
   4. Supervision

5. Which should the manager do **first** to overcome resistance to change?
   1. Ensure that the planned change is within the current beliefs and values of the group.
   2. Provide incentives to encourage commitment of participants to the change.
   3. Implement change by employing small steps rather than large steps.
   4. Use influence power to ensure that goals of change are met.

6. When considering the autocratic leadership style, an "autocratic" leader is to an "authoritarian" leader as a "democratic" leader is to which type of leader?
   1. Directive
   2. Permissive
   3. Oppressive
   4. Consultative

7. Which nursing-care delivery model is based on case management?
   1. Client classification system
   2. Diagnosis Related Groups
   3. Critical pathways
   4. Primary nursing

8. Which statement is **most** significant in relation to the concept of change theory in the health-care environment?
   1. Stages of change are predictable.
   2. Risks and benefits of change must be weighed.
   3. Activities that are new result in positive outcomes.
   4. Changes that are large are easier to adapt to than multiple smaller changes.

9. Several nurses complain to the nurse manager that one of the nursing assistants constantly takes extensive lunch breaks. Which should the nurse manager do?
   1. Convene a group meeting of all the nursing assistants to review their responsibilities related to time management.
   2. Talk with the nursing assistant to explore the reasons for the behavior and review expectations.
   3. Arrange a meeting with the nurses so that they can confront the nursing assistant as a group.
   4. Document the nursing assistant's behavior and place it in the aide's personnel file.

10. Which should the nurse do to ensure efficiency when managing a daily assignment?
    1. Give care to a client in isolation first.
    2. Plan activities to promote nursing convenience.
    3. Organize care around legally required activities.
    4. Perform routine bed baths between breakfast and lunch.

11. A supervisor communicates expectations about a task to be completed and then delegates the task. Which management function is being implemented by the supervisor?
    1. Planning
    2. Directing
    3. Organizing
    4. Controlling

12. A first-year nursing student in the clinical area is given an appropriate client assignment by the instructor. Which should the student nurse do?
    1. Complete the care indicated on the client's plan of care.
    2. Accept the role of leader of the client's health-care team.
    3. Assume accountability for the tasks that are assigned by the instructor.
    4. Help other students to complete their assigned tasks whenever necessary.

13. Which statement is significant in relation to the concept of change theory in the health-care environment?
    1. Barriers to change can be overcome by embracing new ideas uncritically.
    2. Change generates anxiety by moving away from the comfortable.
    3. Behaviors are easy to change when change is supported.
    4. Change is effective when spontaneous.

14. Which is the major task of a nurse manager?
    1. Accomplishing an objective
    2. Empowering others
    3. Problem solving
    4. Planning

15. A staff nurse must solve a complex problem. Which is the nurse's **most** effective resource?
    1. Organizational chart of the institution
    2. Nursing procedure manual
    3. Unit's nurse manager
    4. Nursing supervisor

16. When delegating a specific procedure to a client care aide, the aide refuses to perform the procedure. Which should the nurse do **first**?
    1. Assign the procedure to another client care aide.
    2. Explain that it is part of the client care aide's job description.
    3. Explore why the client care aide refused to perform the procedure.
    4. Send the client care aide to the procedure manual to review the procedure.

17. Which is the **first** thing the nurse should do when planning to apply for a new position within an agency?
    1. Review the job description.
    2. Provide at least several positive references.
    3. Identify if power is associated with the position.
    4. Locate the position on the agency's table of organization.

18. Which is the **most** important reason why a nursing assistant must fully understand how to implement a delegated procedure?
    1. Be capable of completing the procedure safely.
    2. Be proficient enough to perform the procedure quickly.
    3. Have the knowledge to explain the procedure to a client.
    4. Have the correct information when teaching the procedure to another nursing assistant.

19. A nursing team leader delegates a wound irrigation to a Licensed Practical Nurse (LPN). It has been a long time since the LPN performed this procedure. Which should the nursing team leader do to ensure client safety?
    1. Verbally describe how to perform the procedure to the LPN.
    2. Have the LPN demonstrate how to perform the procedure.
    3. Assign another LPN to assist with the procedure.
    4. Delegate the procedure to another LPN.

20. A nurse manager is informed that a large number of clients will be admitted in response to a terrorist attack. Which type of leadership style is appropriate to use in this situation?
    1. Collaborative
    2. Authoritarian
    3. Laissez-faire
    4. Democratic

21. A nurse manager is experiencing staff resistance when implementing change. Which is the **most** important action by the nurse manager to overcome resistance to change?
    1. Identify the reason for the resistance.
    2. Restate the purpose of the change concisely.
    3. Modify the goals to appeal to more key people.
    4. Emphasize the positive consequences of the planned change.

22. Which is the major focus of leadership?
    1. Inspiring people
    2. Initiating change
    3. Controlling others
    4. Producing a product

23. Which factor associated with a manager differentiates the role of a manager from a leader?
    1. Vision
    2. Charisma
    3. Confidence
    4. Responsibility

24. Which situation is reflective of the saying "A stitch in time saves nine"?
    1. Obtaining the vital signs of clients on the unit during a specified time frame
    2. Collecting equipment for a procedure before entering the room
    3. Delegating some interventions to the Licensed Practical Nurse
    4. Documenting the nursing care given every few hours

25. A Registered Nurse delegates a procedure to a Licensed Practical Nurse. Which is the purpose for delegating the procedure to the Licensed Practical Nurse?
    1. Create change.
    2. Establish a network.
    3. Improve productivity.
    4. Transfer accountability.

26. A nurse manager plans to provide feedback to a subordinate who needs a change in behavior. Which is the **first** intervention by the nurse manager?
    1. Be assertive.
    2. Explore alternatives.
    3. Identify the unacceptable behavior.
    4. Document the content of the counseling session.

27. Which is the main reason a nurse manager achieves a consensus when making a decision within a group?
    1. Explore possible alternative solutions.
    2. Demonstrate that staff members are flexible.
    3. Facilitate cooperative effort toward goal achievement.
    4. Ensure the use of effective autocratic decision making.

28. A nurse manager evaluates the performance of a subordinate. Which management function is being implemented by the nurse manager?
    1. Planning
    2. Directing
    3. Organizing
    4. Controlling

29. Which of the following is related to systems theory?
    1. End result
    2. Linear format
    3. Trial and error
    4. Cyclical process

30. Which activity does a nurse manager engage in that values the importance of positive role modeling? **Select all that apply.**
    1. _____ Counseling subordinates who fail to meet expectations
    2. _____ Holding team meetings to review rules of the agency
    3. _____ Engaging in ongoing quality improvement activities
    4. _____ Reviewing job descriptions with employees
    5. _____ Following the policies of the agency

31. Which premise is basic to the motivation climate of the Theory Y management style associated with human relations-oriented management? **Select all that apply.**
    1. _____ Employees will exercise self-direction when committed to organizational goals.
    2. _____ Employees pursue security above other elements related to work.
    3. _____ Employees generally will accept and even request responsibility.
    4. _____ Employees must be pressured with discipline to achieve goals.
    5. _____ Employees seek direction whenever possible.

32. Lewin's planned change theory progresses through phases. Place these statements by the nurse manager in order as change moves through the process.
    1. "Let's implement a pilot project next week."
    2. "This is a new venture that should be exciting."
    3. "I know it may be difficult, but you are doing a great job."

    Answer: _____

33. Which action is an example of a nurse working independently? **Select all that apply.**
1. _____ Giving a bed bath to a client who is experiencing profuse diaphoresis
2. _____ Assigning another nurse to administer intravenous medications
3. _____ Assessing a client's wound for signs of an infection
4. _____ Elevating a client's arm after an IV site infiltrates
5. _____ Obtaining a client's vital signs

34. A nurse who is a member of a quality improvement committee reviews a chart detailing trends of 4 problem categories identified in Incident Reports over a 3-month period of time. Corrective action plans were implemented to address each problem category. After analyzing the chart documenting tends over the successive months of March, April, and May, which problem category demonstrated the **most** improvement?
1. Falls
2. Medication errors
3. Violations of confidentiality
4. Violations in standards of practice

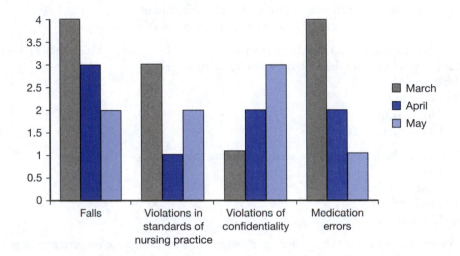

35. A client is to be discharged from the hospital. Which discharge task can be delegated to a nursing assistant? **Select all that apply.**
1. _____ Teaching the client how to measure weight using a standing scale
2. _____ Obtaining the client's temperature, pulse, and respiratory rate
3. _____ Determining if the client knows how to measure fluid intake
4. _____ Demonstrating to the client how to safely use a walker
5. _____ Reviewing foods that are high in vitamin C

36. Place the following steps of the decision-making process in the order in which they should be implemented by a nurse.
1. Identify possible solutions to the problem.
2. Gather relevant information.
3. Identify the problem.
4. Evaluate the result.
5. Test a solution.

Answer: _____

37. A nurse and a nursing assistant are working together on a surgical unit. Which activity should the nurse assign to the nursing assistant? **Select all that apply.**
1. _____ Taking vital signs of clients who are stable
2. _____ Delivering meal trays to clients who are in isolation
3. _____ Explaining to a client how to use an incentive spirometer
4. _____ Changing the linens on beds that are occupied by clients who are on bedrest
5. _____ Emptying a urine collection bag that is attached to continuous bladder irrigation

38. The department of outpatient services of an agency is converting from paper charting to electronic charting. The nurse in charge of one of the clinics is responsible for implementing the change on the unit. Identify the **most** significant barrier to change based on the statements by upper-level managers, the nurse in charge, and staff nurses.
   1. The upper-level managers have given an ultimatum about the change.
   2. The nurse in charge has a negative attitude toward the change.
   3. A staff nurse does not know how to use a computer.
   4. A staff nurse is anxious about the change.

Nurse in Charge
"Come to me if you have concerns about this change."
"I don't think that this is the way to go but it is something we have to do."
Staff Nurses
"I don't know how to use a computer."
"I feel uncomfortable trying something new."
"Maybe in the long run it will make our job easier."
Upper-level Managers
"The nursing education department will provide classes on how to use a computer."
"We must switch to electronic records because it is a requirement of our regulating agencies."

39. The nursing team consists of a nurse in charge, a Registered Nurse, and a nursing assistant. Which task should be delegated to the Registered Nurse rather than the nursing assistant? **Select all that apply.**
   1. _____ Obtaining routine vital signs
   2. _____ Providing discharge teaching
   3. _____ Ambulating a stable client in the hall
   4. _____ Administering a cleansing enema to a client
   5. _____ Transporting a client to another location for an x-ray examination

40. Based on Kurt Lewin's Change Theory, place an X on the box in which change takes place.

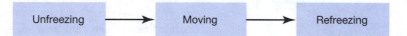

1. 1. **Effective management depends on careful planning. Planning activities include deciding what is to be done, when to do it, where and how to do it, and who will do it and with what level of assistance. Planning is multifaceted and involves establishing goals, identifying interventions based on priorities, and determining how outcomes will be evaluated. What occurs during planning affects all subsequent steps of management activities.**

   2. Getting the work accomplished (directing) is associated with just one step in the management process and does not drive the process of effective management.

   3. Managing human and economic resources to achieve organizational goals (organizing) is associated with just one step in the management process and does not drive the process of effective management.

   4. Measuring goal achievement, ensuring ongoing evaluation, and implementing corrective action when necessary (controlling) are associated with just one step in the management process and do not drive the process of effective management.

2. 1. **Strong communication skills are an essential competency of a nurse manager. Research demonstrates that 80% to 90% of a manager's day is spent communicating verbally and in writing. Managers must express their thoughts clearly, concisely, and accurately.**

   2. Although confrontation may be used occasionally, it is not as important as a competency identified in another option.

   3. Although knowledge of the role of change agent is important, it is not as important as a competency identified in another option.

   4. Recognition by peers as a leader is not as important as a competency identified in another option. A person generally is promoted to a management position because upper management recognizes leadership qualities. As a nurse manager grows into the role, peers will recognize the leadership ability of the nurse manager.

3. 1. This is not an example of influence power. Influence power is the use of persuasion and communication skills to exercise power informally without using the power associated with formal authority.

   2. This is not an example of coercive power. The leader bases coercive power on the fear of retribution or the punitive withholding of rewards.

   3. This is not an example of referent power. Referent power is associated with respect for the leader because of the leader's charisma and prior successes.

   4. **This is an example of expert power. Expert power is the respect one receives based on one's ability, skills, knowledge, and experience.**

4. 1. The right place is not one of the Five Rights of Delegation.

   2. The right route refers to the Five Rights of Medication Administration, not the Five Rights of Delegation.

   3. Feedback is part of communication, which is one of the Five Rights of Delegation already cited in the stem of the question.

   4. **The one who delegates a task is responsible for ensuring that the task is performed safely and according to standards of practice.**

5. 1. **Change that is consistent with current values and beliefs is easier to implement than change that is inconsistent with current values and beliefs. Values and beliefs are difficult to change.**

   2. This is not the priority intervention. Although incentives might motivate some individuals, they do not motivate all because some people have an internal rather than an external locus of control.

   3. Although small steps are more effective than large steps because they are easier to achieve and, once achieved, are motivating, this approach is not the first thing the nurse should do to overcome resistance to change.

   4. Although one person sharing explanations with another (influence power) is helpful when trying to change behavior, it is not the most effective type of power to use when trying to effect change. Another option identifies an action that the nurse should do first.

6. 1. The word *directive* refers to the autocratic, not democratic, leadership style.

   2. The word *permissive* refers to the laissez-faire, not democratic, leadership style.

   3. *Oppressive* is the way some people refer to the autocratic, not democratic, leadership

style. There is little freedom and a large degree of control by the autocratic leader, which frustrates motivated, professionally mature staff members.

4. **The word *consultative* is the word most closely related to the democratic leadership style. Democratic leaders encourage discussion and decision making within the group. The leader facilitates the work of the group by making suggestions, offering constructive criticism, and providing information.**

7. 1. Client classification systems are not a nursing-care delivery model based on case management. Client classification systems are designed to assign an acuity level to clients based on their needs for the purpose of determining the number of nursing care hours required to provide care.
   2. Diagnosis Related Groups (DRGs) are not a nursing-care delivery model based on case management. Diagnosis Related Groups are a prospective reimbursement plan in which clients are grouped based on medical diagnoses for the purposes of reimbursing the cost of hospitalization.
   3. Critical pathways are not just a nursing-care delivery model based on case management but are tools used in managed care that are sets of concurrent and sequential actions by nurses as well as other health-care professionals to achieve a specific outcome. They represent specific practice patterns in relation to specific medical/surgical populations.
   4. **Primary nursing is a case management approach in which one nurse is responsible for a number of clients 24 hours a day, 7 days a week. It is a way of providing comprehensive, individualized, and consistent nursing care.**

8. 1. The stages of change are not always predictable. Although effective change moves through three zones according to Lewin's Change Theory (unfreezing [comfort], moving [discomfort], and refreezing [new comfort]), what happens in each zone is not always predictable, and change is not always successfully achieved. Change is dynamic and the stages are not rigid.
   2. **Risks and benefits must be carefully analyzed before initiating change. Some change is not worth the risk, because the consequences of failure are greater than the benefits.**
   3. Outcomes of new changes can be positive or negative. Sometimes well-planned

change meets with resistance and the effort to change can result in a loss of credibility, lack of achieving the goal, and confusion.

4. Small goals are easier to achieve than large goals. Small goals generally are designed to ensure achievement, which is motivating.

9. 1. It is the nursing assistant who is late and takes extensive lunch breaks who needs to review the responsibilities related to time, not the nursing assistants who follow the rules.
   2. **Recognition of a problem is the first step in the problem-solving process. Once the unacceptable behavior is identified and acknowledged, then the reasons for the problem can be explored, solutions suggested, and expectations reinforced.**
   3. It is not the responsibility of others to confront the employee who is late for work and takes extensive lunch breaks. The employee reports to the nurse manager, who is superior in the chain of command of the organization. The nurse manager should meet with the employee. In addition, counseling sessions with employees should be confidential and conducted in private.
   4. This is premature. The nurse manager first should implement an action identified in another option.

10. 1. This may not be possible, depending on the needs of clients.
    2. Client needs are the priority, not the convenience of the nurse.
    3. **Legally required activities must be accomplished because they are dependent functions that support the medical regimen of care. Although legally required activities should be accomplished first, many independent actions by the nurse also must be implemented to maintain a basic standard of care and client safety. Some nursing interventions, which are not essential, can be implemented after the required activities.**
    4. This may not be possible, depending on the needs of clients.

11. 1. This scenario is not an example of the planning function of management. Planning involves establishing goals, designing interventions based on the priority identified, and determining how outcomes will be evaluated.

2. **This scenario is an example of the directing function of management. Directing involves getting the work accomplished; it includes activities such as assigning and communicating tasks and expectations and guiding, teaching, and motivating staff members in meeting organizational goals.**

3. This scenario is not an example of the organizing function of management. Organizing activities include obtaining and managing human and economic resources and include identifying the chain of command, determining responsibilities, and ensuring that policies and procedures clearly describe standards of care and expected outcomes.

4. This scenario is not an example of the controlling function of management. Controlling activities use outcome criteria to measure the performance of staff members, identify effectiveness in goal achievement, ensure ongoing evaluation, and implement corrective action when necessary.

12. 1. Although students are expected to complete all planned care, the client's condition can change or some unforeseen event may interfere with the plan. The student must keep the instructor or preceptor informed about the client's condition and use the instructor or preceptor as a resource person when the unexpected occurs or guidance is needed.

2. Students are assigned to care for clients for a specific time period and generally are included as members, not leaders, of the nursing team, particularly beginning nursing students.

3. **Students are accountable for the tasks assigned by the instructor or preceptor. As part of accountability, students are obligated to keep the instructor or preceptor informed about the status of the client, how the assignment is progressing, and whether all interventions are implemented as planned.**

4. Students should not help other students unless specifically assigned to do so by the instructor or preceptor. An exception occurs when assistance is needed to ensure client safety in an emergency.

13. 1. All barriers to change may not be overcome (e.g., financial limitations). Before initiating change, barriers should be anticipated and addressed. All aspects of

the new idea are best accomplished when critically analyzed.

2. **Change causes one to move from the comfortable to the uncomfortable and is known as unfreezing in Lewin's Change Model. It involves moving away from that which is known to the unknown, from the routine to the new, and from the expected to the unexpected. The unknown, new, and unexpected can be threatening, which can increase anxiety.**

3. Behaviors are not easy to change even when supported. Most people do not like to function in an unfamiliar environment. In addition, change challenges one's comfort zone in each level of Maslow's Hierarchy of Needs.

4. Planned, not spontaneous, change is most effective because it is organized, systematic, and purposeful.

14. 1. **Although planning, problem solving, and empowering others are tasks of a manager, the bottom line is for the manager to accomplish the work of the organization.**

2. Although empowering others is one of the tasks of a manager, the major task is identified in another option.

3. Although problem solving is one of the tasks of a manager, the major task is identified in another option.

4. Although planning is one of the tasks of a manager, the major task is identified in another option.

15. 1. The organizational chart schematically plots the reporting relationship of every position within the organization. It does not help a staff nurse identify a solution to a complex problem.

2. The nursing procedure manual is not designed to help a staff nurse identify a solution to a complex problem. The nursing procedure manual contains details of policies relative to nursing practice and nursing procedures along with the purpose and all the steps that one must follow to implement the procedure safely.

3. **Generally, in the chain of command of an organization, the staff nurse works under the direction of and reports to the unit's nurse manager. The nurse manager generally is an experienced nurse and is the primary resource person for the staff nurse. The staff nurse should seek guidance from the nurse**

manager when assistance is needed to solve a complex problem.

4. The nursing supervisor is higher up the chain of command in a Table of Organization than another employee who is the best person for the staff nurse to seek assistance from when needing help to solve a complex problem.

16. 1. Assigning the procedure to another staff member is premature. Another option has priority.

2. The employee may be fully aware of the requirements of the job description and not need to have them described. Even though a task is within one's job description, a person can refuse to perform a procedure because of a reason that is considered acceptable.

3. The nurse must first explore the reason for the nurse aide's refusal to perform the procedure. The employee may have an acceptable reason for refusing to comply. When the reason is identified, then the nurse manager can take an informed action.

4. The reason for refusal may have nothing to do with the lack of understanding of the procedure.

17. **1. This is one of the most important actions by the nurse seeking a new position. The job description provides an overview of the requirements and responsibilities of the role. Job descriptions include factors such as educational and experiential requirements, job responsibilities, subordinates to be supervised, and to whom one reports in the chain of command.**

2. Requesting references protects the hiring agency, not the nurse. This is not the most important thing the nurse should do when applying for a new position within an agency.

3. Although understanding the power of the position may help a person meet the responsibilities associated with the job description, it is not the priority when applying for a new position.

4. Although it is important to recognize where the new position fits into the agency's table of organization, it is not the priority when applying for a new position. A table of organization schematically plots the reporting relationship of every position within the organization.

18. **1. Safety of the client is the priority. The nursing assistant must perform only the skills that are within the legal role of the nursing assistant; understood; practiced; and performed correctly on a return demonstration.**

2. Although this may be desirable, it is not the priority.

3. Although this is important, it is not the priority.

4. Nurse aides are trained and supervised by the nurse, not other nurse aides.

19. 1. Providing just a verbal description is unsafe. This does not ensure that cognitive information can be converted to a psychomotor skill.

2. Demonstration is the safest way to assess whether a person has the knowledge and skill to perform a procedure safely. A superior delegating care is responsible for ensuring that the person implementing the care is legally qualified and competent.

3. A peer should not be held responsible for the care assigned to another team member. The Registered Nurse who delegates a procedure to a subordinate is directly responsible for ensuring that the care is safely delivered to clients.

4. This intervention does not address the original Licensed Practical Nurse's need to know how to perform the procedure safely. This procedure is within the legal scope of practice of a Licensed Practical Nurse.

20. 1. Collaborative is not a classic leadership style. Collaborative refers to the democratic leadership style. Democratic leaders encourage discussion and decision making within the group, which requires collaboration, coordination, and communication among group members.

2. The Authoritarian leadership style is the appropriate style to use in a crisis when urgent decisions are necessary. In a crisis, one person must assume the responsibility for decisions. Autocratic leaders give orders and directions and make decisions for the group.

3. The Laissez-faire leadership style is not the appropriate style to use in a crisis when urgent decisions are necessary. Laissez-faire leaders are nondirective and permissive, which allows for self-regulation, creativity, and autonomy but limits fast-acting efficiency.

4. The Democratic leadership style is not the appropriate style to use in a crisis when urgent decisions are necessary. Democratic leaders encourage discussion and decision making within the group, which takes time.

21. 1. **This is essential to overcome resistance to change. There are many different reasons people resist change. Each person will respond to different strategies. There are four different types of interventions to overcome resistance: providing information, disproving currently held beliefs, maintaining psychological safety, and administrating an order or command.**
    2. Although it is important to state the purpose of the change clearly and concisely, another option is a more important action that can be implemented by the nurse manager to overcome resistance to change.
    3. Modifying a goal compromises the integrity of the planned change. All ramifications associated with the change should be explored before beginning and all contingencies planned for so that modifying a goal will be unnecessary.
    4. Although emphasizing the positive consequences of the planned change might be done, another option is a more important action that can be implemented by the nurse manager to overcome resistance to change.

22. 1. **Leaders can inspire others with their vision and gain cooperation through their persuasion and communication skills (influence power), the respect others have for their knowledge and abilities (expert power), and their charisma and prior success (referent power).**
    2. Initiating change is the major function of a change agent, not a leader. Change agents are often managers rather than leaders because managers have responsibility for ensuring that the work of the organization is done.
    3. Controlling others is a function of a manager, not a leader.
    4. Producing a product is a function of a manager, not a leader. A manager is responsible for ensuring that the work of the organization is done, and this often requires the development of such things as a policy or procedure, management reports, and work schedules.

23. 1. Effective leaders and managers both should have vision.
    2. Effective leaders and managers both should have charisma.
    3. Effective leaders and managers both should have confidence.
    4. **Managers, not leaders, have organizational responsibility because of their job description. Leaders are not assigned to direct others. They are viewed as leaders by the members of the group because of their experience, vision, charisma, confidence, expertise, or age.**

24. 1. Taking the vital signs of all the clients on the unit at the same time is called functional nursing and is unrelated to the adage in the question.
    2. **This action is an appropriate example of the adage "A stitch in time saves nine." It means that if you sew a tear when it is small, you need fewer stitches and time to repair it than when it is large. The same adage can be applied to the collection of equipment before a procedure. If the nurse has all the equipment that is needed before beginning a procedure, less time is used than when forgotten equipment is obtained later. Every time the nurse leaves the room for forgotten equipment, the client is inconvenienced and time is wasted.**
    3. Delegation is related to the efficient use of staff and is unrelated to the adage in the question.
    4. This example is unrelated to the adage in the question.

25. 1. Delegation is unrelated to creating change. Delegation is the transfer of responsibility for the performance of a task to another while remaining accountable for the actions of the person to whom the task was delegated. Creating change is associated with responding to a stressor that is either planned or unplanned, which results in change that is positive or negative.
    2. Delegation is unrelated to networking. Networking occurs when a person makes connections with others for sharing ideas, knowledge, information, and professional support.
    3. **Delegation allows the Registered Nurse to assign tasks to various individuals on the nursing team who are best qualified to complete them. In**

today's health-care environment, nursing team members have different levels of educational preparation. The Registered Nurse must take into account the qualifications and scope of practice of each professional and non-professional nursing team member and assign tasks accordingly. When this is done, each person's skills and abilities are used most appropriately and pro-ductivity increases.

4. The person who is assigned a task is responsible for the outcome of the assigned task. However, the Registered Nurse delegating the task is not relieved of accountability but is responsible for the actions of the person to whom the task was delegated as well as the outcome of the intervention.

26. 1. The nurse manager can provide negative feedback that is firm without being assertive. Not yielding under pressure (firm) is less confrontational than being confident in a persistent way (assertive).
   2. When providing negative feedback, the exploration of alternative solutions is performed later in the counseling session.
   3. **Problem recognition is the first step in the problem-solving process. Once the unacceptable behavior is identified and acknowledged, then the reasons for the problem can be explored, solutions suggested, and expectations reinforced.**
   4. Although documenting the content of the counseling session should be done, it is not feedback. Feedback is necessary for the subordinate to recognize one's offending behavior. In addition, documentation is the last, not the first, step in the counseling process.

27. 1. Exploring possible alternative solutions occurs before achieving a consensus. A consensus is achieved when all, or most, agree or have the same opinion.
   2. Consensus, not flexibility, is the goal. However, some members of the group may be flexible and change their opinion to ensure the achievement of a consensus.
   3. **Cooperation and teamwork are essential for the achievement of any goal. If a consensus is achieved about the value of the expected outcome, people are more likely to work together constructively.**

4. Autocratic decision making does not seek a consensus when making a decision within a group. Autocratic leaders give orders and directions and make decisions for the group. There is little freedom within the group.

28. 1. Evaluating the performance of a subordinate does not fall under the planning function of management. Planning involves establishing goals, designing interventions based on the priority identified, and determining how outcomes will be evaluated.
   2. Evaluating the performance of a subordinate does not fall under the directing function of management. Directing involves getting the work accomplished; it includes activities such as assigning and communicating tasks and expectations and guiding, teaching, and motivating staff members in meeting organizational goals.
   3. Evaluating the performance of a subordinate does not fall under the organizing function of management. Organizing activities include obtaining and managing human and economic resources and include identifying the chain of command, determining responsibilities, and ensuring that policies and procedures clearly describe standards of care and expected outcomes.
   4. **The controlling function of management includes the evaluation of staff members. Controlling activities also include measuring effectiveness of goal achievement, ensuring ongoing evaluation, and implementing corrective action when necessary.**

29. 1. There is no end to a system. Individual parts of a system are interrelated, and the whole system responds in an integrated way to changes within a part.
   2. Systems do not function in a linear (straight-line) format. Systems are complex.
   3. The trial and error method is unrelated to systems theory. It is a problem-solving method in which a number of solutions are tried until one solves the problem.
   4. **Systems theory is a cyclical process in which a whole is broken down into parts and the parts are studied individually as well as how they work together within the system. Every system consists of matter, energy, and communication. Because each part of a system**

is interconnected, the whole system reacts to changes in one of its parts. The concept of treating a client holistically is based on an understanding of systems theory.

30. 1. Counseling subordinates who fail to meet expectations is not an example of role modeling from among the options presented.
    2. Holding team meetings to review rules of the agency is not an example of role modeling from among the options presented.
    3. **When a nurse manager engages in ongoing quality improvement activities, the manager is demonstrating behavior that is expected. The nurse manager also should encourage nursing team members to participate in quality improvement activities.**
    4. Reviewing job descriptions with employees is not an example of role modeling from among the options presented.
    5. **When a nurse manager follows policies and procedures, the manager is demonstrating behavior that is expected. Role modeling is more effective than telling as a teaching strategy.**

31. 1. **This statement is associated with the motivational climate of the Theory Y management style. Managers who adopt premises associated with Theory Y believe that workers are responsible and accountable and strive to achieve organizational objectives to which they are committed.**
    2. Employees who pursue security above other elements related to work are associated with the climate of the Theory X management style. Managers who adopt premises associated with Theory X believe that workers generally display little ambition and mainly are interested in the security provided with employment.
    3. **This statement is associated with the motivational climate of the Theory Y management style. Managers who adopt premises associated with Theory Y believe that workers will be self-directed when a manager assists, supports, and rewards inspired workers.**
    4. Employees who require the pressure of discipline to achieve goals are associated with the motivational climate of the Theory X management style. Managers who adopt premises associated with Theory X

believe that workers will generally evade work and must be controlled with the threat of punishment to achieve organizational goals.
    5. Employees who seek constant direction are associated with the motivational climate of the Theory X management style. Managers who adopt premises associated with Theory X believe that workers will generally evade work and therefore constant supervision is essential for productive workers.

32. 2. **The first phase is called "unfreezing" and is concerned with identifying the need for change, exploring alternative solutions, and stimulating enthusiasm.**
    1. **The second phase is called "moving/changing" and is concerned with creating actual visible change.**
    3. **The third phase is called "refreezing" and is concerned with providing feedback, encouragement, and constructive criticism to reinforce new behavior.**

33. 1. **Providing hygiene (e.g., bathing, grooming, and oral care) is an independent function of the nurse that does not require a prescription from a primary health-care provider.**
    2. **Delegating tasks within the scope of nursing practice is an independent function of the nurse and does not require a primary health-care provider's prescription.**
    3. **Assessing a client's wound for signs of an infection is within the scope of nursing practice and does not require a primary health-care provider's prescription.**
    4. **Elevating a client's arm after an IV site infiltrates does not require a prescription from a primary health-care provider and is an independent function of the nurse. Applying a warm soak over the infiltrated IV site would require a prescription from a primary health-care provider and would be a dependent function of the nurse.**
    5. **Collecting data about clients is part of the assessment step of the nursing process and is an independent function of the nurse.**

34. 1. Although *Falls* demonstrate a downward trend of the number of falls from 4 in March, to 3 in April, and to 2 in May, another category demonstrates a greater degree of improvement.

2. *Medication errors* demonstrate the most improvement in decreasing errors from 4 in March, to 2 in April, and to 1 in May. This demonstrates the most significant downward trend of the number of events for all 4 categories.

3. *Violations of confidentiality* demonstrate an increase in the number of events from 1 in March, to 2 in April, and 3 in May. This is a serious concern because the number of events progressively increased in spite of the implementation of a corrective action plan.

4. *Violations in standards of nursing practice* initially demonstrate an improvement in the number of violations from 3 in March to 1 in April; however, the number increased to 2 in May. This demonstrates a lesser degree of improvement than another category.

35. 1. Teaching a client how to obtain a body weight requires the knowledge and judgment of a Registered Nurse. Teaching requires a complex level of interaction with the client, problem solving, and innovation in the form of an individually designed teaching plan of care that addresses the specific learning needs of the client. In addition, the outcome is unpredictable, and it has the potential to cause harm if the skill is taught incorrectly.

2. **Obtaining vital signs can be delegated to a nursing assistant because it is not a complex task. It requires simple problem-solving skills and a simple level of interaction with the client. Although this task has the potential to cause harm if the critical elements of the skill are not implemented appropriately, it is within the scope of practice of a nursing assistant. It does not require the more advanced competencies of a Registered Nurse.**

3. Assessing a client's level of understanding is a complex task that requires knowledge and judgment and is within the scope of practice of a Registered Nurse. This task requires a complex level of interaction with the client, problem solving, and innovation in the form of an individually designed teaching plan of care that addresses the specific learning needs of the client.

4. Teaching a client how to use a walker requires the knowledge and judgment of a Registered Nurse. Teaching requires a complex level of interaction with the

client, problem solving, and innovation in the form of an individually designed teaching plan of care that addresses the specific learning needs of the client. In addition, the outcome is unpredictable, and it has the potential to cause harm if the skill is taught incorrectly.

5. Reviewing foods that are high in vitamin C requires the knowledge and judgment of a Registered Nurse. Teaching requires a complex level of interaction with the client and is beyond the educational preparation of a nursing assistant.

36. 3. **The first step in the decision-making process is defining and describing the problem.**

2. **The second step in the decision-making process is gathering significant information associated with the problem.**

1. **The third step of the decision-making process is identifying promising strategies to resolve the problem.**

5. **The fourth step of the decision-making process is implementing an action to address the problem.**

4. **The fifth step of the decision-making process is evaluating the results by comparing the actual outcomes to the expected outcomes of the employed solution to the problems.**

37. 1. **Taking vital signs of clients who are stable is within the scope of practice of a nursing assistant. Determining the significance of the results of routine vital signs requires the expertise of a Regietered Nurse.**

2. **Delivering meal trays to clients who are in isolation is within the scope of practice of a nursing assistant. Nursing assistants are taught how to use personal protective equipment.**

3. Client teaching is within the legal scope of a Registered Nurse, not a nursing assistant. Teaching requires a complex level of interaction with the client, problem solving, and innovation in the form of an individually designed teaching plan of care that addresses the specific learning needs of the client. In addition, the outcome is unpredictable and it has the potential to cause harm if the skill is taught incorrectly.

4. **Changing the linens on beds that are occupied by clients who are on bedrest is within the scope of practice of a**

nursing assistant. The activity is simple and repetitive.

5. **Emptying and recording the volume of output collected from a urine collection bag is within the legal role of a nursing assistant. The nurse will then calculate the volume of urine by deducting the volume of irrigating solution instilled from the total output. Calculating the actual urine output is an assessment that requires the skill of a Registered Nurse.**

38. 1. An ultimatum can be viewed as a challenge, requirement, stipulation, or demand. The need to convert from paper charting to electronic charting is a requirement of the facility's regulating agencies. The upper-level managers identified the change that must be made and the purpose for the change, which is reasonable. The upper-level managers will be providing classes to assist the nurses in achieving this change, which demonstrates support for the nurses.

2. **Although the nurse in charge appears to be supportive in stating "Come to me if you have concerns about this change," it is better to discuss initial concerns as a group. Specific concerns can be addressed individually later. The statement "I don't think that this is the way to go, but it is something we have to do" is a personal attitude that sets a negative tone regarding the change that ultimately may be destructive to achieving the goal of converting from paper charting to electronic charting.**

3. Change may require the learning of new skills. The staff nurse's statement, "I don't know how to use a computer," is an issue that must be addressed. The upper-level managers have indicated that the nursing education department will provide classes on how to use a computer.

4. Change can precipitate anxiety because it involves the process of transforming, modifying, or doing something different. Anxiety is related to that which is unknown. Therefore, goals and objectives must be identified and educational classes provided to help the staff nurses achieve the conversion from paper charting to electronic charting. The upper-level managers will be providing classes to assist the nurses in achieving this change, which demonstrates support for the nurses.

39. 1. Taking routine vital signs is not complex, has little potential for harm, requires only simple problem-solving skills, involves a simple level of interaction with the client, and is within the scope of practice of a nursing assistant. Taking vital signs requires the more advanced competencies of a Registered Nurse when previous vital signs have been outside the expected range, the client is unstable, or the client is transferred from one service/unit to another.

2. **Discharge teaching requires the knowledge and judgment of a Registered Nurse. It requires synthesizing and summarizing information as well as coordinating a variety of community health-care services to meet client needs.**

3. Ambulating a stable client in the hall is within the scope of practice of a nursing assistant and does not require the educational skill of a Registered Nurse.

4. Administering an enema is not a complex task. It requires simple problem-solving skills, involves a predictable outcome, and employs a simple level of interaction with the client. It does not require the more advanced competencies of a Registered Nurse.

5. Transporting a client is not a complex task. It requires simple problem-solving skills and involves a predictable outcome and a simple level of interaction with the client. It does not require the more advanced competencies of a Registered Nurse.

40. **Change takes place when one is moved out of one's comfort zone and into a discomfort zone. The moving stage causes discomfort as goals and objectives are developed and solutions are implemented. Unfreezing occurs before one enters into the moving stage. Unfreezing is the stage where one is aware of a problem and deciding whether or not improvement is possible. During unfreezing, one is still within one's comfort zone. Refreezing is the stage where the change becomes a part of the work setting and environment. A new comfort zone is developed as one becomes familiar with the change and incorporates the change into daily practice.**

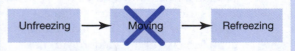

Health-Care Delivery

The following words include nursing/medical terminology, concepts, principles, and information relevant to content specifically addressed in the chapter, or information associated with topics presented in it. English dictionaries, nursing textbooks, and medical dictionaries, such as *Taber's Cyclopedic Medical Dictionary,* are resources that can be used to expand your knowledge and understanding of these words and related information.

Acuity

Advocate

ANA's Principles for Health System
  Transformation 2016

Baby boomers

Burnout

Career ladder

Case management, case manager

Client classification system

Continuity of care

Cost containment

Counselor

Critical pathways

Demographics

Diagnosis Related Groups (DRGs)

Functional nursing

Health-care team members:

  Activity Therapist

  Certified Social Worker

  Client

  Client's family members

  Clinical Nurse Specialist

  Licensed Practical Nurse

  Nurse Anesthetist

  Nursing Assistant (also known as
    Certified Nursing Assistant, Patient
    Care Assistant, Patient Care Techni-
    cian, or Nurse Aide depending on
    educational preparation)

  Nurse Midwife

  Nurse Practitioner

  Occupational Therapist

  Pastoral care provider, clergy

  Physical Therapist

  Physician

  Physician's Assistant

  Registered Dietitian

  Registered Nurse

  Speech Therapist

Health-care settings:

  Acute care hospitals

Ambulatory care centers

Assisted-living residence

Clinics

Day-care centers

Extended care

Home health services

Hospice (inpatient, residential, in the
  home)

Industrial or occupation settings

Life-care community

Long-term care nursing homes

Mental health facilities

Neighborhood community health center

Physicians' offices

Rehabilitation centers

School settings

Urgent care centers

Health Maintenance Organization

Levels of health care delivery:

  Primary health care

  Secondary health care

  Tertiary health care

Managed care

Medicaid

Medicare

Multidisciplinary

Preauthorization

Preferred Provider Organization

Primary nursing

Prospective payment system

Reengineering

Reimbursement

Resource Utilization Groups (RUGs)

Sandwich generation

Third-party payers

Types of agencies:

  Official—governmental

  Proprietary—for profit

  Voluntary—not for profit

Undocumented immigrants

HEALTH-CARE DELIVERY: QUESTIONS

1. Which health-care team member can provide independent health care with third-party reimbursement in the emerging health-care delivery system in the United States?
   1. Licensed Registered Nurse
   2. Clinical Nurse Specialist
   3. Physician's Assistant
   4. Nurse Practitioner

2. Which does critical pathways in health care refer to?
   1. Educational career ladders for health-care professionals
   2. Multidisciplinary plans with predetermined client outcomes
   3. Times during life when certain health problems are more likely to occur
   4. Organizations that provide services that progress from acute care to long-term care

3. Which setting is the organizational center of the United States health-care system?
   1. Clinic setting
   2. Acute care setting
   3. Community setting
   4. Long-term care setting

4. A nurse is explaining mammography screening to a client. Which level of health-care delivery does this diagnostic test reflect?
   1. Secondary
   2. Tertiary
   3. Primary
   4. Acute

5. When should a nurse begin a client's rehabilitative care?
   1. When the client is conscious
   2. After the client begins walking
   3. Once the medical diagnosis is made
   4. Just before discharge from the hospital

6. A nurse case manager is counseling an older adult client about resources available to assist with the cost of health care. Which organization that provides the majority of the health-care costs for people older than 65 years of age should the nurse inform the client about?
   1. Medicare
   2. Medicaid
   3. Blue Cross
   4. Blue Shield

7. Which result of reengineering in hospital settings has raised the greatest concerns for client safety?
   1. Decreased hospital occupancy rates
   2. Increased acuity of hospitalized clients
   3. Hospitals merging with larger institutions
   4. Substitution of less skilled workers for nurses

8. A client is discharged from the hospital 3 days after abdominal surgery because of the influence of Diagnosis Related Groups (DRGs). Which should the nurse performing the discharge teaching be **most** concerned about?
   1. Providing for continuity of care
   2. Ordering equipment to be used in the home
   3. Accepting discharge by the client and family
   4. Verifying that the client has insurance to cover hospital costs

9. Together, the nurse and client are setting a goal during health-care planning. Which factor generates the **most** anxiety for a client with this process?
   1. Role
   2. Values
   3. Beliefs
   4. Change

10. Three hospitals agree to work collectively to provide a full range of health-care services in their neighborhoods. Which type of relationship has been entered into by these hospitals?
    1. Integrated health-care service network
    2. Third-party reimbursement system
    3. Health Maintenance Organization
    4. Diagnosis Related Groups

11. A nurse is planning actions that address a client's health-care needs. Which statement is important for the nurse to consider?
    1. Health and illness clearly are separated at the middle of the health-illness continuum.
    2. Demographics of the population of the United States are changing drastically.
    3. External factors mainly are the cause of most illnesses.
    4. Most people view health as the absence of disease.

12. Which action is common to the majority of Registered Nurse positions in different settings in which nurses work?
    1. Assisting a primary health-care provider
    2. Serving in an administrative capacity
    3. Developing client plans of care
    4. Providing direct physical care

13. A nurse is planning a community outreach program about the variety of health-care professionals and the services they provide. Which members of the health-care team should the nurse indicate are the largest group of health-care personnel in the United States?
    1. Nursing assistants
    2. Social workers
    3. Physicians
    4. Nurses

14. Which is the **major** factor that limits the overhaul of the health-care delivery system of the United States?
    1. Elected officials who do not respond to the pressure of their political constituencies
    2. Explosion of technical advances within the profession of medicine
    3. Complexity of the problems associated with health-care reform
    4. Resistance of physicians to reform

15. Which is emphasized in the traditional health-care delivery system in the United States?
    1. Health promotion
    2. Illness prevention
    3. Diagnosis and treatment
    4. Rehabilitation and long-term care

16. At the end of a shift, the nurse in charge must evaluate each client in relation to the agency's client classification system. Which is the purpose of this client classification system?
    1. Document resource needs for the purpose of establishing reimbursement.
    2. Provide data about client acuity to help assign nursing staff.
    3. Establish that quality standards have been met.
    4. Identify standardized expected outcomes.

17. Which health-care professional is **best** prepared to track a client's progress through the health-care system?
1. Case manager
2. Primary nurse
3. Nurse manager
4. Home-care nurse

18. A nurse is reviewing a variety of surveys regarding the delivery of health care within the United States. Which statement reflects a significant change in the thinking of the general public about concepts related to health-care delivery?
1. "Institutional-based care will have to be increased as baby boomers age."
2. "More services must address the secondary health-care needs of the community."
3. "Individuals can influence their own health through behavior and lifestyle changes."
4. "Health-care providers should be primarily responsible to provide appropriate health-care services."

19. Which should a nurse conclude is the main cause of the shift of health-care delivery from the hospital to the home?
1. Use of Resource Utilization Groups to categorize needs of clients
2. Need for hospital beds to be available for the acutely ill
3. Limits on length of stay by reimbursement sources
4. Shortage of qualified licensed nurses

20. A client asks the nurse, "What is the difference between Medicare and Medicaid?" Which response by the nurse describes the Medicaid program?
1. "A retrospective health-care reimbursement program that pays for costs incurred by health-care agencies for the care of the indigent"
2. "A state program requiring primary health-care providers to deliver care to people living below the designated poverty level"
3. "A federally funded health insurance program for individuals with minimal incomes"
4. "A federally funded health insurance program for people age 65 years or older"

21. A client is told that preauthorization is required before surgery can be performed. The client asks the nurse, "What does preauthorization mean?" Which is an accurate response to the client's question?
1. "Third-party payers have approved the surgery, and the facility will be reimbursed for costs."
2. "The preoperative checklist has been completed and verified by a nurse."
3. "Required preoperative diagnostic tests have been performed."
4. "You have signed the legal consent form for the surgery."

22. A client is to return from the postanesthesia care unit to a semiprivate room. Which is the **most** significant factor concerning the postoperative client's potential room-mate that will influence the nurse's decision to transfer the postoperative client to this room?
1. Emotionally fragile
2. Able to communicate
3. In the bed by the window
4. Physiologically compatible

23. A client with an infection receives medical intervention and nursing care in a hospital setting. Which level health-care has been provided in this situation?
1. Emergency
2. Secondary
3. Tertiary
4. Primary

24. Which is the cornerstone of *Nursing's Agenda for Health Care Reform?*
1. A standardized package of health-care services must be provided by organizations within the federal government.
2. Health-care services should be provided in environments that are accessible, familiar, and friendly.
3. Advanced practice nurses should play a prominent role in the provision of primary health care.
4. Nursing must provide for the central focus of the health-care delivery system.

25. A home health-care nurse is functioning as a case manager for a client recently discharged from the hospital. Which is the **primary** role of the nurse when functioning as a case manager?
1. Coordinator
2. Counselor
3. Provider
4. Teacher

26. Which is the **best** example of an inpatient care setting where nursing care is delivered?
1. Ambulatory care center
2. Extended-care facility
3. Day-care center
4. Hospice

27. Which change identified by the nurse will **most** affect health-care delivery in the United States in the future?
1. Less emphasis will be placed on prolonging life.
2. The proportion of older adults in society will increase.
3. More people will seek health care in an acute care setting.
4. Genetic counseling will dramatically decrease the number of ill infants born.

28. Diagnosis Related Groups (DRGs) were instituted by the federal government mainly to reduce which of the following?
1. Number of professionals working in hospitals
2. Severity of needs of hospitalized clients
3. Fragmentation of care
4. Cost of health care

29. Which characteristic is unique to the nurse-client relationship?
1. Client's needs are satisfied.
2. There is a social component.
3. Both are working toward a common goal.
4. The nurse is the leader of the health team.

30. A recently licensed Registered Nurse is working the night shift on an active medical unit in a hospital. Which is the **best** way that this nurse can prevent professional burnout?
1. Challenge the how and why of one's role.
2. Get adequate sleep and exercise each day.
3. Clarify expectations, strengths, and limitations.
4. Seek a balance among seriousness, humor, and aloofness.

31. Which intervention is likely to have the **most** impact on decreasing the nursing shortage?
1. Providing stress reduction programs to address needs of nurses experiencing burnout
2. Offering bonuses to entice nurses close to retirement to work longer
3. Developing initiatives to fund the education of nursing faculty
4. Increasing the recruitment of foreign registered nurses

32. A client receiving a special diet is given a meal tray that does not contain a food requested by the client. Place the following interventions in the order that they should be implemented by the nurse.
1. Check the dietary manual.
2. Schedule a conference with the dietitian.
3. Verify the primary health-care provider's dietary prescription.
4. Explore with the primary health-care provider the possibility of including this food preference in the diet.

Answer: _____

33. Which is an example of an official agency? **Select all that apply.**
1. _____ American Cancer Society
2. _____ Veterans Affairs Hospital
3. _____ American Heart Association
4. _____ National League for Nursing
5. _____ Nonprofit community hospital

34. An older adult woman, who was incoherent, wandering, and wearing inadequate clothing for the cold weather, was found by a police officer at night. The woman was admitted to the hospital for dehydration and mild hypothermia. The next afternoon, a nurse assesses the client, interviews the client's daughter, and considers the health-care services within the community. Which health-care service should the nurse explore with the daughter?
1. Respite care center
2. Home health aide several hours a day
3. Full-day older adult day-care program
4. Long-term care facility with assistive living services

CLIENT'S CLINICAL RECORD

Client's History
Client lives with daughter and attends a half-day older adult day-care program. She experiences episodes of confusion and generally recognizes her family members but has issues with judgment. She has not attended the day-care program for the past month.

Client Assessment
Vital signs are all within expected limits, including the temperature, which is 97.8°F; knows her name but at this time does not recognize her daughter or grandchildren; moved to room across from the nurses' station for constant observation because client attempted to wander off the unit.

Interview With Daughter
Daughter states her mother's abilities have progressively declined the last several months. "I am a single mom of three kids ages 5, 8, and 10, and I work part-time. Lately, my mom has episodes of not knowing who we are. I was shocked when the police called and said they found her last night. I am exhausted. I don't think that I can keep doing this much longer."

35. Which factor that is increasing and that is associated with older adults has an impact on the delivery of health care to this population within the United States? **Select all that apply.**
1. _____ Accidental falls
2. _____ Misuse of alcohol
3. _____ Presence of cognitive deficits
4. _____ Number of persons living longer
5. _____ Existence of multiple health problems

36. A nurse is a member of an agency's Health Care Research and Quality Committee. The nurse reviews the following bar graph regarding client satisfaction with the hospital experience after implementation of a 3-month initiative to improve client satisfaction related to four quality indicators. Identify which quality indicator related to client satisfaction exhibits the **most** significant improvement between January and March.
1. Satisfaction with educational information
2. Satisfaction with pain management
3. Satisfaction with nursing care
4. Satisfaction with overall care

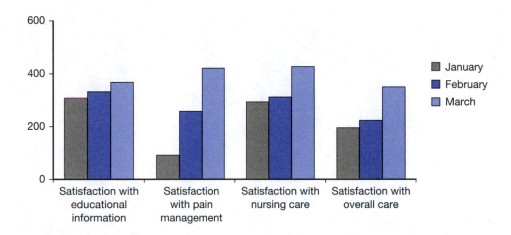

37. Which nursing activity reflects care on the primary level of health-care delivery? **Select all that apply.**
1. _____ Arranging for hospice services
2. _____ Presenting a class on a healthy diet
3. _____ Providing emergency care at a local hospital
4. _____ Encouraging attendance at a Smoke Enders' meeting
5. _____ Administering an immunization to prevent a childhood disease

38. A nurse is considering the services within the community that can meet clients' activities of daily living and health-care needs. Place these services in order beginning with the one in which the client requires the least assistance to the one in which the client receives the most assistance.
1. An intermediate care setting that provides health-care services to individuals who are not acutely ill
2. An assisted-living setting that provides meals and minimal help with activities of daily living
3. An independent care setting that provides meals and housekeeping services
4. A long-term care facility that provides skilled nursing care
5. A subacute unit in a skilled nursing facility

Answer: _____

39. A nurse is functioning as a client advocate. Which word **best** describes this nursing role? **Select all that apply.**
1. _____ Provider
2. _____ Nurturer
3. _____ Protector
4. _____ Evaluator
5. _____ Supporter

40. Identify which of the following individuals are nursing team members. **Select all that apply.**
1. _____ Client
2. _____ Hospice Nurse
3. _____ Registered Nurse
4. _____ Nursing Assistant
5. _____ Licensed Practical Nurse

1. 1. Licensed Registered Nurses do not receive third-party reimbursement for their services.

2. Clinical Nurse Specialists are not health-care professionals who receive third-party reimbursement. Clinical Nurse Specialists have been involved in health-care delivery since the 1960s. They are master's-prepared nurses with a specialty in certain areas (e.g., medical-surgical nursing, pediatrics, mental health), or they may have advanced education and experience in caring for individuals with special needs (e.g., wound care, enterostomal care, or care of the client with diabetes).

3. Physician's Assistants are not health-care professionals who receive third-party reimbursement directly. They work under the supervision of a physician in many different settings and are paid by the physician in private practice or by the organization that hired them. They assist physicians by carrying out common, routine medical treatments, and they have prescriptive authority.

4. **This is a relatively new trend in health-care delivery. Nurse Practitioners generally are master's-prepared individuals who work independently or collaboratively with physicians to provide primary health-care services. Nurse Practitioners work independently under their own license, are accountable for their own practice, have prescriptive authority, and receive third-party reimbursement, depending on the state in which they work. In the states that do not permit this level of health-care delivery, Nurse Practitioners work under the license of a physician who supervises their practice.**

2. 1. Critical pathways are not an educational career ladder for health-care professionals. A career ladder is the organization of educational experiences so that professional growth progresses in a planned manner.

2. **Critical pathways are a case management system that identifies specific protocols and timetables for care and treatment by various disciplines that are designed to achieve expected client outcomes within a specific time frame.**

3. This statement is a definition of critical time, not critical pathways.

4. This statement is unrelated to critical pathways.

3. 1. The clinic setting is not the organizational center of the United States health-care system.

2. **The acute care setting is the organizational center of the United States health-care system today. Specialized services (tertiary level of care) and emergency, critical care, and intense diagnosis and treatment (secondary level of care) of illness and disease are provided for in hospitals (acute care setting). In 1991, the American Nurses Association published *Nursing's Agenda for Health Care Reform*, which made recommendations for health-care reform in many areas. The major trend identified as a result of implementation of the recommendations is a shift of the focus of health care from illness and cure to one of wellness and care. If this occurs, the health-care system of the United States will shift eventually from the acute care setting to the home and community.**

3. The community setting is not the organizational center of the United States health-care system at this time.

4. The long-term care setting is not the organizational center of the United States health-care system.

4. 1. **Screening surveys and diagnostic procedures are examples of secondary health-care delivery. Secondary health-care delivery is associated with early detection, early and quick intervention, health maintenance, and prevention of complications. There are three levels of health-care delivery: primary (avoiding disease through health promotion and disease prevention); secondary (early detection and treatment); and tertiary (reducing complications, rehabilitation, and restoration and maintenance of optimal function).**

2. This scenario is not an example of tertiary health-care delivery. Tertiary care begins after a situation is stabilized, and the focus is on rehabilitation and restoration within the limits of the disability.

3. This scenario is not an example of primary health-care delivery. Primary care is associated with activities that promote health and protect against disease.

4. Acute is not one of the levels of health-care delivery. The word *acute* refers to the type of care that is provided on the secondary level of health-care delivery.

5. 1. Rehabilitation interventions begin whether the client is conscious or unconscious.
2. Rehabilitation interventions begin whether the client is ambulatory or nonambulatory.
3. **As soon as a client is diagnosed with a problem, rehabilitation interventions begin. Care should be present and future oriented.**
4. This is too late to begin rehabilitation interventions.

6. 1. **Medicare has two parts, Part A and Part B. Most people enroll in Part A when they reach 65 years of age. It covers costs if one is admitted to a hospital, hospice, or skilled nursing facility for other than custodial care. Individuals must pay a deductible each year, and those who worked less than 10 years in the United States must pay a monthly fee. Part B covers outpatient care, including primary-care provider visits, physical therapy, diagnostic tests, vaccines, and some medical supplies. Individuals pay a monthly fee, a deductible, and 20% of the Medicare-approved amount for some types of care.**
2. Medicaid is not a program that pays for the majority of health-care costs of people older than 65 years of age. Medicaid is a U.S. federal program that is state operated and provides medical assistance for people with low incomes.
3. Blue Cross is a not-for-profit medical insurance plan that pays for hospital services for people of all ages, not just people older than 65 years of age.
4. Blue Shield is a not-for-profit medical insurance plan that pays for care provided by health-care professionals for all age groups, not just for people older than 65 years of age.

7. 1. Reengineering has not reduced hospital occupancy rates. Decreased hospital occupancy rates are related directly to Diagnosis Related Groups and the resultant decrease in lengths of stay. The concerns about a decrease in occupancy rates are not related to client safety but rather fiscal issues.
2. Although the increased acuity of hospitalized clients is a real concern when providing for client safety, safety should not be

an issue if a unit is adequately staffed with the appropriate mix of nurses to ancillary staff.
3. Hospital mergers and the resulting reengineering should not have an impact on client safety if professional practice standards are maintained.
4. **Reengineering in relation to the delivery care is concerned with training a less educationally prepared nursing assistant to implement nursing tasks that were formerly associated with the practice of nursing. This trend poses a serious threat to the safety and welfare of clients because tasks requiring the complex skills of a nurse are being delegated to minimally prepared individuals. This is dangerous in the present health-care environment, in which hospitalized clients are more acutely ill than ever before.**

8. 1. **Providing for continuity of care is the major concern with early discharge as a result of DRGs. It requires careful planning to ensure that services, personnel, and equipment are provided in a timely and comprehensive manner and care is not fragmented and disorganized.**
2. Although this is a concern for some individuals, if the discharge planner plans early for the client's discharge, all equipment should be in place before the client is discharged.
3. Although this is a concern for some individuals, if clients receive supportive emotional intervention and are prepared for discharge from the first day of admission, clients generally would rather be at home than in the hospital.
4. It is not within the scope of nursing practice to ensure that clients have insurance to cover the cost of services rendered.

9. 1. A role is a set of expectations about how one should behave. Although a health-care goal may conflict with a role one sets for oneself, another option has greater ability to contribute to anxiety than one's role.
2. A value is an enduring attitude about something that is cherished and held dear to one's heart and should not generate anxiety. People generally set health-care goals that do not conflict with their values.
3. A belief is an opinion or a conclusion that one accepts as true and may be based on faith, facts, or both. It should not generate anxiety. People generally set health-care goals that do not conflict with their beliefs.

4. **Change almost always causes anxiety because it requires one to move from that which is comfortable and familiar to that which is uncomfortable, unfamiliar, unpredictable, and threatening.**

10. 1. **This is an example of an integrated health-care service network. Hospitals are joining networks to decrease costs and increase reimbursement. This is accomplished by expanding the breadth of services while avoiding duplication of services, keeping people within the network, negotiating the price of supplies and equipment, and centralizing departments (e.g., administration, staff education, and human resources), which results in fewer personnel.**
    2. This is not an example of a third-party reimbursement system. Third-party reimbursement refers to someone other than the receiver of health care (generally an insurance company) paying for the services provided.
    3. This is not an example of a health maintenance organization (HMO). An HMO is an organization that provides primary health care for a preset fee.
    4. Diagnosis Related Groups (DRGs) are pretreatment diagnoses reimbursement categories designed to decrease the average length of a hospital stay, reducing costs.

11. 1. There is no clear separation between health and illness on the health-illness continuum. Each individual's personal perceptions of multiple factors determine where a person places himself or herself on the health-illness continuum.
    2. **Demographics are changing rapidly in the United States as we become a more heterogeneous, multicultural, multiethnic society. Because of the increasing diversity of the population of the United States, nurses must use transcultural knowledge in a skillful way to provide culturally appropriate, competent care.**
    3. Internal as well as external factors are the cause of illness.
    4. Most people do not view health as the absence of disease. There is no one definition of health because there are so many different factors that affect one's definition of health. Therefore, a definition of health depends on each individual person's own perspective.

12. 1. The majority of nurses' time is concerned with implementing independent and dependent functions within the scope of nursing practice, not spent assisting a primary health-care provider. In most settings, the nurse and the primary health-care provider work in a collaborative relationship to help clients cope with human responses to illness and disease.
    2. Only nursing management positions contain an administrative component.
    3. **Nurses work in a variety of settings; however, a component that is common to all settings is the use of critical thinking to develop client plans of care.**
    4. Not all Registered Nurse positions include direct physical care of clients. For example, many positions in home care, clinics, industry, and schools focus on case finding, ongoing monitoring of progress, and teaching rather than direct physical care.

13. 1. Nursing Assistants are not health-care professionals.
    2. Social workers are not the largest group of health-care professionals in the United States.
    3. Physicians are not the largest group of health-care professionals in the United States.
    4. **Nurses comprise the largest group of health-care professionals in the United States. There are not enough Registered Nurses to meet the present demand. The Bureau of Labor Statistics Employment Projections 2014 to 2024 identified the need for 1.2 million more nurses to replace retiring nurses and meet the increased need for health care related to the aging population. Jobs for Registered Nurses are projected to increase 16% from 2014 to 2024.**

14. 1. Most elected officials recognize the need for health-care reform but generally want to support reform that reflects the desires of their political constituencies. This requires negotiations within the political system that can be prolonged and contentious.
    2. This is not the major factor that limits the overhaul of the health-care delivery system of the United States.
    3. **Health-care delivery in the United States is an extremely complex service industry consisting of public, voluntary,**

and proprietary businesses with multiple disciplines of health-care workers represented. The system is influenced by federal, state, and local social, economic, ethical, and consumer-driven issues.

4. Physician input is only one factor that may prevent an overhaul of the health-care delivery system of the United States. Although the American Medical Association has a strong political action committee, it was unable to prevent the institution of prospective reimbursement systems that in many ways dramatically changed the work world of the physician as well as placing limits on financial compensation for medical services provided.

15. 1. Health promotion is not emphasized in the traditional health-care delivery system in the United States. However, in 1992, the National League for Nursing predicted that, in the future, health care in the United States will move from the traditional hospital setting to the community with an emphasis on health promotion. Although traditional health-care delivery centers on activities associated with diagnosing, treating, and curing illness and disease, more care is delivered in the community setting and a greater emphasis is on health promotion today than in 1992.

2. Illness prevention is not emphasized in the traditional health-care delivery system in the United States. In 1992, the National League for Nursing predicted that in the future, health care in the United States will move from the traditional hospital setting to the community with an emphasis on illness prevention. Although traditional health-care delivery centers on activities associated with diagnosing, treating, and curing illness and disease, more care is delivered in the community setting and a greater emphasis is on health promotion today than in 1992.

3. **Traditional health-care delivery in the United States is centered on activities associated with diagnosing, treating, and curing illness and disease. In addition, hospitals account for the largest proportion of money spent on health care and employ the largest number of health-care workers.**

4. Rehabilitation and long-term care are not emphasized in the traditional health-care delivery system in the United States.

16. 1. This statement does not reflect the purpose of a client classification system.

2. **A client classification system, or acuity report, is designed to rate clients in terms of high or low acuity; the level of acuity is based on the amount of time and nursing resources that are needed to care for the client. A client who is unstable and requires constant monitoring and nursing intervention will be rated a higher acuity score than a client who is stable and relatively self-sufficient in activities of daily living.**

3. Ongoing quality improvement programs are designed to establish whether standards of care have been met and are not a client classification system.

4. Standardized expected outcomes are established by professional educational and practice organizations, credentialing bodies, and critical pathways, not by a client classification system.

17. 1. **A case manager coordinates and links health-care services to clients and their families at single levels of care (e.g., during hospitalization) and across levels of care (e.g., progression through hospitalization, extended-care facilities, and home care).**

2. A primary nurse has total responsibility for the planning and delivery of nursing care to a specific client for the duration of the client's hospitalization. Primary nursing is a nursing care delivery system that attempts to prevent fragmentation of care and ensure a comprehensive, consistent approach to meeting a client's needs while in the hospital.

3. A nurse manager's job is to ensure that the objectives and goals of the organization are met appropriately, efficiently, and in a cost-effective manner.

4. A home-care nurse provides and coordinates health services in the home.

18. 1. Studies and position papers from all segments of the health-care industry indicate the need to provide more health-care services in the community and not institutional settings. To meet the health-care needs of older adults in the future, efforts have to begin now to provide more community-based support services so that people can remain in their own homes and not have to move to an institutional setting.

2. More services need to address the primary, not secondary, health-care needs of the community. Secondary health-care services include emergency care, acute care, diagnosis, and complex treatment. The present health-care system has an infrastructure that supports the delivery of secondary health-care services. More emphasis must be placed on providing services that meet the primary health-care needs of society, which include health promotion, illness prevention, health education, and environmental protection.

3. **Consumers are more aware than ever before that change in their own behavior and lifestyle will have a major influence on their own health status. Public health service announcements, community health education programs, and even television programs and media print materials (e.g., newspapers and magazines) have improved consumer awareness.**

4. Consumers, not health-care providers, should be charged with the primary responsibility for providing appropriate health-care services. As individuals or as groups, consumer demands and expectations will have the greatest impact on the delivery of health care.

19. 1. Resource Utilization Groups (RUGs) is the client classification system used to determine reimbursement rates to nursing homes and is unrelated to the shift of health-care delivery from the hospital to the home.

2. The need for hospital beds to be available for the acutely ill is not the reason for the shift of health-care delivery from the hospital to the home. As a result of Diagnosis Related Groups, many hospitals are downsizing to reduce costs and do not need more hospital beds.

3. **Limits on length of stay by reimbursement sources is the reason for the shift from the hospital to the home because clients are discharged earlier in an effort to reduce the cost of health care. Usually it is less expensive to support a person in the home than in a health-care facility.**

4. Although there is a national shortage of licensed nurses, this has not caused a shift of health-care delivery from the hospital to the home. It is predicted that if the demand for nurses continues at the present rate, and even if the present rate of

graduating nurses increases slightly each year, by the year 2020 the nation's supply of registered nurses will meet only 72% of the demand.

20. 1. Health-care reimbursement in the hospital setting in the United States is based on a prospective, not retrospective, reimbursement formula. Diagnosis Related Groups is a predetermined hospital reimbursement rate based on a medical problem.

2. Participation in programs providing care to people living below the designated poverty level is voluntary, not mandatory.

3. **Medicaid is a federally funded, but state-regulated, health insurance program for individuals with low incomes.**

4. This statement describes Medicare, not Medicaid.

21. 1. **To maintain quality control and cost containment, third-party payers have preauthorization criteria for surgery that may include requirements such as second opinions and initial conservative therapies.**

2. A preoperative checklist is unrelated to preauthorization. A checklist summarizes the client's preoperative preparation to ensure that all significant activities and safety precautions have been completed before surgery.

3. Diagnostic tests are not related to the concept of preauthorization. Diagnostic tests are performed to identify actual or potential health problems that may influence, or be affected by, the surgery.

4. An Informed Consent is unrelated to preauthorization. Informed Consent is a legal document giving permission for surgery, including the procedure, surgical site, and surgeons.

22. 1. Many hospitalized clients may be emotionally fragile because of the stress of the experience. It is only when clients are a threat to themselves or others that they should not be placed with another client and should be under constant supervision.

2. The ability to communicate is not a requirement for roommates. A client does not have to converse with, or be responsible for, another client.

3. The location of a bed within a room is insignificant. When two beds are available, the choice may be left to client preference.

4. **One client's physical condition should not interfere with another client's physical condition. For example, a**

client with a communicable disease should be in a private room, whereas a client with an incision or an open wound should not be in a room with a client with an infection.

23. 1. Emergency care is a type of health-care service, not a level of health-care delivery. Emergency care is a description of one type of service provided in secondary health-care services.
    2. **This scenario is an example of secondary health-care services. Secondary health care is associated with intense and elaborate diagnosis and treatment of disease or trauma and includes critical care and emergency treatment. Health-care services have three levels of health care that describe the scope of services and settings where health care is provided: primary, secondary, and tertiary.**
    3. This scenario is not an example of tertiary health-care services. Tertiary health care is associated with the provision of palliative care and rehabilitation.
    4. This scenario is not an example of primary health-care services. Primary health care is associated with the promotion of health and protection against disease.

24. 1. Although a standardized package of health-care services is a component of *Nursing's Agenda for Health Care Reform*, it is not the cornerstone of the document.
    2. **This statement reflects the cornerstone of *Nursing's Agenda for Health Care Reform*. All people have a right to receive health care, but this right is useless unless the care is easily reached and used.**
    3. Although a prominent role for advanced practice nurses is a component of *Nursing's Agenda for Health Care Reform*, it is not the cornerstone of the document.
    4. Although this is a component of *Nursing's Agenda for Health Care Reform*, it is not the cornerstone of the document.

25. 1. **The primary role of a case manager is to coordinate the activities of all the other members of the health-care team and ensure that the client is receiving care in the most appropriate setting.**
    2. Counseling is not the primary role of a case manager. When counseling, the nurse helps a client recognize and cope with emotional stressors, improve relationships, and/or promote personal growth.

3. Providing care is not the primary role of a case manager. When providing care, the nurse is in the direct caregiver role. Caregiving involves identifying and meeting the client's needs by helping the client regain health through the caring process.
    4. Teaching is not the primary role of a case manager. When teaching, the nurse helps the client learn about health and health-care practices.

26. 1. Ambulatory care centers are not an inpatient care setting. Although some may be located in a hospital, they are more often in convenient locations, such as a shopping mall or storefront. They provide services such as emergency walk-in care, ambulatory surgery, and health prevention and health promotion interventions.
    2. **An extended-care facility is an inpatient setting where a client lives while receiving subacute medical, nursing, or custodial care. It includes facilities such as intermediate care and skilled nursing facilities (nursing homes), assisted living centers, rehabilitation centers, and residential facilities for the mentally or developmentally disabled.**
    3. Day-care centers are not examples of inpatient care settings. Day-care centers provide care for people who arrive in the morning and go home at the end of the day. They provide care for healthy children or older adults so that significant others can work, or they provide specialized services to specific populations, such as individuals with neuromuscular or mental health problems.
    4. Although hospice services may be provided in a hospital, a nursing home, or a residential hospice setting, the majority of hospice services are provided in the home. Hospice agencies provide multiple specialized services to support the dignity and quality of life of individuals who are dying and their family members.

27. 1. Although this remains to be seen, the explosion in knowledge and technology usually results in treatments that prolong life.
    2. **The percentage of older adults in the United States is expected to increase to 20% by the year 2050. Because chronic illness is more prevalent among older adults, additional health-care services will be needed in the future, raising costs.**

3. More people will seek health care in the home and community, not the acute care setting. In 1992, the National League for Nursing predicted that home care will become the center of health care and that community nursing centers and community health programs will focus on illness prevention and health promotion.

4. This may or may not occur because of a multiplicity of factors, such as religious beliefs, unplanned pregnancies, multiple births, and a lack of seeking genetic counseling.

28. 1. This is not the reason why DRGs were instituted. In addition, the DRGs have increased the acuity of hospitalized clients, requiring a lower ratio of nurses to clients, which necessitates the need to hire more nurses. However, many hospitals have not increased the number of nurses because of reengineering and the lack of available qualified nurses.

2. Reducing the severity of needs of hospitalized clients is not why DRGs were instituted. The severity of needs of hospitalized clients increases, not decreases, with DRGs because clients are discharged earlier, making beds available for more acutely ill clients.

3. DRGs were not instituted to solve fragmentation of care. Fragmentation of care generally is caused by overspecialization and caregivers failing to address clients' needs holistically and comprehensively.

4. **The DRGs, pretreatment diagnoses reimbursement categories, were designed to decrease the average length of a hospital stay, reducing costs.**

29. 1. Because of circumstances, a nurse's intervention may not always be able to meet a client's perceived needs.

2. The nurse-client relationship is a therapeutic, not social, relationship.

3. **When planning client care, the nurse and client work together to identify appropriate goals and interventions to facilitate goal achievement.**

4. The client, not the nurse, is the leader of the health-care team.

30. 1. How one practices nursing and why one is a nurse are based on enduring values and beliefs. Although it is important to be aware of how one practices nursing and why one is a nurse, confronting, taking exception to, and calling into question

one's enduring values are not where the problem of burnout lies.

2. Although it is important to get adequate sleep and exercise each day to reduce the effects of stress, these approaches do not reduce the contributing factors that cause stress.

3. **When faced with any stressful situation that can lead to feelings of burnout, the nurse must begin with self-awareness and identify personal expectations, strengths, and limitations associated with the job. After the assessment is complete and problems are identified, the nurse can explore options to reduce factors contributing to job-related stress. Burnout generally occurs because nurses are unable to practice nursing as they were taught based on principles and standards of practice. Nurses experience stress because of such factors as understaffing, increased client care assignments, shift work, excessive mandatory overtime, inadequate support, and caring for more clients who are critically ill and dying. The nurse must employ strategies to manage stress to prevent the physical and emotional exhaustion associated with burnout and not wait until these responses occur.**

4. Although humor may temporarily defuse a stressful situation, it is not an effective strategy to cope with the major issues that contribute to burnout. The nurse should not be distant from the client.

31. 1. Although nurses are leaving the profession because it is stressful, physically strenuous, and demanding work, it is not the major reason for the nurse shortage.

2. A bonus to entice nurses close to retirement age to work longer is a short-term and limited response to the need for more nurses. Retirement of nurses is not the major cause of the nursing shortage.

3. **Programs to fund the education of nursing educators will most likely have the greatest impact on reducing the nursing shortage. Many nursing schools are unable to accept eligible applicants to nursing programs each year because of the shortage of faculty. The American Association of Colleges of Nursing report on *Enrollment and Graduations in Baccalaureate and Graduate Programs of Nursing* (2016–2017) indicated that nursing**

schools turned away 64,067 eligible candidates to baccalaureate and graduate nursing programs mainly as a result of insufficient faculty in addition to other constraints such as insufficient clinical sites, classrooms, and preceptors as well as budget constraints.

4. Hiring foreign nurses is not a long-term strategy to increase the number of nurses. It will worsen the shortage in their own countries, because the nursing shortage is a global problem, and it will raise concerns regarding effects on salaries, adequacy of education, and quality care here in the United States.

32. **3. Providing a special diet is a dependent function of the nurse. The primary health-care provider's prescription should be verified first.**
1. **The dietary manual should be reviewed to determine if the requested food is permitted on the prescribed diet.**
2. **If the requested food is not indicated on the diet in the dietary manual, the nurse should collaborate with appropriate dietary resources (e.g., nutritionist, dietitian).**
4. **If the food is not permitted on the diet, the nurse can function as a client advocate by collaborating with the primary health-care provider to determine if an occasional concession can be made regarding a client's food preference.**

33. 1. The American Cancer Society is a voluntary not-for-profit organization, not an official organization.
2. **A Veterans Affairs Hospital is an official organization because it is a part of the Department of Veterans Affairs, which is under the umbrella of federally supported/operated facilities and is financed by taxation.**
3. The American Heart Association is a voluntary not-for-profit organization, not an official organization.
4. The National League for Nursing (NLN) is a not-for-profit organization founded in 1952 to foster the development and improvement of nursing education and services. It is not an official organization.
5. Nonprofit community hospitals are voluntary, not official, organizations.

34. 1. The daughter needs more than a brief period of relief from caring for her mother. She is a single mother working part-time and caring for three small children.
2. A home health aide several hours a day is an inadequate level of care to keep the client safe.
3. A full-day older adult day-care program may be capable of meeting the client's needs during the day. However, the client also needs supervision during the night, which may be beyond what the daughter can provide.
4. **The client requires assistance with the activities of daily living and supervision 24 hours a day to prevent wandering and promote safety.**

35. 1. **The Centers for Disease Control and Prevention (CDC) reported in 2014 that falls have become the leading cause of fatal and nonfatal injuries for older adults. The CDC stated that 28.7% of older adults reported falling for an estimated 28 million falls in the preceding 12 months with a projection of 48 million falls by 2030. In 2015, the cost of medical care for individuals experiencing falls was 31 billion dollars. Falls are a major factor that has significant impact on the delivery of health care within the United States as the number of individuals 65 years of age and older increases as baby boomers age.**
2. **A study from JAMA Psychiatry (reported September 2017) presented the following data: the proportion of high-risk drinking jumped 65% to 3.8% of the older population; older people engaging in high-risk drinking will increase as baby boomers age; older adults have a reduced ability to metabolize alcohol and aging brains that are more sensitive to sedative properties of alcohol; and older adults who misuse alcohol are subject to falls and aggravation of common chronic diseases, such as hypertension, heart disease, diabetes, brain attack, etc. All of these factors will increase the demand for the delivery of health care in the United States.**
3. **The percentage of older adults experiencing cognitive deficits varies depending on the agency compiling the research. The Centers for Disease Control and Prevention identified that in 2013, 5 million Americans age**

65 years or older had Alzheimer's disease. It was predicted that this number could increase to 13.8 million individuals by 2050. This is a major factor that has significant impact on the delivery of health care within the United States as the number of individuals 65 years of age and older increases as baby boomers age. The Alzheimer's Association predicts that by 2025, 7.1 million people will be affected by Alzheimer's dementia, a rise of 35% above the 5.3 million affected in 2017. The Alzheimer's Association predicts that by 2050, 13.8 million people will be diagnosed with Alzheimer's disease.

4. **Thirteen percent of the population was 65 years of age and older in 2010 (40.3 million people). The U.S. Census Bureau predicts that in 2050 there will be an increase to 80 million older adults, accounting for 24% of the population. This is a major factor that has significant impact on the delivery of health care within the United States as the number of individuals 65 years of age and older increases as baby boomers age.**

5. **The CDC reports that 75% of Americans age 65 and older have multiple chronic health problems, and approximately 71% of the total health care spending in the United States is related to clients with multiple chronic health problems. As the number of older people increases, the need for health care services will also increase.**

36. 1. Although satisfaction with educational information improved between January and March, the improvement was not as significant as improvement in another option.

2. **Although all four quality indicators related to client satisfaction demonstrated a positive trend toward greater satisfaction, satisfaction with pain management increased most dramatically from January to March.**

3. Although satisfaction with nursing care improved between January and March, the improvement was not as significant as improvement in another option.

4. Although satisfaction with overall care improved between January and March, the improvement was not as significant as improvement in another option.

37. 1. Arranging for hospice services is an example of care associated with the tertiary level of health-care services. Tertiary care is associated with long-term, chronic, and hospice care and specialized services.

2. **Presenting a class on a healthy diet is an example of the primary level of health-care services. Primary care is associated with activities that promote health and protect against disease.**

3. Providing emergency care at a local hospital is an example of care on the secondary level of health-care services. Secondary care (acute care) includes emergency treatment, critical care, and care associated with intensive and elaborate diagnosis and treatment.

4. **Encouraging attendance at a Smoke Enders' meeting is an example of the primary level of health-care services. Primary care is associated with activities that promote health and protect against disease.**

5. **Administering an immunization to prevent a childhood disease is an example of the primary level of health-care services. Primary care includes activities that protect a person from contracting a disease.**

38. 3. An independent care setting provides personal space (e.g., one-bedroom apartment, studio apartment) as well as services such meals, housekeeping, and van rides to stores or appointments. Individuals living in this type of setting must be self-sufficient, cognitively competent, and capable of meeting their own physical needs.

2. **In addition to the services provided in an independent care setting, an assisted-living setting provides help with some of the activities of daily living, such as dressing, bathing, and ambulating.**

1. **An intermediate care setting provides health-care services to individuals who require lifelong assistance with the activities of daily living, such as individuals who are cognitively impaired or disabled. These settings provide custodial care and function as the individual's home.**

5. **A subacute unit in a skilled nursing facility provides care to individuals with an acute illness, injury, or exacerbation of a disease process that requires skilled health-care services but**

does not require hospitalization to an acute care facility. The services include activities such as occupational therapy, physical therapy, and learning self-care of a newly created colostomy.

4. Skilled nursing care that must be provided for an extended period of time, frequently for the rest of the person's life, is often provided in a long-term care facility. Examples of clients residing in this type of long-term care setting include people with spinal cord injuries, clients in a coma, clients on mechanical ventilation, and people receiving enteral nutrition via a surgically implanted gastrointestinal tube.

39. 1. When functioning as a *provider*, the nurse is in the caregiver, not advocate, role. Caregiving involves identifying and meeting the client's needs by helping the client regain health through the caring process.

2. When functioning as a *nurturer*, the nurse is in the caregiver, not advocate, role. Nurture means to encourage, foster, and promote, all of which are components of caregiving.

3. The word *protector* describes the role of the nurse when functioning as the client's advocate. In the role of advocate, the nurse supports clients' rights and assists in asserting those rights when clients are unable to defend themselves.

4. Evaluation is the last step in the nursing process; it involves a determination of whether the client's goals are achieved. The word *evaluator* is not synonymous with the word *advocate*.

5. The word *supporter* describes the role of the nurse when functioning as the client's advocate. In the role of advocate, the nurse protects clients' rights and assists in asserting those rights when clients are unable to defend themselves.

40. 1. The client is the center of the health team as well as the nursing team. The client is the most important member of these teams.

2. A Hospice Nurse is a member of the nursing team who provides nursing care to meet the needs of dying clients and their family members.

3. A Registered Nurse is a member of the nursing team. A Registered Nurse provides direct nursing care and supervises other members of the nursing team such as Licensed Practical Nurses and Nursing Assistants.

4. A Nursing Assistant is a member of the nursing team who provides uncomplicated direct care to clients, such as bathing, feeding, dressing, and ambulating.

5. A Licensed Practical Nurse is a member of the nursing team who provides uncomplicated direct client care and works in a structured environment under the direction of a Registered Nurse.

Community-Based Nursing

KEYWORDS

The following words include nursing/medical terminology, concepts, principles, and information relevant to content specifically addressed in the chapter, or information associated with topics presented in it. English dictionaries, nursing textbooks, and medical dictionaries, such as *Taber's Cyclopedic Medical Dictionary,* are resources that can be used to expand your knowledge and understanding of these words and related information.

Case management
Community
Demographics
Epidemiology
Health-care reform
Health-care settings:
  Acute care hospitals
  Ambulatory care centers
  Assisted-living residences
  Clinics
  Day-care centers
  Extended care facilities
  Home health services
  Hospice (inpatient, residential, in the
    home)
  Industrial or occupation settings
  Life-care communities
  Long-term care nursing homes
  Mental health facilities
  Neighborhood community health
    centers
  Physicians' offices
  Rehabilitation centers
  School settings
  Urgent care centers

Healthy People 2020
Holistic
Levels of health-care delivery:
  Primary health care
  Secondary health care
  Tertiary health care
Managed care
Metropolitan
Nursing's Agenda for Health Care Reform
Occupational nurse
Outreach
Population
Primary care
Public health nurse
Quality improvement, quality management
Respite care
Rural
Self-help group
Suburban
Urban
Vulnerable populations
Wellness

COMMUNITY-BASED NURSING: QUESTIONS

1. A family member requests relief from caring for a relative who has a history of excessive intake of alcohol and a rapidly debilitating malignancy. To which resource should the nurse refer the family member for respite care?
   1. Hospice
   2. Meals on Wheels
   3. Ambulatory care center
   4. Substance misuse treatment center

2. Which role of the nurse takes on more emphasis in the delivery of health care in the home than in the acute care setting?
   1. Coordinating the efforts of the health-care team
   2. Delivering skilled nursing care
   3. Providing for healthy meals
   4. Modifying the environment

3. Which is unique to the home-care setting that is different in the acute care setting?
   1. Client is the center of the health-care team.
   2. Nurse functions as an advocate for the client.
   3. Nurse is responsible for coordinating the efforts of the client's health-care team.
   4. Client is not discharged until teaching regarding self-care activities is completed.

4. After arriving at a home location that has a history of domestic violence, a home-care nurse believes that the environment may be unsafe. Which is the **best** nursing action?
   1. Leave the home immediately.
   2. Defuse the situation in the home.
   3. Call the police for a personal escort.
   4. Complete the visit quickly while remaining alert.

5. When do nursing activities related to community nursing begin?
   1. On the first contact with the client
   2. After the client is admitted to the hospital
   3. At the time referrals are made to community resources
   4. When the primary health-care provider writes discharge prescriptions

6. A nurse must collect information about a community to identify its needs. Which is the **most** significant assessment by the nurse?
   1. The demographics of the community
   2. What the community thinks is important
   3. How many support services are available
   4. Environmental data as they relate to public safety

7. A home-care nurse is caring for a variety of clients in their homes. Which individual identified by the nurse will have the **most** difficult time adjusting to a prescribed regimen of long-term home health care?
   1. Middle school–age child
   2. Preschool-age child
   3. Adolescent
   4. Older adult

8. Which is unique to the home-care setting that is different in the acute care setting?
   1. Nurses work more independently.
   2. Nurses require excellent communication skills.
   3. Clients must be taught how to care for themselves.
   4. Clients have needs that require less technical nursing skills.

9. A woman is concerned about her children accidentally ingesting her husband's prescribed medications. Where should the home-care nurse teach the mother to keep medications?
1. On a high shelf
2. In a locked cabinet
3. In a medicine cabinet in the bathroom
4. On a shelf in the back of the refrigerator

10. Who is the **most** important health-care team member in an assisted-living facility?
1. Occupational Therapist
2. Nursing Assistant
3. Client
4. Nurse

11. A client's contract for home-care services is about to end, but the client still requires care. On which factor will the continuation of services **initially** depend?
1. Nursing documentation of the need for care
2. Retrospective audits of quality management
3. Client satisfaction with the care being provided
4. Presence of a primary health-care provider's prescription

12. Which factor is **essential** to the health of a community?
1. Availability of medical specialists
2. Individuals having health insurance
3. Everyone having access to health care
4. Public Health Nurses working in the community

13. A nurse identifies the health-care needs of the members of a community. Which is the nurse's **most** efficient initial approach to meet these needs?
1. Involve community leaders to work within the political arena to obtain funding for programs.
2. Write research grants to explore the community's health needs in more detail.
3. Design educational programs that address the identified community needs.
4. Make clients aware of the resources in the community.

14. A home-care nurse is performing an initial client and home assessment. Which is the **most** essential assessment that must be made by the nurse?
1. Can the home environment support the safety of the client?
2. Is the family willing to participate in the client's recovery?
3. Does the client have the potential for self-care?
4. Can the client participate in the plan of care?

15. During the process of performing a community assessment, the nurse invites members of the community to come to a meeting and share opinions and concerns about a particular issue. Which is this method of data collection?
1. An opinion survey
2. A community forum
3. A demographic assessment
4. An observation of participants

16. Which is **most** important when a nurse works in the home-care setting?
1. Case management
2. Discharge planning
3. Enlisting family support
4. Modifying client values

17. A nurse is preparing a client for discharge from the hospital. Which is designed primarily to provide for a continuum of comprehensive health care after discharge?
1. Primary health-care providers' offices
2. Home-care agencies
3. Urgent care centers
4. Respite programs

18. A nurse must conduct a community assessment. Which information should the nurse collect **first**?
1. General health of community members
2. Characteristics of community members
3. Physical environment of the community
4. Social services available in the community

19. A nurse in a home-care agency is providing an orientation program to a group of newly hired client companions. Which should the nurse teach them about families in the United States?
1. Families are groups of people related by blood, marriage, adoption, or birth.
2. Families are made up of fathers, mothers, and their children.
3. Families vary based on their structural composition.
4. Families live in the same household.

20. A home-care nurse is providing care for a family supporting a client with a chronic illness. Which is the **most** important factor the nurse should teach caregivers who care for a family member who has a stable but chronic illness and is living in the home?
1. Have extra equipment and supplies for emergencies.
2. Plan a daily and monthly schedule of activities.
3. Keep a daily journal of the client's status.
4. Tend to themselves as well as the client.

21. Which of the following falls within the category of tertiary health-care services?
1. Critical care
2. Long-term care
3. Diagnostic care
4. Preventive care

22. A person at home is recovering from an illness that has caused functional deficits. Which support service identified by the nurse will provide the **most** benefit for this person?
1. Hospice services
2. Church outreach program
3. Home health-care agency
4. Meals on Wheels program

23. A nurse is providing information about taking medication in the home. Which is a feature common to **most** containers for prescription medications that should be discussed?
1. Drip-proof tops
2. Unit dose packages
3. Sun-repellent plastic
4. Child-resistant covers

24. A nurse must initiate nursing services in the home setting. Which is an important factor that the nurse must consider to ensure third-party reimbursement?
1. The client must be able to perform some self-care.
2. The family has the financial resources to pay for the care.
3. Additional family members need to be available for support.
4. Intervention must be prescribed by a provider with a prescriptive license.

25. Which client, who has bilateral long leg casts that must be in place for 3 months, probably will require a setting other than the home to recover?
1. Adolescent living in a nuclear family
2. Middle-age married man
3. Older adult living alone
4. Infant with two parents

26. In which setting is it **most** essential for the nurse to assume multiple roles?
1. Rehabilitation facilities
2. Acute care hospitals
3. Rural communities
4. Urban centers

27. Which factor is **essential** to promote healthy lifestyles and behaviors within the community setting?
1. An entire family must be committed to making changes.
2. There must be resources available to support the desired changes.
3. The focus must be on the community as a whole, not on individuals.
4. A primary health-care provider's prescription is necessary before care can be provided.

28. A group of nurses is discussing various concerns about health care in the community setting in the United States. Which of the following should they include in the discussion because it has demonstrated a noticeable decline?
1. Public health organizations
2. At-risk client groups
3. Cost of health care
4. Self-help groups

29. A community health nurse is to care for a client who was just discharged from an acute care facility after receiving initial medical care for tuberculosis. The family recently immigrated to the United States from another country. Place the following interventions in the order in which they should be performed by the nurse.
1. Explore community resources that can help support the client and family.
2. Perform an assessment of the client and home environment.
3. Meet with the client and family in their home.
4. Review the client's medical record.
5. Identify client and family needs.

Answer: _____

30. Which statement reflects hospice care in the health-care delivery system? **Select all that apply.**
1. _____ Clients predicted to have less than half a year to live receive services.
2. _____ It assists families to care for their dying relatives at home.
3. _____ Care is less expensive than in the acute care setting.
4. _____ Support is given to the client and family members.
5. _____ Hospice is a method of care rather than a location.

31. Identify the nursing intervention that reflects tertiary health-care delivery. **Select all that apply.**
1. _____ Providing emotional support to family members after the death of a relative
2. _____ Teaching a client how to use a wheelchair after a stroke
3. _____ Implementing a prescribed hemodialysis treatment
4. _____ Administering an influenza vaccine
5. _____ Changing a dressing after surgery

32. Which activity is an example of an intervention associated with secondary health-care delivery? **Select all that apply.**
1. _____ Conducting a cardiac risk assessment for middle-age adults
2. _____ Teaching a low-fat diet to a person with high cholesterol
3. _____ Immunization of a child during the first year of life
4. _____ Providing a class on smoking cessation
5. _____ Monthly breast self-examinations

33. Which statement accurately reflects a concept about a healthy community? **Select all that apply.**
1. _____ Health of a community is based on the sum of the health of its people.
2. _____ The main focus in community health is on the health of each member of society.
3. _____ A healthy community seeks to make community resources available to all members.
4. _____ The focus of community health mainly is on healing the sick and preventing disease.
5. _____ Promotion of health is one of the most important components of community health practice.

34. Which indictor is among the 10 leading health indicators identified by *Healthy People 2020*? **Select all that apply.**
1. _____ Overweight and obesity
2. _____ Substance misuse
3. _____ Older adults
4. _____ Diabetes
5. _____ Vision

35. An older adult woman who has left-sided paralysis because of a brain attack is being cared for by a daughter in the home in which the daughter lives with her husband. The home-care nurse interviews each member of the family separately. Based on the significant information in each interview, which is the **most** important initial nursing intervention?
1. Be sensitive to the client's cultural beliefs.
2. Arrange respite care for the client's daughter.
3. Reinforce the daughter's responsibility to care for her mother.
4. Encourage the husband to help his wife with the care of his mother-in-law.

Interview With the Client
"I am thankful that my daughter is caring for me. I took care of my parents, and now it is my daughter's turn. Someday my daughter's children will be responsible for caring for her. I want to start acupuncture because I think it will help."

Interview With the Daughter
"Initially, I took several months off from work to care for my mother. I know it is my responsibility to care for her, but it is difficult because I work full-time. She has me doing old-fashioned traditional remedies that take time, and I don't even know if they will help."

Interview With the Daughter's Husband
"My mother-in-law came to live with us after her husband died. Since her recent discharge from the hospital, my wife has been giving her heat and cold applications to promote physiological harmony. It doesn't make any sense to me, but my mother-in-law believes it works. I worry about my wife doing too much."

1. 1. **A hospice program is an example of an agency that may provide or arrange for respite care in a health care facility or in the home. The caregiving role is physically and emotionally grueling, and family members may need relief from the caregiving role or a break to attend a family function or go on vacation.**
   2. Meals on Wheels does not provide respite care. It provides nutritious, low-cost meals for homebound people so that they can remain in their own homes.
   3. Ambulatory care centers do not provide respite care. Ambulatory care centers provide care for people with conditions that do not require hospitalization. Services may include diagnosis and treatment of disease and illness, as well as simple surgical procedures in which the client returns home the same day.
   4. A substance misuse treatment center does not provide respite care. It provides a specialized service in the care and treatment of individuals who misuse alcohol or drugs.

2. 1. Coordinating the efforts of the health-care team is an important responsibility of the nurse in all settings in which nurses work.
   2. Delivering skilled nursing care is an important responsibility of the nurse in all settings in which nurses work.
   3. Ensuring that clients receive healthy meals is an important responsibility of the nurse in all settings in which nurses work.
   4. **The hospital environment rarely requires modification because it is designed to provide for the safety needs of clients. However, in the home setting, a home hazard assessment must be implemented to identify potential problems with walkways, stairways, floors, furniture, bathrooms, kitchens, electrical and fire protection, toxic substances, communication devices, and issues associated with medications and asepsis. Although the nurse may not be able to change a client's living space and lifestyle, recommendations can be made that will minimize or eliminate risks.**

3. 1. The client is the center of the health-care team in all settings.
   2. The nurse functions as an advocate for the client in both the acute care and home-care settings. The role of advocate is important in all settings because in this role the nurse protects and supports clients' rights.
   3. The nurse is responsible for coordinating the efforts of the members of the health-care team in both the acute care and home-care settings.
   4. **Because of the shorter length of hospital stays, clients are being discharged before all teaching and counseling are completed. However, in the home-care setting, clients are provided with appropriate care until they are able to care for themselves.**

4. 1. **Nurses must remove themselves immediately from any environment that they believe is unsafe.**
   2. Attempting to defuse the situation may make the situation worse and place the nurse at additional risk.
   3. Calling the police may inflame the situation and/or take too long for an officer to arrive.
   4. Attempting to complete the visit may place the nurse at additional risk.

5. 1. **As soon as contact with the client is made, planning and teaching should begin so the client is prepared to provide self-care in the home.**
   2. The nurse does not have to wait until the client is admitted to the hospital to begin preparing for the client's return to the community.
   3. At the time referrals are made to community resources is too late. The need for referrals to community agencies can be anticipated in most situations.
   4. Waiting until the primary health-care provider writes discharge prescriptions is too late to prepare the client for self-care in the community.

6. 1. This is not as important as an assessment presented in another option. The demographics of a community are only one component of a community assessment.
   2. **The members in the community are the primary source of data about the community and its needs. Just as the client is the center of the health-care team when caring for an individual, the collective membership of a community is the center of the health-care team when caring for the health-care needs of a community.**

3. This does not help to identify the needs of a community. After the needs of the community are identified, then the ability of the health-care system to deliver the necessary services is assessed.

4. This is not as important as an assessment presented in another option. Environmental data make up only one component of a community assessment.

7. 1. A middle school–age child has to cope with the developmental conflict of Industry versus Inferiority. Tasks associated with this age, such as deriving pleasure from accomplishments and developing a sense of competence, can be facilitated in the home setting. Although a middle school–age child will have to adjust to the need for long-term home health care, there are fewer crises occurring during the middle school years that have an impact on development than the number of crises occurring in a group in another option.

2. A preschool-age child is dependent on a parent to provide for basic human needs and coping with the developmental conflict of Initiative versus Guilt. Tasks associated with this age, such as the development of confidence in ability and having direction and purpose, can be facilitated in the home setting. Although a preschool-age child will have to adjust to the need for long-term home health care, there are fewer crises occurring during the preschool years that have an impact on development than the number of crises occurring in a group in another option.

3. **Adolescents struggle with the developmental conflict of Identity versus Role Confusion. The adolescent generally will have the hardest time adjusting to the need for long-term home health care than any other stage of development. Adolescents experience multiple and complex physiological, psychological, and social developmental milestones. Adolescents want to be attractive to others, similar to their peers, and accepted within a group. It is common for adolescents to experience mood swings, make decisions without having all the facts, challenge authority, and assert the self. Being relatively isolated in the home for an extended period will pose serious stressors associated with adjustment,** which can dramatically influence the outcome of the developmental tasks of adolescence.

4. The developmental conflict of Ego Integrity versus Despair challenges older adults to understand their worth and accept the approaching end of life. Although older adults will have the second-hardest time adjusting to the need for long-term home health care of the options offered, there are fewer crises occurring during the older adult years that have an impact on development than the number of crises occurring in a group in another option.

8. 1. **In the home setting, clients tend to have fewer health-care providers' prescriptions, and therefore nurses work more independently. In addition, the roles of the nurse in community-based practice today are expanding dramatically. The major predictions influencing nurse accountability included the following: nurses will become community leaders; community-nursing centers will expand and focus on preventing disease and promoting health; and the center of health care will shift to the home setting. Nurses already work independently in such programs as community outreach, nursing centers, nurse-sponsored wellness and health promotion programs, and independent practice. These roles require the nurse to utilize nursing theory and skills that are within the scope of the legal definition of nursing practice and do not require dependence on a primary health-care provider's prescriptions.**

2. Excellent communication skills are essential in both the acute care and community-based settings.

3. Teaching occurs in both the acute care and community-based settings. In addition, some clients may never be able to care for themselves.

4. Excellent technical skills are essential in both the acute care and community-based settings. Clients at home receive highly technical therapy such as hemodialysis, intravenous therapy, wound care, and ventilator support.

9. 1. A high shelf is not a safe place to keep medications. Children have natural curiosity, problem-solving abilities, and the agility to climb to a top shelf.

2. **A locked area is the safest place to store prescribed as well as over-the-counter medications to prevent accidental ingestion by children.**

3. A medicine cabinet in the bathroom is not a safe place to keep medications. Children have natural curiosity, problem-solving abilities, and the agility to climb up to a medicine cabinet.

4. A shelf in the back of the refrigerator is not a safe place to keep medications. Children have natural curiosity and problem-solving abilities and could get to the back of a shelf in a refrigerator.

10. 1. The Occupational Therapist (OT) is not the most important member of the health-care team in an assisted-living facility. An Occupational Therapist generally is not a member of the health-care team in an assisted-living residence. On occasion, a primary health-care provider may prescribe occupational therapy, and either the client will go to an Occupational Therapist to receive therapy or one will come to the client and provide therapy.

2. Although Nursing Assistants, under the direction of a Registered Nurse, are the people who provide care related to activities of daily living needed by clients in an assisted-living residence, they are not as important as another member of the health-care team.

3. **The client is always the center of the health-care team in every setting and is the most important member of the team.**

4. The nurse is not the most important health-care team member in an assisted-living facility. An assisted-living residence (i.e., apartment, villa, or condominium) provides limited assistance with activities of daily living, meal preparation, laundry services, transportation, and opportunities for socialization, not extensive nursing services.

11. 1. **Case management by the nurse in the home-care setting includes determining whether a client is ready for discharge or requires a continuation of services. The nurse must document objectively the status of the client to convince those making the decision (e.g., primary health-care provider, insurer, agency manager) that the client requires a continuation of services. Nursing documentation is the initial**

intervention that supports the decision to continue home-care services.

2. Quality management activities are unrelated to whether a client is to receive a continuation of services or is to be discharged from a home health-care program. Ongoing quality management programs are designed to monitor the quality of care being delivered and identify problem areas so that efforts can be employed to improve care.

3. Dissatisfaction with the services of a home health agency may influence whether or not the client and/or family wants a continuation of services. However, satisfaction or dissatisfaction should not influence whether the client still needs the services of the home health-care agency.

4. Ultimately, a primary health-care provider's prescription is necessary to initiate home-care services, continue health-care services, and identify interventions to be performed by nurses that are within the scope of nursing practice. However, the health-care provider's prescriptions take into consideration nursing documentation of the need for care and input from agency managers and the client's insurer.

12. 1. Although it is important to have access to medical specialists, another option has priority. In addition, the availability of primary health-care providers, not specialists, is more essential because primary health care addresses health promotion, illness prevention, and entry into secondary health care (diagnosis and treatment of illness and disease).

2. Although individuals with health insurance have better access to health-care services, it is not essential to have health insurance to receive health care. People can pay privately or, if indigent, they can apply for various government and nonprofit-supported programs that provide basic care. In addition, hospital emergency departments, by law, cannot turn away clients who need emergency care.

3. **For a healthy community, all members of the community must have access to health care. The health of a community depends on each member of the community having appropriate and comprehensive health care.**

4. Public Health Nurses work for only the federal, state, or local governments

implementing programs supported by taxes. These programs are only a small percentage of the multitude of programs and services that are designed to support community health.

13. 1. This is not the most efficient approach. This may be necessary if present resources are not available to meet the needs of the community.
    2. The health needs of the members of the community are identified already. Further study at this time does not appear to be appropriate.
    3. Designing educational approaches is not the most efficient approach. This may eventually be done after an action in another option is implemented first.
    4. **This is the most efficient initial approach to meeting the identified needs of the members of the community. The use of currently available resources is more efficient than the other options presented.**

14. 1. **The first and most important assessment made by the home-care nurse focuses on determining whether the client's home environment is safe. Safety and security are one of the more basic needs identified by Maslow's Hierarchy of Needs.**
    2. Although it is often helpful when family members participate in a home-care client's recovery, it is not necessary.
    3. A client's potential for self-care is not a criterion for receiving home-care services. Clients who have little or no potential for self-care receive home-care services.
    4. Clients who are unable to participate in the plan of care because they are mentally, emotionally, or physically disabled are still eligible for home care.

15. 1. This scenario is not an example of an opinion survey. An opinion survey is designed to collect each individual person's perspective about the problem being studied. Results are tallied to identify the major concerns. Opinion surveys generally are questionnaires.
    2. **A forum is defined as an opportunity for open discussion. Inviting people from the community to share opinions and concerns about a particular issue for the purpose of collecting data is called a community forum.**
    3. This scenario is not an example of a demographic assessment. A demographic assessment is the quantitative study of the characteristics of a population. A demographic assessment might include information such as distribution of the population by gender, size, growth, density, and ethnicity.
    4. This scenario is not an example of an observation of participants. Direct observation is a method of data collection that may be used to determine whether individuals follow a specific procedure or behave in an expected manner.

16. 1. **Case management is a major role of the nurse in the home-care setting. The nurse engages in activities such as assessing, planning, coordinating nursing care and professional services, making referrals, monitoring medical progress, maintaining documentation, evaluating and monitoring outcomes, determining closure, and facilitating discharge of the client after goal achievement.**
    2. Although discharge planning is a component of the role of the nurse in the home-care setting, it is not the role with the highest priority. Traditionally, discharge planning was focused on moving a person from the hospital to the home. However, in the present health-care environment, discharge planning is conducted when moving a client from one level of care to another, which occurs in many settings.
    3. Although family support is helpful, the client's interest and motivation in achieving expected outcomes are the most important contributing factors to success.
    4. The role of the nurse is to help the client achieve expected outcomes that are within the client's present value and belief systems. Although a client might be healthier if other behaviors were adopted, it is difficult, and sometimes impossible, to change or modify a person's values and beliefs.

17. 1. Primary health-care providers' offices are the traditional primary care setting for ambulatory care. Clients go to primary health-care providers' offices for routine physicals and the diagnosis and treatment of routine illnesses or diseases. Follow-up visits to primary health-care providers are only one aspect of comprehensive health care.
    2. **Home-care agencies are responsible for coordinating and providing for a**

continuum of comprehensive health-care services after a client is discharged from the hospital. Because of the decreased length of stay in the hospital setting, clients are being discharged sooner than ever before and are in need of home-care services.

3. Urgent visit centers are designed to diagnose and treat noncritical health problems, such as infections, minor injuries, and physical responses to disease or illness as well as primary care services.

4. Respite programs provide for short-stay, intermittent, inpatient, or day-care services to clients who generally are cared for at home. This service provides a rest period for family members who have the responsibility of sustained caregiving.

18. 1. Although the general health of members of a community is important, it is not the first information that the nurse should collect when assessing a community.

2. Clients are the center of all health care, including community health care. Acquiring core information about the people in the community is the first stage in assessing a community. Core characteristics about the members of a community include information such as vital statistics, values and beliefs, demographics, religious groups, and so on.

3. Although a community's physical environment (e.g., information such as whether it is rural, suburban, or urban, physical boundaries, density, size, types of lodgings, and incidence of crime) is important to know, it is not the first information that the nurse should collect when assessing a community.

4. Although it is important to know information such as agencies and services available, the accessibility to health-care services, sources of health information, transportation services, routine caseloads, and so on, it is not the first information that the nurse should collect when assessing a community.

19. 1. Families are not limited to individuals who are related by blood, marriage, adoption, or birth.

2. A father, mother, and their children are an example of a nuclear family and is only one example of a family structure.

3. A family is defined as a social group whose members are closely related by

blood, marriage, or friendship. Today, family structure is diverse and includes types such as traditional nuclear families, single-parent families, blended families, cohabitating families, families with foster children, and single people living alone but who are part of an extended family.

4. Family members remain connected by their relationships, not because they all live in the same household.

20. 1. Although this is a good idea, it is not the most important factor a home-care nurse can convey to a person caring for a family member in the home.

2. Although this might contribute to efficiency as well as gaining a feeling of control over the activities that must be accomplished, it is not the most important factor a home-care nurse can convey to a person caring for a family member in the home.

3. A daily journal of the client's status is unnecessary when a client is in stable condition. If the client experiences an acute episode, then a record of the client's daily status could be helpful in monitoring progress or lack of progress.

4. Caregiver role strain experienced by a family member is a serious concern of home-care nurses. Caregivers often fail to address their own health needs because of the extraordinary burden of the caregiver role, which can jeopardize their own health and well-being. Caregivers should be encouraged to delegate responsibilities to other family members; get adequate sleep, rest, and nutritional intake; seek assistance from agencies that provide respite services; take time for leisure activities and a vacation; and join a caregiver support group.

21. 1. Critical care lies in the category of secondary, not tertiary, level of health-care services. The secondary level of health-care services is associated with acute care, complex diagnosis, treatment of disease and illness, and emergency care.

2. Long-term care lies in the category of tertiary level of health-care services. The tertiary level of health-care services is associated with rehabilitation, care of the dying, and long-term care.

3. Diagnostic care lies in the category of secondary, not tertiary, level of health-care services.

4. Preventive care lies in the category of primary, not tertiary, level of health-care services. Primary health-care services are concerned with promoting health and preventing disease.

22. 1. Hospice services are designed to assist clients who have less than 6 months to live and who prefer palliative care and support of quality of life. Hospice care and limited medical intervention are not mutually exclusive. Some Hospice programs provide additional supportive services such as intravenous fluids, parenteral nutrition, and antibiotics. The concept underlying inclusion of limited medical interventions is supportive, not curative. Hospice programs also provide support services to members of the client's family as well as bereavement care for significant others after the death of the client.

2. Although church outreach programs may be able to provide some support services, generally they are not able to provide the multiple services needed or to coordinate the continuum of comprehensive services that a person with functional deficits will require. Many church outreach programs generally serve as a source of information about services and programs available in the community, and they provide additional support that augments home-care services.

3. **A home health-care agency is designed to coordinate the comprehensive services that a client may need to recover from an illness that has caused functional deficits. This person may require help in areas such as assistance with activities of daily living, physical and occupational rehabilitation, direct nursing care, counseling, and so on.**

4. Meals on Wheels provides for only the nutritional needs of a client.

23. 1. This is not common to all medication containers. Only medications in liquid form should have drip-proof tops.

2. Most prescribed medications for home use are in multidose containers.

3. Not all medications must be protected from the sun.

4. **All prescribed medications for home use are dispensed in containers with child-resistant tops, as required by law. If a person has a physical limitation, such as arthritis, that interferes with his or her ability to open a medication**

container, the person can request that a nonsafety top be provided. The pharmacy generally will document the request in its computer and may even require that a waiver be signed and witnessed for the record.

24. 1. The ability to provide some self-care is not necessary. In some instances, family members provide total care with no help from the client.

2. A person does not have to have adequate financial resources to receive nursing services in the home. For example, Medicare, Medicaid, or private health-care insurance plans assume some of the costs of care provided in the home.

3. The presence of family members is not a requirement for home-care services. However, if it is unsafe for the client to be home alone or unattended for long periods, the home may not be the most appropriate setting. In addition, clients who have no family support may rely on a friend, neighbor, or volunteers from a neighborhood outreach group to help in a supportive way.

4. **Health-care professionals who have prescriptive licenses (e.g., physicians, nurse practitioners, physician's assistants) must prescribe home-care nursing services. A prescription from a provider with a prescriptive license is required if a home-care agency is to receive reimbursement from third-party sources (e.g., government, medical insurance plans). Prescriptions written by these professionals direct the medical plan of care.**

25. 1. A nuclear family of siblings and parents should be able to provide an adolescent with the assistance needed to meet basic human needs and probably will not need a setting other than the home to recover.

2. A middle-age married man should be able to rely on his spouse to provide the needed assistance to meet basic human needs and probably will not require a setting other than the home to recover.

3. **A person with bilateral long leg casts for 3 months will have to rely on others to provide for one's basic needs, such as food and assistance with activities of daily living. An independently living older adult probably will not have the daily assistance needed to recover at home and therefore is a**

candidate for a setting that provides assistance with activities of daily living.

4. The infant should be able to depend on the parents to provide for basic human needs and therefore probably will not need a setting other than the home to recover.

26. 1. Of the options presented, nurses working in a rehabilitation setting are less likely to assume multiple roles. Generally, nurses working in a rehabilitation setting have specific roles and responsibilities.

2. Of the options presented, nurses working in the acute care setting are less likely to assume multiple roles. Generally, nurses working in acute care settings have specific roles and responsibilities.

3. **Nurses working in rural communities wear many hats. The adage "wear many hats" refers to someone with many different roles and responsibilities. Rural refers to the country or the farm, where communities are less populated and are a great distance from primary health-care providers and health-care services. Because of the uneven distribution of health-care professionals and services in rural areas versus urban areas, nurses working in a rural area will assume many different roles and perform a variety of tasks.**

4. Of the options presented, nurses working in urban centers are less likely to assume multiple roles. Urban centers refer to cities with a population of more than 50,000 individuals, and they tend to have a concentration of specialized services where nurses have specific roles and responsibilities.

27. 1. Each individual person is responsible for his or her own health-seeking actions and behavior. It is ideal if all members of a family are interested and motivated to promote a healthy lifestyle; however, not all members of a family are committed to this value.

2. **Resources that support health promotion, health protection, and preventive health services are essential if one expects members of the community to engage in healthy lifestyles and behaviors. Resources, such as availability of health professionals, sites for primary health prevention programs for**

meetings and provision of services, consumables in the form of equipment and medications (e.g., immunizations), and so on, must be available to promote and support health.

3. Although programs are designed to meet the needs of groups in a community, each individual must be reached and influenced when promoting healthy lifestyles and behaviors.

4. Educational intervention is an independent function of the nurse and does not require a primary health-care provider's prescription.

28. 1. **Public health agencies established at the federal, state, and local levels to safeguard and improve the physical, mental, and social well-being of an entire community are on the decline. In an effort to reduce the escalating rise in the budgets of public health agencies, programs and services have been reduced or terminated.**

2. The number of client groups at risk is increasing, not declining; for example, it includes groups such as older adults, the homeless, the uninsured, people living below the poverty level, single-parent families, and immigrants.

3. The cost of health care in the United States is dramatically increasing, not declining. In 2017, 20% of the gross domestic product was spent on health-care costs. It is predicted that by 2040, it will be 26% to 30% of the gross domestic product.

4. The number of self-help groups is increasing, not declining. A few sources claim that there are 500,000 to 750,000 self-help groups internationally. Groups represent almost all the major health problems, life events, or crises. The National Self-Help Clearinghouse provides information about existing groups and guidelines on how to begin a new group. Consumer access to the World Wide Web and the Internet has disseminated information about self-help groups.

29. 4. **Before meeting with the client and family, the nurse should obtain as much information about the client as possible.**

3. **An assessment of the home environment can be performed only in the home. The client's family members should be included when feasible**

because they may provide emotional support and/or be involved with physical care of the client.

2. A health history and physical assessment of the client should be performed by the community health nurse. The information on the client's clinical record may not reflect the client's current status. The home must be assessed to ensure that it is a safe environment for the client and that care can be delivered adequately to meet the client's needs.

5. The nurse, in conjunction with the client (and family members when appropriate), must identify present needs. Once this is accomplished, then goals and objectives can be identified and a plan of care formulated.

1. Once a plan of care is formulated, then the nurse, in conjunction with the client (and family members when appropriate), can identify community resources that may assist them in attaining the goals and objectives of the plan of care.

30. 1. To be eligible for hospice services, individuals are predicted to have less than 6 months to live. It is a service to support clients and their families through the process of dying.

2. Most hospice care is delivered in clients' homes supported by a team of health-care providers and volunteers. However, there are inpatient hospice programs, palliative care units in hospitals, and residential hospice settings.

3. The majority of hospice care is provided in the home. The home is a less expensive setting than other health-care settings because family members provide most of the care, supported by a team of professionals, nonprofessionals, and volunteers.

4. Hospice services provide supportive care, physical care, and promotion of the quality of life for the terminally ill client and family members. In addition, hospice care assists family members with bereavement and adjustment after the death of the client.

5. Hospice is not a location but a concept. It provides supportive, palliative services that focus on managing pain, treatment of symptoms, and helping clients maintain their quality of life so they

can live the remainder of their lives to the fullest.

31. 1. Providing bereavement services is an example of a tertiary health-care service. Tertiary care is associated with rehabilitation, long-term care, and care of the dying. Health-care delivery includes primary, secondary, and tertiary care.

2. Teaching a client how to use a wheelchair after a stroke is an example of a tertiary health-care service. Tertiary services provide care related to rehabilitation.

3. Implementing a prescribed hemodialysis treatment is an example of tertiary health care. Tertiary health care includes providing palliative care and supporting comfort and quality of life as well as maximizing abilities in light of chronic or irreversible conditions.

4. Immunizations are an example of primary, not tertiary, health-care delivery. Primary health care is concerned with promoting health, preventing disease, and providing environmental protection and health education.

5. Changing a dressing after surgery is care associated with the secondary, not tertiary, level of health-care delivery. Secondary health care is associated with acute care, complex diagnosis and treatment of disease and illness, and emergency care.

32. 1. This is a primary, not secondary, health-care delivery. Risk assessments for specific diseases are included in primary health-care services. Primary health-care services are concerned with generalized health promotion and specific protection against disease.

2. A low-fat diet generally is part of a medical management program for a person who is overweight or who has high cholesterol. This is a tertiary, not secondary, health-care service. Tertiary health-care services are associated with attempts to reduce the extent and severity of a health problem in an effort to limit disability as well as restore and maintain function.

3. Administering an immunization is a primary, not secondary, health-care service. Primary health-care services include protecting people from disease.

4. Providing a class on smoking cessation is associated with primary, not secondary,

health care. Primary health care is associated with health promotion and illness prevention.

5. Monthly breast self-examinations are associated with secondary health-care services because they are concerned with detection of breast cancer.

33. 1. This statement does not accurately reflect a concept about a healthy community. A healthy community seeks to provide infrastructure, resources, and activities that support a healthy community and is not just reflective of the health of its members.
    2. This is not an accurate statement. Community health focuses on families, groups, and the community, not just individuals.
    3. A healthy community is concerned about all members of the community and works to ensure that all members have access to all of the system's resources.
    4. This statement focuses on illness and is too limited in relation to community health.
    5. Health promotion has taken on new meaning as consumers take more responsibility for their health status. Teaching about promoting health is a more positive perspective than teaching about preventing illness, which is a negative perspective.

34. **1. Overweight and obesity is one of the 10 leading health indicators identified by *Healthy People 2020*. The other nine topics are physical activity, substance misuse, tobacco use, responsible sexual behavior, mental health, injury and violence, environmental quality, immunization, and access to health care.**

2. **Substance misuse is one of the 10 leading health indicators identified by *Healthy People 2020*. The other nine topics are physical activity, overweight and obesity, tobacco use, responsible sexual behavior, mental health, injury and violence, environmental quality, immunization, and access to health care.**
   3. Older adults is not one of the 10 leading health indicators, but it is one of the 42 topic areas.
   4. Diabetes is not one of the 10 leading health indicators, but it is one of the 42 topic areas.
   5. Vision is not one of the 10 leading health indicators, but it is one of the 42 topic areas.

35. **1. Beliefs and values usually are held long term and are engrained within one's view of self. It is essential that nurses respect a client's beliefs and values, particularly for nontraditional healing practices, as long as they are not harmful to the client. Demonstrating respect and a nonjudgmental attitude will help promote a trusting nurse-client relationship.**
    2. Arranging respite care for the daughter is premature at this time. This may eventually become necessary.
    3. This is an inappropriate intervention by the nurse. Only the daughter can come to the conclusion that it is her responsibility to care for her mother.
    4. This is not the priority. This intervention may be done after a discussion with the client, daughter, and husband.

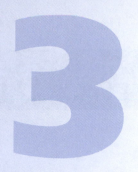

Psychosociocultural Nursing Care

Nursing Care Across the Life Span

KEYWORDS

The following words include nursing/medical terminology, concepts, principles, and information relevant to content specifically addressed in the chapter or associated with topics presented in it. English dictionaries, nursing textbooks, and medical dictionaries, such as *Taber's Cyclopedic Medical Dictionary,* are resources that can be used to expand your knowledge and understanding of these words and related information.

Adolescent (teenager)

Ageism

Attachment, bonding

Brazelton, Berry—Neonatal Behavioral Assessment Scale

Cephalocaudal

Congenital anomalies

Critical time

Developmental:
  Milestones
  Stressor
  Task

Egocentrism

Erikson, Erik—Theory of Personality Development

Failure to thrive

Fetus

Fowler, James—Theory of Faith Development

Freud, Sigmund—Psychoanalytical Theory

Genetics

Havighurst, Robert—Developmental Task Theory of Development

Infancy, infant, neonate, newborn

Kohlberg, Lawrence—Theory of Moral Development

Life cycle

Low birth weight

Maslow, Abraham—Hierarchy of Basic Human Needs

Menarche

Menopause

Middle adulthood

Midlife crisis

Moral reasoning

Older adult

Organogenesis

Piaget, Jean—Cognitive Development Theory

Premenopausal, postmenopausal

Preschool-age child

Preterm

Proximodistal

Psychosocial development

Puberty

Regression

Retirement

Role reversal

Sandwich generation

School-age child

Senescence

Sibling rivalry

Teratogenic

Toddler

Young adulthood

NURSING CARE ACROSS THE LIFE SPAN: QUESTIONS

1. A nurse is administering medication to an older adult. For which response to medication that occurs **most** frequently in older adults should the nurse assess the client?
   1. Toxicity
   2. Side effects
   3. Hypersensitivity
   4. Idiosyncratic effects

2. A nurse in a clinic is caring for clients in a variety of age groups. Which age group should the nurse anticipate will have the **highest** potential to demonstrate regression when ill?
   1. Infants
   2. Toddlers
   3. Adolescents
   4. Young adults

3. When the nurse assesses an adult client, which client behavior may indicate an unresolved developmental task of infancy?
   1. Avoiding assistance from others
   2. Rationalizing unacceptable behaviors
   3. Being overly concerned about cleanliness
   4. Apologizing constantly for small mistakes

4. Which client should the nurse identify is at the **highest** risk when taking a drug that has a high teratogenic potential?
   1. Older adult man
   2. Pregnant woman
   3. Four-year-old child
   4. One-month-old infant

5. A nurse in the emergency department is assessing clients of various ages. Which age group should the nurse anticipate will have the **most** individual differences in appearance and behavior?
   1. Adolescents
   2. Older adults
   3. Middle-age adults
   4. School-age children

6. A 70-year-old client tells the nurse about experiencing problems with sleep and requests sleeping medication. Which concept associated with drug therapy and quality of sleep is important for the nurse to explain when providing nursing care for this client?
   1. "Sedatives are not well tolerated by older adults."
   2. "Antianxiety drugs are the least helpful to support sleep."
   3. "Effectiveness of hypnotics increases with prolonged use."
   4. "Melatonin is the drug of choice for long-term use in sleep disorders."

7. Which concept is reflective of Erik Erikson's Theory of Personality Development?
   1. Defense mechanisms help people to cope with anxiety.
   2. Moral maturity is a central theme in all stages of development.
   3. Achievement of developmental goals is affected by the social environment.
   4. Two continual processes, assimilation and accommodation, stimulate intellectual growth.

8. A nurse in the clinic is monitoring clients for iron-deficiency anemia. Which group of individuals should the nurse anticipate to be at the **highest** risk?
   1. Postmenopausal women
   2. Older adults
   3. Teenagers
   4. Infants

9. Which group of individuals should the nurse anticipate is at the **highest** risk for constipation?
   1. Inactive school-age children
   2. Middle-age adults
   3. Bottle-fed infants
   4. Older-age adults

10. A parent tells the nurse in the well-child clinic that their 2-year-old is trying to eat with a spoon and is making a mess. Which should the nurse encourage the parent to do?
    1. Praise and encourage the child while eating.
    2. Provide finger foods until the child is older.
    3. Feed the child along with the child's attempts at eating.
    4. Take the spoon and feed the child until the child is more capable.

11. One of the participants attending a parenting seminar asks the nurse teaching the class, "What is the leading cause of death during the first year of life?" Besides exploring the person's concerns, what should the nurse respond?
    1. Sudden infant death syndrome
    2. Congenital malformations
    3. Unintentional injuries
    4. Short gestation

12. Which individual does the nurse anticipate has the **highest** risk for problems with regulating body temperature?
    1. Toddler
    2. Teenager
    3. Older adult
    4. School-age child

13. A pediatric nurse is caring for children of a variety of ages. Which group should the nurse anticipate will have the **most** problems sleeping as a result of multiple complex developmental factors?
    1. Infants
    2. Toddlers
    3. Adolescents
    4. Preschoolers

14. Which is a person referring to when during an interview the person says, "I am a member of the *sandwich generation*"?
    1. Cares for children and aging parents at the same time
    2. Has reversed roles between parents and self
    3. Assists own parents and spouse's parents
    4. Has both older and younger siblings

15. A nurse is planning a teaching session for an older adult about a prescribed medication regimen. Which is a major concern about older adults that the nurse should consider?
    1. They experience an increase in absorption of drugs from the gastrointestinal tract.
    2. They are less motivated to follow a prescribed drug regimen.
    3. They are less likely to learn due to a decline in intelligence.
    4. They have a decreased risk for adverse reactions to drugs.

16. A nurse is caring for several children on a pediatric unit. Children in which age group should the nurse expect will be **most** unstable and challenging with regard to the development of a personal identity?
    1. Toddlerhood
    2. Adolescence
    3. Childhood
    4. Infancy

17. A nurse is caring for clients of a variety of ages. Which individual should the nurse anticipate will have the **highest** risk for complications during the perioperative period?
    1. Middle-age adult
    2. Pregnant woman
    3. Adolescent
    4. Infant

18. Which word describes the process of growth and development?
    1. Fast
    2. Simple
    3. Limiting
    4. Individual

19. A hospice nurse is providing emotional support for eight young children of a dying mother. At which age do children **first** recognize that death is irreversible, universal, and natural?
    1. 9 years of age
    2. 6 years of age
    3. 15 years of age
    4. 12 years of age

20. A school nurse is teaching a class of adolescents about nutrition. Which age group should the nurse identify as having the **highest** energy expenditure and nutrient requirements?
    1. End of the life cycle
    2. Middle adult years
    3. Early adult years
    4. First year of life

21. A nurse determines that according to Erikson, establishing relationships based on commitment mainly occurs in which stage of psychosocial development?
    1. Middle-age adulthood
    2. Young adulthood
    3. Adolescence
    4. Infancy

22. Which age group should the nurse identify as being reflected in the following statement? "More time is spent in bed, but less time is spent asleep."
    1. 2-year-olds
    2. 40-year-olds
    3. 70-year-olds
    4. 14-year-olds

23. A nurse is teaching a parenting class at a local community health center. Which common stressor associated with the developmental stage of early childhood (1 to 3 years) should the nurse include?
    1. Accepting limited dietary choices
    2. Adjusting to a change in physique
    3. Responding to a life-threatening illness
    4. Resolving conflicts concerning independence

24. A nurse is providing dietary teaching to a group of adolescents recently diagnosed with diabetes mellitus. Which factor should the nurse consider that frequently influences food choices by adolescents?
    1. Taste
    2. Routine
    3. Pressure
    4. Preference

25. Which common physiological change associated with aging should the nurse assess for in an older adult? **Select all that apply.**
    1. _____ Increase in sebaceous gland activity
    2. _____ Deterioration of joint cartilage
    3. _____ Loss of social support system
    4. _____ Decreased hearing acuity
    5. _____ Increased need for sleep

26. A nurse is facilitating a mothers' class, and the women begin discussing experiences that reflect the intellectual development of their children. Each woman describes a situation that reflects one of the stages of Jean Piaget's theory about logical thinking. Place the situations described in order, beginning with the sensorimotor stage and ending with formal operations.
    1. "My son touched the radiator and got burned. He'll never do that again."
    2. "My son is learning math and is getting 100s on his tests. He is so smart."
    3. "My daughter is on the debating team in school. We go to interschool meets."
    4. "My daughter asked an obese lady if she had a baby in her stomach. I was so embarrassed."

    Answer: _____

27. A nurse identifies that an older adult has successfully resolved the developmental conflict associated with aging. Which ability of the person **supports** this conclusion? **Select all that apply.**
    1. _____ Accepting social isolation
    2. _____ Regretting past life events
    3. _____ Managing the change in social roles
    4. _____ Associating with members of every age group
    5. _____ Increasing the number of meaningful relationships

28. An older adult is admitted to the intensive care unit. For which common adaptation to sensory overload should the nurse monitor the client? **Select all that apply.**
    1. _____ Tachycardia
    2. _____ Restlessness
    3. _____ Confusion
    4. _____ Irritability
    5. _____ Fatigue

29. A nurse identifies which word as being related to a principle of growth and development? **Select all that apply.**
    1. _____ Predictable
    2. _____ Sequential
    3. _____ Integrated
    4. _____ Complex
    5. _____ Static

30. A nurse identifies that a client in middle adulthood is experiencing a developmental crisis. Which of the person's behaviors **supports** this conclusion? **Select all that apply.**
    1. _____ Unable to mentor children in the next generation
    2. _____ Difficulty in developing peer relationships
    3. _____ Inability to achieve feelings of success
    4. _____ Incapable of delaying satisfaction
    5. _____ Failure to face eventual death

31. A school nurse is assessing several school-age children between the ages of 6 and 12 years. Which child requires a further assessment?
    1. 7-year-old boy
    2. 9-year-old girl
    3. 11-year-old boy
    4. 12-year-old girl

CLIENT'S CLINICAL RECORD

7-Year-Old Boy
Grew 1 inch in the last year
Gained 15 pounds in the last year

9-Year-Old Girl
Concerned about achieving acceptable grades in school
Identifies with other girls in her grade

11-Year-Old Boy
Appears clumsy
Is tall and thin

12-Year-Old Girl
Concerned about her physical appearance
Interested in boys

32. A nurse is caring for a variety of individuals across the life span. Which age group generally demonstrates an inefficiency of adaptation? **Select all that apply.**
    1. _____ Older than 60 years
    2. _____ 40 to 60 years
    3. _____ 12 to 19 years
    4. _____ 3 to 11 years
    5. _____ 0 to 1 year

33. A nurse identifies that an adult has an unresolved developmental conflict associated with adolescence. Which behavior **supports** this conclusion? **Select all that apply.**
    1. _____ Being overly concerned about following daily routines
    2. _____ Requiring excessive attention from others
    3. _____ Relying on oneself rather than others
    4. _____ Failing to express a sense of self
    5. _____ Lacking goals in life

34. Which family member's comment about an older adult member of the family demonstrates ageism? **Select all that apply.**
    1. _____ "She has outlived her usefulness."
    2. _____ "She is elderly, but she is so cute."
    3. _____ "She reads the newspaper with difficulty."
    4. _____ "He reminisces about his past work experience."
    5. _____ "He is happiest when working in his home workshop."

35. A nurse is assessing a 4-year-old child's growth and development. Which activity should the nurse expect the child to be capable of performing? **Select all that apply.**
    1. _____ Dresses self
    2. _____ Uses toy tools
    3. _____ Hops on one foot
    4. _____ Rides a two-wheel bicycle
    5. _____ Swims using the freestyle stroke

1. 1. **This is a serious concern because of a decrease in efficiency of hepatic metabolism and renal excretion of drugs in older adults; as a result, accumulation of the drug occurs, resulting in toxicity.**
   2. Although side effects are a concern in older adults, another option is a greater concern.
   3. Although hypersensitivity is a concern in older adults, another option is a greater concern.
   4. Although idiosyncratic effects are a concern in older adults, another option is a greater concern.

2. 1. Infants already demonstrate behavior on the most basic level.
   2. **Toddlers are less able to understand and interpret what is happening to them when ill; therefore, they commonly regress to a previous level of development in an attempt to reduce anxiety.**
   3. Adolescents generally want to behave in an adult manner and therefore demonstrate a controlled behavioral response to illness.
   4. Although some young adults may regress to an earlier level of development as a coping strategy, regression commonly is not used as a defense mechanism when coping with illness.

3. 1. **People who avoid help from others and who would rather do things themselves generally have not completely resolved the developmental task of Trust versus Mistrust during infancy.**
   2. Rationalizing unacceptable behaviors is a defense mechanism, not an indication of an unresolved developmental task of infancy. Rationalization is used to justify in some socially acceptable way ideas, feelings, or behavior through explanations that appear to be logical.
   3. This behavior relates more to the Anal Stage of Freud's Psychosexual Theory of Development. Freud believed that when toilet training is approached in a rigid and demanding manner, a child develops into an adult who is overly concerned with orderliness and cleanliness.
   4. This may indicate an unresolved conflict of Autonomy versus Shame and Doubt associated with the 18-month- to 3-year-old age group. One of the developmental tasks of this age group is learning right from

wrong. When parents are overly critical and controlling, a child may be overly self-judgmental and become an adult who feels the need to apologize for small mistakes constantly.

4. 1. An older adult man is not at risk when receiving a medication that has a teratogenic effect.
   2. **A pregnant woman is at risk. Teratogenic refers to a substance that can cross the placental barrier and interfere with growth and development of the fetus.**
   3. A 4-year-old child is not at risk when receiving a medication that has a teratogenic effect.
   4. A newborn is not at risk when receiving a medication that has a teratogenic effect.

5. 1. Although adolescents (12 to 20 years) may be viewed as different from the norms of their parents, they are similar to their peers. In their search for self-identity, adolescents experience role confusion. Adolescents are attracted to and conform to peer groups to control anxiety with role confusion. This provides a sense of security.
   2. Although there is diversity in the older adult group (65 years or older), individuals have to adjust to common experiences, such as physical decline, retirement, multiple losses, and changes in social roles. Older adults commonly seek out people of the same age to share similar interests and find status among their peers.
   3. **Middle-age adults (40 to 60 years) are in a time of transition between young adulthood and older adulthood. Therefore, individuals in this group, more so than in any other age group, have the greatest individual differences in appearance and behavior because they span the norms seen in young adulthood, middle adulthood, and older adulthood.**
   4. School-age children (6 to 12 years) tend to have fewer differences in appearance and behavior from their peers. These children begin to be involved with formalized groups where conformity is expected.

6. 1. **Sedatives are not well tolerated by older adults because a decrease in the metabolism and excretion of the drug can result in toxicity. In addition, older adults may**

experience idiosyncratic effects (e.g., un-expected or opposite to desired effect).

2. Antianxiety drugs depress the central nervous system and therefore are helpful in supporting sleep.
3. The effectiveness of hypnotics decreases, not increases, with prolonged use. They should be used only as a short-term inter-vention because tolerance and rebound insomnia occur in approximately 4 weeks.
4. Although melatonin demonstrates promise as a drug to support sleep, it is not the drug of choice because its safety and efficacy for long-term use are not yet established.

7. 1. Sigmund Freud, not Erik Erikson, identified that defense mechanisms are used to reduce anxiety by preventing conscious awareness of threatening thoughts or feelings.
2. Lawrence Kohlberg, not Erik Erikson, es-tablished a framework for understanding the development of moral maturity, which is the ability to recognize independently what is right and what is wrong.
3. **Erik Erikson expanded on Freud's The-ory of Personality Development by giv-ing equal emphasis to the influence of a person's social and cultural environment. He stressed that psychosocial develop-ment depends on an interactive process between the physical and emotional variables during a person's life at eight distinct stages. Each stage requires reso-lution of a developmental conflict that has opposite outcomes and that requires interaction within the self and with oth-ers in the environment.**
4. Assimilation and accommodation of new in-formation necessary to stimulate intellectual growth comprise a concept basic to Jean Piaget's Theory of Cognitive Development, not Erikson's Theory of Personality Devel-opment. Assimilation involves the process of organizing new information into one's present body of knowledge, and accommo-dation involves rearranging and restructur-ing thought processes to deal with the imbalance caused by new information and thereby increase understanding.

8. 1. Cessation of estrogen and progesterone production during menopause does not contribute to iron-deficiency anemia.
2. Although older adults are at risk for iron-deficiency anemia because of decreased intake and less efficient absorption of nutri-ents, they are not at as high a risk as an age group in another option.
3. Although teenagers are at risk for iron-deficiency anemia because of rapid growth and diets high in fat and low in vitamins, they are not at as high a risk as an age group in another option.
4. **Infants are at the highest risk for iron-deficiency anemia because of the in-creased physiological demand for blood production during growth, inadequate solid food intake after 6 months of age, and formula not fortified with iron. In addition, preterm or multiple-birth infants are at special risk because of inadequate stores of iron during the end of fetal development.**

9. 1. Although inactivity may promote consti-pation, there are no physiological changes in school-age children that will compound the risk for constipation.
2. Although middle-age adults experience slower gastrointestinal motility than when they were younger, they are not at as great a risk for constipation as an age group in another option.
3. Constipation in infants is uncommon except when they are weaned from for-mula to cow's milk or when their diet is mismanaged.
4. **Older adults are at the greatest risk for constipation because of decreases in activity levels, in intake of high-fiber foods, in peristalsis, in digestive enzymes, and in fluid intake.**

10. 1. **From 18 months to 3 years of age (Autonomy versus Shame and Doubt), the child strives for independence. Attempts to self-feed should be encouraged and enthusiastically praised even though the child may make a mess. They allow the child to practice and perfect new skills, help to develop fine-motor skills, and support control of the self and the environment.**
2. Although finger foods help to avoid a mess during mealtime, the child must learn how to use utensils when eating. This intervention interferes with the achievement of the task associated with this age group.
3. Feeding the child along with the child's at-tempts at eating should be avoided. When children are made to feel that the job they are doing is not good enough, it conveys a sense of shame and doubt and will make them feel inadequate.

4. Feeding the child until the child is more capable is discouraging to the child and may precipitate feelings of inadequacy, shame, and doubt. When caregivers always do what children should be learning, children are not permitted to learn for themselves.

11. 1. The most recent statistics from the National Center for Health Statistics indicate that sudden infant death syndrome (SIDS) is ranked as the third leading cause of all infant deaths.
    2. The most recent statistics (2015) from the National Center for Health Statistics indicate that congenital malformations are ranked first as the leading cause of all infant deaths.
    3. The most recent statistics from the National Center for Health Statistics indicate that unintentional injuries are ranked as the fifth leading cause of all infant deaths. Maternal complications associated with pregnancy are ranked as the fourth leading cause of all infant deaths.
    4. The most recent statistics from the National Center for Health Statistics indicate that short gestation and low birth weight are ranked as the second leading cause of all infant deaths.

12. 1. Toddlers generally are able to regulate body temperature as long as they are basically healthy.
    2. Adolescents generally are able to regulate body temperature as long as there are no coexisting health problems.
    3. Regulation of body temperature depends on the ability to dilate or constrict blood vessels and control the activity of sweat glands. In the older adult, the production of sweat glands decreases, reducing a person's ability to perspire and resulting in risk for heat exhaustion. Decreased amounts of muscle mass and subcutaneous fat lead to increased susceptibility to cold. Inefficient vasoconstriction occurs in response to cold, and inefficient vasodilation occurs in response to heat. There is also a diminished ability to shiver.
    4. School-age children generally are able to regulate temperature as long as there are no other underlying medical conditions.

13. 1. Infants initially sleep 17 to 20 hours a day and, by the end of the first year, are sleeping 12 to 16 hours a day. Infants generally do not have problems sleeping.

2. Toddlers (18 months to 3 years) generally sleep 12 to 15 hours a day with one or two naps. Toddlers occasionally will awaken during the night because of teething pains, illness, separation anxiety, and loneliness; awakening during the night is not unusual in the toddler. If caregivers establish regular bedtime routines and provide emotional comfort, sleep problems are minimal during this age group.
    3. Adolescents (12 to 20 years) have more multiple and complex milestones than individuals in any other stage of development. These milestones are physiological (e.g., puberty), psychological (e.g., self-identity and independence issues), and social (e.g., peer pressure, altered roles, and maturing relationships). Anxiety associated with all of these stressors contributes to altered sleep patterns and sleep deprivation. Adolescents generally need 8 to 10 hours of sleep a day; however, adolescents' sleep needs vary widely.
    4. Preschoolers (3 to 5 years) have well-established sleep-wake cycles; they sleep 10 to 12 hours a day, and daytime napping decreases. Dreams and nightmares, which can awaken the child, can occur but are not considered abnormal. Establishing consistent rituals that include quiet time helps to minimize nighttime awakening.

14. **1. When middle-age adults are caring for their children and their aging, dependent parents at the same time, they are referred to as the sandwich generation. Their parents and children represent the bread, and they are the meat in between.**
    2. Role reversal is not a definition of the sandwich generation.
    3. Assisting both sets of parents is not a definition of the sandwich generation.
    4. Being a middle child between older and younger siblings is not the definition of the sandwich generation.

15. 1. Older adults experience decreased, not increased, absorption of drugs from the gastrointestinal tract.
    2. The literature documents that older adults are at high risk for nonadherence to a medication regimen because of its complexity. The larger the number of medications and the larger the number of doses per day, the higher the risk of nonadherence. One study indicated that the adherence rate was

87% for daily dosing, 81% for doses twice a day, 77% for doses three times a day, and 39% for doses four times a day. Other reasons for not fully adhering to a drug regimen include inconvenience, side effects, financial limitations, and/or perceived ineffectiveness of the drugs.

3. Older adults do not experience a decline in intelligence due to aging. Although some older adults may experience a decline in short-term memory, they are not less intelligent. When older adults experience a decline in sensory function (e.g., vision, hearing), they may feel ashamed or frustrated, causing withdrawal. Behaviors reflective of withdrawal may be misperceived as a decline in intelligence.

4. Older adults have an increased, not decreased, risk for adverse reactions to drugs. Adverse effects are any effects that are not therapeutic. Adverse effects can be side effects that are minor and tolerable or serious, requiring discontinuation of the drug.

16. 1. Although toddlers (18 months to 3 years; early childhood—Autonomy versus Shame and Doubt) experience a number of developmental milestones, toddlerhood is not as unstable or complex as another stage of development. Toddlers explore and test the environment, develop independence, and have a beginning ability to control the self.

2. **Adolescents (12 to 20 years—Identity versus Role Confusion) have more multiple and complex milestones than individuals in any other stage of development. These milestones are physiological (e.g., puberty), psychological (e.g., self-identity and independence), and social (e.g., peer pressure, altered roles, and maturing relationships) The multiplicity of these stressors can have a major impact on the development of the adolescent's personal identity and sense of self.**

3. Although children in early childhood or toddlerhood (18 months to 3 years—Autonomy versus Shame and Doubt) and late childhood (3 to 6 years—Initiative versus Guilt) experience a number of developmental milestones, their development is not as unstable or complex as that of another age group. The main tasks of childhood are achievement of self-control, initiation of one's own activities, and development of purpose and competence.

4. Although infants (birth to 18 months—Trust versus Mistrust) experience a number of developmental milestones, their development is not as unstable or complex as that of another age group. The main tasks of infancy are to adjust to living in and responding to the environment and to develop trust.

17. 1. Middle-age adults usually do not have complications during the perioperative period.

2. Although a pregnant woman has unique needs during the perioperative period, as long as the mother's cardiovascular and fluid and electrolyte statuses are maintained, the fetus and the mother are supported and safe.

3. Although the adolescent has needs related to body image and separation from friends, the physiological risk for complications during the perioperative period is not increased.

4. **Infants are at risk for fluid volume depletion because of a small blood volume and limited fluid reserves. In addition, immature liver and kidneys affect the ability to metabolize and eliminate drugs, an undeveloped immune system increases the risk of infection, and immature temperature-regulating mechanisms increase the risk of hyperthermia and hypothermia.**

18. 1. Some stages are faster and some are slower, depending on the person and the developmental level.

2. The growth and development process is complex and influenced by many different factors.

3. Just the opposite is true; the growth and development process helps people to extend themselves to be the most that they can be.

4. **Although people follow a general pattern, they do not grow and develop at exactly the same rate or extent.**

19. 1. **A 9-year-old child has a more realistic understanding of death than a younger child and recognizes that death is universal, irreversible, and natural. A 9-year-old child has a beginning knowledge of his or her own mortality and may fear death.**

2. A 6-year-old child is developing an understanding of the differences among the concepts of past, present, and future. A 6-year-old child believes that death is

temporary, can be caused by bad thoughts, and may be a punishment and that magic can make the dead person alive.

3. Recognizing that death is irreversible, universal, and natural occurs at an earlier age than 15 years.

4. Recognizing that death is irreversible, universal, and natural occurs at an earlier age than 12 years.

20. 1. Older adults experience decreases in basal metabolic rate, lean body mass, and physical activity that contribute to a decrease in caloric needs.

2. Energy expenditure decreases and nutritional needs stabilize during the middle adult years. People in other age groups have greater needs for nutrients to meet physiological demands than do those in the middle adult years.

3. Although young adults tend to be active and require nutrients adequate to meet high energy expenditure, physical growth slows and the basal metabolic rate begins to stabilize, so they require fewer calories than do other age groups.

4. During the first year of life, nutritional needs per unit of body weight are the greatest in comparison to any other time during the life span. Birth weight generally doubles in 4 to 6 months and triples by the end of the first year.

21. 1. Middle-age adults (25 to 45 years—Generativity versus Stagnation) strive to fulfill life goals associated with family, career, and society, as well as to give to and care for others.

2. Young adults (18 to 25 years—Intimacy versus Isolation) strive to establish mature relationships, commit to suitable partners, and develop social and work roles acceptable to society. Unsuccessful resolution results in self-absorption, egocentricity, and emotional isolation.

3. Adolescents (12 to 20 years—Identity versus Role Confusion) strive to make the transition from childhood to adulthood with a sense of personal self.

4. Infants (newborn to 18 months—Trust versus Mistrust) strive to have their needs met through interacting with others. When their needs are consistently met, they develop a sense of trust in their caregivers.

22. 1. Toddlers are active once awake and rarely spend much time in bed when not sleeping. Toddlers sleep 12 to 14 hours a day, including one or two daytime naps.

2. Middle-age adults sleep 6 to 8 hours a day. Although middle-age adults spend more time in bed awake than when they were younger, they spend less time in bed awake than an age group in another option.

3. Older adults still need 7 to 9 hours of sleep daily but often receive less because of difficulty falling asleep and more frequent awakening. They often go to bed earlier in an effort to get more sleep and end up spending more time in bed awake. Sleeping difficulties are attributed to a decrease in melatonin, less deep sleep, a decrease in exercise, more naps, movement disorders, sleep apnea, and medical and psychological problems.

4. Adolescents sleep 8 to 10 hours a day. Adolescents generally have high activity levels and stay up late. It may seem as though adolescents are always sleeping because they sleep later in the morning, but generally they go to bed much later at night.

23. 1. Accepting limited dietary choices might be required of an older adult who is learning to adjust to a therapeutic diet. More often, people in the older age group need to adapt to the stress of a declining ability to ingest, digest, and/or absorb particular food.

2. Adjusting to a change in physique is an expected developmental task of adolescence, not early childhood. Many bodily changes occur in this transitional period, such as a growth spurt and sexual maturity.

3. Responding to a life-threatening illness is not an expected developmental stressor of this age group. Only a small percentage of the population of 18-month-old to 3-year-old children faces the challenge of a life-threatening illness.

4. During early childhood, the child gains independence through learning right from wrong. Independence occurs with guidance from parents as the child learns self-control without feeling shame and doubt. When parents are overly protective or critical, feelings of inferiority will develop.

24. 1. Although taste influences choices of foods ingested by adolescents, a factor identified in another option generally has more influence over what adolescents eat.

2. Adolescents tend to have few rigid routines because of their busy schedules. A factor identified in another option generally has more influence over what adolescents eat than do routines.

3. Peers often dictate the dietary choices of adolescents. Fad dieting and demands of socialization that generally involve fast food are common among adolescents.

4. Although personal preferences may influence choices of foods ingested by adolescents, a factor identified in another option generally has more influence over what adolescents eat.

25. 1. Although sebaceous glands increase in size with age, the amount of sebum produced decreases, hastening the evaporation of water from the stratum corneum and resulting in cracked, dry skin.

   2. Older adults generally experience a deterioration of the hyaline cartilage surface of joints, which tears, allowing bones to be in direct contact with each other. Often, this results in the formation of spurs, or projecting points, that limit joint motion.

   3. Loss of a social support system is a psychosocial, not physiological, change commonly experienced by older adults.

   4. Hearing acuity decreases, particularly in relation to high-pitched sounds, because of atrophy in the organ of Corti and cochlear neurons, loss of sensory hair cells, and degeneration of the stria vascularis.

   5. Older adults have the same need for sleep as younger individuals. However, it is more difficult for older adults to obtain the quality and quantity of sleep desired. Chemical, structural, and functional changes in the nervous system disrupt circadian rhythms and sleep.

26. **1. The sensorimotor stage (birth to 2 years) is governed by sensations in which simple learning takes place. It progresses from reflex activity through repetitive behaviors to imitative behavior. These children are curious, experiment, and learn primarily through trial and error.**

   4. The preoperational stage (2 to 7 years) involves thinking that is concrete and tangible; these children cannot reason beyond the observable. Also, their thinking is transductive; that is,

knowledge of one characteristic is transferred to another.

   2. The concrete-operational stage (7 to 11 years) reflects an increasing ability to use symbols and understand relationships between things and ideas. Judgments are made based on what they reason (conceptual thinking) rather than just what they see (preoperational thinking). Also, they develop the concept of conservation; that is, physical factors (e.g., volume, weight, and number) remain the same even though outward appearances may change.

   3. The formal operational stage (11 to 15 years) involves thinking that is abstract, theoretical, philosophical, and hypothetical. Thinking is characterized by flexibility, adaptability, and drawing logical conclusions.

27. 1. Although social isolation is a risk for some older adults because of declining health, death of family members and friends, fear of crime, or injury precipitating a desire not to leave the house, most older adults seek opportunities to maintain and build social contacts via the telephone, Internet, community groups, senior centers, life-care communities, and so on.

   2. Older adults who have a sense of loss or regret about past life events are struggling to complete a successful life review. A successful life review results in accepting past life events for what they were, and the individual views life as meaningful, respects the self, and feels respect from others.

   3. The older adult needs to adjust to multiple changes in social roles to emerge emotionally integrated with an intact ego and a sense of wholeness. Changes in social roles are often dramatic as the result of retirement, the death of significant others, changing responsibilities within the extended family structure, moving to different living quarters, and decreasing finances.

   4. Although older adults associate with members of all age groups, they generally establish an explicit affiliation with select members of their own age group. This supports a sharing of common interests and concerns, as well as meeting belonging and self-esteem needs as older adults seek status among their peers.

5. Older adults do not always have the energy or stamina needed to invest in increasing the number of new meaningful relationships. In addition, they tend to experience a decrease, not an increase, in meaningful relationships because of the death of members of their circle of friends and relatives.

28. **1. If sensory overload precipitates anxiety and the autonomic nervous system is stimulated by the fight-or-flight mechanism, tachycardia will occur.**
2. **Sensory overload generally precipitates anxiety, resulting in agitation and restlessness.**
3. **Confusion is a common response to sensory overload. Because of excessive sensory stimulation, a person is unable to perceive the environment accurately or respond appropriately.**
4. **Excessive sensory stimulation from the environment can overwhelm an individual's nervous system, resulting in irritability.**
5. **Excessive sensory input stimulates the autonomic nervous system, interfering with rest and sleep and resulting in fatigue.**

29. **1. Growth and development comprise an orderly process that follows a predictable path. There are three predictable patterns: cephalocaudal— proceeding from head to toe; proximodistal—progressing from gross-motor to fine-motor movements; and symmetrical—both sides developing equally. Growth is marked by measurable changes in the physical aspects of the life cycle, and development is marked by behavioral changes that occur because of achievement of developmental tasks and their resulting functional abilities and skills.**
2. **Growth and development follow a sequential timetable whereby multiple dynamic changes occur in a systematic and orderly manner.**
3. **Individuals grow and develop in the physiological, cognitive, psychosocial, moral, and spiritual realms in an integrated way, with each one influencing the others.**
4. **Growth and development comprise a complex process that involves multiple influencing variables, such as genetics,**

experience, health, culture, and environment.
5. The word *static* means stationary, stagnant, or fixed. Growth and development are dynamic and progressive.

30. **1. A task associated with middle adulthood is sharing of self and performing activities that promote the growth of others, particularly those in the next generation.**
2. Developing peer relationships is one of the developmental tasks of the 6- to 12-year-old child and adolescent, not the middle-age adult.
3. **A major task of middle adulthood is successfully fulfilling lifelong goals that involve family, career, and society. If these goals are not achieved, a crisis often is precipitated.**
4. Delaying satisfaction is one of the developmental tasks of the 18-month- to 3-year-old child, not the middle-age adult.
5. Facing death is one of the developmental tasks of the 65-year-old and older adult, not the middle-age adult.

31. **1. During the school-age years, children usually grow approximately 2 inches a year and gain 4.5 to 6 pounds a year. This child should be assessed further because of the potential for obesity. Obesity in children is increasing in the United States.**
2. Age-appropriate psychosocial development in school-age children includes associating with peers of the same gender and desiring peer approval. This age group also is developing personal and interpersonal competence; they are conscientious and industrious.
3. Children approaching 10 to 12 years of age often appear awkward and lanky. They tend to be uncoordinated as muscle and bone growth advances; they are adjusting to these physical changes.
4. Children approaching 10 to 12 years begin to develop a self-image and a body image. They have increasing concerns about their appearance and begin to become interested in children of the opposite gender.

32. **1. When a person reaches 60 years of age and older, all physiological systems are less efficient, which reduces compensatory reserve.**
2. In the 40- to 60-year-old age group, a person will begin to see the earliest signs of

aging. Changes are gradual and insidious and generally do not have an impact on function.

3. In the 12- to 19-year-old age group, the adolescent is experiencing rapid growth and a beginning transition to adulthood, not a decline in the ability to adapt.

4. In the 3- to 11-year-old age group, children are growing at a continuous pace in their ability to adapt to the world around them, not declining in their ability to adapt.

5. **Infants have immature immune systems and body systems that are still developing. Also, the physiological processes of an infant's body have a limited experiential background on which to draw responses to new stressors. These issues result in an inefficiency of adaptation.**

33. 1. This relates to Freud's Anal Stage of development (1 to 3 years). According to Freud, if a parent is strict, overbearing, and oppressive during toilet training, the child may develop traits of an anal-retentive personality (e.g., obsessive-compulsive tendencies, rigid thought patterns, stinginess, and/or stubbornness).

2. Seeking excessive attention from others is most likely the result of an unresolved task of the 6- to 12-year-old age group (school age), Industry versus Inferiority. Seeking attention often is an attempt to increase self-esteem.

3. People who have difficulty accepting help from others or who would rather do things themselves generally have not completely resolved the developmental task of infancy, Trust versus Mistrust.

4. **A main developmental task of adolescence is being capable of determining "who you are." An inability to express a sense of self later in life reflects an unresolved conflict of Identity versus Role Confusion.**

5. **A main developmental task of adolescence is forming a sense of personal identity as a foundation for the tasks of young adulthood, making decisions regarding career choices, and selecting a mate. An adult who has difficulty setting**

goals in life indicates an unresolved conflict of Identity versus Role Confusion.

34. 1. **This statement is a clear example of ageism, whereby older adults are systematically stereotyped and discriminated against because they are old. This is a form of prejudice, an unfavorable opinion without concrete information about the individual. Ageism is based on the misconceptions that older adults are no longer productive, are narrow minded, are unable to learn, are dependent, experience memory loss, live in a nursing home, are ill, are boring, and so on.**

2. **The word *elderly* has a negative connotation. It implies that the person is different from other human beings and is frail, weak, or disabled. To call an adult *cute* is demeaning because it may imply that the person is childlike.**

3. This is not a discriminatory statement indicative of ageism.

4. This is not a discriminatory statement indicative of ageism.

5. This is not a discriminatory statement indicative of ageism.

35. 1. **Preschool-age children have the fine-motor skills to open and close zippers and buttons.**

2. **Preschool-age children have the motor skills necessary to manipulate a toy tool, such as a hammer.**

3. **Preschool-age children have the gross-motor skills and balance to be able to hop and skip on one foot, balance on one foot, and perform a broad jump.**

4. Preschool-age children do not have the strength and balance to ride a two-wheel bicycle. A preschooler usually can ride a tricycle. School-age children, not preschool-age children, usually are able to ride a two-wheel bicycle.

5. Preschool-age children do not have the strength and coordination to swim using the freestyle stroke. Some preschool-age children are able to do the "doggie paddle." School-age children, not preschool-age children, usually are able to swim using the freestyle stroke.

Communication

KEYWORDS

The following words include nursing/medical terminology, concepts, principles, or information relevant to content specifically addressed in the chapter or associated with topics presented in it. English dictionaries, nursing textbooks, and medical dictionaries, such as *Taber's Cyclopedic Medical Dictionary,* are resources that can be used to expand your knowledge and understanding of these words and related information.

Assertive skills
Barriers to communication:
  Advising
  Direct questions
  Disapproving
  False reassurance
  Moralizing
  Patronizing
  Probing
Body language
Communication process:
  Channels of communication:
    Auditory
    Kinesthetic
    Visual
  Decoding by receiver
  Encoding by sender
  Feedback
  Message
Confidential, confidentiality
Confrontation
Congruence
Content themes
Conversation
Empathy, empathetic, empathic
Group dynamics
Interaction
Interpersonal communication
Interview:
  Informal
  Formal

Intrapersonal communication
Nonverbal
Rapport
Space:
  Intimate
  Personal
  Public
  Social
Territoriality
Therapeutic communication skills:
  Active listening
  Clarifying
  Exploring
  Focusing
  Indirect question
  Open-ended question
  Paraphrasing
  Reflection
  Responding
  Silence
  Summarizing
  Touching
  Validating
Therapeutic relationship, phases:
  Orientation
  Termination
  Working
Verbal

COMMUNICATION: QUESTIONS

1. A nurse is collecting data from a client for an admission nursing history. Which question by the nurse is **best** to open the discussion?
   1. "What brought you to the hospital?"
   2. "Would it help to discuss your feelings?"
   3. "Do you want to talk about your concerns?"
   4. "Would you like to talk about why you are here?"

2. A nurse must conduct a focused interview to complete an admission history. Which interviewing technique should the nurse use?
   1. Probing
   2. Clarification
   3. Direct questions
   4. Paraphrasing statements

3. Which statement about communication should the nurse consider to be accurate?
   1. Verbal communication is essential for human relationships.
   2. Hands are the most expressive part of the body.
   3. Behavior clearly reflects feelings.
   4. Communication is inevitable.

4. A client is extremely upset and mentions something about a work-related issue that the nurse cannot understand. Which is the nurse's **best** response?
   1. "It's natural to worry about your job."
   2. "Your job must be very important to you."
   3. "Calm down so that I can understand what you are saying."
   4. "I'm not quite sure I heard what you were saying about your work."

5. Which is the purpose of the use of humor by a nurse when interacting with a client?
   1. Diminish feelings of anger
   2. Refocus the client's attention
   3. Maintain a balanced perspective
   4. Delay dealing with the inevitable

6. A nurse is caring for a client who is blind in the left eye and visually impaired in the right eye. Which actions should the nurse employ to promote communication with this client?
   1. Touch the client's left arm before initiating a conversation.
   2. Ensure that the door to the client's room is on the client's left side.
   3. Close the window curtains and dim the lights before speaking with the client.
   4. Knock on the door and request permission to enter before approaching the client.

7. A client is admitted to the hospital with cirrhosis of the liver caused by long-term alcohol misuse. Which is the **best** response by the nurse when the client says, "I really don't believe that my drinking a couple of beers a day has anything to do with my liver problem"?
   1. "You find it hard to believe that beer can hurt the liver."
   2. "How long is it that you have been drinking several beers a day?"
   3. "Each beer is equivalent to one shot of liquor, so it's just as damaging to the liver as hard liquor."
   4. "Do you believe that beer is not harmful even though research shows that it is just as bad for you as hard liquor?"

8. Which is being communicated when the nurse leans forward during a client interview?
   1. Aggression
   2. Anxiety
   3. Interest
   4. Privacy

9. Which statement describes the following proverb? *What you do speaks so loudly I cannot hear what you say.*
   1. Hearing ability is an important factor in communicating.
   2. Nonverbal messages are often more meaningful than words.
   3. Listening to what people say requires attention to what is being said.
   4. When people talk too loudly, it is hard to understand what is being said.

10. A mother whose young daughter has died of leukemia is crying and is unable to talk about her feelings. Which is the **best** response by the nurse?
1. "Everyone will remember her because she was so cute. She was one of our favorites."
2. "As hard as this is, it is probably for the best because she was in a lot of pain."
3. "She put up the good fight, but now she is out of pain and in heaven."
4. "It must be hard to deal with such a precious loss."

11. A young adult who had a leg amputated because of trauma says, "No one will ever choose to love a person with one leg." Which is the **best** response by the nurse?
1. "You are a good-looking person, and you will have no trouble meeting someone who cares."
2. "You may feel that way now, but you will feel differently as time passes."
3. "Do you feel that no one will marry you because you have one leg?"
4. "How do you see your situation at this point?"

12. A nurse is changing a client's dressing over an abdominal wound. Which level of space around the client is entered during the dressing change?
1. Public
2. Social
3. Intimate
4. Personal

13. Which stage of an interview establishes the relationship between the nurse and the client?
1. Preinteraction stage
2. Orientation stage
3. Examining stage
4. Working stage

14. A client is exhibiting anxious behavior and states, "I just found out that I have cancer everywhere, and I don't have very long to live. My life is over." Which is the **best** response by the nurse?
1. "It might be good if your family were here right now. Shall I call them?"
2. "What might be the best way to approach this terrible news?"
3. "That is so sad. You must feel like crying."
4. "It sounds like you feel hopeless."

15. Which interviewing skill is used when the nurse says, "You mentioned before that you are having a problem with your colostomy"?
1. Focusing
2. Clarifying
3. Paraphrasing
4. Acknowledging

16. A client says, "I am really nervous about having a spinal tap tomorrow." Which is the **best** response by the nurse?
1. "I'll ask the doctor for a little medication to help you relax."
2. "Clients who have had a spinal tap say it is not that uncomfortable."
3. "It's all right to be nervous, and I don't remember anyone who wasn't."
4. "Your physician is excellent and is very careful when spinal taps are done."

17. A client with chest pain is being admitted to the emergency department. When asked about next of kin, the client states, "Don't bother calling my daughter; she is always too busy." Which is the **best** response by the nurse?
1. "Your daughter might be upset if you don't call."
2. "What does your daughter do that makes her so busy?"
3. "Is there someone else besides your daughter that I can call?"
4. "I think that your daughter would want to know that you are sick."

18. Which is the nurse doing when using the interviewing technique of *attentive listening*?
   1. Identifying the client's concerns and exploring them with "why" questions
   2. Determining the content and feeling of the client's message
   3. Employing silence to encourage the client to talk
   4. Using verbal skills to obtain information

19. A client who has had postoperative complications appears upset and agitated yet withdrawn. Which is the **most** appropriate statement by the nurse?
   1. "You seem distressed. Tell me why you are upset."
   2. "You've been having a pretty rough time recovering since surgery."
   3. "It's not uncommon to have complications after the kind of surgery that you had."
   4. "I'm not sure that I know everything that has been happening. Tell me what has happened to you since surgery."

20. A nurse is admitting a client to the unit who was transferred from the emergency department. Which should the nurse do to facilitate communication?
   1. Ensure that the client has an effective way to communicate with health-care team members.
   2. Use interviewing techniques to control the direction of the client's communication.
   3. Minimize energy spent by the client on negative feelings and concerns.
   4. Refocus to the positive aspects of the client's situation and prognosis.

21. A nurse is caring for a very confused client with a diagnosis of dementia of the Alzheimer's type. Which should the nurse say when assisting the client to eat?
   1. "Please eat your meat."
   2. "It's important that you eat."
   3. "What would you like to eat?"
   4. "If you don't eat, you can't have dessert."

22. A client states, "Do you think I could have cancer?" The nurse responds, "What did the doctor tell you?" Which interviewing approach did the nurse use?
   1. Paraphrasing
   2. Confrontation
   3. Reflective technique
   4. Open-ended question

23. A nurse is developing a therapeutic relationship with a client with emotional needs. Which nursing intervention is **essential** during the working stage of the relationship?
   1. Establish a formal or informal contract that addresses the client's problems.
   2. Implement nursing actions that are designed to achieve expected client outcomes.
   3. Develop rapport and trust so the client feels protected and an initial plan can be identified.
   4. Clearly identify the role of the nurse and establish the parameters of the professional relationship.

24. A nurse uses reflective technique when communicating with an anxious client. On which does the nurse focus when using reflective technique in this situation?
   1. Feelings
   2. Content themes
   3. Clarification of information
   4. Summarization of the topics discussed

25. A client states, "My wife is going to be very upset that my prostate surgery probably is going to leave me impotent." Which is the **best** response by the nurse?
1. "I'm sure your wife will be willing to make this sacrifice in exchange for your well-being."
2. "The surgeons are getting great results with nerve-sparing surgery today."
3. "Your wife may not put as much emphasis on sex as you think."
4. "Let's talk about how you feel about this surgery."

26. A client states, "I think that I am dying." The nurse responds, "You believe that you are dying?" Which interviewing approach did the nurse use?
1. Focusing
2. Reflecting
3. Validating
4. Paraphrasing

27. A nurse plans to foster a therapeutic relationship with a client. Which is important for the nurse to do?
1. Sympathize with the client when the client communicates sad feelings.
2. Demonstrate respect when discussing emotionally charged subjects.
3. Use humor to defuse emotionally charged topics of discussion.
4. Work on establishing a friendship with the client.

28. A client appears tearful and is quiet and withdrawn. The nurse says, "You seem very sad today." Which interviewing approach did the nurse use?
1. Examining
2. Reflecting
3. Clarifying
4. Orienting

29. A client is admitted to the hospital with a tentative medical diagnosis, and multiple diagnostic tests are performed. Where in the client's medical record can the nurse find documentation about the current medical diagnosis after the diagnostic test results are reviewed by the primary health-care provider?
1. Progress Notes
2. Admission Sheet
3. History and Physical
4. Social Service Record

30. Which nursing action should the nurse implement when speaking with an older adult whose hearing is impaired? **Select all that apply.**
1. _____ Limit background noise.
2. _____ Enunciate words without exaggeration.
3. _____ Use gestures to augment communication.
4. _____ Stand directly in front of the client when speaking.
5. _____ Talk in a normal rate and volume when speaking with the client.

31. A client with a newly created colostomy wants to learn how to irrigate the colostomy. The nurse provides this teaching by developing a therapeutic nurse-client relationship and implementing teaching strategies. Identify the statement that is included in the working stage of this therapeutic relationship. **Select all that apply.**

1. _____ "How do you feel about doing this procedure?"
2. _____ "Would you like to try to insert the cone yourself today?"
3. _____ "You did a great job managing the instillation of fluid today."
4. _____ "I am here to help you learn how to irrigate your colostomy."
5. _____ "I'll arrange for a home-care nurse to visit you in your home when you are discharged."

32. A risk manager is conducting a retrospective audit of a client's clinical record to identify the use of unacceptable abbreviations. Which abbreviation did the risk manager identify that is on The Joint Commission's official *Do Not Use List*? **Select all that apply.**

1. _____ U
2. _____ ml
3. _____ mg
4. _____ MS
5. _____ QOD
6. _____ 0800 hour

CLIENT'S CLINICAL RECORD

Medication Administration Record
MS 4 mg subcutaneous at 1400 hour and client expressed relief within 15 minutes. Client's serum glucose was 180 at 1700 hour; 4 U regular insulin administered subcutaneously as prescribed.

Intake and Output Record
0800 hour: Milk 60 ml, orange juice 120 ml; coffee 120 ml

Progress Note
Client to be discharged in a.m. and will receive physical therapy QOD.

---

33. A nurse is attempting to develop a helping relationship with a client who was recently diagnosed with cancer. Which factor is unique to this helping relationship? **Select all that apply.**

1. _____ The client should always assume the dominant role.
2. _____ The nurse and the client equally share information.
3. _____ The interaction is specific to the client.
4. _____ The interaction is guided by a purpose.
5. _____ The needs of both participants are met.

34. A nurse is using military time when entering information into a client's clinical record. For example, the clock below indicates that the time is 0708 a.m. Which number in military time should the nurse enter to document a wound irrigation that was implemented at 9 p.m.?
1. 0900
2. 1900
3. 2100
4. 2300

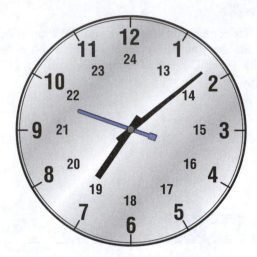

35. An agitated 80-year-old client states, "I'm having trouble with my bowels." Which response by the nurse incorporates the interviewing skill of paraphrasing? **Select all that apply.**
1. _____ "Tell me what you mean by having trouble."
2. _____ "It sounds like your bowels are causing you problems."
3. _____ "You sound upset that your bowels are causing difficulties."
4. _____ "It's common to have problems with the bowels at your age."
5. _____ "When did you first notice having trouble with your bowels?"

36. A client states, "I am surprised that I couldn't even eat half my breakfast." Which statement by the nurse uses the interviewing skill of reflection? **Select all that apply.**
1. _____ "Let's talk about your inability to eat."
2. _____ "What part of your breakfast were you able to eat?"
3. _____ "You appear startled that you did not finish your tray of food."
4. _____ "How long have you been unable to eat most of your breakfast?"
5. _____ "You seem surprised that you were unable to eat all your breakfast."

37. A nurse in a subacute unit in a skilled nursing facility is caring for a client who recently had the surgical creation of a colostomy. Place the following nursing actions in the order that reflects the nurse-client therapeutic relationship, beginning with the first stage and progressing to the last stage.
1. Provide positive feedback to the client for successful performance of a colostomy irrigation.
2. Assist the client to learn how to perform colostomy self-care.
3. Review all the information on the client's clinical record.
4. Explore the reasons for the nurse-client interaction.
5. Summarize the goals and objectives achieved.
6. Introduce self to the client.

Answer: _____

38. Which ability of the nurse is important to achieve effective therapeutic communication? **Select all that apply.**
   1. _____ Using interviewing skills
   2. _____ Remaining nonjudgmental
   3. _____ Sending only verbal messages
   4. _____ Being assertive when collecting data
   5. _____ Displaying sympathy when communicating

39. A client is to have arthroscopic surgery of the knee to repair a torn tendon. The client says, "I don't know if I'll make it through this surgery." Which response by the nurse may block further communication by the client? **Select all that apply.**
   1. _____ "The type of surgery you are having is minor."
   2. _____ "Surgery often can be frightening."
   3. _____ "Everything will be all right."
   4. _____ "You are not going to die."
   5. _____ "You sound scared."

40. Which should a nurse never do when documenting information on a client's electronic medical record? **Select all that apply.**
   1. _____ Leave the client's medical record open on the computer screen when entering the client's room to administer a medication.
   2. _____ Share information verbally about a client with another nurse who is also caring for the client.
   3. _____ Document nursing care administered to a client immediately after it is completed.
   4. _____ Give a personal access code to another member of the health-care team.
   5. _____ Document exact quotes of a client's subjective information.

1. 1. **This is a focused, open-ended statement that invites the client to communicate while centering on the reason for seeking health care.**
   2. This direct question can be answered with a "yes" or "no" response. If the response is "no," then communication will be cut off.
   3. This direct question can be answered with a "yes" or "no" response, which may limit communication.
   4. This direct question can be answered with a "yes" or "no" response. The client may not like to talk, but the client may need to talk.

2. 1. Probing questions violate the client's privacy, may cut off communication, and are inappropriate even in a focused interview. Probing interviewing occurs when the nurse persistently attempts to obtain information even after the client indicates an unwillingness to discuss the topic or the nurse pursues information out of curiosity rather than because the information is significant.
   2. Although clarification may be used during a focused interview to understand what the client is saying, it is not the primary technique used for seeking specific information.
   3. **A focused interview explores a particular topic or obtains specific information. Direct questions meet these objectives and avoid extraneous information.**
   4. Paraphrasing may be used during a focused interview to redirect ideas back to the client so that the client can verify that the nurse received the message accurately or to allow the client to hear what was said. However, it is not a technique that obtains specific information quickly.

3. 1. All communication, not just verbal communication, is essential for human relationships.
   2. The face, not the hands, is the most expressive part of the body.
   3. Behavior may imply, not clearly reflect, feelings. The nurse should obtain verbal feedback from the client regarding assumptions about behavior.
   4. **Theory indicates that all behavior has meaning, people are always behaving, and we cannot stop behaving or communicating; therefore, communication is inevitable.**

4. 1. This response may or may not be an accurate assumption.
   2. This response makes an assumption that may be erroneous.
   3. This patronizing response treats the client in a condescending manner. The client cannot calm down.
   4. **This response requests additional information in an attempt to clarify an unclear message.**

5. 1. Humor used inappropriately can cause anger to be increased, suppressed, or repressed. Anger should be expressed safely, not diminished.
   2. The focus should be on the client's concerns.
   3. **Humor is an interpersonal tool and a healing strategy. Humor releases physical and psychic energy, enhances well-being, reduces anxiety, increases pain tolerance, and places experiences within the context of life.**
   4. Coping strategies should not be delayed because delay increases stress and anxiety and prolongs the process.

6. 1. Touching a client with a visual impairment before speaking is an intrusive action and may startle the client.
   2. A door to the room on the client's left side will require the client to completely turn the head to the left so that the client can use the right eye to view a person entering the room. The door should be on the client's right side.
   3. Clients with visual impairments may still have some sight. Adequate lighting facilitates nonverbal communication.
   4. **Knocking on the door before entering the room alerts the client that someone is at the door, and requesting permission to enter the room demonstrates respect and provides for privacy.**

7. 1. **This is an example of paraphrasing. It repeats the content in the client's message in similar words to provide feedback to let the client know whether the message was understood and to prompt further communication.**
   2. This response does not address the content or emotional theme of the client's statement. In addition, this probing question may be a barrier to further communication.
   3. Although factual, this response is confrontational. This nurse's statement may put the client on the defensive and inhibit further communication.

4. This assertive, confronting, judgmental response may put the client on the defensive and cut off communication.

8. 1. Piercing eye contact, increased voice volume, challenging or confrontational conversation, invasion of personal space, and inappropriate touching convey aggression, which is a hostile, injurious, or destructive action or manner.
   2. A closed posture, avoidance of eye contact, increased muscle tension, and increased motor activity convey anxiety.
   3. **Leaning forward is a nonverbal behavior that conveys involvement. It is a form of physical attending, which is being present to another.**
   4. Privacy is not reflected by leaning forward during an interview. Privacy is facilitated by pulling a client's curtain or finding a separate room or quiet space to talk.

9. 1. Although hearing, one aspect of decoding a message, is an important factor in the communication process, it is unrelated to the stated proverb.
   2. **Nonverbal communication (e.g., body language) conveys messages without words and is under less conscious control than verbal statements. When a person's words and behavior are incongruent, nonverbal behavior most likely reflects the person's true feelings.**
   3. Although this true statement reflects active listening, it is unrelated to the stated proverb.
   4. This statement is unrelated to the stated proverb. The volume of a message may or may not influence understanding of the message. The volume of a message occurs on the physiological level, whereas understanding a message occurs on the cognitive level.

10. 1. This response is not therapeutic because it focuses on the nurse rather than on the mother.
    2. The first part of this response minimizes the loss. The second part of the response focuses on the pain experienced by the child, which may increase the mother's grief.
    3. This response minimizes the loss and focuses on the pain experienced by the child, which may increase the mother's grief. Also, the mother may not believe in heaven.
    4. **The nurse's response is empathetic. The response focuses on the feelings surrounding the loss and provides an**

opportunity for the mother to express feelings.

11. 1. This negates the client's concerns and provides false reassurance. The client needs to focus on the "negative" before focusing on the "positive." In addition, only the future will tell if the client meets someone who cares.
    2. This is false reassurance. There is no way the nurse can ensure that this belief will change.
    3. **This is an example of paraphrasing, which restates the client's message in similar words. It promotes communication.**
    4. This statement is unnecessary. The client has already stated a point of view.

12. 1. Touching is not used with public distance. Public space (12 feet and beyond) is effective for communicating with groups or the community. Individuality is lost.
    2. Invasive touching does not occur with social distance. Social space (4 to 12 feet) is effective for more formal interactions or group conversations.
    3. **Physically caring for a client involves inspection and touch that invades the instinctual, protective distance immediately surrounding an individual. Intimate space (physical contact to 1½ feet) is characterized by body contact and visual exposure.**
    4. "Laying on of the hands" does not occur with personal distance. Personal space (1½ to 4 feet) is effective for communicating with another. It is close enough to imply caring and is not extended to the distance that implies lack of involvement.

13. 1. The preinteraction stage occurs before the nurse meets the client. During this stage, the nurse gathers information about the client.
    2. **The purposes of the orientation stage of an interview are to establish rapport and orient the interviewee. A relationship is established through a process of creating goodwill and trust. The orientation stage focuses on explaining the purpose and nature of the interview and what is expected of the client.**
    3. There is no stage called the examining stage in an interview. Examining takes place during a physical assessment, when specific skills are used to collect data systematically to identify health problems.

4. This is not the purpose of the working stage. In the working stage (also called the body stage) of an interview, clients communicate how they think, feel, know, and perceive in response to questions by the nurse.

14. 1. This response abdicates the nurse's responsibility to explore the client's concerns immediately. In addition, it could be an erroneous assumption.
    2. The client is in the shock and disbelief mode of coping and will not be able to explore approaches to coping. In addition, using the words "terrible news" may increase anxiety and hopelessness.
    3. This response imposes the nurse's feelings and own coping skills into the situation.
    4. **This is an example of reflective technique because the nurse incorporated the client's feelings into the response. When no solutions to a problem are evident, a person becomes hopeless (i.e., despairing, despondent).**

15. 1. **This example of focusing helps the client explore a topic of importance. The nurse selects one topic for further discussion from among several topics presented by the client.**
    2. This is not an example of clarifying, which lets the client know that a message was unclear and seeks specific information to make the message clearer.
    3. This is not an example of paraphrasing, which is restating the client's message in similar words.
    4. This is not an example of acknowledging, which is providing nonjudgmental recognition for a contribution to the conversation, a change in behavior, or an effort by the client.

16. 1. This statement avoids the client's feelings and fails to respond to the client's need to talk about concerns. It cuts off communication.
    2. This is a generalization that minimizes the client's concern and should be avoided.
    3. **This statement is therapeutic. It recognizes the client's feelings, gives the client permission to feel nervous, and reassures the client that one's behavior is not unusual. This statement sets the groundwork for the next statement, such as, "Let's talk a little bit about the spinal tap and the concerns you may have."**

4. This is false reassurance, which discourages discussion of feelings and should be avoided.

17. 1. This may be a false assumption by the nurse. This response will put the client on the defensive and jeopardize the nurse-client relationship.
    2. This response requires the client to rationalize the daughter's behavior and focuses on information that is not significant at this time.
    3. **This response lets the client know that the message has been heard and moves forward to meet the need to notify a different significant other of the client's situation.**
    4. This provides false reassurance. Only the daughter can convey this message.

18. 1. "Why" statements are direct questions that tend to put the client on the defensive and cut off communication.
    2. **Attentive listening is the active use of all the senses to comprehend and appreciate the client's verbal and nonverbal thoughts and feelings.**
    3. Silence is a passive interaction. Silence allows the client time for quiet contemplation of what has been discussed.
    4. Using verbal skills to obtain information is an interview. The nurse is talking instead of listening.

19. 1. The first part of this statement uses the therapeutic interviewing technique of reflection, which identifies the underlying feelings of the client and is appropriate. However, the second half of the statement is asking for an explanation, which is inappropriate. Clients often interpret "why" questions as accusations, which can cause resentment and mistrust and should be avoided.
    2. **This is an example of the therapeutic interviewing skill of an open-ended statement. It demonstrates that the nurse recognizes what the client is going through, and the statement encourages the client's expression of feelings. At the very least, it demonstrates caring and concern.**
    3. This statement minimizes the client's feelings and is not supportive.
    4. This statement will not inspire confidence in the nurse. Nurses should know what is happening if care is to be comprehensive and client centered.

20. 1. **Communication between the client and health-care providers is essential, particularly for obtaining subjective data and feedback. Speech, pantomime, writing, touch, and picture boards are examples of channels of transmission (i.e., method used to convey a message).**
    2. The client, not the nurse, should direct the flow of communication.
    3. Negative feelings or concerns must be addressed. Both physical and psychic energy are used when coping with stress.
    4. The focus must be on the client's present concerns before refocusing to other issues because anxiety increases if immediate concerns are not addressed. Focusing on the negative sometimes is necessary before focusing on the positive.

21. 1. **Very confused clients more easily understand simple words and sentences.**
    2. This statement may not be understood by a very confused client because the word "important" involves a conceptual thought. These clients respond better to concrete communication.
    3. A very confused client may not be able to make a decision.
    4. This statement is a threat and should be avoided when talking with all clients. Also, it involves interpreting a "cause and effect" relationship.

22. 1. The nurse's response is not an example of paraphrasing, which is restating the client's basic message in similar words.
    2. The nurse's response is not an example of confrontation. A confronting or challenging statement fails to consider feelings, puts the client on the defensive, and is a barrier to communication.
    3. The nurse's response is not an example of reflective technique, which is referring back the basic feelings underlying the client's statement.
    4. **This open-ended statement invites the client to elaborate on the expressed thought with more than a one- or two-word response.**

23. 1. Formal or informal contracts are established during the introductory (orientation), not working, stage of a therapeutic relationship.
    2. **During the working stage of the therapeutic relationship, nursing interventions have a twofold purpose: assisting clients to explore and understand their thoughts and feelings and facilitating**
    and supporting clients' decisions and actions. Both of these help the client achieve expected outcomes.
    3. The development of trust is the primary goal of the introductory (orientation), not working, stage of a therapeutic relationship. Trust is achieved through respect, concern, credibility, and reliability.
    4. These tasks are achieved during the introductory (orientation), not working, stage of a therapeutic relationship.

24. 1. **Reflective technique requires active listening to identify the underlying emotional concerns or feelings contained in clients' messages. These feelings are then referred back to clients to promote a clearer understanding of what they have said.**
    2. Content themes are referred back to clients through paraphrasing, which is a restatement of what was said in similar words.
    3. When seeking clarification, the nurse can indicate confusion, restate the message, or ask the client to elaborate in an attempt to make the client's message more clearly understood.
    4. Summarization is not reflective technique. Summarization reviews the significant points of the discussion to reiterate or clarify information.

25. 1. This response is false reassurance. Only the wife can make this statement.
    2. Although a true statement, this response negates the client's concerns and cuts off communication.
    3. This may or may not be a true statement. Only the wife can make this statement.
    4. **The client may be using projection to cope with the potential for impotence. This response indicates that it is acceptable to talk about sexuality and invites the client to express concerns.**

26. 1. This is not an example of focusing, which centers on the key elements of the client's message in an attempt to eliminate vagueness. It keeps a rambling conversation on target to explore the major concern. The client was not rambling.
    2. This is not an example of reflecting, which focuses on feelings.
    3. This is not an example of validating. Consensual validation, a form of clarification, verifies the meaning of specific words rather than the overall meaning of the message. This ensures that both client and

nurse agree on the meaning of the words used.

4. **The nurse's response is an example of paraphrasing because it uses similar words to restate the client's message.**

27. 1. Sympathy denotes pity, which should be avoided. The nurse should empathize, not sympathize, with the client.

2. **Emotionally charged topics should be approached with respectful, sincere interactions that are accepting and nonjudgmental and that will promote further expression of feelings.**

3. Humor with emotionally charged issues may be viewed as minimizing concerns or being frivolous and could be a barrier to communication.

4. The nurse should maintain a professional relationship with the client. Nurses may be "friendly" toward clients but should not establish a "friendship" with a client.

28. 1. Examining is not an interviewing technique.

2. **Reflective technique refers to feelings implied in the content of verbal communication or in exhibited nonverbal behaviors. Clients who are crying, quiet, and withdrawn often are sad.**

3. This is not an example of clarifying, which is the use of a statement to understand a message better when communication is unclear, rambling, or garbled.

4. This is not an example of orienting. Reality orientation is a nursing technique used to assist clients in restoring an awareness of what is actual, authentic, or real.

29. 1. **Generally, the Progress Notes contain documentation by all members of the health-care team. After a client is admitted and diagnostic tests are completed, the client's medical diagnosis may change. The ongoing changes and current status of the client are documented in the Progress Notes.**

2. The Admission Sheet is the best source for identifying the client's admitting medical diagnosis, but it will not contain the current medical diagnosis if the diagnosis changed after completion of diagnostic tests.

3. The History and Physical Examination contain a history of the client, results of the physical examination, and a list of the medical problems on the day of admission

to the hospital. The admission medical diagnosis may be different after diagnostic tests are completed.

4. The client's medical diagnosis may or may not be documented on the client's Social Service Record; it is not the major source for this information.

30. 1. **Limiting competing stimuli promotes reception of verbal messages.**

2. **Clear enunciation permits lip reading by the client. Overexaggeration of lip movements may be demeaning and interfere with lip reading.**

3. **Use of gestures and facial expressions supplements verbal messages.**

4. **Standing directly in front of the client when speaking helps to focus the client's attention on the nurse. A hearing-impaired individual must be aware that a message is being sent before the message can be received and decoded.**

5. **Talking in a normal rate and volume promotes communication. Raising the volume of the voice is demeaning and may be viewed by the client as aggressive behavior.**

31. 1. This statement reflects the orientation stages of a therapeutic relationship. Although exploration of feelings is done throughout the stages, the primary goal of the orientation stage is the establishment of trust. Trust is promoted when the nurse focuses on the client's emotional needs, is respectful, and individualizes care.

2. **This statement reflects the working stage of a therapeutic relationship. It involves completing interventions that address expected outcomes, such as learning how to perform a colostomy irrigation.**

3. **This statement reflects the working stage of a therapeutic relationship. It includes providing feedback and encouragement.**

4. This statement reflects the orientation stage of a therapeutic relationship. The nurse and the client make a verbal agreement to work together to assist the client to achieve a goal.

5. This statement reflects the termination stage of a therapeutic relationship. It focuses on summarizing what has transpired and been accomplished and looks to the future.

32. 1. The abbreviations U and u for *units* are on The Joint Commission's official *Do Not Use List*. These abbreviations may be mistaken for the number 0, the number 4, or cc. The word *unit* should be written out in full.

2. An abbreviation for *milliliter* is ml. The abbreviation ml is not on The Joint Commission's official *Do Not Use List*.

3. The use of the abbreviation mg for *milligram* is not on The Joint Commission's official *Do Not Use List*.

4. **The abbreviation MS for *morphine sulfate* is on The Joint Commission's official *Do Not Use List*. MS can be mistaken for *morphine sulfate* or *magnesium sulfate*. The name of the medication should be spelled out in full.**

5. **The use of the abbreviation QOD for every other day is on The Joint Commission's official *Do Not Use List*. Other abbreviations for every other day include qod, q.o.d., and Q.O.D., and they also are on The Joint Commission's official *Do Not Use List*. "Every other day" should be written out in full.**

6. The use of 0800 represents 8 a.m. in military time. This reflects acceptable documentation.

33. 1. There are times when the nurse, not the client, must assume a dominant role; examples include when the client is unconscious, out of touch with reality, in a crisis, or experiencing panic.

2. In a therapeutic relationship, the focus is on the client, not the nurse.

3. **The helping relationship (interpersonal relationship, therapeutic relationship) is a personal, client-focused, process. The client is the center of the health team and therefore the focus of any nurse-client interaction.**

4. **Nursing interventions should be designed to achieve desirable client outcomes. Nursing care is purposeful and goal directed.**

5. The purpose of a therapeutic relationship is to focus on and meet the needs of the client, not the nurse.

34. 1. 0900 is 9 a.m.
2. 1900 is 7 p.m.

3. 2100 is 9 p.m. The large font numbers reflect a.m. The small font numbers reflect p.m.
4. 2300 is 11 p.m.

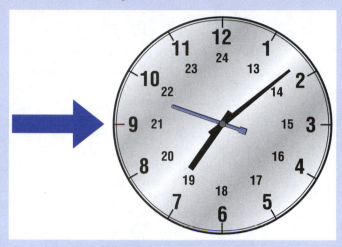

35. 1. This response is an example of clarification. The nurse wants the client to elaborate in an effort to obtain more information about the word "trouble."

2. **The nurse's statement substitutes the word *problems* for *trouble*, which paraphrases the client's comment.**

3. This is not an example of paraphrasing. This statement uses the interviewing technique of reflection because it focuses on feelings rather than words.

4. This negates the client's concern and shuts off communication.

5. This is not an example of paraphrasing; it is a direct question (focused assessment) that collects specific information.

36. 1. The nurse's response does not employ reflective technique. This open-ended statement invites the client to explore factors that may be influencing eating.

2. This response is an example of a direct question, not the use of reflective technique. It elicits a minimal amount of information about only one aspect of eating.

3. **This statement is an example of reflective technique because it focuses on the feeling of disbelief.**

4. This response is an example of a direct question (focused assessment), not the use of reflective technique.

5. **This statement is an example of reflective technique because it focuses on the feeling of disbelief.**

37. **3.** During the *preinteraction stage* of the nurse-client therapeutic relationship, the nurse gathers information about the client. This stage occurs before meeting the client.

6. During the *orientation stage* of the nurse-client therapeutic relationship, the nurse introduces himself or herself to the client and begins to establish a rapport with the client.

4. During the *orientation stage* of the nurse-client therapeutic relationship, the nurse and the client exchange information, clarify roles, and identify goals and objectives of the interaction.

2. During the *working stage* of the nurse-client therapeutic relationship, the nurse and client work toward meeting the client's needs. The nurse may function as a caregiver, counselor, teacher, resource person, etc.

1. During the *working stage* of the nurse-client therapeutic relationship, the nurse provides feedback about the client's performance.

5. During the *termination stage* of the nurse-client therapeutic relationship, the nurse summarizes what has been accomplished, reinforces past learning, arranges for available resources, and concludes the interpersonal relationship.

38. **1.** Communication is facilitated by interviewing techniques that elicit client attitudes, behaviors, and verbal messages. Interviewing skills promote therapeutic communication because they are client centered and goal directed.

2. A nonjudgmental attitude communicates acceptance to the client, which provides emotional support and precipitates further communication.

3. Communication involves both verbal and nonverbal messages. Often, nonverbal messages carry more meaning than verbal messages because actions speak louder than words.

4. Assertiveness when collecting data may be perceived by the client as aggression, which is a barrier to communication.

5. A therapeutic relationship should avoid sympathy because it implies pity. The nurse should empathize, not sympathize, with clients.

39. **1.** This response minimizes the client's concerns. It is major, not minor, surgery for this client.

2. This example of reflective technique focuses on feelings, which promotes communication.

3. This response is false reassurance. It denies the client's concerns about survival and does not invite the client to elaborate.

4. This response denies the client's feelings and is false reassurance. Also, it closes communication and does not provide the client with an opportunity to discuss concerns.

5. This example of reflective technique identifies feelings, which promotes communication.

40. **1.** Leaving the client's medical record open on the computer screen violates client confidentiality as well as leaves the file vulnerable to another person contaminating the information in the file.

2. A nurse should communicate, verbally and in writing, important information to other members of the health-care team responsible for caring for the client. Valuable time may lapse before other members of the team read the client's electronic medical record.

3. Documenting care immediately after it is administered ensures that the information is in the client's medical record. Also, delaying documentation may result in the nurse's forgetting to include pertinent information.

4. A nurse should never share a personal access code. This ensures that only the nurse assigned the code can insert information into the electronic medical record via that code. This protects the nurse who has the code.

5. Inclusion of exact client statements prevents the nurse from including personal interpretations that may not be accurate.

Psychological Support

The following words include nursing/medical terminology, concepts, principles, and information relevant to content specifically addressed in the chapter or associated with topics presented in it. English dictionaries, nursing textbooks, and medical dictionaries, such as *Taber's Cyclopedic Medical Dictionary,* are resources that can be used to expand your knowledge and understanding of these words and related information.

Anxiety:
  Mild
  Moderate
  Panic, panic attack
  Severe
Behavior modification
Beliefs
Bereavement
Body image
Confusion
Conscious, unconscious, subconscious
Coping
Crisis:
  Adventitious/unpredictable events
  Developmental/maturational
  Situational
Crisis intervention
Defense mechanisms:
  Compensation
  Conversion
  Denial
  Depersonalization
  Dissociation
  Identification
  Intellectualization
  Introjection
  Minimization
  Projection
  Rationalization
  Reaction formation
  Regression
  Repression
  Sublimation
  Substitution
  Suppression
Delirium
Delusions
Dementia
Dependence
Depression
Desensitization
Ego integrity

Egocentric
Empathy, empathetic, empathic
Freudian terms:
  Ego
  Id
  Superego
Grieving:
  Anticipatory
  Dysfunctional
  Stages of grieving (Kübler-Ross):
    Denial
    Anger
    Bargaining
    Depression
    Acceptance
Guided imagery
Hallucinations
Hopelessness
Meditation
Memory
Midlife crisis
Personal identity
Positive mental attitude
Powerlessness
Progressive relaxation
Psychodynamic
Psychosocial development
Psychotherapy
Role:
  Role ambiguity
  Role conflict
  Role strain
Self-concept
Self-esteem
Social isolation
Spirituality, spiritual distress
Suicide, suicidal
Sympathy
Transference/countertransference
Trust
Values

PSYCHOLOGICAL SUPPORT: QUESTIONS

1. A client with a terminal illness tells the nurse, "I have lived a long life. I am ready to go." Which is the nurse's **best** response?
   1. Offer the client a back rub.
   2. Sit quietly by the client's bedside.
   3. Tell the family about the client's statement.
   4. Discuss with the client how dying is part of the life cycle.

2. A man with a heart condition continues to perform strenuous sports against medical advice. Which defense mechanism does the nurse identify the client is using?
   1. Denial
   2. Repression
   3. Introjection
   4. Dissociation

3. To provide appropriate nursing care, which concept about anxiety is important to consider?
   1. Panic attacks related to anxiety, which generally have a slow onset, can be prevented if identified early.
   2. One can conceptualize anxiety as being similar to the health-illness continuum.
   3. People who lead healthy lifestyles rarely experience anxiety.
   4. Anxiety is an abnormal reaction to realistic danger.

4. Which word reflects the ability of a nurse to perceive a client's emotions accurately?
   1. Autonomy
   2. Sympathy
   3. Empathy
   4. Trust

5. What is the consequence when the nurse denies a client the use of a defense mechanism?
   1. Causes more anxiety
   2. Precipitates withdrawal
   3. Facilitates effective coping
   4. Encourages emotional growth

6. Which defense mechanism is being used when a client who has just been diagnosed with terminal cancer calmly says to the nurse, "I'll have to get on the Internet to assess my options"?
   1. Intellectualization
   2. Introjection
   3. Depression
   4. Denial

7. A client is told that surgery is necessary. The client begins to experience elevations in pulse, respirations, and blood pressure. Which stage of anxiety is indicated by these nursing assessments?
   1. Mild
   2. Moderate
   3. Severe
   4. Panic

8. A nurse concludes that a woman is remembering only the good times after the death of her husband. Which defense mechanism is the woman using?
   1. Compensation
   2. Minimization
   3. Repression
   4. Regression

9. A client strongly states the desire to go to the hospital coffee shop for lunch regardless of hospital policy. Which does the nurse conclude that this behavior **most** likely reflects?
   1. Anger with the policies of the hospital
   2. Dissatisfaction with hospital meals
   3. The need to regain a little control
   4. A desire for a change of scenery

10. A nurse is teaching a client about the positive effects of exercise to reduce anxiety. Which client comment about how exercise reduces anxiety indicates that the client understands the nurse's teaching?
    1. "It interferes with the ability to concentrate."
    2. "It stimulates the production of endorphins."
    3. "It reduces the metabolism of epinephrine."
    4. "It decreases the acidity of blood."

11. A primary health-care provider informs a client that the diagnosis is inoperable cancer and the prognosis is poor. After the primary health-care provider leaves the room, the client begins to cry. Which should the nurse do?
    1. Touch the client's hand to provide support.
    2. Leave the room to give the client privacy to cry.
    3. Telephone the client's family to inform them of the diagnosis.
    4. Ask the client questions to encourage an expression of feelings.

12. A nurse is caring for a client who is scheduled for IV chemotherapy for cancer. Which defense mechanism is being used when the client says to the daughter, "Be brave"?
    1. Rationalization
    2. Minimization
    3. Substitution
    4. Projection

13. A client says to a nurse, "I'm the same age as my father when he died. Am I going to die of my cancer?" Which is the appropriate inference about what the client is experiencing?
    1. Grieving associated with the potential for death
    2. Powerlessness associated with feelings of being out of control
    3. Fear associated with the perceived threat to biological integrity
    4. Impaired coping associated with inadequate psychological resources

14. A client who is withdrawn says, "When I have the opportunity, I am going to commit suicide." Which is the **best** response by the nurse?
    1. "You have a lovely family. They need you."
    2. "You must feel overwhelmed to want to kill yourself."
    3. "Let's explore the reasons you have for wanting to live."
    4. "Suicide does not solve problems. Tell me what is wrong."

15. Which situation identified by the nurse reflects the defense mechanism of displacement?
    1. A woman is very nice to her mother-in-law, whom she secretly dislikes.
    2. A man says that he is not so bad, so don't believe what they say about him.
    3. An adolescent puts a poor grade on a test out of her mind when at her after-school job.
    4. An older man gets angry with friends after family members attempt to talk with him about his illness.

16. A client is scheduled for an elective abortion. Which is the **best** way for the nurse to reinforce this client's self-esteem needs?
    1. Supporting the use of defense mechanisms
    2. Encouraging social interaction with others
    3. Providing a nonjudgmental environment
    4. Employing a positive mental attitude

17. A nurse identifies that a client is mildly anxious. Which assessment of the client **supports** this conclusion?
    1. Preoccupied
    2. Forgetful
    3. Fearful
    4. Alert

18. A client expresses a sense of hopelessness. Which concern identified by the nurse is the **priority**?
    1. Risk for self-harm
    2. Inability to cope
    3. Powerlessness
    4. Fatigue

19. When assessing a client for anxiety, which characteristic about anxiety should the nurse consider?
    1. It is triggered by a known stressor.
    2. It occurs simultaneously with fear.
    3. It is a response that is avoidable.
    4. It is a universal experience.

20. A woman with diabetes does not follow her prescribed diet and states, "Everyone with diabetes cheats on their diet." Which defense mechanism does the nurse identify this client is using?
    1. Rationalization
    2. Sublimation
    3. Undoing
    4. Denial

21. A nurse is caring for a client who is being admitted for a cardiac catheterization. The client tells the nurse, "I am so stressed out." Which question should the nurse ask when assessing the effectiveness of the client's coping ability?
    1. "How do you feel when you are stressed?"
    2. "How have you coped with similar stressors before?"
    3. "Did you receive treatment for any stress-related problems in the past?"
    4. "What has been the most stressful event that you have ever had before?"

22. A confused client becomes extremely upset. Which is the **best** action by the nurse?
    1. Speak louder with a lower-pitched voice.
    2. Use touch to communicate caring and concern.
    3. Talk to the client in a way that is simple and direct.
    4. Administer medication to minimize the client's anxiety.

23. Which statement by a dying client reflects Kübler-Ross's stage of depression in the grief process?
    1. "I am upset that I will not be here for my daughter's wedding."
    2. "I wrote a letter to be read by my daughter on the day of her wedding."
    3. "I just need to get a little stronger so I can go to my daughter's wedding."
    4. "I don't care if I die as long as I live long enough to see my daughter married."

24. A client says, "I have something important to tell you, but you have to promise me that you will not tell anyone." Which is the **best** response by the nurse?
    1. "I will share everything you tell me with the health team, because we are here to help you."
    2. "Something is clearly upsetting you for you to place such a restriction on our interaction."
    3. "Whatever you tell me is between us, because your personal information is confidential."
    4. "You will have to trust that I will maintain your confidentiality as long as it will not cause harm to you or others."

25. A bathrobe is draped over a chair near a client in the hospital who is confused. The client tells the nurse, "Tell that scary man to get out of my chair." Which is the **best** response by the nurse?
    1. "People in an unfamiliar environment sometimes think that they see things that are not really there."
    2. "I understand you are afraid, but there is no one there. Your bathrobe on the chair may look like a person."
    3. "The medication is making you confused. There is nobody sitting in the chair."
    4. "Tell me more about the scary man that you see sitting in the chair."

26. A woman comes to the emergency department with multiple traumas from a suspected assault by a boyfriend. The client indicates an unwillingness to talk about what happened. Which is the **best** statement by the nurse?
    1. "Did your boyfriend do this to you?"
    2. "You really got beat up pretty bad this time."
    3. "Would you like to talk about how this happened to you?"
    4. "Sometimes people are reluctant to share information about their situation."

27. A nurse is providing emotional support to a client who is upset. Which action depicted in this photograph is a therapeutic communication technique? **Select all that apply.**
    1. _____ Making eye contact
    2. _____ Holding the client's hand
    3. _____ Leaning toward the client
    4. _____ Sitting at the client's eye level
    5. _____ Maintaining personal distance from the client

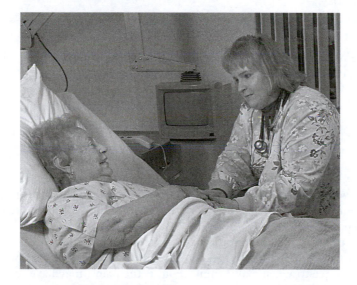

28. Which client statement **supports** the nurse's conclusion that the client with a newly diagnosed tumor of the lung may be experiencing denial? **Select all that apply.**

1. _____ "It's hard for me to ask other people for help."
2. _____ "I really think that this is just a cold."
3. _____ "I don't care what you do to me."
4. _____ "It's not so bad; I'll get over it."
5. _____ "I feel like I'm losing it."

29. A male client is diagnosed with hypertension. The nurse reviews the primary health-care provider's prescriptions, obtains the client's vital signs, and interviews the client and the client's wife. Which should the nurse do?

1. Obtain the client's vital signs again in one hour.
2. Explain to the wife that garlic will not help lower her husband's blood pressure.
3. Explore with the couple the idea that prayer will not lower a person's blood pressure.
4. Accept the couple's decision about consuming a clove of garlic and the juice of a lemon daily.

CLIENT'S CLINICAL RECORD

Primary Health-Care Provider's Prescriptions
2-gram sodium diet
Vital signs every 4 hours
Hydrochlorothiazide (HCTZ) 25 mg by mouth once a day
Furosemide 20 mg by mouth once a day

Client's Vital Signs
Temperature: 98.8°F, orally
Pulse: 88 beats per minute, bounding
Respirations: 22 breaths per minute, unlabored
Blood pressure: 160/94 mm Hg

Client and Spouse Interview
Client: "I am going to pray because God has kept me healthy up to now."
Client's Wife: "We decided that my husband will eat a clove of garlic and drink the juice from a lemon every day."

---

30. When the nurse analyzes a client's statements, which statement **best** reflects the dimension of self-esteem? **Select all that apply.**

1. _____ "I really like the me that I see."
2. _____ "What do I want to achieve?"
3. _____ "How do I appear to others?"
4. _____ "I like things my way."
5. _____ "I'm OK, you're OK."

31. Anxiety can progress through levels of severity from mild to panic. The client's level of anxiety will influence how the nurse approaches the client situation. Place these client statements in order as anxiety progresses from mild to moderate to severe and, finally, to panic.

1. "I want to know more about the surgery I am having tomorrow."
2. "I don't think I am going to make it through the surgery tomorrow."
3. "I can't concentrate, and all I think about is the pain I may have tomorrow."
4. "I get butterflies in my stomach when I think about having surgery tomorrow."

Answer: _____

32. A nurse is caring for a client who has problems comprehending the spoken word. Which should the nurse do to **support** this client? **Select all that apply.**
1. _____ Use simple words and sentences.
2. _____ Speak directly in front of the client.
3. _____ Encourage the client to request that unclear words be repeated.
4. _____ Paraphrase statements when they are not understood by the client.
5. _____ Employ facial expressions and gestures to enhance communication.

33. Which nursing action demonstrates **support** of human dignity in the practice of nursing? **Select all that apply.**
1. _____ Maintaining confidentiality of information about clients
2. _____ Supporting the rights of others to refuse treatment
3. _____ Obtaining sufficient data to make inferences
4. _____ Calling clients by their preferred name
5. _____ Staying at the scene of an accident

34. A preoperative client is anxious about pending elective surgery. Which nursing intervention will help the client reduce the anxiety? **Select all that apply.**
1. _____ Involve significant others.
2. _____ Use distraction techniques.
3. _____ Explore identified concerns.
4. _____ Foster expression of feelings.
5. _____ Use progressive desensitization strategies.

35. A dying client is withdrawn and depressed. Which nursing action is therapeutic? **Select all that apply.**
1. _____ Assisting the client to focus on positive thoughts daily
2. _____ Explaining that the client should focus on future goals
3. _____ Remaining available in case the client wants to talk
4. _____ Involving the client in conversations during the day
5. _____ Offering the client advice when appropriate

1. 1. Although a back rub may provide physical comfort, at this time the client requires psychosocial comfort. Offering to provide a back rub changes the subject and may cut off further communication.
   2. **Sitting quietly by the client's bedside conveys nonjudgmental acceptance of the statement and provides emotional support. Silence may precipitate further communication.**
   3. Telling the family about the client's statement is a violation of confidentiality.
   4. This is not an appropriate time to initiate an intellectual discussion (cognitive domain). The client's needs are in the psychosocial domain (affective domain).

2. 1. **This scenario is an example of denial. Denial is being used when a person ignores or refuses to acknowledge something unacceptable or unpleasant.**
   2. This scenario is not an example of repression. Repression is an unconscious mechanism whereby painful or unpleasant ideas are kept from conscious awareness.
   3. This scenario is not an example of introjection. Introjection is the taking into one's personality the norms and values of another as a means of reducing anxiety.
   4. This scenario is not an example of dissociation. Dissociation occurs when a person segregates a group of thoughts from consciousness or when an object or idea is segregated from its emotional significance in an effort to avoid emotional distress.

3. 1. Panic attacks cannot be prevented if identified early, and they do not have a slow onset. Panic attacks usually occur suddenly and spontaneously, build to a peak in 10 minutes or less, and last from several minutes to as long as an hour.
   2. **People can experience anxiety along a continuum from no anxiety to mild, moderate, severe, or panic, just as health is viewed along a continuum from illness to health.**
   3. Anxiety is a universal response to a threat. Healthy people experience anxiety when exposed to a physical threat (e.g., potential change in health status) or emotional threat (e.g., potential alteration in self-identity or self-esteem).
   4. A realistic danger triggers fear, not anxiety.

4. 1. Autonomy is being self-directed, not being able to perceive another person's emotions.

2. Sympathy is more than expressing concern and sorrow for a client but also contains an element of pity. When sympathetic, the nurse may let personal feelings interfere with the therapeutic relationship, which can impair judgment and limit the ability to identify realistic solutions to problems.
3. **Empathy is a person's ability to have insight into the feelings, emotions, and behavior of another person.**
4. Trust is not the nurse's perceiving the client's emotions accurately. Trust is established when a client has confidence in the nurse because the nurse demonstrates competence and respect for the client and behaves in a predictable way.

5. 1. **Defense mechanisms are used to reduce anxiety and achieve or maintain emotional balance. If a nurse identifies reality and does not recognize the client's need to use defense mechanisms, the client will become more anxious, even to the point of panic.**
   2. Denying the use of a defense mechanism usually does not precipitate withdrawal. Behavioral responses usually include irritability, increased motor activity, and even anger.
   3. Denying a client the use of a defense mechanism will contribute to ineffective coping, not facilitate effective coping.
   4. Denying the use of a defense mechanism will not encourage emotional growth. Emotional growth develops as a result of gaining insight into behavior, recognizing reality, and addressing problems constructively.

6. 1. **This scenario is an example of intellectualization. Intellectualization is the use of reasoning to avoid facing unacceptable stimuli in an effort to protect the self from anxiety.**
   2. This scenario is not an example of introjection. Introjection is the taking into one's personality the norms and values of another as a means of reducing anxiety.
   3. This scenario is not an example of depression. Depression is not a defense mechanism; it is an altered mood indicated by feelings of sadness, discouragement, and loss of interest in usual pleasurable activities.
   4. This scenario is not an example of denial. Denial is ignoring or refusing to acknowledge something unacceptable or unpleasant.

7. 1. During mild anxiety, the pulse, respirations, and blood pressure remain at the resting rate.
  2. During moderate anxiety, the pulse, respirations, and blood pressure are slightly elevated in response to the stimulation of the autonomic nervous system.
  3. During severe anxiety, the pulse, respirations, and blood pressure are more than just slightly elevated. The pulse and respirations are rapid and may be irregular, and the blood pressure is high, not just slightly elevated.
  4. During a panic attack, the pulse and respirations are very rapid and may be irregular, the blood pressure will be high, and the client may hyperventilate. If a panic attack is extreme, the blood pressure may suddenly drop and cause fainting.

8. 1. This scenario is not an example of compensation. Compensation is making an attempt to achieve respect in one area as a substitute for a weakness in another area.
  2. This scenario not an example of minimization. Minimization is not admitting to the significance of one's own behavior, thereby reducing one's responsibility.
  3. This scenario is an example of repression. Repression is an unconscious mechanism in which painful or unpleasant ideas are kept from conscious awareness.
  4. This scenario is not an example of regression. Regression is resorting to an earlier, more comfortable pattern of behavior that was successful in earlier years but is now inappropriate.

9. 1. Clients generally follow hospital policies because they recognize that they are designed to keep clients safe. When they do not follow rules, usually it is for a reason other than because they are angry.
  2. Clients have an opportunity to choose foods they like from the menu, to request alternative meals if they are unhappy with the food that arrives, and to ask family members to bring in food as long as the food is permitted on the prescribed diet.
  3. All behavior has meaning. Acting-out behaviors that reflect attempts to control events often are covert expressions of feeling powerless.
  4. Most hospital units have a lounge that supports clients' needs to have a change of scenery from their rooms.

10. 1. Exercise improves, not interferes with, one's ability to concentrate and solve problems by increasing circulation, which facilitates oxygenation of brain cells.
  2. Exercise stimulates endorphin production, which promotes a sense of well-being and euphoria. Also, endorphins act as opiates and produce analgesia by modulating the transmission of pain perception.
  3. Exercise promotes, not reduces, metabolism of epinephrine, thereby minimizing autonomic arousal and decreasing vigilance associated with the anxious response.
  4. The acidity of blood is increased, not decreased, by exercise. This improves digestion and metabolism and thereby increases one's energy level.

11. **1. Touching the client conveys concern and caring and is supportive. Quiet support provides a nonjudgmental environment in which the client is allowed to cry, which is the expression of a feeling.**
  2. Leaving abandons the client at a time when the client needs emotional support.
  3. Conveying this information to the client's family is a violation of confidentiality.
  4. Exploring the client's feelings is premature. The client requires time to cry as a way to express sad feelings.

12. 1. This scenario is not an example of rationalization. Rationalization is used to justify in some socially acceptable way ideas, feelings, or behavior through explanations that appear to be logical.
  2. This scenario is not an example of minimization. Minimization is not admitting to the significance of one's own behavior, thereby reducing one's responsibility.
  3. This scenario is not an example of substitution. Substitution is replacement of an unattainable, unavailable, or unacceptable goal, emotion, or motive with one that is attainable, available, or acceptable in an effort to reduce anxiety, frustration, or disappointment.
  4. This scenario is an example of projection. Projection is attributing thoughts, emotions, motives, or characteristics within oneself to others.

13. 1. A characteristic of grieving is that the person must express distress regarding a loss or potential loss. This client is asking questions, not displaying distress related to a perceived impending death.

2. This statement does not reflect powerlessness. People who are powerless usually do not ask questions.

3. This statement supports the concept that the client is experiencing fear. A characteristic of fear is the expression of feelings of apprehension and alarm related to an identifiable source.

4. This statement does not indicate that the client is coping ineffectively or has inadequate psychological resources. The client is gathering data by appropriately asking questions, which is an effective, task-oriented action in the coping process.

14. 1. This statement is inappropriate; the client is unable to cope, is selecting the ultimate escape, and is not capable of meeting the needs of others; this response also may precipitate feelings such as guilt.

2. This statement identifies feelings and invites further communication; it uses the interviewing technique of reflection.

3. This denies the client's feelings; the client must focus on the negatives before exploring the positives.

4. This is a judgmental response that may cut off communication. This response is too direct, and the client may not consciously know what is wrong.

15. 1. This scenario is an example of reaction formation, not displacement. Reaction formation is when a person develops conscious attitudes, behaviors, interests, and feelings that are the exact opposite of unconscious attitudes, interests, and feelings.

2. This scenario is an example of minimization. Minimization allows a person to decrease responsibility for one's own behavior.

3. This scenario is an example of suppression, not displacement. Suppression is a conscious attempt to put unpleasant thoughts out of the conscious mind to be dealt with at a later time.

4. This scenario is an example of displacement. Displacement is the transfer of emotion from one person or object to a person or an object that is more acceptable and less threatening.

16. 1. The support of a defense mechanism results in reality distortion. The use of defense mechanisms should be accepted, not supported. The nurse should recognize when defense mechanisms are being used because all behavior has meaning.

2. This may or may not support self-esteem needs. The benefit of this intervention

depends on the relationships that develop and whether they promote self-worth.

3. When the nurse establishes a nonjudgmental environment; functions without biases, preconceptions, or stereotypes; and avoids challenging a client's values and beliefs, a client's self-esteem is supported.

4. The nurse's personal attitudes should not be imposed on the client. An attitude is a mental position or feeling toward a person, an object, or an idea.

17. 1. Preoccupation reflects moderate, not mild, anxiety. People with moderate anxiety tend to focus on one issue and use selective attention.

2. Forgetfulness reflects moderate, not mild, anxiety. With moderate anxiety, the person has a narrowed focus of attention and may become forgetful because of an inability to focus attention.

3. Fearfulness is not a response to anxiety. Fearfulness is a response to an identifiable source, whereas anxiety is caused by an unidentifiable source.

4. Increased alertness occurs when one is mildly anxious. Alertness and vigilance are the result of an increase in one's perceptual field and state of arousal in response to the stimulation of the autonomic nervous system when one feels threatened.

18. **1. Risk for self-harm takes priority over the other three concerns because of the potential for suicide.**

2. Although a person who expresses hopelessness also may demonstrate an inability to manage stressors because of inadequate physical, psychological, behavioral, or cognitive resources, another option identifies a concern that has a higher priority.

3. Although a person who expresses hopelessness also may perceive a lack of personal control over events or situations, another option identifies a concern that has a higher priority.

4. Although a person who expresses hopelessness also may experience an overwhelming sense of exhaustion unrelieved by rest, another option identifies a concern that has a higher priority.

19. 1. Anxiety is triggered by an unknown, not known, stressor.

2. Anxiety and fear do not occur simultaneously. Anxiety is precipitated by an

unknown stressor, while fear is precipitated by a known stressor.

3. Anxiety cannot be avoided. It is an expected aspect of everyday living.

4. **Anxiety is a common and universal response. Anxiety is a psychosocial response to an unknown stressor; it may range from a vague sense of apprehension (at one extreme) to impending doom (at the other extreme).**

20. 1. **This statement is an example of rationalization. Rationalization is used to justify in some socially acceptable way ideas, feelings, or behavior through explanations that appear to be logical.**

2. This statement is not an example of sublimation. Sublimation is the channeling of primitive sexual or aggressive drives into activities or behaviors that are more socially acceptable, such as sports or creative work.

3. This statement is not an example of undoing. Undoing is use of actions or words in an attempt to cancel unacceptable thoughts, impulses, or acts. This reduces feelings of guilt through atonement or retribution.

4. This statement is not an example of denial. Denial is an unconscious protective response that involves a person's ignoring or refusing to acknowledge something unacceptable or unpleasant to reduce anxiety.

21. 1. This question explores the client's feelings, rather than coping abilities, when stressed.

2. **This question identifies how the client coped in the past, whether the client's strategy was problem focused (taking action to improve a situation) or emotion focused (thoughts and actions to relieve emotional distress), and whether the strategy was effective or ineffective. This information helps the nurse because the client may respond to the present situation in a similar manner.**

3. Although this information may be helpful to include in the health history, it does not address the client's present ability to cope with stress.

4. This question assesses the presence of past stressors, not the client's coping abilities.

22. 1. A confused client may interpret a loud voice as aggression. A confused client does not necessarily have a hearing problem.

2. A confused client might interpret touch as an aggressive act and respond by being frightened or agitated.

3. **Simple, direct statements are messages that require minimal effort and time to decode, resulting in better understanding by the confused client.**

4. Medication is used as a last resort. Nursing interventions often can calm an upset and confused client.

23. 1. **This statement characterizes the depression stage in the grieving process. The person grieves over what will not happen.**

2. This statement characterizes the acceptance, not depression, stage in the grieving process. During acceptance, the person may make funeral plans, complete final arrangements regarding personal belongings, and write letters to family members to be read in the future.

3. The statement about needing to get a little stronger characterizes the bargaining, not depression, stage in the grieving process. The client is bargaining for more time.

4. The statement about wanting to live to attend the daughter's wedding characterizes the bargaining, not depression, stage in the grieving process and is an attempt to barter for more time. The client is saying, "Yes, me, but..."

24. 1. This statement is a barrier to communication. Most information communicated by the client can remain confidential.

2. This open-ended statement invites the client to continue talking; however, it does not set up the parameters of the therapeutic relationship.

3. Personal information remains confidential even if significant other members of the health team are informed of the information. This is known as the *circle of confidentiality*. However, this response does not clarify that confidential information can be shared with other members of the health team.

4. **This statement is an open, honest response and sets up the parameters of the therapeutic relationship. The nurse must be credible—that is trustworthy, reliable, caring, supportive, and honest.**

25. 1. This statement minimizes concerns and dismisses the client's fear response. It is a statement that demonstrates lack of real interest in the needs of the client.

2. **This statement is therapeutic. The nurse first recognizes that the client is afraid and addresses the fear. In the second half of the statement, the nurse**

explains what might be contributing to a misinterpretation of environmental stimuli (illusion).

3. A person who is confused may not be able to recognize cause and effect. In addition, to point out to the client that one is confused because of medication may be frightening and contribute to an increase in the client's anxiety.

4. The client is experiencing an illusion. The nurse needs to orient the patient to reality and not add credibility to the misinterpretation of the environment.

26. 1. This probing question attempts to seek information about a topic the client is unwilling to explore. This direct question may put the client on the defensive and further close communication.

2. This judgmental statement may further close communication.

3. This direct question will probably elicit a response of "No," because the client appears reluctant to talk.

4. **This statement identifies a common reaction to an emotionally charged situation. It is an accepting, open-ended remark that provides an opportunity for the client to talk with the nurse.**

27. 1. **Maintaining eye contact is a therapeutic communication technique that communicates personal interest in the client and conveys that communication is an open channel.**

2. **Holding the client's hand is the therapeutic communication technique of touch. Touch conveys caring, concern, and comfort.**

3. **Leaning toward the client conveys interest.**

4. **Sitting at the client's eye level indicates that communication is an open channel and that the nurse intends to stay awhile.**

5. **The nurse is maintaining an intimate distance from the client. Intimate distance involves physical contact to within 18 inches of the client during an interaction.**

28. 1. This statement is not denying the presence of a problem. The inability to ask for help is a characteristic of ineffective coping.

2. **This statement indicates that the client denies that the source of the problem could be a tumor of the lung.**

3. This statement reflects apathy, a characteristic of powerlessness, not denial.

4. **This statement indicates that the client is minimizing and denying the seriousness of the diagnosis of a lung tumor, which is a serious threat to life.**

5. This statement is not denying the presence of a problem. Expressing an inability to cope is a characteristic of ineffective coping.

29. 1. It is unnecessary to obtain the client's vital signs in 1 hour. Although the blood pressure is increased, it is not at a dangerous level. The primary health-care provider prescribed that vital signs be obtained every 4 hours.

2. Garlic has hypolipemic and antiplatelet properties that can help lower blood pressure.

3. Prayer, meditation, and biofeedback exercises can help lower the vital signs, especially heart rate and blood pressure.

4. **The nurse should accept the client's decision to consume a clove of garlic and the juice of a lemon daily. Some cultural groups believe illness is caused by an imbalance in hot and cold principles. Hypertension is considered a "hot" illness and therefore should be treated with "cold" therapies. Cold therapies include the ingestion of foods such as citrus fruits, garlic, and bananas.**

30. 1. **This statement best reflects the dimension of self-esteem. Self-esteem is a person's self-evaluation of one's own worth or value. A person whose self-concept comes close to one's ideal self generally will have a high self-esteem.**

2. This statement reflects one's self-expectations, not self-esteem. Establishing expectations contributes to the composition of the ideal self.

3. This statement reflects self-concept, not self-esteem. Self-concept is an individual's knowledge about oneself. Self-concept is derived from all the collective beliefs and images about oneself as a result of interaction with the environment, society, and feedback from others.

4. This statement is a reflection of a client's need to be autonomous and self-reliant. Having confidence in one's ability to complete a task is only one component of self-concept.

5. **This statement reflects the dimension of self-esteem. By stating "I'm OK," the person demonstrates self-acceptance.**

31. 1. Mild anxiety is a slightly aroused state that enhances perception, learning, and performance of activities.
    4. Moderate anxiety increases the arousal state that precipitates feelings of tension and nervousness. The heart and respiratory rates increase, and the person may have mild gastrointestinal symptoms, such as a feeling of butterflies in the stomach.
    3. Severe anxiety consumes the person's physical and emotional energy. Perceptions are decreased, and the person focuses on limited aspects of what is precipitating the anxiety.
    2. Panic is an overwhelming state where the person feels out of control. Perceptions may be distorted and exaggerated, and the person may have feelings of impending doom.

32. 1. Simple words and sentences are easier to process and comprehend than complex words and sentences.
    2. Speaking directly in front of the client focuses the attention of both the client and the nurse that communication is occurring. Words may be heard more clearly, and lip movements by the nurse may facilitate interpretation of the sounds received by the client. The use of two senses, sight and hearing, may facilitate receiving and decoding of verbal messages.
    3. Requesting that unclear words be repeated allows the client an opportunity to attempt to decode the words a second time. In addition, it sends a message to the nurse that the message was not understood.
    4. Paraphrasing a message uses different words that the client may understand, promoting decoding of the message and improving comprehension.
    5. Facial expressions and gestures may be easier to decode because they are not as complex as the spoken word.

33. 1. Confidentiality respects the client's right to privacy, which is a component of human dignity.
    2. This supports the right of a client to self-determination, which is based on the concept of freedom, not human dignity.
    3. This reflects the nurse's attempt to seek the truth, not support human dignity.
    4. Calling clients by their given name demonstrates respect for the individual. Avoid names such as "dear," "sweetie," "honey," and "grandma," or "grandpa," because they are demeaning and disrespectful.
    5. This reflects a nurse's attempt to be responsible and accountable, not support human dignity.

34. 1. Significant others generally are as anxious as the client because anxiety is contagious. Anxious significant others bring to the discussion their own emotional problems that can misdirect the focus from the client as well as compound the problem.
    2. Distraction techniques, such as guided imagery, can help manage stress, thus reducing anxiety.
    3. Exploring identified concerns individualizes the nurse's interventions. Specific issues can be addressed and knowledge deficits corrected.
    4. Using interviewing techniques encourages the client to express feelings and explore concerns, which reduces anxiety. Expression of feelings uses energy, makes concerns recognizable, and promotes problem-solving.
    5. Anxiety is not something one can desensitize oneself to by increasing exposure to the stressor. With anxiety, the stressor is unknown.

35. 1. Focusing on positive thoughts is inappropriate because it denies the client's feelings; the client needs to focus on the future loss.
    2. Focusing on future goals is inappropriate because it denies the client's feelings; the client needs to focus on the impending death.
    3. Remaining available to the client indicates that the nurse is not abandoning the client. The nurse's presence provides quiet support without intruding on the client's coping.
    4. Depression is the fourth stage of grieving according to Kübler-Ross; clients become withdrawn and noncommunicative when feeling a loss of control and recognizing future losses. The nurse should accept the behavior and not attempt to involve the client in conversation during the day.
    5. It is never appropriate to offer advice; people must explore their alternatives and come to their own conclusions.

Teaching and Learning

KEYWORDS

The following words include nursing/medical terminology, concepts, principles, and information relevant to content specifically addressed in the chapter or associated with topics presented in it. English dictionaries, nursing textbooks, and medical dictionaries, such as *Taber's Cyclopedic Medical Dictionary,* are resources that can be used to expand your knowledge and understanding of these words and related information.

Behavior modification

Continuing education program

Feedback

Focus group

Inservice education program

Learning domains:

   Affective

   Cognitive

   Psychomotor

Locus of control:

   External

   Internal

Motivation

Orientation program

Pre-test, post-test

Readiness

Reading level

Reinforcement

Teaching:

   Formal

   Informal

Teaching methods:

   Active learning

   Audiovisual aids

   Case study

   Computer-assisted instruction

   Demonstration

   Discussion

   Lecture

   Programmed instruction

   Return demonstration

   Role-playing

   Simulation

   Written material

TEACHING AND LEARNING: QUESTIONS

1. A nurse is caring for a client who has type 1 diabetes and an ulcer on the big toe of the right foot. The nurse plans to review how to perform self-blood glucose monitoring, self-administer an injection, and apply a sterile dressing to the ulcer on the toe. The nurse identifies that the client is a kinesthetic learner. Which teaching strategy is **most** appropriate for the nurse to use with this client?
   1. Give verbal instructions and encourage a discussion.
   2. Provide occasions to touch and handle equipment.
   3. Present pictures and illustrations.
   4. Use models and videos.

2. A nurse is assessing a client to determine educational needs. Which is **most** important for the nurse to consider?
   1. Make no assumptions about the client.
   2. Teaching may be informal or formal in nature.
   3. The teaching plan should be documented on appropriate records.
   4. A copy of the teaching-learning contract should be given to the client.

3. Which is the **primary** reason why nurses attend continuing education programs?
   1. Update professional knowledge.
   2. Network within the nursing profession.
   3. Fulfill requirements for an advanced degree.
   4. Graduate from an accredited nursing program.

4. A nurse is designing a teaching-learning program for a client who is to be discharged from the hospital. After developing a nurse-client relationship, which should the nurse do **next?**
   1. Identify the client's locus of control.
   2. Use a variety of teaching methods appropriate for the client.
   3. Formulate an achievable, measurable, and realistic client goal.
   4. Assess the client's current understanding of the content to be taught.

5. A nurse is teaching an older adult how to perform a dressing change. Which nursing action is **most** important to address a developmental stress of older adults?
   1. Speak loudly when talking to the client.
   2. Use terminology understandable to the client.
   3. Have the client provide a return demonstration.
   4. Allow more time for the client to process information.

6. A nurse is planning a weight-reduction program with an obese client. Which should the nurse anticipate will be the **most** important component that will determine the success or failure of this program?
   1. Rewarding compliant behavior with favorite foods
   2. Encouraging at least 1 hour of exercise daily
   3. Using an 800-calorie daily dietary regimen
   4. Setting realistic goals

7. A nurse is teaching a client recently diagnosed with diabetes mellitus the step-by-step procedure of administering an insulin injection by using an orange. However, after two sessions of practice, the client is still reluctant to self-administer the insulin. Which should the nurse do?
   1. Keep reinforcing the principles that have been presented.
   2. Have the client administer the injection to an orange again.
   3. Give the client an opportunity to explore concerns about the injection.
   4. Determine if a member of the family is willing to administer the insulin.

8. Every person who attended a smoking cessation educational program completed a questionnaire. What is the name for this type of evaluation?
   1. Survey
   2. Post-test
   3. Case study
   4. Focus group

9. A nurse educator designed various educational programs that employ role-playing as a teaching strategy. Which group of people should the nurse anticipate will benefit the **most** from role-playing?
   1. Older adults preparing to retire from the workforce
   2. Men unwilling to admit that they have a drinking problem
   3. Adolescents learning to abstain from recreational drug use
   4. Middle-age adults preparing for total-knee replacement surgery

10. To be **most** effective, at which grade reading level should the nurse prepare written educational medical material?
    1. Fourth-grade
    2. Eighth-grade
    3. Tenth-grade
    4. Sixth-grade

11. A nurse uses computer-assisted instruction as a strategy when providing preoperative teaching. Which should the nurse explain to preoperative clients is the **best** advantage of computer-assisted instruction?
    1. Learners can progress at their own rate.
    2. It is the least expensive teaching strategy.
    3. There are opportunities for pre- and post-testing.
    4. Information is presented in a well-organized format.

12. A nurse is teaching a preschool-age child. Which teaching method is **most** appropriate for the nurse to use when teaching a child in this age group?
    1. Demonstrations
    2. Coloring books
    3. Small groups
    4. Videos

13. A nurse is attending a class about a new infusion pump presented by the hospital staff education department. What type of educational program is this?
    1. Continuing education program
    2. Inservice education program
    3. Certification program
    4. Orientation program

14. A nurse is planning to teach weight-reduction strategies for an obese client. Which should the nurse assess **first** before implementing the teaching plan?
    1. Intelligence
    2. Experience
    3. Motivation
    4. Strengths

15. A nurse is planning to engage a client in a program to learn about a newly diagnosed illness. Which psychosocial response to the illness will have the **most** impact on the client's future success of learning?
    1. Fear
    2. Denial
    3. Fatigue
    4. Anxiety

16. A nurse must implement a teaching plan for a client recently diagnosed with heart failure. Which should the nurse do **first**?
    1. Identify the client's level of recognition of the need for learning.
    2. Frame the goal within the client's value system.
    3. Determine the client's preferred learning style.
    4. Assess the client's personal support system.

17. Which of the following teaching-learning concepts that moves from one extreme to the other is basic to all teaching plans?
    1. Cognitive to the affective domain
    2. Formal to the informal
    3. Simple to the complex
    4. Broad to the specific

18. A nurse is teaching a postoperative client deep breathing and coughing exercises. Which method of instruction is **most** appropriate in this situation?
    1. Explanation
    2. Demonstration
    3. Video presentation
    4. Brochure with pictures

19. A nurse is teaching a client colostomy care in relation to the affective domain. Which teaching method is **most** effective for this situation?
1. Discussing a pamphlet about colostomy care from the American Cancer Society
2. Exploring how the client feels about having a colostomy
3. Providing a demonstration on how to do colostomy care
4. Showing a videotape demonstrating colostomy care

20. A school nurse is teaching a class of adolescents about avoiding smoking and includes role-playing as a creative learning activity. Which is the **primary** reason for using role-playing?
1. Provides more fun than other methods
2. Eliminates the need for media equipment
3. Requires active participation by the learner
4. Gives the learner the opportunity to be another person

21. A client who is learning how to use a syringe to self-administer insulin says, "This is so complicated. I'm never going to learn this." Which is an appropriate response by the nurse?
1. "A lot of people feel that way in the beginning."
2. "Let's have a family member give you your insulin."
3. "Most people learn how to do this well. It just takes a little time."
4. "Let's take one step at a time and master each step before we go on to the next."

22. A nurse is planning to teach a client how to self-administer a colostomy irrigation. Place the following actions that the nurse should employ in the order in which they should be implemented.
1. Identify the client's readiness to learn.
2. Involve the client in learning activities.
3. Identify the client's motivation to learn.
4. Repeat essential concepts to reinforce learning.
5. Evaluate the client's learning versus desired outcomes.

    Answer: _____

23. A nursing instructor is evaluating a student nurse's knowledge. Which student behavior indicates that learning has occurred in the highest level of learning in the cognitive domain? **Select all that apply.**
1. _____ Identifies the expected properties of urine
2. _____ Explains the importance of producing urine
3. _____ Recognizes when something is contaminated
4. _____ Compares achieved outcomes with planned outcomes
5. _____ Contrasts laboratory results of urine testing against the expected range

24. A nurse is to teach a client how to change a dressing and irrigate a wound that resulted from the separation of wound edges of an incision and that is healing by secondary intention. The nurse reviews the primary health-care provider's prescriptions, obtains the client's vital signs, and assesses the client. Which should the nurse do **next**?
1. Administer the prescribed pain medication, and reassess the client in 30 minutes.
2. Teach the client how to irrigate the wound and change the dressing.
3. Notify the primary health-care provider of the client's status.
4. Wait 15 minutes, and retake the client's vital signs.

CLIENT'S CLINICAL RECORD

Primary Health-Care Provider's Prescriptions
Irrigate abdominal wound with 0.9% sodium chloride and apply a wet to damp dressing twice a day.
Oxycodone 7.5 mg every 6 hours prn for incisional pain

Client's Vital Signs
Temperature: 100.2°F, orally
Pulse: 98 beats per minute
Respirations: 20 breaths per minute
Blood pressure: 140/90 mm Hg

Client Interview
Client is quiet and responding with one-phrase answers. States pain is 7 on a scale of 0 to 10. Transferred from chair to bed while bent over and holding abdomen. Client states, "I can't wait to learn how to do this dressing so that I can go home."

25. A nurse is providing health teaching for a client with a cognitive deficit. Which intervention by the nurse will **support** this client's learning? **Select all that apply.**
1. _____ Using simple vocabulary and syntax
2. _____ Establishing a structured environment
3. _____ Asking that unclear words be repeated
4. _____ Speaking directly in front of the client
5. _____ Making a referral for a hearing evaluation

26. A unit secretary tells the nurse that the primary health-care provider has just prescribed a low-calorie diet for a client who is overweight. Place these nursing interventions in the order in which they should be implemented.
1. Determine food preferences.
2. Verify the dietary prescription.
3. Teach specifics about a low-calorie diet.
4. Review a meal plan designed by the client.
5. Assess the client's motivation to follow the diet.

Answer: _____

27. Which describes a client with an external locus of control? **Select all that apply.**
1. _____ Behaves appropriately to obtain the right to watch a television program
2. _____ Is self-motivated when implementing health promotion behaviors
3. _____ Adheres to a weight-loss diet in order to feel better
4. _____ Understands the expected outcome of therapy
5. _____ Is a self-actualized adult

28. A nurse is teaching a client with a hearing impairment. Which should the nurse do to facilitate the teaching-learning process? **Select all that apply.**
    1. _____ Limit educational sessions to ten minutes.
    2. _____ Provide information in written format.
    3. _____ Use at least two teaching methods.
    4. _____ Face the client when talking.
    5. _____ Teach in group settings.

29. A nurse formulates teaching goals using action verbs. Which word is an example of a verb employed in a learning outcome in the psychomotor domain? **Select all that apply.**
    1. _____ Accepts
    2. _____ Explains
    3. _____ Performs
    4. _____ Assembles
    5. _____ Demonstrates

30. A nurse is assessing the results of dietary teaching for a client with diabetes mellitus. Which client behavior indicates that learning occurred in the affective domain? **Select all that apply.**
    1. _____ Discusses which food on the prescribed diet must be avoided
    2. _____ Eats only food approved on the prescribed special diet
    3. _____ Lists foods that are permitted on the diet
    4. _____ Asks about which foods can be eaten
    5. _____ Identifies foods that are high in sugar

31. A community health nurse is caring for a client who has a pressure ulcer and requires assistance with bathing, grooming, and toileting. Docusate sodium, daily weights, and a dressing change of the wound twice a day are prescribed. Which nursing intervention should the nurse perform while educating the client about docusate sodium? **Select all that apply.**
    1. _____ Bathing
    2. _____ Toileting
    3. _____ Daily weights
    4. _____ Wound treatment
    5. _____ Medication administration

32. After assessing a client's learning needs, abilities, and motivation and identifying client goals, the nurse must formulate a teaching plan. Place the following steps in the order in which they should be implemented.
    1. Choose teaching strategies to be employed.
    2. Evaluate the effectiveness of the teaching plan.
    3. Identify the information that the learner must learn.
    4. Organize the information in the sequence that information is to be presented.
    5. Develop instructional materials that will reinforce and supplement information provided in the class.

    Answer: _____

33. A nurse is planning a teaching plan for an older adult. Which common factor among older adult clients must be considered? **Select all that apply.**
    1. _____ Sensory decline occurs as one ages.
    2. _____ Learning may require more energy.
    3. _____ Intelligence decreases as people age.
    4. _____ Older adults rely more on visual rather than auditory learning.
    5. _____ Older adult clients are more resistant to change that accompanies new learning.

34. A nurse is teaching a client who has impaired vision to self-inject insulin. Which should the nurse do to facilitate the teaching-learning process? **Select all that apply.**

1. _____ Obtain a prescription for automatic-stop syringes.
2. _____ Provide written information in large print.
3. _____ Use audio learning materials.
4. _____ Speak in a normal volume.
5. _____ Talk at a regular rate.

35. A nurse educator is teaching a class on problem-solving and reinforces the concepts of inductive and deductive reasoning using the attached illustration. Which is the **most** important reason why the nurse educator presented this illustration?

1. It appeals to students who are visual learners.
2. It employs the concept of positive reinforcement.
3. It stimulates learning in students with an internal locus of control.
4. It improves students' conceptual understanding of complex content.

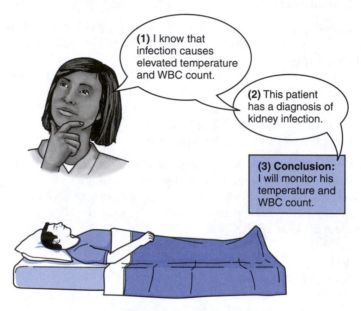

Deductive Reasoning

1. 1. Verbal instructions and discussions are most appropriate to use with clients who are auditory, not kinesthetic, learners. Auditory learners learn best by processing information when listening to words.

2. **Kinesthetic learners learn best when processing information by doing. Kinesthetic learners should be engaged in physical activities that allow them to touch and handle equipment.**

3. Pictures and illustrations are most appropriate to use with clients who are visual, not kinesthetic, learners. Visual learners learn best by processing information with the eyes.

4. Models and videos are most appropriate to use with clients who are visual, not kinesthetic, learners. Visual learners learn best by processing information with the eyes.

2. 1. **Many variables influence an individual's willingness and ability to learn (e.g., readiness, motivation, physical and emotional abilities, education, age, cultural and health beliefs, cognitive abilities). Because everyone is unique with individual needs, the nurse must avoid making assumptions and generalizations.**

2. The client's needs must be identified before teaching formats and strategies are designed.

3. The client's needs must be identified before the teaching plan is designed, implemented, and documented.

4. The client's needs must be identified before a plan is designed and a contract is written.

3. 1. **Continuing education programs are formal learning experiences designed to update and enhance professional knowledge or skills. This is necessary because of the explosion in information and technology within health care. Some states require evidence of continuing education units (CEUs) for license renewal.**

2. Although nurses who attend continuing education programs have the opportunity to network professionally with other nurses, it is not the main purpose of attending a continuing education program.

3. Continuing education programs do not fulfill requirements for an advanced degree. Master's and doctoral programs grant advanced degrees in specialty areas (e.g., parent-child health, mental health, medical-surgical nursing, and gerontology)

and practice roles (e.g., nurse practitioner, education, and administration).

4. Continuing education programs do not prepare a person to graduate from an accredited nursing degree program. Associate degree programs, baccalaureate degree programs, and diploma schools of nursing prepare graduates to take the NCLEX-RN® examination.

4. 1. Determining the client's locus of control will influence whether the client will be motivated by rewards from outside the self (external locus of control) or by personally identified rewards within the self (internal locus of control). This information should influence the nurse's teaching-learning plan. However, it is not the first thing the nurse should do from the options presented.

2. Although a variety of teaching methods should be used so that all the senses are engaged in learning, it is not the first thing the nurse should do from the options presented.

3. Goal setting is accomplished after the nurse gathers essential information that will influence the goal, particularly in relation to the achievable and realistic factors of a goal.

4. **Learners bring their own lifetimes of learning to the learning situation. The nurse must customize each teaching plan, capitalize on the client's previous experience and knowledge, and identify what the client still needs to know before teaching can begin.**

5. 1. Speaking loudly can be demeaning. A normal volume of speaking is appropriate.

2. Using understandable terminology is a teaching principle common to all age groups, not just older adults.

3. Obtaining a return demonstration is a teaching principle common to all age groups, not just older adults. This ensures that the learner has learned all the critical elements associated with the skill.

4. **Reaction time will slow as one ages; therefore, older adults need more time to process and respond to information or perform a skill. In addition, some older adults may have less energy, experience more fatigue, and may need shorter, frequent learning sessions.**

6. 1. Learning is encouraged when positive behaviors are reinforced with a reward. However, food as a reward should be avoided in this scenario because it may foster old habits that contributed to the original weight gain. For people with an internal locus of control, rewards should center on recognition of personal achievement, such as pleasing oneself, returning to a usual lifestyle, avoiding complications, and, in this scenario, losing weight. For the person with an external locus of control, rewards might center on privileges or praise received from pleasing significant others or members of the health-care team.

2. Although exercise is an important component of any weight-loss program, exercise alone will not determine the success or failure of a weight-loss program.

3. This is a dependent function of the nurse and requires a primary health-care provider's prescription. In addition, an 800-calorie diet is too few calories to acquire basic nutrients to maintain adequate health. Weight-loss diets should be between 1,200 and 1,500 calories for women and between 1,500 and 1,800 calories for men.

4. **Setting realistic goals is important to the success of a weight-loss program. Because achieving success is dependent largely on motivation, the teacher and the client should design goals that demonstrate immediate progress or growth. One strategy is to design numerous realistic short-term intermediary goals that are achieved more easily than one long-term goal.**

7. 1. The nurse has been doing this, and it has not been effective. A reassessment is necessary.

2. The client already knows the technique of how to administer the injection. The issue is that the client is reluctant to self-administer the injection.

3. **When a teaching plan is ineffective, the nurse must gather more data and revise the teaching plan to achieve the desired goal.**

4. This promotes dependency and prevents the client from becoming self-sufficient.

8. 1. **The terms questionnaire and survey are used interchangeably to describe a type of evaluation tool designed to gather data about a topic. This method is used to obtain information, such as feedback regarding an educational program.**

2. A post-test is not a questionnaire. A post-test is an examination given to assess cognitive learning after an educational program is completed.

3. A case study is not a questionnaire. A case study is a teaching tool that presents a scenario and a sequence of data to which the learner is required to analyze and respond.

4. A focus group is not a questionnaire. A focus group is designed to gather opinions and suggestions from a group of people about a particular topic using a discussion format, not a survey format.

9. 1. The role-playing technique is unlikely to be used by adults preparing to retire. Role-playing is most often used when learning parenting and other interpersonal skills.

2. Men who are unwilling to admit that they have a drinking problem are not demonstrating readiness to learn. In addition, role-playing requires a person to assume a role for the purpose of learning a new behavior. These men are demonstrating an unwillingness to learn a new behavior.

3. **A group of adolescents learning how to abstain from recreational drug use should benefit most from role-playing. Role-playing provides a safe environment in which to practice interpersonal skills. It enables individuals to rehearse what should be said, learn to respond to the emotional environment, and experience the pressures of the person playing the peer using drugs.**

4. The role-playing technique is unlikely to be used by adults preparing for knee replacement surgery. Role-playing is used most often when learning parenting and other interpersonal skills.

10. 1. The fourth-grade reading level is too low for medical material. Research demonstrates that the average reading level is higher than fourth grade.

2. The eighth-grade reading level is too high a reading level for educational medical material. Randomized studies demonstrate that only 22% of individuals requiring health teaching are able to profit from written health materials on the eighth-grade reading level.

3. The 10th-grade reading level is too high a reading level for educational medical material. Twenty percent of Americans read at or below the fifth-grade reading level and are considered functionally illiterate.

4. **Randomized studies demonstrate that the average reading level of individuals who need health teaching is at six to seven grades of schooling.**

11. 1. **Learners progress through a program at their own pace in viewing informational material, answering questions, and receiving immediate feedback. Some programs feature simulated situations that require critical thinking and a response. Correct responses are rationalized, praise is offered, and incorrect responses trigger an explanation of why the wrong answer is wrong and offer encouragement to try again. This is a superior teaching strategy for the learner who may find that group lessons are paced either too fast or too slowly for effective learning.**

2. Computer-assisted instruction (CAI) is not the least inexpensive teaching strategy. CAI requires a computer, a keyboard, and a station; software; technical support to install, maintain, and repair equipment; and a computer-literate teaching staff to preview, select, and implement CAI programs.

3. Although individual CAI programs often include pre- and post-testing components, this is not the greatest advantage of CAI as a teaching strategy.

4. Although CAI programs generally are well organized in a programmed instruction (step-by-step) format, this is not the greatest advantage of using CAI as a teaching strategy.

12. 1. Demonstrations generally are used for teaching a skill. Skills involve learning about equipment, rationales, and sequencing multiple steps and are too cognitively complex for the developmental abilities of a preschooler. A teaching method in another option is more age appropriate for a preschooler.

2. **Coloring books are the best approach because they require preschoolers to be active participants in their own learning and the child has a product to keep and be proud of. The use of coloring books reduces anxiety associated with learning because coloring is an activity most preschoolers are familiar with and the coloring task falls within a preschooler's cognitive level.**

3. Preschoolers are just beginning to interact with peers, have a short attention span, and get distracted easily; therefore, they need a one-on-one relationship with the teacher. The teacher facilitates the learning specifically for the individual, keeps the learner focused, and provides reinforcement on the learner's cognitive level.

Other age-specific strategies include using games; storybooks; dolls, puppets, or toys; and role-playing.

4. A video requires concentration and an attention span that may be beyond the developmental abilities of a preschooler.

13. 1. This scenario is not an example of a continuing education program. Continuing education refers to formal professional development experiences designed to enhance the knowledge or skills of the learner.

2. **Inservice programs generally are provided by health-care agencies to reinforce current knowledge and skills or provide new information about such issues as policies, theory, skills, practice, or equipment.**

3. This scenario is not an example of a certification program. The American Nurses Association has a certification program in which nurses can demonstrate minimum competence in specialty areas. Achievement of certification demonstrates advanced expertise and a commitment to ensuring competence.

4. This scenario is not an example of an orientation program. An orientation program is provided by a health-care agency to introduce new employees to the policies, procedures, departments, services, table of organization, expectations, equipment, and so on, within the agency.

14. 1. Assessing intelligence by a nurse is a subjective assessment that is difficult to perform. Declining functional abilities, debilitating diseases, pain, and stress may impair the intellectual functioning of some individuals.

2. Although it is important to assess a client's experience before implementing a teaching plan, of the options presented, it is not the first thing the nurse should do.

3. **If the client does not recognize the need to learn or value the information to be learned, the client will not be ready to learn.**

4. Although it is important to assess a client's strengths before implementing a teaching plan, of the options presented, it is not the first thing the nurse should do.

15. 1. Although fear will affect the success of a teaching program, will need to be assessed, and modifications to accommodate it will need to be employed, it is not the factor that will have the greatest impact on

the future success of a teaching program. Fear initially causes change; however, as fear subsides, a person often returns to the previous behavior.

2. Of all the options presented, the client in denial is the person least ready and motivated to learn. The client in denial is unable to recognize the need for the learning.

3. Fatigue is a physiological, not psychosocial, response to an illness. When teaching, the nurse must assess the client's stamina and modify the teaching program so as not to unduly strain the client and yet meet the objectives.

4. Although assessing for anxiety is important, it is not the factor that has the greatest impact on the future success of a teaching program. Mild anxiety is motivating. Moderate anxiety will motivate a client to learn but may require the nurse to keep concepts and approaches simple. The person with moderate anxiety may need to be refocused and have distractions minimized to facilitate learning. If severe anxiety or panic is present, the teaching program will have to be postponed until the client is less anxious.

16. **1. The learner must recognize that the need exists and that the material to be learned is valuable. Motivation is the most important factor influencing learning.**

2. Although setting goals within the client's value system is important, it is not the first thing the nurse should do before implementing a teaching plan.

3. Although the teacher should identify a client's learning style, a variety of teaching methods, not just the client's preference, should be used. This ensures that as many senses as possible are stimulated when learning, thereby increasing the probability of a successful outcome to the learning.

4. Although supportive individuals (e.g., family members and friends) can assist in helping the client maintain a positive mental attitude and reinforce learning, another option has a higher priority.

17. 1. Teaching and learning involve one or all domains of learning (e.g., cognitive, affective, and psychomotor) and do not move from one to the other in a progressive order.

2. Teaching methods that are formal or informal are equally effective. The key is to select the approach that is most likely to be effective for the individual learner. This depends on a variety of factors, such as intelligence, content to be taught, learning style preferences, available resources, reading level, and so on.

3. **When moving from the simple to the complex, a person works at integrating and incorporating the less complex, new learning into one's body of knowledge and understanding before moving on to more complex information. Complex material is best learned when easily understood aspects of the topic are presented first as a foundation for the more complex aspects.**

4. There is no documented principle that supports the need to present content in the direction of broad to specific rather than specific to broad. Each individual client and the information to be taught will influence the direction in which content is taught.

18. 1. An explanation is not the best approach to teach a psychomotor skill. An explanation uses words to describe a behavior that the learner then has to attempt to perform.

2. **A demonstration is the best strategy for teaching a psychomotor skill. A demonstration is an actual performance of the skill by the teacher, who is acting as a role model. A demonstration usually is followed by a return demonstration. The learner can imitate the teacher during a return demonstration, ask questions, and receive feedback from the instructor.**

3. Although a video provides a realistic performance of the skill, it does not allow for questions or feedback.

4. A brochure with pictures is too static and one-dimensional for teaching a psychomotor skill.

19. 1. This option reflects learning in the cognitive domain. Cognitive learning involves the intellect and requires thinking.

2. **This option reflects learning in the affective domain. Affective learning is concerned with feelings, emotions, values, beliefs, and attitudes about the colostomy.**

3. Providing a demonstration on colostomy care is an example of a teaching strategy in the psychomotor domain. The psychomotor domain is related to mastering a skill and requires the use of physical and motor activity.

4. Showing a videotape demonstrating colostomy care is an example of a teaching strategy in the psychomotor domain. It reflects a beginning awareness of the objects needed and steps to be implemented in a skill.

20. 1. Role-playing is no more or less fun than many other active and creative learning strategies.
2. This is not the reason for using role-playing. Media equipment can be used with role-playing.
3. **Learning activities that actively engage the learner have been shown to be more effective as well as more fun than methods that do not actively engage the learner. When learners are actively involved, they assume more responsibility for their own learning and develop more self-interest in learning the content.**
4. Role-playing is designed to support rehearsing a desired behavior in a safe environment. Although it may involve an opportunity to play another person, which allows one to view a situation from another vantage point, it is not the most important reason why role-playing is effective.

21. 1. This response minimizes the client's concern and cuts off communication.
2. This response does not focus on the client's concern. Also, it promotes dependence.
3. This response is false reassurance, minimizes the client's concern, and cuts off communication.
4. **This response addresses the client's immediate concern, plans to break the task into manageable steps, and ensures mastery of each step so that the client does not feel overwhelmed. In addition, it communicates to the client that the nurse is there for the client and that they will tackle the problem together.**

22. 3. **The first step of the options presented involves determining the client's desire to learn. If the client does not recognize that the learning is important, the client will not be invested in the learning process.**
1. **The second step of the options presented is determining if the client is ready to learn. The client may be**

motivated to learn, but if the client is in pain or fatigued, the client may not be able to focus on the learning.
2. **The third step of the options presented is to implement a teaching plan by engaging the client in planned learning activities.**
4. **The fourth step of the options presented is related to the concept of repetition of essential concepts to facilitate retention of learned information. Practice of psychomotor skills along with feedback from the nurse strengthens the learning and encourages independence.**
5. **The fifth step of the options presented is the evaluation of the client's performance in light of stated goals. When evaluating a psychomotor skill, the nurse observes the client's implementation of the skill to ensure that steps in the skill (e.g., collects necessary equipment, follows standards of asepsis and safety, and recognizes and responds to problems associated with the procedure) are implemented according to principles.**

23. 1. Identifying the expected properties of urine reflects learning on the knowledge level, which is the first of six levels of complexity in the cognitive domain.
2. Explaining the importance of producing urine reflects learning on the comprehension level, which is the second of six levels of complexity in the cognitive domain.
3. Recognizing when something is contaminated reflects learning on the application level, which is the third level of six levels of complexity within the cognitive domain.
4. **When a learner compares achieved outcomes with planned outcomes, the learner is evaluating the effectiveness of the learning. This activity is evaluation, which is the highest level of the cognitive domain. It requires the nurse to compare, contrast, and differentiate information.**
5. **This is the highest level of learning in the cognitive domain. Contrasting laboratory results of urine testing with the expected range reflects learning on the evaluation level, which is the sixth and highest level of learning in the cognitive domain.**

24. 1. **The client's pulse, respirations, and blood pressure are all slightly increased. These adaptations probably are being caused by the release of catecholamines resulting from the pain the client is experiencing. Moderate to severe pain will interfere with learning. The client will have difficulty concentrating on the task at hand. The nurse should postpone the teaching session, administer the prescribed pain medication, and reassess the client in 30 minutes. The teaching session can be reinstituted after the pain is reduced.**

2. Teaching at this time is an inappropriate intervention.

3. Notifying the primary health-care provider is unnecessary. The client's adaptations are common responses to the client's physical status.

4. Waiting will delay meeting the client's physical needs.

25. 1. **Using a simple vocabulary with as few syllables as possible, along with using short, simple sentences, is less confusing for a client with a comprehension deficit.**

2. **For people who have a cognitive deficit, participating in a learning program often makes them feel overwhelmed and threatened. The teacher should provide a structured environment in which variables are controlled to reduce anxiety and support comprehension. The nurse should minimize ambiguity, provide a familiar environment, teach at the same time each day, limit environmental distractions, and provide simple learning materials.**

3. **Clarifying unclear words stated by the client helps the nurse understand what the client is saying. Client concerns and questions must be addressed by the nurse.**

4. Speaking directly in front of the client helps the client with impaired hearing, not the client who has a cognitive deficit.

5. The client does not need a hearing evaluation. The client's problem is a cognitive deficit, not a hearing loss.

26. 2. **Verifying the prescription should be done first because a diet requires a primary health-care provider's prescription; following a specific diet is a dependent function of the nurse.**

5. **Assessing motivation is one of the most important factors influencing learning. The learner must recognize that the need exists and that the need will be addressed through the learning.**

1. **Determining food preferences is part of nursing assessment. Food preferences can then be included in the teaching plan about the low-calorie diet.**

3. **Details of the diet can be taught after the prescription is verified, motivation is determined, preferences and needs are identified, and a teaching plan is formulated.**

4. **Evaluation is the final step of teaching. A meal plan designed by the client requires not just an understanding of the information but an ability to apply the information.**

27. 1. **The person with an external locus of control is motivated by rewards that center on privileges, incentives, or praise received from pleasing significant others or members of the health-care team. Watching television is a privilege in this situation.**

2. Self-motivated behavior indicates an internal, not external, locus of control. People with an internal locus of control are motivated by personal internal rewards such as achieving a personal goal, pleasing oneself, returning to a usual lifestyle, and avoiding complications.

3. Adhering to a weight-loss diet to feel better is a behavior that reflects an internal, not external, locus of control. People with an internal locus of control are motivated by personal internal rewards such as achieving a personal goal, pleasing oneself, returning to a usual lifestyle, and avoiding complications.

4. Understanding the expected outcome of therapy is associated with recognizing the goal one is working to achieve; it does not describe an external locus of control.

5. A self-actualized adult is motivated by an internal locus of control. According to Maslow, the self-actualized person is an individual who has a need to develop to one's maximum potential and personally realize one's qualities and abilities.

28. 1. Limiting the length of sessions is unnecessary. Hearing is the problem, not fatigue.

2. Written materials augment verbal teaching. The client can review the written materials during and after the teaching session.

3. Varieties of teaching methods facilitate learning because multiple senses are stimulated. When we see, hear, and touch, learning is more effective than when we see or hear alone. In addition, research demonstrates that we remember only 10% of what we read, 20% of what we hear, 30% of what we see, 50% of what we see and hear, and 80% of what we say and do.

4. Some clients who are hearing-impaired lip-read. Facing the client enables the client to see the nurse's lips clearly.

5. A group setting is the least desirable teaching format for hearing-impaired individuals. One-on-one learning sessions limit background noise and distractions that hinder learning. In addition, a one-on-one session allows for individual feedback that ensures that the message is received as intended.

29. 1. Accepting something indicates learning in the affective, not psychomotor, domain. Learning in the affective domain includes things such as feelings, emotions, and attitudes.

2. Explaining something indicates learning in the cognitive, not psychomotor, domain. Learning in the cognitive domain is reflected in the ability to understand the meaning of learned content.

3. Performing an activity indicates learning in the psychomotor domain. Learning in the psychomotor domain is related to mastering a skill and requires motor activity.

4. Assembling something indicates learning in the psychomotor domain. Learning in the psychomotor domain is related to mastering a skill and requires motor activity.

5. Demonstrating something indicates learning in the psychomotor domain. Learning in the psychomotor domain is related to mastering a skill and requires motor activity.

30. 1. This behavior is an example of learning in the cognitive, not affective, domain. Cognitive learning involves the intellect and requires thinking.

2. Eating food on the prescribed diet is an example of learning in the affective domain. When learning is incorporated into the learner's behavior because it is perceived as important, learning has occurred in the affective domain. Affective learning involves the expression of feelings and the changing of beliefs, attitudes, or values.

3. Compiling a list of permitted foods is an example of learning in the cognitive, not affective, domain. Cognitive learning involves the intellect and requires thinking.

4. Asking questions is not an outcome demonstrating learning. This is an example of a question a learner might ask when learning content in the cognitive domain. Cognitive learning involves the intellect and requires thinking.

5. Identifying foods high in sugar is an example of learning in the cognitive, not affective, domain. Cognitive learning involves the intellect and requires thinking.

31. 1. Docusate sodium is a stool softener and is unrelated to the activity of bathing. Teaching the client about skin assessment and skin care is best performed during a bath.

2. An excellent time for the nurse to teach the client about docusate sodium, a medication that promotes bowel elimination, is when the client is being assisted to the toilet.

3. Docusate sodium is a stool softener and is unrelated to the activity of monitoring a client's daily weight. Daily weights are taken to assess fluid balance.

4. Docusate sodium is a stool softener and is unrelated to a dressing change of a pressure ulcer.

5. During medication administration is a perfect time for the nurse to educate a client about the medications that the client is receiving.

32. 3. The first step in designing a teaching plan is to identify the information that the learner must acquire. This step is accomplished by formulating realistic, measurable learning goals.

4. The second step in designing a teaching plan is organizing the information in an appropriate sequence to be presented.

1. The third step in designing a teaching plan is the selection of the teaching strategies to be employed based on the advantages and disadvantages of each strategy and which is best to achieve the learning goals.

5. The fourth step in designing a teaching plan is to develop instructional materials that will reinforce and supplement information provided in the class.

2. The teacher should develop a method to evaluate whether learning goals are met. Post-tests, written exercises, questionnaires, surveys, and direct observation of performance are some examples of evaluation methods.

33. 1. Sensory impairment results from the aging process, which must be considered when planning a teaching plan for an older adult. Aging causes such changes as a reduced ability to focus or accommodate because of reduced elasticity of the lens of the eye; a narrowing of the visual field; increased opacification of the lens, which causes cataracts, with accompanying blurring of vision and increased sensitivity to glare; a decrease in the ability to hear high-frequency sounds; and an increase in the keratin content of cerumen that causes an accumulation of cerumen in the middle ear and thus endangers hearing.

2. Various physiological changes of aging have an impact on the rate of learning (e.g., declines in sensory perception and speed of mental processing and more time needed for recall). These changes require the use of multisensory teaching strategies and a repetitive approach. In addition, older adults may have less physical and emotional stamina because of more chronic illnesses, so they may require shorter and more frequent learning sessions.

3. Although some older adults may experience a decline in short-term memory, they are not less intelligent. When older adults experience a decline in sensory function (e.g., vision, hearing), they may feel ashamed or frustrated, causing withdrawal. Behaviors reflective of withdrawal may be misperceived as a decline in intelligence.

4. This is not necessarily true. Individuals usually have learning preferences that persist throughout life.

5. Older adults generally are not resistant to change. Some older adults may be less motivated to learn if they believe that

death is near. However, in this situation, when older adults are shown how learning will improve their quality of life and independence, they are motivated to learn.

34. 1. An automatic-stop syringe ensures that an appropriate dose of insulin can be prepared despite a client's vision impairment.

2. Large print magnifies the written information to a size that may facilitate reading by the client who is vision impaired.

3. Audio learning materials use the sense of hearing rather than sight to promote the teaching-learning process.

4. Speaking in a normal volume is an appropriate intervention for a client who has a vision impairment. The client is visually impaired, not hearing impaired.

5. A client who has a visual impairment is able to follow a conversation spoken at a normal rate (not too fast or slow). Talking slowly is an appropriate intervention for a client who has a hearing, not a vision, impairment.

35. 1. Although an illustration appeals to visual learners, this is not the primary reason why the nurse educator decided to present this illustration to reinforce content presented in the lecture.

2. The concept of positive reinforcement is not associated with presenting an illustration to reinforce learning. Positive reinforcement is associated with using praise and encouragement to enhance motivation. Research by Ivan Pavlov and B. F. Skinner presented the theory of positive reinforcement.

3. An internal or external locus of control is associated with motivational theory and is unrelated to the rationale for using graphics to explain complex information.

4. Research demonstrates that when illustrations are used in conjunction with reading content, learners outperform students who just read the content. Illustrations attract attention, facilitate retention of information, and improve understanding of complex content by creating a context.

Diversity and Spirituality

KEYWORDS

The following words include nursing/medical terminology, concepts, principles, and information relevant to content specifically addressed in the chapter or associated with topics presented in it. English dictionaries, nursing textbooks, and medical dictionaries, such as *Taber's Cyclopedic Medical Dictionary,* are resources that can be used to expand your knowledge and understanding of these words and related information.

Acculturation
Assimilation
Beliefs
Bias
Chauvinism, chauvinistic
Culture
Discrimination
Diversity
Ethnicity
Ethnocentrism, ethnocentric
Immigrant
Misogyny, misogynist, misogynism

Prejudice
Race
Racism
Religion
Sexism
Socialization
Spiritual distress
Spiritual well-being
Spirituality
Stereotype
Value
Xenophobia

DIVERSITY AND SPIRITUALITY: QUESTIONS

1. A nurse is caring for a client for the first time. Which is the **initial** intervention that should be performed by the nurse before planning to meet the hygiene needs of this client?
   1. Determine the client's preferences about hygiene practices.
   2. Assess the client's ability to assist with hygiene activities.
   3. Collect the client's toiletries needed for the bath.
   4. Ensure the client's bathroom will be available.

2. A home-care nurse working in a rural community determines that there is an underutilization of services by the members of the community. Which does the nurse conclude is the **most** common cause for the underutilization of services?
   1. The culture of independence
   2. The varieties of ethnicity
   3. A decreased intelligence
   4. A disinterest in health

3. A home-care nurse is assessing a client and family members from a cultural perspective. Which is **most** important for the nurse to do?
   1. Recall experiences of caring for clients with a similar background.
   2. Recognize beliefs common to the client's ethnic group.
   3. Interview the members of the client's family.
   4. Use the client as the main source of data.

4. A nurse is caring for several clients who state that they faithfully practice the religion of either Orthodox Judaism or Islam. Which food custom common to both Islam and Orthodox Judaism should the nurse consider when meeting these clients' nutritional needs?
1. Pork is prohibited in the diet.
2. Meat cannot be eaten on Fridays.
3. Special cookware is used for different meals.
4. Meat and dairy products are served at different meals.

5. A 4-year-old boy is admitted to the emergency department and diagnosed with leukemia. The parents are informed that their child has an excellent prognosis if treated with chemotherapy. The parents adamantly refuse drug therapy because it is not consistent with their religious beliefs. They believe that prayer can cure everything. Which should the nurse do?
1. Encourage the parents to seek the prayers of one of their church's clergy.
2. Explain to the parents how the chemotherapeutic regimen will cure the leukemia.
3. Talk with the nursing supervisor about referring this situation to the ethics committee.
4. Accept the decision based on the First Amendment of the Constitution of the United States.

6. A nurse is caring for a client who recently was diagnosed with a terminal illness. The client says to the nurse, "I was told this morning that I have 3 to 6 months to live. I have to just keep the faith." Which response by the nurse is appropriate when considering the needs of this client?
1. "You have a few months left. It's important that you make the most of the days you do have."
2. "I am sorry to hear about your terminal illness. Let's talk about what the future holds for you."
3. "You should get a second opinion. There may be additional medical interventions that can help you."
4. "Some people express spiritual needs. Let me know if there is some way that I can help you meet similar needs."

7. A nurse is teaching an older adult who immigrated to the United States 10 years ago about foods that are low in sodium. Which is **most** important when teaching this client?
1. Encourage the asking of questions.
2. Seek feedback that is measurable.
3. Use humor when appropriate.
4. Observe family interactions.

8. A client who has a sorrowful and dejected facial expression says to the nurse, "I am very sorry for some of the things that I did in my early life." Which is the **best** response by the nurse?
1. "That was a long time ago, and it seems as though you have done many good things in your later life."
2. "God is total love and forgives our past transgressions."
3. "You seemed very sad as you shared that with me."
4. "I want to do something to make you feel better."

9. A nurse is caring for a woman who on admission stated that she belongs to a church that traditionally prohibits blood transfusions. However, the woman agreed to receive packed red blood cells as part of her medical regimen. The husband says to the nurse in the hall, "I can't believe that she is having packed red blood cells. We both have attended our church our whole lives, and now she is going against the convictions that we have had faith in for over 30 years." What is the **best** response by the nurse?
   1. "Do you think you could be as supportive as you can possibly be?"
   2. "This is a difficult topic. However, let's sit down and talk about it."
   3. "How do you feel about your wife's willingness to have a transfusion?"
   4. "Men don't always understand what women are going through. Ask her about how she feels."

10. A nurse overhears two health-care personnel having a conversation. One person says to the other, "I think that turning that Muslim woman's bed toward mecca is bizarre." Which specific barrier to culturally competent care is demonstrated by the statement?
    1. Ethnocentrism
    2. Chauvinism
    3. Racism
    4. Sexism

11. A nurse is caring for four clients who each engage in one of the following behaviors. Which of the following is based on a religious belief?
    1. Drinks lemon juice to treat hypertension
    2. Wears an amulet to chase away bad spirits
    3. Massages a foot to relieve migraine headache pain
    4. Brushes the teeth after every meal to prevent tooth decay

12. A culturally competent nurse is planning to teach a client about a new regimen of self-care. Which must the nurse assess **first** about the client before implementing the teaching plan?
    1. Religious affiliation
    2. Support system
    3. National origin
    4. Health beliefs

13. A nurse is caring for a client who recently immigrated to the United States and who is not completely fluent in English. The nurse is discussing options for continuity of care after the client is discharged from the hospital. Which is the **most** appropriate response by the nurse after presenting various options?
    1. "Which seems to be the option that best meets your needs as you see them?"
    2. "Do you have any questions regarding any of the options that we discussed?"
    3. "In light of your values and beliefs, I believe that home care might be the best option."
    4. "I think that you should take some time to discuss these options with your family members."

14. A nurse is assisting a client with morning care. Which is **most** important for the nurse to do when assisting the client with care of the hair?
    1. Use rubbing alcohol to remove tangles.
    2. Ensure that the client's hair is left dry, not wet.
    3. Ask the client what should be done with the hair.
    4. Comb hair from the proximal to distal end of the hair shaft.

15. A nurse is planning care in the spiritual realm for clients with a variety of ages. Which age group should the nurse identify generally is more involved with expanding and refining spiritual beliefs?
    1. Adolescents
    2. Older adults
    3. Young adults
    4. Middle-age adults

16. A male client refuses to have a male nurse as a caregiver. The client tells the nurse in charge, "I don't want a man for a nurse. Nursing is a woman's job; they are great." Which of the following can be attributed to the client based on his statement?
    1. Racism
    2. Sexism
    3. Chauvinism
    4. Misogynism

17. A young adult who is receiving chemotherapy for cancer says to the nurse, "I was brought up as a Christian by my parents, but since I have been on my own I have not practiced my religion. I guess I should get more involved again." Which is the **best** response by the nurse?
    1. "Which religion do you belong to?"
    2. "How long has it been since you went to church?"
    3. "What can I do to support your religious endeavors?"
    4. "When do you want me to call your spiritual advisor to come visit you?"

18. A dying client says to the nurse, "I know I am dying, and what scares me the most is I don't know what is going to happen on the other side. Do you believe that there is a heaven and a hell?" Which is an appropriate response by the nurse? **Select all that apply.**
    1. _____ "What do you think about heaven and hell?"
    2. _____ "I really don't know; I have not thought about it."
    3. _____ "Does your religion have theories about heaven and hell?"
    4. _____ "This is a topic you should explore with your spiritual advisor."
    5. _____ "I practice a religion that supports concepts about heaven and hell."

19. A nurse is caring for a male client who is dying of AIDS and weighs less than 100 pounds as a result of the disease. The client lives with his spouse, and both are members of the Alliance for Gay, Lesbian, Bisexual, Transgender, and Questioning Youth. The client's spouse and parents visit daily, and a male friend visits once a week. The nurse documents the following conversation with the client's family members and best friend. Which person expressed a bias against gay individuals?
    1. Mother
    2. Spouse
    3. Friend
    4. Father

CLIENT'S CLINICAL RECORD

Nurse's Progress Note: 1600, 11/8/18
Client was admitted to the hospital a week ago for rehydration therapy and pain management. A few days ago, the client decided that after his pain was manageable, he wanted to be transferred to a hospice facility rather than going home. He said that he did not want to be a burden to his family. Yesterday, the spouse shared the following comment, "I can't stand the way he looks. He is wasting away. This AIDS disease is devastating," and the mother responded, "I love my son, but I dislike his being gay because it has made his life so difficult." A meeting is planned for tomorrow to discuss a discharge plan with family members.

Nurse's Progress Note: 1200, 11/9/18
With the client's permission, I had a conversation with the client's spouse, parents, and the client's best friend regarding the client's plan for transfer to a hospice facility. The client did not want to be present, so he was off the unit having physical therapy. The father stated, "We should have expected this. This is what always happens when you live that kind of lifestyle." The mother asked the friend about how he felt about her son being gay. The friend responded, "Being gay is not for me. It is against my religion." After discussing all aspects of the plan and reviewing the plan with the client, which he approved, he will be transferred tomorrow to hospice.

20. A primary health-care provider prescribes a regular diet for a client who follows a kosher diet. Which meal arranged by the nurse is culturally appropriate? **Select all that apply.**
    1. _____ Chicken lo main, fried rice, pineapple chunks, and tea
    2. _____ Sliced beef, mixed vegetables, baked potato, and cola
    3. _____ Hamburger on a bun, potato chips, and milk
    4. _____ Curried shrimp, egg noodles, and coffee
    5. _____ Eggs, buttered roll, and orange juice
    6. _____ Oatmeal, toast, and hot chocolate

21. A family from another country immigrates to the United States. Which of the following reflects the concept of acculturation? **Select all that apply.**
    1. _____ The husband is attending school to learn English.
    2. _____ The family members celebrate Christmas together.
    3. _____ The parents expect their children to attend college.
    4. _____ The wife prepared a meal with turkey on Thanksgiving.
    5. _____ The grandparents live in the same house as the rest of the family.

22. A nurse must provide culturally competent nursing care to a client. Place the following in the order in which they should be performed.
1. Provide care that incorporates the client's specific beliefs, values, and health-care practices.
2. Recall the beliefs, values, and health-care practices associated with the client's culture.
3. Explore the client's specific beliefs, values, and health-care practices.
4. Explore own beliefs, values, and health-care practices.

Answer: _____

23. A nurse is caring for a client who belongs to a church that traditionally prohibits blood transfusions. The client is to have a total hip replacement and states, "I cannot have a blood transfusion." Which should be implemented by the nurse? **Select all that apply.**
1. _____ Teach the client about non-blood plasma expanders.
2. _____ Inform the client about intraoperative blood salvaging.
3. _____ Explain the benefits of a blood transfusion in the event of surgical bleeding.
4. _____ Tell the client about the option of preoperative autologous blood transfusions.
5. _____ Describe how whole blood can be treated to retrieve just the red blood cells for a transfusion.

24. A nurse is caring for a group of clients who have diverse religious affiliations. The nurse is planning a class on what foods constitute a nutritious diet. When preparing for class, which religion should the nurse recognize that traditionally prohibits the ingestion of pork and products made of pork? **Select all that apply.**
1. _____ Islam
2. _____ Jewish
3. _____ Mormon
4. _____ Jehovah's Witness
5. _____ Seventh-day Adventist

25. A client who has a diagnosis of a terminal illness asks the nurse to pray together for a recovery from the illness. Which response by the nurse will provide spiritual **support** for the client? **Select all that apply.**
1. _____ "I will see if the social worker is able to meet with you to help you with your religious needs."
2. _____ "I am uncomfortable with prayer, but if it is alright with you, I will refer you to the chaplain."
3. _____ "We are unable to change some things, and we just have to move forward as best we can."
4. _____ "I think it is better if you pray with members of your family."
5. _____ "You sound as though you feel hopeless."

1. 1. **Hygiene is a personal matter determined by individual beliefs, values, and practices. Hygiene practices are influenced by culture, religion, environment, age, health, and personal preferences. When personal preferences are supported, the client has a sense of control and usually is more accepting of care.**
   2. Although identifying the client's ability to assist in hygiene activities is significant in relation to the extent of self-care that may be expected, it is not the initial assessment.
   3. This intervention is premature. Collecting the client's toiletries is done after several other considerations and just before actually beginning the bath.
   4. Arranging access to the client's bathroom is premature.

2. 1. **Rural communities are more isolated from services, stores, and resources, and therefore people tend to be self-sufficient, independent, and autonomous.**
   2. Although culture and the inability to speak English may be a factor in underutilization of services in rural communities, it is not the main reason services are underutilized. In addition, there are more ethnic neighborhoods in urban and suburban, not rural, areas. Ethnic neighborhoods are groups within a social system that have common traits or characteristics, such as language or religion.
   3. Intelligence is not a factor in underutilization of health-care services in rural communities. People in rural areas are no less intelligent than city dwellers.
   4. Interest is not a factor in underutilization of health-care services in rural communities. People in rural areas are no less interested in health and health care than people who live in other areas of the country.

3. 1. This denies the individuality of the client. The nurse's experiential background may be limited and is influenced by personal views that may not be accurate.
   2. Each client is an individual, and generalizations should not be made based on a person's ethnic or cultural group. Generalizations often are based on stereotypes that are preconceived and untested beliefs about people based on their culture, race, and/or ethnic backgrounds.
   3. Family members provide only their own views, which are not the most important when assessing variables that affect a client from a cultural perspective.
   4. **The client is the center of the health-care team and is the most important source of information about his or her perspective.**

4. 1. **All pork and pork products are prohibited by the religions of Orthodox Judaism and Islam. The dietary laws of Orthodox Judaism are known as the Rules of Kashruth.**
   2. Abstinence from meat on Fridays is a traditional tenant of Catholicism, not Orthodox Judaism or Islam.
   3. In just Orthodox Judaism, meat and dairy products cannot be prepared using the same cookware.
   4. In just Orthodox Judaism, dairy products and meat cannot be eaten at the same meal or prepared and served with the same pots, dishes, or utensils.

5. 1. Although prayer can be powerful, it alone will not cure leukemia.
   2. This is an inappropriate intervention at this time. The parents are steadfastly and obstinately refusing drug therapy for their child. This response also provides false reassurance because not all children with leukemia experience a cure after undergoing chemotherapy.
   3. **This is an ethical dilemma because the client is a minor and the parents are refusing standard medical treatment for their child. An ethics committee is an advisory body with a multidisciplinary composition that facilitates the exploration and resolution of ethical issues that occur within the facility.**
   4. The U.S. court system can intervene on the behalf of infants and children when parents refuse lifesaving treatments. Accepting the parents' decision to forgo standard medical treatment is not being an advocate for the child in this situation.

6. 1. This statement is a reflection of the values of the nurse, not the client, and should be avoided.
   2. This statement is inappropriate. This statement unnecessarily reinforces that the client has a "terminal illness" and may have "little time left." Also, the nurse is not able to know "what the future holds" for the client.

3. This statement is inappropriate because it may undermine the confidence that the client has in the primary health-care provider and should be avoided.

4. This statement is an appropriate response by the nurse. The client did bring up the concept of "keep the faith." The nurse's response provides an opportunity for the client to discuss spiritual needs if desired.

7. 1. Although encouraging the asking of questions should be done, it is not as important as a factor in another option.

2. Seeking feedback that is objective and measurable is essential because a person from another culture may nod, smile, and say "yes, I understand" even when information is not understood in an effort to save face. Also, a person may be embarrassed to ask questions or believe that it will embarrass the nurse if a question is asked. Seeking careful feedback enables the nurse to determine if learning objectives are met or not met and is the most important factor of the options presented.

3. Humor should be avoided. Humor does not always translate well because of implications, subtexts, or culture-specific context; it may be misunderstood.

4. Observing family interaction may be done for many different reasons (e.g., seeking congruence of the client's values and desires with family members, determining who is the decision maker in the family); however, it is not as important as a factor in another option.

8. 1. This statement minimizes the client's concern for past actions and cuts off communication.

2. This statement minimizes the client's concern for past actions, offers false reassurance, and cuts off communication.

3. Pointing out nonverbal behavior may help a client to recognize feelings. Only a client knows if he or she has feelings such as sadness, grief, or remorse and requires absolution or forgiveness. Eventually, the nurse can help the client contact a chosen religious representative who can provide the spiritual support that the client needs.

4. This statement focuses on the nurse rather than the client. Only the client can assume responsibility to feel better.

9. 1. This response focuses on the wife's needs and ignores the husband's concerns.

2. This response acknowledges that the husband is in a dilemma, and it offers an opportunity to explore the situation. Validation and an invitation to talk provide emotional support.

3. This question is too direct. The husband's statement already indicates that he is surprised and upset with his wife's decision.

4. This response is condescending and focuses on the wife's, not the husband's, needs.

10. **1. The statement in the stem is an example of ethnocentrism. Ethnocentrism is when people embrace the values and beliefs of their ethnicity and culture as right and those of others as wrong or unacceptable. Also, referring to the woman as a "Muslim woman" rather than a "woman who is Muslim" can be considered degrading and insensitive. The statement by the health-care professional may also reflect an irrational dislike or fear (xenophobia) of a person who is a Muslim.**

2. The statement in the stem is not an example of chauvinism. Chauvinism is the assumption of supremacy of one's group over another. For example, the group can be male, female, a religion, a political party, or those who are financially successful.

3. The statement in the stem is not an example of racism. Racism is a form of prejudice and discrimination (unjust treatment) perpetrated on people who share genetically transmitted physical characteristics, a common history, a nationality, or a geographical location. The perpetrators of racism feel superior to the targeted group. Discrimination against people whose background is not white in American history demonstrates racial divisiveness, which is present even today.

4. The statement in the stem is not an example of sexism. Sexism is demonstrated when people of one sex believe that they are superior to those of another sex. For example, some people believe that women should not become police officers.

11. 1. Drinking lemon juice to treat high blood pressure is a naturalistic or holistic belief that health is a balance between "hot" and "cold"; it is not an action based on a religious belief. Hypertension is considered a

"hot" illness by some cultures and therefore is treated with a "cold" remedy, lemon juice.

2. **Wearing an amulet to chase away bad spirits is a religious belief that illness is caused by supernatural forces and that the wearing of amulets or talismans and performing rites can prevent or restore health by supernatural forces.**

3. Massaging a foot to relieve migraine headache pain is a form of folk healing and is not based on a religious belief. This form of folk healing or alternative therapy is reflexology.

4. Brushing the teeth after every meal to prevent tooth decay is a scientifically based belief and is not based on a religious belief. If the benefit can be proved by scientific research, then it is accepted as truth.

12. 1. Although religious affiliation may be important to know, it is only one part of a client's sociocultural makeup. Another option has a higher priority.

2. Although the level of support is important to know, it is only one part of a client's sociocultural makeup. Another option has a higher priority.

3. Although national origin is important to know, it is only one part of a client's sociocultural makeup. In addition, nurses have to be careful not to make generalizations and stereotype an individual because of national origin; each person is an individual.

4. **Not all members of a culture have the same beliefs. Individuals have their own beliefs associated with cultural health practices, faith, diet, illness, death and dying, lifestyle, and faith, which all have a major impact on health beliefs. The nurse should understand that faith is an unshakable trust in something for which there is no proof.**

13. 1. This statement is premature. Another statement is the priority.

2. **This question should be asked first. The nurse must have feedback to ensure that the client understands the options for continuity of care after discharge from the hospital before a decision can be made by the client.**

3. This statement is inappropriate. The nurse should leave the decision to the client and not impose personal opinions.

4. Although this might be suggested by the nurse, it is not the priority.

14. 1. A small amount of a lubricant, not alcohol, applied to the hair will facilitate the combing out of tangles.

2. After shampooing a client's hair, it may be dried or just toweled dry until it is free of excess moisture.

3. **The appearance of one's hair is an extension of self-image. Therefore, the client's personal preferences should be considered before grooming the hair.**

4. Combing or brushing should progress from the ends of the hair, then from the middle to the ends, and finally from the scalp to the ends (distal to proximal). This technique limits discomfort and prevents broken ends and damaged hair shafts.

15. 1. During adolescence, the individual is beginning to question life-guiding values such as spirituality. However, it is not uncommon for the adolescent to turn away from religious practices as part of dealing with role confusion and exploration of self-identity. Faith becomes centered on the peer group and away from the parents. This stage is called Synthetic-Conventional Faith by James Fowler.

2. People expand and refine spiritual beliefs at an earlier stage of development than older adulthood.

3. Young adults are just beginning to think about spirituality more introspectively at this age. Young adults generally enter a reflective period as a discovery of values in relation to social goals is explored within their own frame of reference rather than from the peer group frame of reference (as during adolescence). This stage is called Individuative-Reflective Faith by James Fowler.

4. **Middle-age adults tend to engage in refining and expanding spiritual beliefs through questioning. Middle-age adults are reported to have greater faith, have more reliance on personal spiritual strength, and be more flexible in spiritual beliefs. Middle-age adults integrate other viewpoints about faith, which introduces tension while working toward resolution of spiritual beliefs. This stage is called Conjunctive Faith by James Fowler.**

16. 1. Racism does not reflect the basis of this client's statement. A racist is a person who is prejudiced against people who share a different common history, nationality, geographic area, or genetically transmitted

physical characteristics. Racists feel superior to the targeted group.

2. Sexism reflects the basis of this client's statement. A sexist is a person who has opinions that stereotype social roles based on gender.

3. Chauvinism does not reflect the basis of this client's statement. A chauvinist adopts the view that the group to which one belongs is superior to other groups. The client is male and is making an implied comment about other men.

4. Misogynism does not reflect the basis of this client's statement. A misogynist is a person who has contempt for women. The client thinks that nurses, who are women, are great.

17. 1. This is a probing response. This information may be shared by the client at a future time.

2. This is a probing response. It is insignificant information that should not influence further nursing care.

3. This response reaches out to the client in a supportive manner. It gives the client control over what is desired.

4. The nurse is dictating to the client what should be done.

18. **1. This response places the emphasis on the client. It is a question that permits the client to explore the concept about heaven and hell in any way desired.**

2. This response sidesteps the question and places the emphasis on the nurse rather than the client.

3. This response assumes that the client has a religion, which may not be true. It places an emphasis on a religion rather than the client. Also, it is a direct question that can be answered with a "yes" or "no" reply, which can cut off further communication.

4. This response cuts off communication and abandons the client. The nurse's message is, "I do not want to talk about this."

5. This response places an emphasis on the nurse rather than the client.

19. 1. The mother was not expressing a bias against gay individuals. She was being empathetic.

2. The spouse was not expressing a bias against gay individuals. The spouse was commenting on the physical effects that AIDS has brought on the partner and the devastating nature of AIDS.

3. The friend was not expressing a bias against gay individuals. The friend shared several personal facts.

4. The father made a negative, judgmental comment about the son's lifestyle. It was a negative expectation about all gay individuals—their lifestyle results in AIDs.

20. **1. All the foods and fluid in this meal are permitted on a kosher diet. Meat from animals that are cloven footed, cud chewing, and slaughtered and prepared following strict laws of Kashruth (kosher diet) are permitted.**

2. All of the foods and fluid in this meal are permitted together on a kosher diet. Beef is from a cow, a cud-chewing animal, which is permitted on a kosher diet as long as it is not served at the same meal as a dairy product.

3. Hamburger is ground beef, and milk is a dairy product. Meat and dairy products cannot be served at the same meal. Each requires separate sets of dishes, pots, pans, and utensils to ensure that they remain separate and do not contaminate each other. Potato chips are permitted with meals that contain meat or dairy products.

4. Only fish that have scales and fins are permitted on a kosher dict. Shcllfish such as shrimp, crab, and lobster are not permitted on a kosher diet.

5. All of the foods and this fluid in this meal are permitted together on a kosher diet. This meal does not contain both dairy and meat products and does not contain pork.

6. All of these foods and this fluid are permitted at the same meal when a person is following a kosher diet. This meal does not contain both dairy and meat products and does not contain pork.

21. **1. An immigrant is a person who moves from one country to remain permanently in another country. Acculturation is the process of an immigrant adapting to a new environment or situation that is different from one's own. Currently, the dominant language in the United States is English. The husband is attempting to adapt to the United States. Assimilation and socialization are additional words to describe the adoption of the characteristics of another culture.**

2. This is not an example of acculturation. Not everyone in the United States celebrates Christmas.
3. This does not reflect acculturation. Not all children in the United States attend college.
4. **Eating turkey on Thanksgiving is a tradition in the United States. The wife's making a turkey on Thanksgiving is incorporating a tradition associated with their new country into the family's practices.**
5. This is not an example of acculturation. Several generations of family members living in the same household is not something that generally is practiced in the United States.

22. 4. **A nurse must know herself or himself before caring for others. Personal values (principle, ideal, tenant), beliefs (viewpoint, faith, conviction), practices, biases (obstruction of open-minded judgment), and prejudices (negative or positive beliefs generalized to a group, race, or religion) must be identified to ensure that they are not imposed on clients.**
2. Often, there are commonalities in the values, beliefs, and practices within a culture. It is important for the nurse to be aware of these commonalities to promote culturally competent nursing care. However, the nurse must be careful not to impose generalizations about a culture on a client. Every client is an individual who brings different elements and experiences (diversity) to a situation.
3. Individuals within a culture do not always ascribe to the beliefs, values, and practices of the collective culture. Preferences must be explored with clients to ensure that nursing care is individualized.
1. Knowing about the beliefs, values, and practices within a culture and specific to an individual is not enough. A nurse must respect and provide care that adheres to the beliefs, values, and practices of each individual to provide culturally appropriate and competent nursing care.

23. 1. Teaching the client who is from a religion that does not permit blood transfusions about non-blood plasma expanders is something the nurse may do. Non-blood expanders basically are sugar molecules that hold water within blood vessels and expand blood volume, which helps to maintain blood pressure.
2. **Informing the client about intraoperative blood salvaging is something the nurse may do when caring for a client who refuses blood transfusions. During surgery, the client's blood is collected, cleaned of impurities, and prepared for reinfusion into the client (commonly called "cell saver").**
3. Explaining the benefit of a blood transfusion denies the client's right to refuse a blood transfusion and may be considered harassment.
4. The option of preoperative autologous blood transfusions (one's own blood collected in advance of the surgery to have on hand in case of need) is also prohibited by some religions that do not permit blood transfusions.
5. A transfusion of red blood cells is a product of whole blood and is prohibited by some religions that do not permit blood transfusions.

24. 1. **In Islam, the prohibition of pork comes from a verse in the *Quran*, "Forbidden to you are: dead meat, blood, the flesh of swine…."**
2. **Several passages in the *Torah* (the first five books of Moses) contain passages that identify *animals that have cloven hoof but do not chew their cud* are prohibited. Pigs have a cloven hoof but do not chew their cud.**
3. The Mormon religion (The Church of Jesus Christ of Latter-day Saints) does not prohibit the ingestion of pork.
4. Jehovah's Witness religion does not prohibit the ingestion of pork as long as the animal is *properly bleed* (drained of blood) when slaughtered. In addition, verses in the New Testament contain information that basically states that all animals are clean.
5. **The Seventh-day Adventist religion prohibits the consumption of pork, shrimp, and other meats designated as unclean in the book of Leviticus.**

25. 1. **This statement is appropriate when meeting a client's spiritual needs if a nurse is uncomfortable about praying with a client. Prayer is a fundamental element of most religions. Religion is the faith or belief in and worship of a**

God or a higher power; religion contains organized attitudes, beliefs, and practices.

2. A nurse who may feel uncomfortable with praying with a client should make arrangements that will help the client to meet spiritual needs.

3. This statement cuts off communication and does not help a client who is experiencing spiritual distress to seek spiritual well-being. Spiritual well-being is the ability to experience and integrate meaning and purpose in life via factors such as self, art, music, literature, nature, or a power greater than oneself.

4. This response cuts off communication and does not provide an avenue of assistance for the client. It abandons the client, who is experiencing spiritual distress. Spiritual distress is a disruption in a person's life principles that transcends one's psychological and biophysical being.

5. Hope inspiration is a form of spiritual support. Hope involves having a positive focus and faith in the future. Determining if a client feels hopeless is important to identify.

Essential Components of Nursing Care

Nursing Process

The following words include nursing/medical terminology, concepts, principles, and information relevant to content specifically addressed in the chapter or associated with topics presented in it. English dictionaries, nursing textbooks, and medical dictionaries, such as *Taber's Cyclopedic Medical Dictionary,* are resources that can be used to expand your knowledge and understanding of these words and related information.

Care plan, types:
  Case management
  Clinical pathway
  Computerized
  Individualized
  Standardized
Clinical record, parts of:
  Admission sheet
  Consents
  Flow sheets
  Health-care provider's prescriptions
  History and physical
  Laboratory/diagnostic test results
  Medication administration
    record
  Progress notes
Data, sources of:
  Primary
  Secondary
Data, types:
  Objective
  Subjective
Data collection methods:
  Auscultation
  Examination
  Inspection
  Interview
  Observation
  Palpation
  Percussion
Functions of the nurse:
  Dependent
  Independent
  Interdependent

Goal, components of:
  Achievable
  Measurable
  Realistic
  Time frame
Inference
Intervention skills:
  Assisting
  Collaborating
  Coordinating
  Managing
  Monitoring
  Protecting
  Supporting
  Sustaining
  Teaching
Nursing diagnosis:
  Diagnostic label
  Related to factors: contributing factors,
    etiology
  As evidenced by: signs and symptoms,
    defining characteristics
Nursing process:
  Assessment
  Analysis
  Planning
  Implementation
  Evaluation
Outcomes:
  Actual
  Expected
Reasoning:
  Deductive
  Inductive

NURSING PROCESS: QUESTIONS

1. A nurse makes a home-care visit for a client who had total hip replacement surgery 1 week ago. During which of the five steps in the nursing process does the nurse determine whether outcomes of care are achieved?
   1. Implementation
   2. Evaluation
   3. Planning
   4. Analysis

2. When considering the nursing process, the word "observe" is to "assess" as the word "explore" is to which of the following words?
   1. Plan
   2. Analyze
   3. Evaluate
   4. Implement

3. Which statement is related to the concept that is central to the nursing process?
   1. It is dynamic rather than static.
   2. It focuses on the role of the nurse.
   3. It moves from the simple to the complex.
   4. It is based on the client's medical problem.

4. Which word **best** describes the role of the nurse when using the nursing process to meet the needs of the client holistically?
   1. Teacher
   2. Advocate
   3. Surrogate
   4. Counselor

5. Which word is **most** closely associated with scientific principles?
   1. Data
   2. Problem
   3. Rationale
   4. Evaluation

6. A pebble dropped into a pond causes ripples on the surface of the water. Which part of the nursing diagnosis is directly related to this concept?
   1. Defining characteristics
   2. Outcome criteria
   3. Etiology
   4. Goal

7. A nurse teaches a client to use visualization to cope with chronic pain. Which step of the nursing process is associated with this nursing intervention?
   1. Planning
   2. Analysis
   3. Evaluation
   4. Implementation

8. A nurse is caring for several clients. Which nursing action reflects the assessment step of the nursing process?
   1. Taking a client's apical pulse rate every 2 hours after the client is admitted for an episode of chest pain
   2. Scheduling a client's fluid intake over 12 hours when the client has a fluid restriction
   3. Examining a client for injury after a fall in the bathroom
   4. Obtaining a client's respiratory rate after a nebulizer treatment

9. A nurse is caring for a client with a fever. Which is a well-designed goal for this client?
   1. "The client will have a lower temperature."
   2. "The client will be taught how to take an accurate temperature."
   3. "The client will maintain fluid intake adequate to prevent dehydration."
   4. "The client will be given aspirin every eight hours whenever necessary."

10. Which should the nurse do during the evaluation step of the nursing process?
    1. Set the time frames for goals.
    2. Revise a plan of care.
    3. Determine priorities.
    4. Establish outcomes.

11. A client is admitted to a postoperative surgical unit after abdominal surgery. During which step of the nursing process does the nurse determine which actions are required to meet the needs of this client?
    1. Implementation
    2. Assessment
    3. Planning
    4. Analysis

12. Which information **supports** the appropriateness of a nursing diagnosis?
    1. Defining characteristics
    2. Planned interventions
    3. Diagnostic statement
    4. Related risk factors

13. Which is the primary goal of the assessment phase of the nursing process?
    1. Build trust
    2. Collect data
    3. Establish goals
    4. Validate the medical diagnosis

14. Which **most** directly influences the planning step of the nursing process?
    1. Related factors
    2. Diagnostic label
    3. Secondary factors
    4. Medical diagnosis

15. A nurse collects information about a client. Which should the nurse do **next**?
    1. Plan nursing interventions.
    2. Write client-centered goals.
    3. Formulate nursing diagnoses.
    4. Determine significance of the data.

16. When two nursing diagnoses appear closely related, which should the nurse do **first** to determine which diagnosis most accurately reflects the needs of the client?
    1. Reassess the client.
    2. Examine the related to factors.
    3. Analyze the secondary to factors.
    4. Review the defining characteristics.

17. Which is the **primary** reason why a nurse performs a physical assessment of a newly admitted client?
   1. Identify if the client is at risk for falls.
   2. Ensure that the client's skin is totally intact.
   3. Identify important information about the client.
   4. Establish a therapeutic relationship with the client.

18. A nurse evaluates a client's response to a nebulizer treatment. To which aspect of the nursing process is this evaluation **most** directly related?
   1. Goal
   2. Problem
   3. Etiology
   4. Implementation

19. A nurse concludes that a client's elevated temperature, pulse, and respirations are significant. Which step of the nursing process is being used when the nurse comes to this conclusion?
   1. Implementation
   2. Assessment
   3. Evaluation
   4. Analysis

20. When the nurse considers the nursing process, the word "identify" is to "recognize" as the word "do" is to which of the following words?
   1. Implement
   2. Evaluate
   3. Analyze
   4. Plan

21. A nurse is collecting subjective data associated with a client's anxiety. Which assessment method should be used to collect this information?
   1. Observing
   2. Inspection
   3. Auscultation
   4. Interviewing

22. A nurse assesses that a client has slurred speech and a retained bolus of food in the mouth. Which additional condition assessed by the nurse should be clustered with these clinical indicators? **Select all that apply.**
   1. _____ Hoarseness
   2. _____ Dyspepsia
   3. _____ Coughing
   4. _____ Drooling
   5. _____ Gurgling
   6. _____ Plaque

23. Nurses use the nursing process to provide nursing care. These statements reflect nursing care being provided to several clients. Place the statements in order as the nurse progresses through the steps of the nursing process, starting with assessment and ending with evaluation.
   1. "Did you sleep last night after I gave you the sleeping medication?"
   2. "The client's clinical manifestations indicate dehydration."
   3. "The client will have a bowel movement in the morning."
   4. "What brought you to the hospital today?"
   5. "I am going to give you an enema."

   Answer: _____

24. A nurse is caring for a client with a urinary elimination problem. Which is an accurately stated goal? **Select all that apply.**
1. _____ "The client will be taught how to use a bedpan while on bedrest."
2. _____ "The client will experience fewer incontinence episodes at night."
3. _____ "The client will transfer from a chair to the toilet independently and safely."
4. _____ "The client will be assisted to the commode every 2 hours and whenever necessary."
5. _____ "The client will experience one or no events of urinary incontinence daily within 6 weeks."

25. Which human response identified by the nurse is an example of objective data? **Select all that apply.**
1. _____ Irregular radial pulse of 50 beats per minute
2. _____ Wheezing on expiration
3. _____ Temperature of 99°F
4. _____ Bradypnea
5. _____ Vomiting

26. Place the following statements that reflect the analysis step of the nursing process in the order in which they should be implemented.
1. Cluster data.
2. Identify conclusions.
3. Interpret clustered data.
4. Communicate conclusion to other health team members.
5. Identify when additional data are needed to further validate clustered data.

Answer: _____

27. Which client statement provides subjective data? **Select all that apply.**
1. _____ "I'm not sure that I am going to be able to manage at home by myself."
2. _____ "I can call a home-care agency if I feel I need help at home."
3. _____ "What should I do if I have uncontrollable pain at home?"
4. _____ "Will a home health aide help me with my care at home?"
5. _____ "I'm afraid because I live alone and I'm on my own."

28. Which nursing action reflects an activity associated with the analysis step of the nursing process? **Select all that apply.**
1. _____ Formulating a plan of care
2. _____ Identifying the client's potential risks
3. _____ Grouping data into meaningful relationships
4. _____ Designing ways to minimize a client's stressors
5. _____ Making decisions about the effectiveness of client care

29. A nurse is interviewing a client. Which client statement is an example of objective data? **Select all that apply.**
1. _____ "I am hungry."
2. _____ "I feel very warm."
3. _____ "I ate half my lunch."
4. _____ "I have a rash on my arm."
5. _____ "I have the urge to urinate."
6. _____ "I vomit every time I eat something."

30. Which statement indicates that the nurse is using inductive reasoning? **Select all that apply.**
    1. _____ A client is admitted with a diagnosis of dehydration, and the nurse assesses the client's skin for tenting.
    2. _____ A nurse observes a client fall out of bed on the right hip and immediately assesses the client for right hip pain.
    3. _____ A client has an elevated white blood cell count and a fever. The nurse concludes that the client may have an infection.
    4. _____ A client who is scheduled for surgery is crying, trembling, and has a rapid pulse. The nurse makes the inference that the client is anxious.
    5. _____ A nurse receives a call from the admission department that a client with hypoglycemia is being admitted to the unit. The nurse plans to assess the client for pale, cool, clammy skin and a low blood glucose level.

31. The following statements reflect steps in the nursing process. Place the statements in order as the nurse advances through the steps of the nursing process, beginning with assessment and ending with evaluation.
    1. "The client is encouraged to attempt to defecate after meals."
    2. "The client reports not having had a bowel movement for 8 days."
    3. "The client has constipation related to immobility and inadequate fluid intake."
    4. "The client will have a bowel movement within 2 days that is of soft consistency."
    5. "The client's stool is still hard and dry 2 days after initiating an increase in fluids and activity."

    Answer: _____

32. A nurse is interviewing a client at the change of shift. Which client statement reflects subjective data? **Select all that apply.**
    1. _____ "When I lift my head up off the bed, I feel like vomiting."
    2. _____ "I just used the urinal, and it needs to be emptied."
    3. _____ "My pain feels like a 5 on a scale of 0 to 5."
    4. _____ "The physician said I can go home today."
    5. _____ "I gained 10 pounds in the last month."

33. A nurse identifies that the client's report of decreased activity and intake of fluids may be the underlying cause of the client's constipation. Place an X over the word that reflects the step of the nursing process that is functioning.

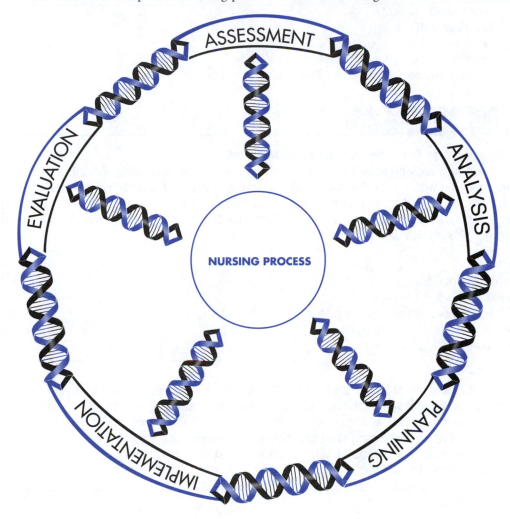

34. A client is transferred from the emergency department to a medical-surgical unit at 6:30 p.m. The nurse arriving on duty at 8 p.m. reviews the client's clinical record. Which information documented in the clinical record reflects the evaluation step of the nursing process?
1. Productive cough
2. No dizziness reported by the client
3. Seek prescription for chest physiotherapy
4. Acetaminophen 650 mg administered at 5 p.m.

CLIENT'S CLINICAL RECORD

Nurse's Transfer Note From the Emergency Department

Client admitted to the emergency department at 3 p.m. stating experiencing shortness of breath that became worse over the last few days. Sputum culture obtained and metabolic panel and complete blood count drawn. Oxygen prescribed at 2 L via nasal cannula, acetaminophen 650 mg PO administered at 5 p.m. Client transferred to 5 South with a diagnosis of rule out pneumonia at 6 p.m.

Vital Signs

Oxygen saturation: 85%
Temperature: 102.4°F, temporal
Pulse: 92 beats per minute, regular rate
Respirations: 28 breaths per minute
Blood pressure: 160/90 mm Hg

Progress Note

7 p.m.: IV 0.45% sodium chloride running at 100 mL per hour. IV site is clean, dry, and intact. Client has a productive cough and excessive respiratory secretions, and respirations are 28 breaths per minute. Called primary health-care provider for a prescription for chest physiotherapy. Client states feeling tired and nauseated. Client had 4 ounces of soup and 3 ounces of water and refused rest of dinner. Client assisted to the bathroom to void; no dizziness reported by the client.

35. The nurse assesses a client and collects a variety of data. Identify the human response that is subjective data. **Select all that apply.**
1. _____ Nausea
2. _____ Jaundice
3. _____ Ecchymosis
4. _____ Diaphoresis
5. _____ Hypotension

1. 1. During the implementation step of the nursing process, outcomes are not determined; instead, planned nursing care is delivered.

2. Evaluation occurs when actual outcomes are compared with expected outcomes that reflect goal achievement. If the goal is achieved, the client's needs are met.

3. During the planning step of the nursing process, expected outcomes are determined, but their achievement is measured in another step of the nursing process.

4. During the analysis step of the nursing process, outcomes are not determined; instead, the nurse identifies human responses to actual or potential health problems.

2. 1. The definitions of the words "observe" and "assess" are similar. Observe means to view something scientifically, and assess means to collect information. The word "plan" does not fit the analogy because the definitions of the words "plan" and "explore" are not similar. Explore means to examine. Plan means to design an intention.

2. The definitions of the words "observe" and "assess" are similar. Observe means to view something scientifically, and assess means to collect information. The word "analyze" fits the analogy. Explore means to examine. Analyze means to investigate.

3. The definitions of the words "observe" and "assess" are similar. Observe means to view something scientifically, and assess means to collect information. The word "evaluation" does not fit the analogy because the definitions of explore and evaluate are not similar. Explore means to examine. Evaluation within the concept of the nursing process means to come to a conclusion about a client's response to a nursing intervention.

4. The definitions of the words "observe" and "assess" are similar. Observe means to examine something scientifically, and assess means to collect information. The word "implement" does not fit the analogy because the definitions of explore and implement are not similar. Explore means to examine. Implement means to carry out an action.

3. 1. **The nursing process is a dynamic five-step problem-solving process (assessment, analysis, planning, implementation, and evaluation) designed to diagnose and treat human responses to health problems.**

2. The nursing process focuses on the needs of the client, not the role of the nurse.

3. Moving from the simple to the complex is a principle of teaching, not the nursing process. The nursing process is a complex, interactive, five-step problem-solving process designed to meet a client's needs. It requires an understanding of systems and information-processing theory and the critical-thinking, problem-solving, decision-making, and diagnostic-reasoning processes.

4. The nursing process is concerned with a person's human responses to actual or potential health problems, not the client's medical problem.

4. 1. Although functioning as a teacher is an important role of the nurse, it is a limited role compared with another option. As a teacher, the nurse helps the client gain new knowledge about health and health care to maintain or restore health.

2. **When the nurse supports, protects, and defends a client from a holistic perspective, the nurse functions as an advocate. Advocacy includes exploring, informing, mediating, and affirming in all areas to help a client navigate the health-care system, maintain autonomy, and achieve the best possible health outcomes.**

3. The word surrogate is not the word that best describes the role of the nurse providing holistic care. The nurse is placed in the surrogate role when a client projects onto the nurse the image of another and then responds to the nurse with the feelings for the other person's image.

4. Although functioning as a counselor is an important role of the nurse, it is a limited role compared with another option. As counselor, the nurse helps the client improve interpersonal relationships, recognize and deal with stressful psychosocial problems, and promote achievement of self-actualization.

5. 1. The word "data" (information) is not associated with the term "scientific principles" (established rules of action).

2. The word "problem" (difficulty) is not associated with the term "scientific principles" (established rules of action).

3. **The word "rationale" (justification based on reasoning) is closely associated with the term "scientific principles" (established rules of action). Scientific principles are based on rationales.**

4. The word "evaluation" (determining the value or worth of something) is not associated with the term "scientific principles" (established rules of action).

6. 1. Defining characteristics do not contribute to the problem statement, but they support or indicate the presence of the nursing diagnosis. Defining characteristics are the major and minor signs and symptoms that support the presence of a nursing diagnosis.
2. Outcome criteria are not a part of the nursing diagnosis. Outcome criteria (goals) are part of the planning step of the nursing process.
3. The etiology (also known as related to or contributing factors) includes the conditions, situations, or circumstances that cause the development of the human response identified in the problem statement of the nursing diagnosis. The etiology precipitates the human response, just as a pebble dropped in a pond causes ripples on the surface of water.
4. Goals are not part of the nursing diagnosis. Goals are the expected outcomes or what is anticipated that the client will achieve in response to nursing intervention.

7. 1. This is not an example of the planning step of the nursing process. During the planning step, the nurse identifies the nursing interventions that are most likely to be effective.
2. This is not an example of the analysis step of the nursing process. During the analysis step, data are critically explored and interpreted, significance of data is determined, inferences are made and validated, signs and symptoms and clusters of signs and symptoms are compared with the defining characteristics of nursing diagnoses, contributing factors are identified, and nursing diagnoses are identified and organized in order of priority.
3. This is not an example of the evaluation step of the nursing process. Evaluation occurs when actual outcomes are compared with expected outcomes that reflect goal achievement.
4. This is an example of the implementation step of the nursing process. It is during the implementation step that planned nursing care is delivered.

8. 1. This action reflects the step of implementation. The nurse puts into action the plan to monitor the client's vital signs after a cardiac event is suspected.
2. This action reflects the planning step of the nursing process.
3. This action reflects the assessment step of the nursing process. Assessment involves collecting data via observation, physical examination, and interviewing.
4. This action reflects the evaluation step of the nursing process. The nurse assesses the client's respiratory rate and effort after a nebulizer treatment to determine if the treatment was effective in reducing airway resistance, thereby improving the client's respiratory rate and reducing respiratory effort.

9. 1. This goal is inappropriate because the word "lower" is not specific, measurable, or objective.
2. This is not a goal. This is an action the nurse plans to implement to help a client achieve a goal.
3. This is a well-written goal. Goals must be client centered, specific, measurable, and realistic and have a time frame in which the expected outcome is to be achieved. The words "adequate" and "dehydration" are based on generally accepted criteria against which to measure the client's actual outcome. The word "maintain" connotes continuously, which is a time frame.
4. This is not a goal. This is an action the nurse plans to implement to help a client achieve a goal.

10. 1. Setting time frames for goals to be achieved is part of the planning, not evaluation, step of the nursing process.
2. Revising a plan of care takes place in the evaluation step of the nursing process. If, during evaluation, it is determined that the goal was not met, the reasons for failure have to be identified and the plan has to be modified.
3. Determining priorities is part of the planning, not evaluation, step of the nursing process. Priority setting is a decision-making process that ranks a client's nursing needs and nursing interventions in order of importance.
4. Establishing outcomes is part of the planning, not evaluation, step of the nursing process.

11. 1. This does not occur during the implementation step of the nursing process. During the implementation step, the nurse puts

the plan of care into action. Nursing interventions include actions that are dependent (requiring a primary health-care provider's prescription), independent (autonomous actions within the nurse's scope of practice), and interdependent (interventions that require a primary health-care provider's prescription but that permit nurses to use clinical judgment in their implementation).

2. This does not occur during the assessment step of the nursing process. During the assessment step, the nurse uses various skills, such as observation, interviewing, and physical examination, to collect data from various sources.

3. **The identification of nursing actions designed to help a client achieve a goal occurs during the planning step of the nursing process.**

4. This does not occur during the analysis step of the nursing process. The nurse identifies the client's human responses to actual or potential health problems during the analysis step of the nursing process.

12. 1. **The defining characteristics are the major and minor cues that form a cluster that supports or validates the presence of a nursing diagnosis. At least one major defining characteristic must be present for a nursing diagnosis to be considered appropriate for the client.**

2. Planned interventions do not support the nursing diagnosis. They are the nursing actions designed to help resolve the "related to" or "contributing to" factors and achieve expected client outcomes that reflect goal achievement.

3. The diagnostic statement cannot support the nursing diagnosis because it is the first part of the nursing diagnosis. A nursing diagnosis is made up of two parts, the diagnostic statement (also known as the problem statement) and the "related to" factors (also known as factors that contribute to the problem or the etiology).

4. Related risk factors cannot support the nursing diagnosis because they are the second part of the nursing diagnosis. A nursing diagnosis is made up of two parts, the diagnostic statement (also known as the problem statement) and the "related to" factors (also known as factors that contribute to the problem or the etiology).

13. 1. Although trust may be established during the assessment phase of the nursing

process, it is not the purpose of this step of the nursing process. The development of trust generally takes time.

2. **The primary purpose of the assessment step of the nursing process is to collect data (information) from various sources using a variety of approaches.**

3. When a five-step nursing process is followed, formulating goals occurs during the planning, not assessment, step of the nursing process.

4. Validating the medical diagnosis is not within a nurse's legal scope of practice.

14. 1. **Related factors (i.e., "contributing to" factors, etiology) contribute to the problem statement of the nursing diagnosis and directly have an impact on the planning step of the nursing process. Nursing interventions are selected to minimize or relieve the effects of the related factors. If nursing interventions are appropriate and effective, the human response identified in the problem statement part of the nursing diagnosis will resolve.**

2. The planning step of the nursing process includes setting a goal, identifying the outcomes that will reflect goal achievement, and planning nursing interventions. Although the wording of the goal is directly influenced by the diagnostic label (problem statement of the nursing diagnosis), the selection of nursing interventions is not.

3. Secondary factors generally have only a minor influence on the planning step of the nursing process.

4. The medical diagnosis does not influence the planning step of the nursing process. The nurse is concerned with human responses to actual or potential health problems, not the medical diagnosis.

15. 1. Nursing care is planned after nursing diagnoses and goals are identified, not immediately after data are collected.

2. Goals are designed after a nursing diagnosis is identified, not after data are collected.

3. Once data are collected, the nurse must first organize and cluster the data to determine significance and make inferences. After all this is accomplished, then the nurse can formulate a nursing diagnosis.

4. **After data are collected, they are clustered to determine their significance.**

16. 1. If a thorough assessment was completed initially, a reassessment should not be necessary.
    2. Establishing which of two nursing diagnoses is most appropriate is not dependent on identifying the factors that *contributed to* (also known as *related to* or *etiology of*) the nursing diagnosis. These factors are identified after the problem statement is identified.
    3. Establishing which of two nursing diagnoses is more appropriate is not dependent on analyzing the *secondary to* factors. *Secondary to* factors generally are medical conditions that precipitate the *related to* factors. The *secondary to* factors are identified after the *related to* factors of the problem are identified.
    4. **The first thing the nurse should do to differentiate between two closely associated nursing diagnoses is to compare the data collected to the major and minor defining characteristics of each of the nursing diagnoses being considered.**

17. 1. Although completing a nursing physical assessment includes an assessment of the risk for falls, it is only one component of the assessment.
    2. Although completing a nursing physical admission assessment includes an assessment of the skin, it is only one component of the assessment.
    3. **This is the primary purpose of a nursing physical assessment. Data must be collected and then analyzed to determine significance and be grouped in meaningful clusters before a nursing diagnosis or plan of care can be made.**
    4. Although completing a nursing physical assessment helps to initiate the nurse-client relationship, it is not the primary purpose of completing a nursing admission assessment.

18. 1. **To evaluate the effectiveness of a nursing action, the nurse must compare the actual client outcome with the expected client outcome. The expected outcomes are the measurable data that reflect goal achievement, and the actual outcomes are what really happened.**
    2. The problem is associated with the first half (problem statement) of the nursing diagnosis, not the evaluation step of the nursing process.

3. Etiology is a term used to identify the factors that relate to or contribute to the problem statement of the nursing diagnosis, not the evaluation step of the nursing process.
    4. Implementation is a step separate from evaluation in the nursing process. Nursing care must be performed before it can be evaluated.

19. 1. This is not an example of the implementation step of the nursing process. It is during the implementation step that planned nursing care is delivered.
    2. This is not an example of the assessment step of the nursing process. Although data may be gathered during the assessment step, the manipulation of the data is conducted in a different step of the nursing process.
    3. This is not an example of the evaluation step of the nursing process. Evaluation occurs when actual outcomes are compared with expected outcomes, which reflect attainment or nonattainment of the goal.
    4. **During the analysis step of the nursing process, data are critically explored and interpreted, significance of data is determined, inferences are made and validated, cues and clusters of cues are compared with the defining characteristics of nursing diagnoses, contributing factors are identified, and nursing diagnoses are identified and organized in order of priority.**

20. 1. **This is the correct analogy. The words "identify" and "recognize" have the same definition. They both mean the same as that which is known. The words "do" and "implement" both have the same definition. They both mean to carry out some action.**
    2. The words "identify" and "recognize" have the same definition. They both mean the same as that which is known. The word "evaluate" does not fit the analogy because the definitions of "evaluate" and "do" are different. The word "evaluate" means to determine the worth of something, whereas the word "do" means to carry into effect or to accomplish.
    3. The words "identify" and "recognize" have the same definition. They both mean the same as that which is known. The word "analyze" does not fit the analogy because the definitions of "analyze" and "do" are different. The word "analyze"

means to investigate the client's human response to an actual or potential health problem. The word "do" means to carry into effect or to accomplish.

4. The words "identify" and "recognize" have the same definition. They both mean the same as that which is known. The word "plan" does not fit the analogy because the definitions of "plan" and "do" are different. The word "plan" means a method of proceeding. The word "do" means to carry into effect or to accomplish.

21. 1. Observing is the deliberate use of all the senses and involves more than just inspection and examination. It includes surveying, looking, scanning, scrutinizing, and appraising. Although the nurse makes inferences based on data collected by observation, this is not as effective as another data collection method to identify subjective data associated with a client's anxiety.

2. Inspection involves the act of making observations of physical features and behavior. Although the nurse observes behaviors and makes inferences based on their perceived meaning, another data collection method is more effective in identifying subjective data associated with a client's anxiety.

3. Auscultation is listening for sounds within the body. This collects objective, not subjective, data, which are measurable.

4. **Interviewing a client is the most effective data collection method when collecting subjective data associated with a client's anxiety. The client is the primary source for subjective data about beliefs, values, feelings, perceptions, fears, and concerns.**

22. 1. **Hoarseness may be a sign of laryngeal inflammation as a result of microaspiration and should be clustered with the group of signs presented in the question.**

2. Epigastric discomfort after eating (dyspepsia) may be symptom of a gastrointestinal problem. Dyspepsia is unrelated to the client's clinical manifestations presented in the question.

3. **The body continuously secretes saliva (approximately 1,000 mL/day) that usually is swallowed. If a client is having difficulty swallowing, the client may aspirate saliva, which can cause**

coughing. **Coughing in addition to the client's other clinical manifestations indicates that the client may have impaired swallowing.**

4. **The body continuously secretes saliva (approximately 1,000 mL/day) that usually is swallowed. When saliva accumulates and is not swallowed, it dribbles out of the mouth (drooling). Drooling in addition to the client's other clinical manifestations indicates that the client may have impaired swallowing.**

5. **The body continuously secretes saliva (approximately 1,000 mL/day) that usually is swallowed. When saliva accumulates and is not swallowed, it makes a bubbling or gurgling sound in the posterior oropharynx as air is inhaled and exhaled.**

6. A thin film of mucin, food debris, and dead epithelial cells on the teeth (plaque) is not related to the client's other clinical manifestations. Plaque is related to the development of dental caries.

23. 4. **Objective and subjective data must be collected, verified, and communicated during the assessment step of the nursing process.**

2. **Data are clustered and analyzed, and their significance is determined, leading to a conclusion about the client's condition, during the analysis step of the nursing process.**

3. **Identifying goals, projecting outcomes, setting priorities, and identifying interventions are all part of the planning step of the nursing process.**

5. **Planned actions are initiated and completed during the implementation step of the nursing process.**

1. **Identifying responses to care, comparing actual outcomes with expected outcomes, analyzing factors that affected outcomes, and modifying the plan of care if necessary are all part of the evaluation step of the nursing process.**

24. 1. This statement is not a goal. This is an action the nurse plans to implement to help a client achieve a goal.

2. This goal is inappropriate because the word "fewer" is not specific, measurable, or objective.

3. This goal statement is incomplete. Although the statement is client-centered, measurable, and realistic, it does not

include a time frame in which the expected goal is to be achieved.

4. This statement is not a goal. This is an action the nurse plans to implement to help a client achieve a goal.

5. **This is a correctly worded goal. Goals must be client-centered, measurable, realistic, and include the time frame in which the expected goal is to be achieved. The words "one or no events … daily" comprise a measurable statement, and the words "within 6 weeks" establish a time frame.**

25. 1. **A radial pulse is objective information. Objective data are measurable and checkable.**

2. **The sound of wheezing is objective data because it can be heard by others. Air becomes turbulent when it moves through narrow passages that cause vibration of airway walls, resulting in high-pitched whistling sounds (wheezing).**

3. **A temperature of 99°F is objective information. Objective data are measurable and can be verified.**

4. **Bradypnea is an example of objective data. Objective data are measurable and can be verified.**

5. **Vomiting is an example of objective data. Objective data are measurable and can be verified.**

26. 1. **The first step in the analysis phase of the nursing process is to group and cluster data that appear to have a relationship. The nurse uses indicative reasoning, moving from the specific to the general.**

5. **The second step in analysis involves gathering additional data to corroborate, substantiate, support, and validate clustered data further.**

3. **The third step in analysis involves interpreting the data. The nurse uses reasoning based on knowing commonalities and differences and a scientific foundation of knowledge and experiential background to determine if the data cluster is significant.**

2. **The fourth step in analysis involves the nurse making a conclusion about the clustered and validated data.**

4. **The fifth step in analysis involves communicating conclusions to other health team members in a nursing plan of care.**

27. 1. **Knowing one's own abilities is subjective information because it is the client's perception and can be verified only by the client. Subjective data are those responses, feelings, beliefs, preferences, and information that only the client can confirm.**

2. This statement is neither subjective nor objective data. It is a statement indicating an understanding of how to seek home-care services after discharge.

3. This statement is neither subjective nor objective data. It is a question indicating that the client wants more information about how to control pain when at home.

4. This statement is neither subjective nor objective data. It is a statement exploring who will provide assistance with care once the client goes home.

5. **Fear is subjective information because it is the client's perception and can be verified only by the client. Subjective data are those responses, feelings, beliefs, preferences, and information that only the client can confirm.**

28. 1. Formulating a plan of care occurs during the planning, not analysis, step of the nursing process.

2. **Potential risk factors are identified during the analysis step of the nursing process. Risk diagnoses are designed to address situations in which clients have a particular vulnerability to health problems.**

3. **Determining which data are significant or insignificant and then categorizing the meaningful data into clusters of data that are related are parts of the analysis step of the nursing process.**

4. This occurs during the planning, not analysis, step of the nursing process.

5. This occurs during the evaluation, not analysis, step of the nursing process.

29. 1. Hunger is an example of subjective, not objective, data. Subjective data are those responses, feelings, beliefs, preferences, and information that only the client can confirm.

2. Feeling warm is an example of subjective, not objective, data. Subjective data are those responses, feelings, beliefs, preferences, and information that only the client can confirm.

3. **The amount of food eaten by a client can be objectively verified. The nurse**

measures and documents the percentage of a meal ingested by a client to quantify the amount of food consumed.

4. **A rash on a client's arm can be objectively verified via inspection.**

5. Having the urge to void is an example of subjective, not objective, data. Subjective data are those responses, feelings, beliefs, preferences, and information that only the client can confirm.

6. **Vomiting is a human response that is observable, and the amount vomited can be measured. Vomiting is objective information.**

30. 1. This statement reflects the nurse using deductive reasoning. It moves from a general premise (the client is dehydrated) to a specific deduction (the client will probably have tenting of the skin, which is a sign of dehydration).

2. This statement reflects the nurse using deductive reasoning. It moves from a general premise (the client may have fractured the head of the femur in the fall) to a specific deduction (the client will probably have pain in the hip if it is fractured).

3. **This statement reflects the nurse using inductive reasoning. It moves from the specific to the general. A pattern of information (an elevated white blood cell count and elevated temperature) leads to a generalization (the client may have an infection).**

4. **This statement reflects the nurse using inductive reasoning. It moves from the specific to the general. A pattern of information (crying, trembling, and a rapid pulse) leads to a generalization (the client may be anxious).**

5. This statement reflects the nurse using deductive reasoning. It moves from a general premise (the client is experiencing hypoglycemia) to a specific deduction (the client

will probably have pale, cool, clammy skin and a low blood glucose level).

31. 2. This statement reflects data collection that occurs in the assessment phase of the nursing process, which is the first step.

3. This statement reflects etiological factors contributing to the nursing diagnosis problem statement, which is "constipation." This step analyzes the data collected in the assessment phase of the nursing process.

4. **This statement is a measurable goal. Identifying goals occurs after the nursing diagnosis is identified.**

1. **This statement indicates implementation of a planned action that is designed to address the problem statement.**

5. **Information about a client's response to nursing care can be used to compare the client's actual outcome with the expect outcome, which is the evaluation phase of the nursing process.**

32. 1. **Feeling like vomiting is something that only the client can perceive. Subjective data are those responses, feelings, beliefs, preferences, and information that only the client can confirm.**

2. This statement reflects objective, not subjective, information. The urine is observable and measurable. Objective data can be verified.

3. **A client's perception about a level of pain is subjective information. Subjective data are those responses, feelings, beliefs, preferences, and information that only the client can confirm.**

4. This information reflects objective, not subjective, data. The statement can be verified.

5. This information reflects objective, not subjective, data. The statement can be verified.

33. Determining relationships of data and their significance are associated with the analysis phase of the nursing process.

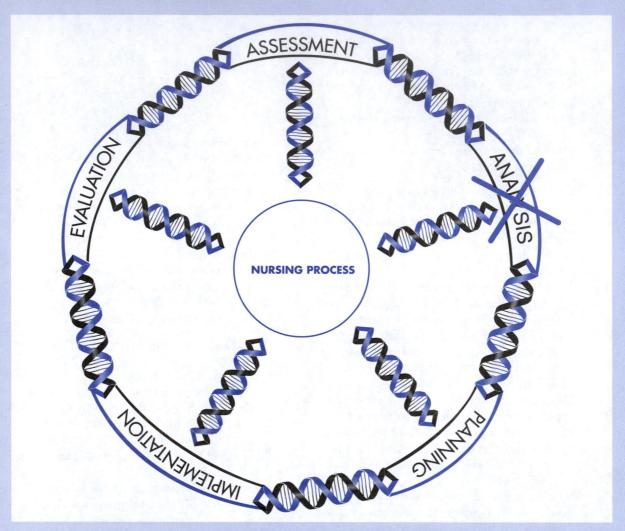

34. 1. A productive cough is information collected during the assessment phase of the nursing process.

 2. This statement reflects an evaluation of the client's response to ambulation.

 3. Seeking a prescription for chest physiotherapy reflects the planning phase of the nursing process.

 4. Administering a prescribed medication reflects the implementation phase of the nursing process.

35. 1. Nausea is an unpleasant, wavelike sensation in the back of the throat, epigastrium, or abdomen that may lead to vomiting. It is considered subjective data because it cannot be measured by the nurse objectively. It is experienced only by the client.

 2. A yellow color of the skin, whites of the eyes, and mucous membranes (jaundice) because of deposition of bile pigments from excess bilirubin in the blood is objective, not subjective, information. Objective data are measurable and checkable.

 3. Ecchymosis is objective data because it is visible on the skin and is measurable and checkable. It is a discoloration of the skin caused by extravasation of blood into subcutaneous tissue from ruptured blood vessels near the surface of the skin. Ecchymosis can be caused by trauma, hematologic disease, or other medical conditions.

 4. Excessive sweating (diaphoresis) is objective, not subjective, information. Objective data are measurable and checkable.

 5. Abnormally low systolic and diastolic blood pressure levels (hypotension) can be measured and verified and therefore are objective data.

Physical Assessment

KEYWORDS

The following words include nursing/medical terminology, concepts, principles, and information relevant to content specifically addressed in the chapter or associated with topics presented in it. English dictionaries, nursing textbooks, and medical dictionaries, such as *Taber's Cyclopedic Medical Dictionary,* are resources that can be used to expand your knowledge and understanding of these words and related information.

Afebrile

Asymptomatic

Autonomic nervous system

Barrel chest

Blood pressure:
  Auscultatory gap
  Korotkoff's sounds
  Pulse pressure
  Systolic/diastolic

Body weight

Borborygmi (bowel sounds)

Breathing:
  Costal (thoracic)
  Diaphragmatic (abdominal)
  Patterns:
    Biot
    Cheyne-Stokes
    Eupnea
    Kussmaul
  Rate:
    Apnea
    Bradypnea
    Tachypnea

Breath sounds:
  Adventitious:
    Crackles (rales)
    Gurgles (rhonchi)
    Pleural friction rub
    Stridor
    Wheeze
  Expected:
    Bronchial
    Bronchovesicular
    Vesicular

Capillary refill

Circadian rhythms, diurnal variations

Clubbing

Cognitive impairment:
  Confusion
  Delirium
  Dementia

Data:
  Objective, subjective
  Primary source of
  Secondary source of

Ecchymosis

Edema:
  Dependent
  Sacral

Erythema

Exacerbation

Fever (pyrexia), stages of:
  Course (plateau phase)
  Onset (cold or chill phase)
  Defervescence (fever abatement, flush phase)

General adaptation syndrome (GAS)

Heart rate:
  Bradycardia
  Irregular rhythm (dysrhythmia)
  Pulse deficit
  Tachycardia

Hirsutism

Hyperemia

Hypertension

Hypotension

Hypovolemic shock

Jaundice

Lesions

Lethargy

Level of consciousness

Local adaptation syndrome (LAS)

Malaise

Memory:
  Long term
  Short term

Mental status

Mobility:
  Balance
  Gait
  Posture
  Strength

Mood
Neuro-checks
Neurovascular assessment
Orientation to time, place, person
Orthostatic hypotension
Pain assessment scales:
    FLACC pain rating scale
    Numerical scales
    Wong-Baker FACES Rating Scale
Parasympathetic nervous system
Physical assessment:
    Auscultation
    Inspection
    Palpation
    Percussion
Pruritus
Pulse sites:
    Apical
    Brachial

Carotid
Femoral
Pedal
Popliteal
Posterior tibial
Temporal
Tibial
Remission
Shivering
Sympathetic nervous system
Temperature sites:
    Axillary
    Oral
    Rectal
    Tympanic
Tremor
Turgor
Urticaria

PHYSICAL ASSESSMENT: QUESTIONS

1. A nurse is assessing a client's bilateral pulses for symmetry. Which pulse site should not be assessed on both sides of the body at the same time?
   1. Radial
   2. Carotid
   3. Femoral
   4. Brachial

2. A nurse is caring for a client who is experiencing an increase in clinical manifestations associated with multiple sclerosis. Which term describes this recurrence of clinical manifestations?
   1. Variance
   2. Remission
   3. Adaptation
   4. Exacerbation

3. When evaluating the vital signs of a group of clients, the nurse takes into consideration the circadian rhythm of body temperature. At which time of day is body temperature usually at its lowest?
   1. 4 p.m. to 6 p.m.
   2. 4 a.m. to 6 a.m.
   3. 8 p.m. to 10 p.m.
   4. 8 a.m. to 10 a.m.

4. Which method of examination is being used when the nurse's hands are used to assess the temperature of a client's skin?
   1. Palpation
   2. Inspection
   3. Percussion
   4. Observation

5. A nurse must assess for the presence of bowel sounds in a postoperative client. Which technique should the nurse employ to obtain accurate results when auscultating the client's abdomen?
   1. Listen for several minutes in each quadrant of the abdomen.
   2. Place a warmed stethoscope on the surface of the abdomen.
   3. Perform auscultation before palpation of the abdomen.
   4. Start at the left lower quadrant of the abdomen.

6. Which assessment requires the nurse to assess the client further?
   1. 18-year-old woman with a pulse rate of 140 after riding 2 miles on an exercise bike
   2. 50-year-old man with a BP of 112/60 mm Hg on awakening in the morning
   3. 65-year-old man with a respiratory rate of 10
   4. 40-year-old woman with a pulse of 88

7. A nurse is monitoring the status of postoperative clients. Which vital sign will change **first** when a postoperative client has internal bleeding?
   1. Body temperature
   2. Blood pressure
   3. Pulse pressure
   4. Heart rate

8. A client has had a 101°F fever for the past 24 hours. How often should the nurse monitor this client's temperature?
   1. Every 2 hours
   2. Every 4 hours
   3. Every 6 hours
   4. Every 8 hours

9. A nurse is unable to palpate a client's brachial pulse. Which pulse should the nurse assess to determine adequate brachial blood flow in this client?
   1. Radial
   2. Carotid
   3. Femoral
   4. Popliteal

10. A nurse is assessing the characteristics of a client's urine. Which of the following can cause urine to appear red?
   1. Beets
   2. Strawberries
   3. Red food dye
   4. Cherry gelatin

11. A nurse is assessing a client's heart rate by palpating the carotid artery. Which action should the nurse implement when assessing a pulse at this site?
   1. Monitor for a full minute.
   2. Palpate just below the ear.
   3. Press gently when palpating the site.
   4. Massage the site before assessing for rate.

12. A nurse obtains the blood pressure of several adults. Which blood pressure result should cause the **most** concern?
   1. 102/70 mm Hg
   2. 140/92 mm Hg
   3. 125/78 mm Hg
   4. 135/85 mm Hg

13. A nurse is planning care for a client who has intolerance to activity. Which is the **first** assessment that should be made by the nurse?
    1. Range of motion
    2. Pattern of vital signs
    3. Impact on functional health patterns
    4. Influence on the other family members

14. A nurse is caring for a client receiving contact isolation. The nurse must take the client's rectal temperature with a plastic thermometer. Which should the nurse do?
    1. Take the temperature for 5 minutes.
    2. Wear gloves throughout the procedure.
    3. Place the client in the right lateral position.
    4. Insert the thermometer 2 inches into the client's anus.

15. Which usually is unrelated to a nursing physical assessment?
    1. Posture and gait
    2. Balance and strength
    3. Hygiene and grooming
    4. Blood and urine values

16. A nurse is performing a psychosocial assessment. Which assessment should be identified as a subtle indicator of depression?
    1. Unkempt appearance
    2. Anxious behavior
    3. Tense posture
    4. Crying

17. A nurse in the emergency department is caring for a client who is diagnosed with hypothermia. Which factor present in the client's history may have precipitated this condition?
    1. Heatstroke
    2. Inability to sweat
    3. Excessive exercise
    4. High alcohol intake

18. Which is common to the collection of all specimens for culture and sensitivity tests regardless of their source?
    1. Preservative media must be used.
    2. Two specimens should be obtained.
    3. Surgical asepsis must be maintained.
    4. A morning specimen should be collected.

19. An adult client's vital signs are: oral temperature 99°F, pulse 88 beats per minute with a regular rhythm, respirations 16 breaths per minute and deep, and blood pressure 182/100 mm Hg. Which sign should cause concern?
    1. Pulse
    2. Respirations
    3. Temperature
    4. Blood pressure

20. A client is admitted to the emergency department with difficulty breathing. Which client response identified by the nurse causes the **most** concern?
    1. Low pulse oximetry
    2. Wheezes on expiration
    3. Shortness of breath on exertion
    4. Use of accessory muscles of respiration

21. When evaluating the vital signs of a group of clients, the nurse takes into consideration the circadian rhythm of body temperature. At which time of day is body temperature usually at its **highest**?
    1. 12 a.m. to 2 a.m.
    2. 6 a.m. to 8 a.m.
    3. 4 p.m. to 6 p.m.
    4. 8 p.m. to 10 p.m.

22. Which physical examination method should a nurse use when assessing a client for borborygmi?
    1. Palpation
    2. Inspection
    3. Percussion
    4. Auscultation

23. Which nursing action is common to all instruments when taking a temperature?
    1. Ensure that the instrument is clean.
    2. Place a disposable sheath over the probe.
    3. Wash with cool soap and water after use.
    4. Check that it is below ninety-six degrees before insertion.

24. A nurse concludes that a client is experiencing pyrexia. Which client assessment precipitated this conclusion?
    1. Mental confusion
    2. Increased appetite
    3. Rectal temperature of 101°F
    4. Heart rate of 50 beats per minute

25. A nurse in the emergency department is engaging in an initial assessment of a client. Which assessment takes **priority**?
    1. Blood pressure
    2. Airway clearance
    3. Breathing pattern
    4. Circulatory status

26. A nurse plans to take a client's radial pulse. Which method of examination should be used by the nurse?
    1. Palpation
    2. Inspection
    3. Percussion
    4. Auscultation

27. The nurse is obtaining a client's blood pressure. Which information is **most** important for the nurse to document?
    1. Staff member who took the blood pressure
    2. Client's tolerance to having the blood pressure taken
    3. Client's body position if the client is not in a sitting position
    4. Which head of a dual-head stethoscope was used to obtain the reading

28. A nurse is teaching a community health class about cancer prevention for people who are asymptomatic and not at risk for cancer. Which screening guideline for this group of people should the nurse include?
    1. Pap smear annually for females 13 years of age and older
    2. Mammogram annually for women 30 years of age and older
    3. Colonoscopy at 50 years of age and every 10 years thereafter
    4. Prostate-specific antigen yearly for men 30 years of age and older

29. A nurse is assessing a client who states, "I feel cold." Which mechanism that helps regulate body temperature will increase body heat?
    1. Vasodilation
    2. Evaporation
    3. Shivering
    4. Radiation

30. Edrophonium IV is administered to a client suspected of having myasthenia gravis. Within 30 seconds after administration of the edrophonium, the client experiences a cholinergic reaction with increased muscle weakness, bradycardia, diaphoresis, and hypotension. The primary health-care provider prescribes atropine sulfate 1 mg IV STAT. The vial of atropine sulfate indicates 0.5 mg/mL. Calculate how many milliliters of atropine sulfate the nurse should administer. **Record your answer using a whole number.**

    Answer: _____ mL.

31. A nurse in the clinic must obtain the vital signs of each client via an electronic thermometer before clients are assessed by the primary health-care provider. Which client characteristic indicates that the nurse should take the client's temperature via the rectal, rather than the oral, route? **Select all that apply.**
    1. _____ Mouth breather
    2. _____ History of vomiting
    3. _____ Presence of confusion
    4. _____ Intolerance of the semi-Fowler position
    5. _____ Intelligence at the level of a seven-year-old child

32. A client with hypertension is given discharge instructions to take the blood pressure every day. A nurse is evaluating a family member taking the client's blood pressure as part of the client's discharge teaching plan. Which behavior indicates that the family member needs additional teaching? **Select all that apply.**
    1. _____ Positions the arm higher than the level of the heart
    2. _____ Places the diaphragm of the stethoscope over the brachial artery
    3. _____ Applies the center of the bladder of the cuff on the lateral aspect of the arm
    4. _____ Releases the valve on the manometer so that the gauge drops 10 mm Hg per heartbeat
    5. _____ Inserts the earpieces of the stethoscope into the ears so that they tilt slightly backward

33. A nurse is caring for a client who sustained trauma in an automobile collision. The nurse makes the following assessments: Does not open the eyes when asked a question but opens eyes and withdraws from painful stimulus when turned and positioned; makes sounds but does not speak words. The nurse uses the Glasgow Coma Scale (GCS) to rate the client's level of consciousness. Which point total on the GCS should the nurse document in the client's clinical record indicating the client's level of consciousness?
    1. 4
    2. 6
    3. 8
    4. 10

GLASGOW COMA SCALE

Eye Opening Points
Eyes open spontaneously: **4 points**
Eyes open in response to voice: **3 points**
Eyes open in response to pain: **2 points**
No eye opening response: **1 point**
Best Verbal Response Points
Oriented (e.g., to person, place, time): **5 points**
Confused, speaks but is disoriented: **4 points**
Inappropriate, but comprehensible words: **3 points**
Incomprehensible sounds, but no words are spoken: **2 points**
None: **1 point**
Best Motor Response Points
Obeys command to move: **6 points**
Localizes painful stimulus: **5 points**
Withdraws from painful stimulus: **4 points**
Flexion, abnormal decorticate posturing: **3 points**
Extension, abnormal decerebrate posturing: **2 points**
No movement or posturing: **1 point**

Total Points
Major Head Injury ≤8
Moderate Head Injury 9–12
Minor Head Injury 13–15

34. A client has a serious vitamin K deficiency. For which clinical manifestation should the nurse assess this client? **Select all that apply.**
    1. _____ Bone pain
    2. _____ Skin lesions
    3. _____ Bleeding gums
    4. _____ Ecchymotic area
    5. _____ Muscle weakness

35. A client has lost approximately 2 units of blood during a vaginal delivery. For which response to this blood loss should the nurse assess this client? **Select all that apply.**
    1. _____ Increased urinary output
    2. _____ Slow, shallow breathing
    3. _____ Hypertension
    4. _____ Tachycardia
    5. _____ Bradypnea

36. A nurse identifies that a client is exhibiting signs of the onset phase (cold or chill phase) of a fever. Which client assessment **supports** this conclusion? **Select all that apply.**

1. _____ Goose bumps on the skin
2. _____ Decreased heart rate
3. _____ Cyanotic nail beds
4. _____ Flushed skin
5. _____ Sweating

37. A nurse is interviewing a newly admitted client. Which word used by the client describes information associated with the defervescence phase (fever abatement, flush phase) of a fever? **Select all that apply.**

1. _____ Cold
2. _____ Achy
3. _____ Warm
4. _____ Sweaty
5. _____ Thirsty

38. A nurse is caring for a client who had surgery for a hysterectomy 2 days ago. After the nurse reviews the client's medical record, which piece of data should cause the nurse the **most** concern?

1. Vomited after eating 6 ounces of soup
2. Respirations: 10 breaths per minute
3. IV infiltration in left hand
4. Temperature: 99.4°F

CLIENT'S CLINICAL RECORD

Primary Health-Care Provider's Prescriptions
Hydromorphone 6 mg PO every 4 hours for severe incisional pain
Acetaminophen 325 mg PO every 4 hours prn for mild incisional pain or 650 mg PO every
   4 hours prn for moderate incisional pain
Diet: Clear liquids, progress to regular as tolerated
Activity: OOB three times a day, ambulate in hallway
Vital signs every 4 hours

Progress Notes
Client progressed to full liquids; full liquids not well tolerated, vomited after eating 6 ounces
of soup; ambulated in hallway 30 feet, tolerated well without signs of activity intolerance.
Administered hydromorphone 6 mg at 4 p.m. for incisional pain reported at level 7 out
of 10. Abdominal dressing dry and intact. IV 0.9% sodium chloride at 100 mL per hour
infiltration in left hand, discontinued and moved to right hand. Warm soak applied
20 minutes to left hand as per protocol.

Vital Signs 6 p.m.
Temperature: 99.4°F, orally
Pulse: 68 beats per minute, regular
Respirations: 10 breaths per minute
Blood pressure: 110/68 mm Hg

39. A nurse concludes that a client has inadequate nutrition. Which client adaptation **supports** this conclusion? **Select all that apply.**
    1. _____ Beefy red and smooth tongue surface
    2. _____ Reddish-pink mucous membranes
    3. _____ Cachectic appearance
    4. _____ Spoon-shaped nails
    5. _____ Shiny eyes

40. A nurse is performing a physical assessment on a newly admitted client. The photograph reflects the condition of the client's tongue. Which nursing intervention should the nurse anticipate will address the origin of this client's problem?
    1. Administering prescribed B vitamins
    2. Providing oral hygiene 4 times a day
    3. Administering prescribed antifungal medication
    4. Encouraging the intake of 3,000 mL of oral fluid daily

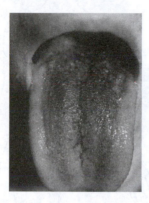

41. A client has an elevated temperature and reports feeling cold. Which additional physical change should the nurse expect during the onset phase (cold or chill phase) of a fever? **Select all that apply.**
    1. _____ Restlessness with confusion
    2. _____ Decreased respiratory rate
    3. _____ Profuse perspiration
    4. _____ Warm skin
    5. _____ Shivering

42. At which day and time did the client have a pulse rate of 75 beats per minute?
    1. 9-9 at 0002
    2. 9-9 at 1800
    3. 9-11 at 0006
    4. 9-10 at 1000

GRAPHIC CHART																							(PT STAMP)
	Date: 9-9						Date: 9-10						Date: 9-11						Date: 9-12				
Hour →	02	06	10	14	18	22	02	06	10	14	18	22	02	06	10	14	18	22	02	06	10	14	18	22

Pulse chart (y-axis Pulse: 60, 70, 80, 90, 100, 110, 120, 130, 140, 150)

43. A nurse is assessing a postoperative client for signs of hemorrhage. Which clinical manifestation is indicative of shock? **Select all that apply.**
1. _____ Hypotension
2. _____ Tachycardia
3. _____ Fast respirations
4. _____ Cold, clammy skin
5. _____ Prolonged capillary refill

44. Place an X over the site in the illustration that is used **most** often by nurses for assessing a client's heart rate.

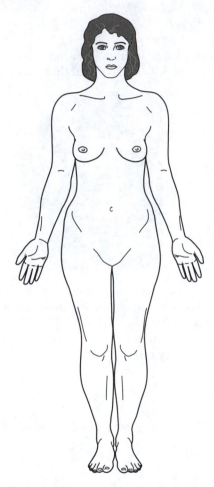

45. A nurse refers to the Glasgow Coma Scale when assessing a client's level of consciousness. Place the following statements related to verbal response in the Glasgow Coma Scale in order from behaviors that support alertness to those that support unresponsiveness.
1. No response
2. Oriented, converses
3. Disoriented, converses
4. Uses inappropriate words
5. Makes incomprehensible sounds

Answer: _____

1. 1. There are no contraindications for palpating both radial arteries at the same time.
   2. **It is unsafe to palpate both carotid arteries at the same time. Slight compression of both carotid arteries can interfere with blood flow to the brain. In addition, excessive compression of the carotid arteries can stimulate the carotid sinuses, which causes a reflex drop in the heart rate.**
   3. There are no contraindications for palpating both femoral arteries at the same time.
   4. There are no contraindications for palpating both brachial arteries at the same time.

2. 1. The word "variance" is not a term that describes recurrence of clinical manifestations of a chronic illness. Variance occurs when there is a deviation from a critical pathway. This occurs when goals are not met or interventions are not performed according to the stipulated time period.
   2. The word "remission" is not a term that describes recurrence of clinical manifestations of a chronic illness. A remission is a period during a chronic illness of lessened severity or cessation of clinical manifestations.
   3. The word "adaptation" is not a term that describes recurrence of clinical manifestations of a chronic illness. An adaptation is a physical or emotional response to an internal or external stimulus.
   4. **An exacerbation is the period during a chronic illness when clinical manifestations reappear after a reduction or absence of clinical manifestations.**

3. 1. Body temperature is rising between 4 p.m. and 6 p.m.
   2. **Diurnal variations (circadian rhythms) vary throughout the day, with the lowest body temperature usually occurring between 4 a.m. and 6 a.m. The metabolic rate is at its lowest while the person is sleeping.**
   3. Body temperature is at its highest between 8 p.m. and 10 p.m.
   4. Body temperature is rising between 8 a.m. and 10 a.m.

4. 1. **Gross temperature assessments (e.g., cold, cool, warm, hot) can be obtained by palpation. Palpation is the examination of the body using the sense of touch. Sensory nerves in the fingers transmit messages through the spinal cord to the cerebral cortex, where they are interpreted by the nurse.**
   2. Inspection cannot assess skin temperature. Inspection uses the naked eye to perform a visual assessment of the body.
   3. Percussion cannot assess skin temperature. Percussion is the act of striking the body's surface to elicit sounds that provide information about the size and shape of internal organs or whether tissue is air filled, fluid filled, or solid.
   4. Observation cannot assess skin temperature. Observation uses the naked eye to perform a visual assessment of the body.

5. 1. This is unnecessary. Bowel sounds may be hyperactive (1 every 3 seconds) or hypoactive (1 every minute). After a few sounds are heard, the stethoscope can be moved to the next site. For sounds to be considered absent, there must be no sounds for 3 to 5 minutes.
   2. This is done for client comfort, not to influence the accuracy of the assessment.
   3. **Bowel sounds are auscultated before palpation and percussion because these techniques stimulate the intestines and thus cause an increase in peristalsis and a false increase in bowel sounds.**
   4. A systematic assessment can begin in any of the four abdominal quadrants. However, many people do begin the systematic four-quadrant assessment in the lower right quadrant over the ileocecal valve, where the digestive contents from the small intestine empty through a valve into the large intestine.

6. 1. This is an acceptable increase in heart rate with strenuous aerobic exercise.
   2. This is an acceptable blood pressure with the body at rest. The expected blood pressure in an adult is a systolic value of less than 120 mm Hg and a diastolic value of less than 80 mm Hg.
   3. **A respiratory rate of 10 is below the expected respiratory rate for an adult and should be assessed further. The expected respiratory rate for an adult is 12 to 20 breaths per minute.**
   4. This is within the expected range of 60 to 100 beats per minute.

7. 1. Although the body temperature decreases as shock progresses because of a decreased metabolic rate, it is not one of the first signs of shock.

2. Two other vital signs will alter before blood pressure as the heart attempts to compensate for decreased circulating blood volume.

3. Although the pulse pressure will narrow during shock, other vital signs will change first. Pulse pressure is the difference between the systolic and diastolic pressures.

4. **The initial stage of shock begins when baroreceptors in the aortic arch and the carotid sinuses detect a drop in the mean arterial pressure. The sympathetic nervous system responds by constricting peripheral vessels and increasing the heart and respiratory rates. During the compensatory stage of shock, the effects of epinephrine and norepinephrine continue with stimulation of alpha-adrenergic fibers, causing vasoconstriction of vessels supplying the skin and abdominal viscera, and beta-adrenergic fibers, causing vasodilation of vessels supplying the heart, skeletal muscles, and respiratory system.**

8. 1. This is too frequent for routine monitoring of body temperature. Although the set-point for body temperature changes rapidly, it takes several hours for the core body temperature to change.

2. **This is an appropriate interval of time for routine monitoring of body temperature. It is frequent enough to identify trends in changes in body temperature while limiting unnecessary assessments.**

3. Every 6 hours is too long an interval for monitoring a client with a fever and is unsafe.

4. Every 8 hours is too long an interval for monitoring a client with a fever and is unsafe.

9. 1. **The brachial artery splits (bifurcates) into the radial and ulnar arteries. When there is an adequate radial pulse, the brachial artery must be patent.**

2. This information will not provide information about brachial artery blood flow. The carotid arteries are in the neck, whereas the brachial arteries are in the arms. A carotid pulse site is located on the neck at the side of the larynx, between the trachea and the sternomastoid muscle.

3. This information will not provide information about brachial artery blood flow. The femoral arteries are in the legs, whereas the brachial arteries are in the arms. A femoral pulse site is in the groin in the femoral triangle. It is in the anterior, medial aspect of the thigh, just below the inguinal ligament, halfway between the anterior superior iliac spine and the symphysis pubis.

4. This information will not provide information about brachial artery blood flow. The popliteal arteries are in the legs, whereas the brachial arteries are in the arms. A popliteal pulse site is in the lateral aspect of the hollow area at the back of the knee (popliteal fossa).

10. 1. **Betacyanin, a pigment that gives beets their purplish red color, is excreted in the urine and feces of some people when it is nonmetabolized (a genetically determined trait). This bright red pigment turns the urine and feces red for several days after eating beets.**

2. Strawberries will not turn the urine red. However, they can cause an allergic reaction (reason is unknown), producing the cellular release of histamine and hives.

3. Red food dye does not turn the urine red. Red dye No. 3, found in foods such as maraschino cherries, is a suspected carcinogen.

4. Red food dye does not turn the urine red. However, red dye No. 3, found in foods such as gelatin desserts and maraschino cherries, is a suspected carcinogen.

11. 1. This is unnecessarily long, and even slight compression can interfere with blood flow to the brain.

2. This is not the site to access the carotid artery. A carotid pulse site is located on the neck at the side of the larynx, between the trachea and the sternomastoid muscle.

3. **The carotid artery should be palpated with a light touch to prevent interference to blood flow to the brain and stimulation of the carotid sinus that can cause a reflex drop in the heart rate.**

4. This is contraindicated. Massage can stimulate the carotid sinus located at the level of the bifurcation of the carotid artery, and this results in a reflex drop in the heart rate.

12. 1. A BP of 102/70 mm Hg is within the acceptable ranges for an adult, which are a systolic of less than 120 mm Hg and a diastolic of less than 80 mm Hg.

2. **A BP of 140/92 mm Hg is considered high-stage II hypertension and is the BP that should cause the most concern. A systolic more than 139 mm Hg or a diastolic more than 89 mm Hg is high-stage II hypertension.**

3. A BP of 125/78 mm Hg is within the parameters of an elevated BP, which is a systolic of 120 to 129 mm Hg and a

diastolic of less than 80 mm Hg. This BP is not as high as a BP in another option.

4. A BP of 135/85 mm Hg is considered high-stage I hypertension. A systolic between 130 and 139 mm Hg or a diastolic between 80 and 90 mm Hg is considered high-stage I hypertension. This is not as high as a BP in another option.

13. 1. Activity intolerance is related to the cardiovascular and respiratory systems, not the nervous and musculoskeletal systems.

2. Activity intolerance is related to the inability to maintain adequate oxygenation to body cells, which is associated with respiratory and cardiovascular problems. Obtaining the vital signs (e.g., pulse, respirations, and blood pressure) will provide valuable information about these systems.

3. Although the impact on functional health patterns might eventually be assessed, it is not the priority.

4. Although the influence on the other family members might eventually be assessed, it is not the priority.

14. 1. A plastic rectal thermometer must remain in place 2 to 4, not 5, minutes to obtain an accurate reading. An electronic thermometer usually will obtain a reading within several seconds.

2. Gloves, personal protective pieces of equipment, are the best way the nurse is protected from contracting or transmitting a pathogen.

3. The left, not right, lateral position is the best position to place a client in when obtaining a rectal temperature because it utilizes the anatomical position of the anus and rectum for safe, easy insertion of the thermometer.

4. Inserting the thermometer 2 inches into the anus can cause damage to the mucous membranes. A lubricated thermometer should be inserted 1.5 inches into the anus to ensure a safe, accurate reading.

15. 1. Assessing posture and gait is within the scope of nursing practice because posture and gait reflect human responses.

2. Assessing balance and strength is within the scope of nursing practice because balance and strength reflect human responses.

3. Assessing hygiene and grooming is within the scope of nursing practice because hygiene and good grooming reflect human responses.

4. Prescribing and assessing urine and blood values are not in the independent practice of nursing. These assessments are dependent or interdependent functions of the nurse and are covered by specific prescriptions or standing prescriptions.

16. **1. When people are depressed, they frequently do not have the physical or psychic energy to perform the activities of daily living and often exhibit an unkempt appearance. A disheveled, untidy appearance is a covert, subtle indication of depression.**

2. Anxious behavior is overt, not covert and subtle.

3. Tense posture is overt, not covert and subtle.

4. Crying is overt, not covert and subtle.

17. 1. Hyperthermia, not hypothermia, is associated with this condition. Heatstroke (heat hyperpyrexia) is failure of the heat-regulating capacity of the body that results in extremely high body temperatures (105°F).

2. Hyperthermia, not hypothermia, can result from the lack of sweat. The inability to perspire does not allow the body to cool by the evaporation of sweat (vaporization).

3. Hyperthermia, not hypothermia, can result from excessive exercise. Exercise increases heat production as carbohydrates and fats break down to provide energy. Body temperature temporarily can increase to as high as 104°F.

4. Excessive alcohol intake interferes with thermoregulation by providing a false sense of warmth, inhibiting shivering, and causing vasodilation, which promotes heat loss. In addition, it impairs judgment, which increases the risk of making inappropriate self-care decisions.

18. 1. This is not necessary for all specimens.

2. Generally, if a specimen is collected using proper technique, one specimen is sufficient for testing for culture and sensitivity.

3. The results of culture and sensitivity tests are faulty and erroneous if the collection container or inappropriate collection technique introduces extraneous microorganisms that falsify and misrepresent results.

Surgical asepsis (sterile technique) must be maintained.
4. This is not necessary for any culture and sensitivity specimen.

19. 1. This is within the expected adult pulse range of 60 to 100 beats per minute and the rhythm is regular; the client should be assessed further and the information compared with the client's baseline data.
2. This is within the expected adult respiratory range of 12 to 20 breaths per minute.
3. This is within the expected adult temperature range of 97.5°F to 99.5°F for an oral temperature.
4. **The blood pressure is more than the expected systolic value of less than 120 mm Hg and a diastolic value of less than 80 mm Hg and, of the options presented, should cause the most concern. A systolic blood pressure of 180 or more and/or a diastolic pressure of 121 or more is in the blood pressure category of Crisis.**

20. 1. **Pulse oximetry is a noninvasive procedure to measure the oxygen saturation of the blood. The expected value is 95% or more. If a client's pulse oximetry result is low, the client is hypoxic and needs medical intervention.**
2. Although wheezing on expiration, which is associated with bronchial constriction, requires continuous monitoring, it is not as critical an assessment as is a clinical manifestation presented in another option. Wheezing on exhalation that increases in severity or wheezing on both inhalation and exhalation becomes a priority in relation to the situation presented.
3. Shortness of breath is an expected response to exertion and is not a cause for concern.
4. Although using accessory muscles of respiration requires monitoring, it is not as critical an assessment as low pulse oximetry. Some people with chronic respiratory problems always use accessory muscles of respiration when breathing.

21. 1. The body temperature is on the decline during this time.
2. The body temperature is just beginning to rise from its lowest level, which occurs between 4 a.m. and 6 a.m.
3. Although the body temperature is rising, it has not reached its peak at this time.

4. **Diurnal variations (circadian rhythms) vary throughout the day, with the highest body temperature usually occurring between 8 p.m. and midnight.**

22. 1. Palpation may stimulate intestinal motility, which increases bowel sounds, but it is not the assessment method used to hear bowel sounds. Palpation is the examination of the body using the sense of touch.
2. Inspection cannot assess bowel sounds. Inspection uses the naked eye to perform a visual assessment of the body.
3. Percussion may stimulate intestinal motility, which increases bowel sounds, but it is not the assessment method used to hear bowel sounds. Percussion is the act of striking the body's surface to elicit sounds that provide information about the size and shape of internal organs or whether tissue is air filled, fluid filled, or solid.
4. **Auscultation is the process of listening to sounds produced in the body. It is performed directly by just listening with the ears or indirectly by using a stethoscope that amplifies the sounds and conveys them to the nurse's ears. Active intestinal peristalsis causes rumbling, gurgling, and tinkling abdominal sounds known as bowel sounds (borborygmi).**

23. 1. **This is an acceptable medical asepsis practice. All instruments, regardless of their type, must be clean before and after use.**
2. This is true only for electronic thermometers and sometimes used for plastic thermometers.
3. This is true only for plastic thermometers.
4. This is not true for all thermometers, such as chemical disposable thermometers, temperature-sensitive tape, and electronic thermometers. This is true for plastic thermometers.

24. 1. Mental confusion is a not a common human response to pyrexia (fever).
2. Loss of appetite (anorexia), not an increased appetite, is a common human response to pyrexia (fever).
3. **A rectal temperature of 101°F (38.3°C) or an oral temperature of 100°F (37.8°C) is a common human response that indicates pyrexia (fever).**
4. An increased heart rate (tachycardia), not a decreased heart rate (bradycardia), is a common human response to pyrexia.

25. 1. Although important, blood pressure is related to circulation, which is not the priority.
2. **Client assessment must always be conducted in order of priority of needs. In an emergency, the ABCs of assessment are airway, breathing, and circulation. A clear airway is essential for life and therefore has priority.**
3. Although important, assessment of a breathing pattern is not the priority.
4. Although important, circulation is not the priority.

26. 1. **Palpation, the examination of the body using the sense of touch, is used to obtain the heart rate at a pulse site. When measuring a pulse, an artery is compressed slightly by the fingers so that the pulsating artery is held between the fingers and a bone or firm structure.**
2. A pulse is not measured by using the sense of sight. Inspection uses the naked eye to perform a visual assessment of the body.
3. Percussion cannot measure a pulse. Percussion is the act of striking the body's surface to elicit sounds that provide information about the size and shape of internal organs or whether tissue is air filled, fluid filled, or solid.
4. Auscultation is used to obtain an apical, not radial, pulse. Auscultation is the process of listening to sounds produced in the body. It is performed directly by just listening with the ears or indirectly by using a stethoscope that amplifies the sounds and conveys them to the nurse's ears.

27. 1. Although this should be done, it is not the most important information.
2. This is necessary only if the client did not tolerate the procedure.
3. **The client's position when the blood pressure is measured may influence results. Generally, systolic and diastolic readings are lower in the horizontal than in the sitting position. There is a lower reading in the uppermost arm when a person is in a lateral recumbent position. A change from the horizontal to an upright position may result in a temporary decrease (5 to 10 mm Hg) in blood pressure; when this decrease exceeds 25 mm Hg systolic or 10 mm Hg diastolic, it is called orthostatic hypotension.**

4. Either the bell or diaphragm of a dual head stethoscope can be used to obtain a blood pressure reading.

28. 1. The American Cancer Society recommends Pap smears screening every 3 years for women between the ages of 21 and 65.
2. The American Cancer Society recommends that women with average breast cancer risk begin yearly mammograms at 45 years of age until 55 years of age and then continue with biennial screening if the client is in good health or has a life expectancy of at least 10 years. However, clients have the option to continue annual screening if desired.
3. **A colonoscopy should be performed at age 50 and every 10 years thereafter for individuals at average risk for developing colorectal cancer. This is the age when the risk for colon cancer increases.**
4. The American Cancer Society recommends that screening for cancer of the prostate be conducted at 50 years of age yearly or on an individual basis. Individuals who are African American or have a family member with the disease before the age of 65 should discuss the need for screening with a primary health-care provider starting at age 40 or 45.

29. 1. Vasodilation brings warm blood to the peripheral circulation, where it is lost through the skin via radiation; this produces heat loss.
2. Evaporation (vaporization) is the conversion of a liquid into a vapor. When perspiration on the skin evaporates, it promotes heat loss.
3. **Shivering generates heat by causing muscle contraction, which increases the metabolic rate by 100% to 200%.**
4. Radiation is the transfer of heat from the surface of one object to the surface of another without direct contact; this produces heat loss.

30. Answer: 2 mL. Solve the question by using ratio and proportion.

$$\frac{\text{Desired}}{\text{Have}} \quad \frac{1\text{mg}}{0.5\text{mg}} = \frac{\text{X mL}}{1\text{mL}}$$
$$0.5\text{x} = 1 \text{ mL}$$
$$\text{x} = 1 \div 0.5$$
$$\text{x} = 2 \text{ mL}$$

31. 1. **Mouth breathing allows environmental air to enter the mouth, which may result in an inaccurately low reading. To take an oral temperature, the**

instrument must remain under the tongue of a closed mouth until the reading is obtained. This can take as little as several seconds (electronic thermometers) or as long as 3 to 4 minutes (plastic thermometers).

2. A history of vomiting does not negate the use of an oral thermometer. If the client should begin to vomit, the nurse can remove the thermometer.

3. **Taking an oral temperature when a client is confused is unsafe. A client who is confused may bite down on an oral thermometer and cause injury to the mouth.**

4. An oral thermometer can be used with a client maintained in any position.

5. A 7-year-old child understands cause and effect and can follow directions regarding the use of an oral thermometer.

32. 1. **A blood pressure reading should be taken with the arm supported at the level of the heart. If the arm is above the level of the heart, the blood pressure reading will be inaccurately decreased, and if the arm is below the level of the heart or not supported, the blood pressure reading will be inaccurately increased.**

2. This is a correct action when obtaining a blood pressure reading. The brachial artery is close to the skin's surface, and the diaphragm of the stethoscope is used for low-pitched sounds of a blood pressure reading.

3. **This is an incorrect placement of the center of the bladder cuff. The bladder of the cuff should be directly over the brachial artery. This ensures an accurate reading because it provides uniform and complete compression of the brachial artery.**

4. This may result in an inaccurate reading. The valve on the manometer should be opened to allow the gauge to drop 2 to 3 mm Hg per heartbeat.

5. **The earpieces of the stethoscope should be placed into the ears so that they tilt slightly forward, not backward. This ensures that the openings in the earpieces of the stethoscope are facing toward the ear canal for uninterrupted transmission of sounds.**

33. 1. The number 4 does not reflect the client's total points on the Glasgow Coma Scale.

2. The number 6 does not reflect the client's total points on the Glasgow Coma Scale.

3. **The number 8 reflects the client's total points on the Glasgow Coma Scale, as demonstrated in the scale below.**

4. The number 10 does not reflect the client's total points on the Glasgow Coma Scale.

GLASGOW COMA SCALE

Eye Opening Points
Eyes open spontaneously: **4 points**
Eyes open in response to voice: **3 points**
Eyes open in response to pain: **2 points**
No eye opening response: **1 point**
Best Verbal Response Points
Oriented (e.g., to person, place, time): **5 points**
Confused, speaks but is disoriented: **4 points**
Inappropriate, but comprehensible words: **3 points**
Incomprehensible sounds, but no words are spoken: **2 points**
None: **1 point**
Best Motor Response Points
Obeys command to move: **6 points**
Localizes painful stimulus: **5 points**
Withdraws from painful stimulus: **4 points**
Flexion, abnormal decorticate posturing: **3 points**
Extension, abnormal decerebrate posturing: **2 points**
No movement or posturing: **1 point**

Total Points 8
Major Head Injury ≤8
Moderate Head Injury 9–12
Minor Head Injury 13–15

34. 1. A deficiency in vitamin D, not vitamin K, causes bone pain associated with osteoporosis.

2. Vitamin K deficiency is not associated with skin lesions. Ascorbic acid (vitamin C) deficiency causes small skin hemorrhages and delays wound healing. Riboflavin (vitamin B_2) deficiency causes lip lesions, seborrheic dermatitis, and scrotal and vulval skin changes.

3. **A disruption in the clotting mechanism of the body can result in bleeding. Vitamin K plays an essential role in the production of the clotting factors II (prothrombin), VII, IX, and X.**

4. **An ecchymotic area is caused by extravasation of blood into skin or mucous membranes. In this client's situation, it is caused by a disruption in the clotting mechanism of the body as a result of a vitamin K deficiency.**

5. A deficiency in thiamine (vitamin B_1), not vitamin K, causes muscle weakness.

35. 1. With a reduction in blood volume, there will be less blood circulating through the kidneys, resulting in a decreased, not increased, urinary output.

2. With a decrease in circulating red blood cells, the respiratory rate will increase to meet oxygen needs.

3. With a reduction in blood volume, the blood pressure will be decreased, not increased.

4. **Tachycardia occurs with hemorrhage as the body attempts to bring more oxygen to cells via the circulation.**

5. Rapid breathing, not bradypnea, occurs with hemorrhage as the respiratory rate increases to meet oxygen needs.

36. 1. **Contraction of the *arrector pili* muscles (goose bumps), an attempt by the body to trap air around body hairs, is associated with the onset phase (cold or chill phase) of a fever. During this phase, the body responds to pyrogens by conserving heat to raise the body's temperature and reset the body's thermostat.**

2. During the onset phase (cold or chill phase) of a fever, the heart and respiratory rates increase, not decrease.

3. **Cyanosis of the nail beds occurs during the onset phase (cold or chill phase) of a fever. Vasoconstriction and shivering are the body's attempt to conserve heat.**

4. Flushed skin occurs during the defervescence phase (fever abatement, flush phase) of a fever as the hypothalamus attempts to lower the body's temperature. Quick vasodilation occurs, which helps to cool the body.

5. Profuse diaphoresis (sweating) occurs during the defervescence phase (fever abatement, flush phase) of a fever as the hypothalamus attempts to lower the body's temperature. During this phase, the fever abates and the body's temperature returns to the expected range.

37. 1. Feeling cold occurs during the onset phase (cold or chill phase) of a fever because of vasoconstriction, cool skin, and shivering.

2. Feeling achy occurs during the course phase (plateau phase) of a fever. Generally, this is the result of extra energy being exerted by the body fighting the infection, as well as a response to activation of the immune system.

3. **Feeling warm is associated with the defervescence phase (fever abatement, flush phase) of a fever because of sudden vasodilation.**

4. **Feeling sweaty occurs during the defervescence phase (fever abatement, flush phase) of a fever because of the body's heat loss response.**

5. Feeling thirsty is associated with the course phase (plateau phase) of a fever because of mild to severe dehydration.

38. 1. Although vomiting is a concern, it is not as important as information presented in another option. The client is receiving 100 mL of fluid hourly; therefore, the client is most likely adequately hydrated.

2. **A respiratory rate of 10 or below is a concern. The client is receiving hydromorphone, an opioid, which depresses the central nervous system. A respiratory rate is depressed when an opioid medication is excessive. The dose of hydromorphone may need to be reduced.**

3. Although an IV infiltration is a concern, it is not as important as data presented in another option. The IV was discontinued and replaced in the other hand, and a warm soak was applied to the site of the infiltration.

4. Although an increase in temperature after surgery is a concern, an oral temperature of 99.4°F is within the expected range of 97.5°F to 99.5°F.

39. 1. The tongue usually is pink, moist, and smooth, with papillae and fissures present. A beefy red or magenta color, smooth appearance, and increase or decrease in size indicate nutritional problems.

2. This is the usual color of mucous membranes because of their rich vascular supply. Pale mucous membranes or the presence of lesions indicates nutritional problems.

3. Cachexia is general ill health and malnutrition marked by weakness and excessive leanness (emaciation).

4. Fingernails that curve inward like spoons can be caused by iron deficiency, vitamin B$_{12}$ deficiency, or anemia.

5. The eyes are always moist and shiny because lacrimal fluid continually washes the eyes. Pale or red conjunctivae, dryness, and soft or dull corneas are signs of nutritional problems.

40. 1. The client is not exhibiting the signs of a vitamin B deficiency. B vitamins treat fissures and cracking at the corners of the mouth (cheilosis) caused by a deficiency of B vitamins.

2. Providing oral hygiene four times a day will not address the origin of this client's problem.

3. The photograph demonstrates a human response to a fungal infection in the oral cavity. When documenting this assessment, the nurse should describe this client's tongue as a "black, hairy tongue," which is characteristic of an oral fungal infection.

4. Encouraging an increase in the intake of oral fluids does not address the origin of this client's problem.

41. 1. Restlessness with confusion may indicate the beginning of delirium associated with high fevers that alter cerebral functioning. Delirium is associated with the course phase (plateau phase) of a fever.

2. During the onset phase (cold or chill phase) of a fever, the pulse and respiratory rates increase as the body attempts to achieve the new set-point.

3. Profuse diaphoresis (sweating) occurs during the defervescence phase (fever abatement, flush phase) of a fever.

4. Pale, cold skin occurs during the onset phase of a fever. Warm skin occurs with flushing due to vasodilation during the defervescence phase (fever abatement, flush phase) of a fever.

5. Shivering occurs during the onset phase (cold or chill phase) of a fever. Fever is caused by the release of inflammatory mediators (pyrogens) that cause the hypothalamus to reset the set-point of temperature. When this happens, the body feels cold, and shivering occurs. Shivering involves muscle contraction that produces heat, which increases the temperature to the new hypothalamic set-point.

42. 1. On 9-9 at 0002, the client's pulse rate was 65 beats per minute.

2. On 9-9 at 1800, the client's pulse rate was 75 beats per minute.

3. On 9-11 at 0006, the client's pulse rate was 65 beats per minute.

4. On 9-10 at 1000, the client's pulse rate was 90 beats per minute.

GRAPHIC CHART																								(PT STAMP)

Date: 9-9						Date: 9-10						Date: 9-11						Date: 9-12					

Hour →	02	06	10	14	18	22	02	06	10	14	18	22	02	06	10	14	18	22	02	06	10	14	18	22

Pulse: 150, 140, 130, 120, 110, 100, 90, 80, 70, 60

43. 1. The circulating blood volume is reduced by 25% to 35% during the compensatory stage of shock and by 35% to 50% during the progressive stage of shock as the peripheral vessels constrict to increase blood flow to vital organs. This shunting of blood causes hypotension.
  2. The heart rate increases (tachycardia) during the compensatory stage of shock to maintain adequate blood flow to body tissues.
  3. During the compensatory stage of shock, the respiratory rate increases to maintain adequate oxygenation of body cells.
  4. With hemorrhage, there is a decrease in blood pressure as a result of hypovolemia, which in turn stimulates the sympathetic nervous system. The sympathetic nervous system stimulates vasoconstriction, which moves blood from the periphery of the body to vital organs. The decrease in circulation to the skin causes it to become cold and clammy.
  5. Prolonged capillary refill occurs with shock because of reduced circulating blood volume (hypovolemia) due to blood loss.

44. The radial pulse is the most easily found and accessible site for routine monitoring of the pulse, and it provides accurate information when the heart rate is regular. The radial pulse site is where the radial artery runs along the radial bone, on the thumb side of the inner aspect of the wrist.

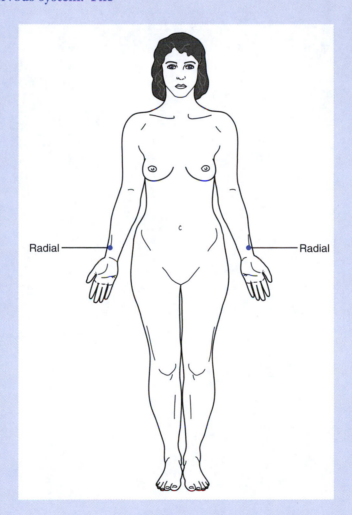

Radial ——   —— Radial

45. 2. *Oriented and converses* is rated 5, the highest level of functioning of the five levels in the Best Verbal Response category of the Glasgow Coma Scale.
3. *Disoriented and converses* is rated 4 out of five levels of functioning and is after *oriented and converses*, level 5 in the Best Verbal Response category of the Glasgow Coma Scale.
4. *Uses inappropriate words* is rated 3 out of five levels of functioning and is after *disoriented and converses*, level 4 in the Best Verbal Response category of the Glasgow Coma Scale.
5. *Makes incomprehensible sounds* is rated 2 out of five levels of functioning and is after *uses inappropriate words*, level 3 in the Best Verbal Response category of the Glasgow Coma Scale.
1. *No response* is rated 1, the lowest level of the five levels of functioning, and is after *makes incomprehensible sounds*, level 2 in the Best Verbal Response category of the Glasgow Coma Scale.

Infection Control

KEYWORDS

The following words include nursing/medical terminology, concepts, principles, and information relevant to content specifically addressed in the chapter or associated with topics presented in it. English dictionaries, nursing textbooks, and medical dictionaries, such as *Taber's Cyclopedic Medical Dictionary*, are resources that can be used to expand your knowledge and understanding of these words and related information.

Afebrile
Antibiotics
Antibody
Antigen
Antimicrobial
Antipyretic
Asepsis:
   Medical
   Surgical
Biohazardous
Chain of infection:
   Infectious agent
   Mode of transmission
   Portal of entry
   Portal of exit
   Reservoir
   Susceptible host
Culture and sensitivity
Débridement
Drainage, exudate:
   Purulent, pus
   Sanguineous
   Serosanguineous
   Serous
Endotoxin
Erythema
Fever (febrile, pyrexia)
General adaptation syndrome (GAS)
Healing:
   Primary intention
   Secondary intention
Hyperthermia

Immune response
Immune system
Immunity
Immunization
Immunocompromised
Immunosuppression
Inflammatory response
Infection, types:
   Health-care–associated infection (HAI)
     (formerly called nosocomial infection)
   Iatrogenic
   Local
   Opportunistic
   Systemic
Leukocytosis
Local adaptation syndrome (LAS)
Microorganisms:
   Bacteria
   Fungi
   Viruses
Neutropenia
Ova and parasites
Pediculosis
Phagocytosis
Pyrogens
Standard precautions
Transmission-based precautions:
   Airborne precautions
   Contact precautions
   Droplet precautions
White blood cell count

INFECTION CONTROL: QUESTIONS

1. Which is the **primary** reason why the nurse should avoid glued-on artificial nails?
   1. They interfere with dexterity of the fingers.
   2. They could fall off in a client's bed.
   3. They harbor microorganisms.
   4. They can scratch a client.

2. A nurse working in a clinic is assessing clients of a variety of ages. Which age group should the nurse particularly assess for subtle clinical manifestations of subclinical infections?
   1. Children of school age
   2. Older adults
   3. Adolescents
   4. Infants

3. Which condition places a client at the **highest** risk for developing an infection?
   1. Implantation of a prosthetic device
   2. Burns over more than 20% of the body
   3. Presence of an indwelling urinary catheter
   4. More than 2 puncture sites from laparoscopic surgery

4. Which does the nurse determine is a specific line of defense against infection?
   1. Mucous membrane of the respiratory tract
   2. Urinary tract environment
   3. Integumentary system
   4. Immune response

5. A nurse is concerned about a client's ability to withstand exposure to pathogens. Which blood component should the nurse monitor?
   1. Platelets
   2. Hemoglobin
   3. Neutrophils
   4. Erythrocytes

6. When brushing a client's hair, the nurse identifies white oval particles attached to the hair behind the ears. Which condition with additional clinical manifestations that support it should lead the nurse to assess the client further?
   1. Pediculosis
   2. Hirsutism
   3. Dandruff
   4. Scabies

7. A nurse educator is evaluating whether a new staff nurse understands the relationship between a fever and an infection. Which statement by the new staff nurse indicates an understanding of this relationship?
   1. "Phagocytic cells release pyrogens that stimulate the hypothalamus."
   2. "Leukocyte migration precipitates the inflammatory response."
   3. "Erythema increases the flow of blood throughout the body."
   4. "Pain activates the sympathetic nervous system."

8. A nurse is caring for a group of clients with infections. Which infection is classified as a health-care–associated infection?
   1. Respiratory infection contracted from a visitor
   2. Vaginal infection in a postmenopausal woman
   3. Urinary tract infection in a client who is sedentary
   4. Wound infection caused by unwashed hands of a caregiver

9. A nurse is caring for a client with a high fever secondary to septicemia. The primary health-care provider prescribes a cooling blanket (hypothermia blanket). Through which mechanism does the hypothermia blanket achieve heat loss?
   1. Radiation
   2. Convection
   3. Conduction
   4. Evaporation

10. Which client condition identified by a nurse is unrelated to infection?
    1. Catabolism
    2. Hyperglycemia
    3. Ketones in the urine
    4. Decreased metabolic activity

11. A nurse is caring for a group of hospitalized clients. Which should the nurse do **first** to prevent client infections?
    1. Provide small bedside bags to dispose of used tissues.
    2. Encourage staff to avoid coughing near clients.
    3. Administer antibiotics as prescribed.
    4. Identify clients at risk.

12. A client has a wound that is healing by secondary intention. Which solution to cleanse the wound and dressing should the nurse expect will be prescribed to **support** wound healing?
    1. Normal saline and a gauze dressing
    2. Normal saline and a wet-to-damp dressing
    3. Povidone-iodine and a dry sterile dressing
    4. Half peroxide and half normal saline and a wet-to-dry dressing

13. A nurse is caring for a group of clients experiencing various medical conditions. Which condition places the client at the **highest** risk for a wound infection?
    1. Surgical creation of a colostomy
    2. First-degree burn on the back
    3. Puncture of the foot by a nail
    4. Paper cut on the finger

14. A school nurse is teaching a class of adolescents about the function of the integumentary system. Which fact about how the skin protects the body against infection is important to include in this discussion?
    1. Cells of the skin are constantly being replaced, thereby eliminating external pathogens.
    2. Epithelial cells are loosely compacted on skin, providing a barrier against pathogens.
    3. Moisture on the skin surface prevents colonization of pathogens.
    4. Alkalinity of the skin limits the growth of pathogens.

15. A client's stool specimen is positive for *Clostridium difficile*. Which isolation precautions should the nurse institute for this client?
    1. Droplet
    2. Contact
    3. Reverse
    4. Airborne

16. Which should the nurse do to interrupt the transmission link in the chain of infection?
    1. Wash the hands before providing care to a client.
    2. Position a commode next to a client's bed.
    3. Provide education about a balanced diet.
    4. Change a dressing when it is soiled.

17. Which client statement indicates that further teaching by the nurse is necessary regarding how to ensure protection from food contamination? **Select all that apply.**
    1. _____ "I should stuff a turkey immediately before putting it in the oven."
    2. _____ "I love juicy, rare hamburgers with onion and tomato."
    3. _____ "I prefer chicken salad sandwiches with mayonnaise."
    4. _____ "I know to spit out food that does not taste good."
    5. _____ "I should defrost frozen food in the refrigerator."

18. A client is admitted to the ambulatory surgery unit for an elective procedure. When performing a physical assessment, the nurse identifies that the client has *Pediculus capitis* (head lice). Place the nurse's interventions in the order in which they should be implemented.
1. Establish contact isolation.
2. Comb the hair with a fine-toothed comb.
3. Notify the provider of the client's condition.
4. Obtain a prescription for a pediculicidal shampoo.
5. Wash the client's hair with a pediculicidal shampoo.

Answer: _____

19. Which primary defense protects the body from infection? **Select all that apply.**
1. _____ Tears in the eyes
2. _____ Healthy, intact skin
3. _____ Cilia of respiratory passages
4. _____ Acidity of gastric secretions
5. _____ Dry environment of the epidermis

20. A nurse is caring for clients with a variety of wounds. Which wound will likely heal by primary intention? **Select all that apply.**
1. _____ Cut in the skin from a kitchen knife
2. _____ Excoriated perianal area
3. _____ Abrasion of the skin
4. _____ Surgical incision
5. _____ Pressure ulcer

21. The nurse seeks to limit the presence of mosquitoes that carry the Zika virus. The nurse teaches strategies to prevent standing water inside and outside of homes of community members. Place an X in the center of the link that is concerned with these strategies.

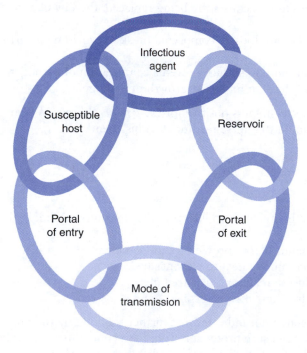

22. A client has a wound infection. Which local human response should the nurse expect to identify? **Select all that apply.**
    1. _____ Leukocytosis
    2. _____ Malaise
    3. _____ Edema
    4. _____ Fever
    5. _____ Pain

23. Which nursing action protects clients as susceptible hosts in the chain of infection? **Select all that apply.**
    1. _____ Wearing personal protective equipment
    2. _____ Administering childhood immunizations
    3. _____ Recapping a used needle before discarding
    4. _____ Instituting prescribed immunoglobulin therapy
    5. _____ Disposing of soiled gloves in a waste container

24. From which type of isolation precaution is this mask designed to protect the nurse?

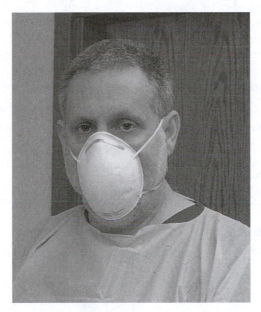

    1. Contact
    2. Airborne
    3. Standard
    4. Protective

25. A client tells the nurse, "I think I have an ear infection." For which objective human response to an ear infection should the nurse assess this client? **Select all that apply.**
    1. _____ Throbbing pain
    2. _____ Purulent drainage
    3. _____ Feeling of pressure
    4. _____ Dizziness when moving
    5. _____ Hearing a buzzing sound

26. Which is an example of a primary defense that protects the body from infection? **Select all that apply.**
    1. _____ Antibiotic therapy
    2. _____ Lysozymes in saliva
    3. _____ The low pH of the skin
    4. _____ The acidic environment of the vagina
    5. _____ Production of mucus by cells in the genitourinary tract

27. A nurse is caring for a client who has a prescription for shortening a Penrose drain 1 inch daily. The nurse washes the hands, removes the soiled dressing, sets a sterile field, dons sterile gloves, and cleans around the drain with sterile saline solution as prescribed. Place the following steps in the order in which they should be implemented by the nurse.
   1. Complete dressing the wound.
   2. Pull the drain out 1 inch, gently and steadily.
   3. Grip the Penrose drain with a pair of sterile forceps.
   4. Remove the pin and reattach it to the drain closer to the surface of the wound.
   5. Cut off the excess drain using sterile scissors, ensuring that 2 inches remain outside the wound.

   Answer: _____

28. Which nursing action protects clients from infection at the portal of entry portion of the chain of infection? **Select all that apply.**
   1. _____ Positioning an indwelling urine collection bag below the level of the client's pelvis
   2. _____ Using sterile technique when administering an intramuscular injection
   3. _____ Enclosing a urine specimen in a biohazardous transport bag
   4. _____ Wearing clean gloves when handling a client's excretions
   5. _____ Washing the hands after removal of soiled gloves
   6. _____ Maintaining a dressing over a surgical incision

29. The nurse is reviewing the clinical record of a newly admitted older adult male client. Which piece of information should cause the **most** concern?
   1. Temperature 103°F
   2. Abdominal cramping
   3. WBC 30,000 cells/mcL
   4. Blood pressure 110/86 mm Hg

CLIENT'S CLINICAL RECORD

Laboratory Results
WBC: 30,000 cells/mcL
Hct: 52%
Hb: 13 g/dL

Emergency Department Nurse's Admission Note
Client reports feeling overwhelming fatigue, anorexia, "high" fevers, burning on urination, "frequently urinating small amounts," and abdominal cramping. States that these signs and symptoms have progressively worsened over the last few days.

Vital Signs
Pulse: 100 beats per minute, regular
Temperature (oral): 103°F
Respirations: 24 breaths per minute
Blood pressure: 110/86 mm Hg

30. A nurse identifies that a client has an inflammatory response. Which localized client response **supports** this conclusion? **Select all that apply.**
   1. _____ Fever
   2. _____ Swelling
   3. _____ Erythema
   4. _____ Bradypnea
   5. _____ Tachycardia

31. A nurse must collect the following specimens. Which specimen does not require the use of surgical aseptic technique? **Select all that apply.**
    1. _____ Stool for occult blood
    2. _____ Stool for ova and parasites
    3. _____ Oropharyngeal mucus for a culture
    4. _____ Urine from a retention catheter for a urinalysis
    5. _____ Exudate from a wound for culture and sensitivity

32. A nurse plans to remove a client's wound dressing. The nurse identifies the client, explains what is going to be done and why, washes the hands, collects equipment, provides for the client's privacy, and places the client in an appropriate and comfortable position. Place the following steps in the order in which they should be implemented when removing the soiled dressing.
    1. Don clean gloves.
    2. Pull the tape away from the skin gently.
    3. Assess the volume, color, and odor of exudate.
    4. Place the soiled dressing and gloves in a biohazardous waste receptacle.
    5. Remove the dressing by lifting the edge of the dressing upward and toward the center of the wound.
    6. Loosen the edges of the tape around the dressing, starting from the outside and moving toward the center of the dressing.

    Answer: _____

33. Which client information collected by the nurse reflects a systemic response to a wound infection? **Select all that apply.**
    1. _____ Increased body temperature
    2. _____ Increased heart rate
    3. _____ Leukocytosis
    4. _____ Fatigue
    5. _____ Chills

34. A nurse is caring for a client who has a prescription for a vacuum-assisted closure device using black foam to facilitate wound healing. The nurse verifies the prescription, explains to the client what is to be done and why, gathers equipment, washes the hands, sets a sterile field, and dons sterile gloves. Place the following steps in the order in which they should be implemented.
    1. Trim the black foam to the size of the wound cavity.
    2. Pinch and cut a 2-cm round hole in the center of the transparent film.
    3. Connect the suction device tubing to the collection canister tubing and pump.
    4. Place the foam in the wound cavity without overlapping onto the surrounding skin.
    5. Place the suction device pad over the hole in the film and apply gentle pressure to the suction device pad.
    6. Apply the transparent film 1 to 2 inches beyond wound edges without stretching or wrinkling the transparent film.

    Answer: _____

35. A primary health-care provider prescribes azithromycin for a client with a diagnosis of chronic bronchitis. Which should the nurse teach the client that is important to know about taking azithromycin? **Select all that apply.**
    1. _____ "Take this medication with food."
    2. _____ "You can discontinue the medication as soon as you feel better."
    3. _____ "Take 500 mg on the first day and then 250 mg for 4 more days, for a total of 1.5 g."
    4. _____ "The first dose should be taken after we notify you of the results of the culture and sensitivity."
    5. _____ "Avoid taking an antacid containing aluminum or magnesium within 2 hours of taking this medication."

1. 1. Artificial nails do not interfere with finger dexterity if kept at a reasonable length (not longer than 1/4 inch beyond the end of the finger).
   2. Although an artificial nail falling off in a client's bed is a concern, it is not the main reason why artificial nails should be avoided.
   3. **Studies have demonstrated that artificial nails, especially when cracked, broken, or split, provide crevices in which microorganisms can grow and multiply and therefore should be avoided by direct care providers.**
   4. When artificial nails are cared for so that they remain intact and free of cracks or breaks, they should not scratch the skin.

2. 1. School-age children generally respond to infections with acute clinical manifestations that are identified easier and earlier than in an age group in another option.
   2. **Infections are more difficult to identify in the older adult because the clinical manifestations are not as acute and obvious as in other age groups. This outcome occurs as a result of the decline in all body systems related to aging.**
   3. Adolescents generally respond to infections with acute clinical manifestations that are identified more easily and earlier than in an age group in another option.
   4. Infants generally respond to infections with acute clinical manifestations that are identified more easily and earlier than in an age group in another option.

3. 1. Although wound infections can occur when prosthetic devices are implanted, they are surgically implanted under sterile conditions to minimize this risk.
   2. **Burns on more than 20% of a person's total body surface generally are considered major burn injuries. When the skin is damaged by a burn, the underlying tissue is left unprotected, and the individual is at risk for infection. The greater the extent and the deeper the depth of the burn, the higher the risk for infection is.**
   3. Although urinary tract infections can occur with an indwelling urinary catheter, these catheters are closed systems in which sterile technique is maintained; this minimizes the risk for infection.

   4. Laparoscopic surgery is performed using sterile technique to minimize the risk of infection.

4. 1. Protective mechanisms in the respiratory tract provide a nonspecific defense against pathogenic microorganisms. Primary defenses are nonspecific immune defenses that are anatomical, mechanical, or chemical barriers. In the respiratory tract, they include intact mucous membranes, mucus, bactericidal enzymes, cilia, sneezing, and coughing.
   2. Protective mechanisms in the urinary tract environment provide a nonspecific line of defense against pathogenic microorganisms. These defenses include intact mucous membranes, urine flowing out of the body, and urine acidity.
   3. Skin provides a nonspecific defense against pathogenic microorganisms. These defenses include intact skin, surface acidity, and the usual flora that is found on the skin.
   4. **The immune response is a specific defense against pathogenic microorganisms. The production of antibodies to neutralize and eliminate pathogens and their toxins (immune response) is activated when phagocytes fail to completely destroy invading microorganisms. The nonspecific defenses (anatomical and physiological barriers, inflammatory response, and vascular and cellular responses) work in harmony with the specific immune response to defend the body from pathogenic microorganisms.**

5. 1. Platelets are essential for blood clotting and are unrelated to an individual's ability to withstand exposure to pathogens.
   2. Hemoglobin is the part of the red blood cell that carries oxygen from the lungs to the tissues and is unrelated to the assessment of an individual's ability to withstand exposure to pathogens.
   3. **Neutrophils, the most numerous leukocytes (white blood cells), are a primary defense against infection because they ingest and destroy microorganisms (phagocytosis). When the leukocyte count is low, it indicates a compromised ability to fight infection.**
   4. Red blood cells (erythrocytes) do not reflect an individual's ability to withstand exposure to pathogens. Erythrocytes transport oxygen via hemoglobin molecules.

6. 1. Pediculosis (*Pediculus humanus capitis*) is characterized by white oval particles attached to the hair. When this condition is identified, the nurse should assess the client further for the presence of scratch marks on the scalp and by asking the client if the head feels itchy. Also, the nurse must assess the extent of infestation and if any other areas of the body are infested with other types of lice (*P. humanus corporis* [body hair] and *Phthirus pubis* [pubic and axillary hair]). A client with this infestation should be on contact isolation to prevent spread of the infestation to others.

2. White oval particles attached to hair are not indicative of hirsutism. Hirsutism is the excessive growth of hair or hair growth in unusual places, particularly in female clients. In female clients, usually it is caused by excessive androgen production or metabolic abnormalities.

3. White oval particles attached to hair are not indicative of dandruff. Dandruff is the excessive shedding of dry white scales as a result of the expected exfoliation of the epidermis of the scalp. Dandruff scales do not attach to the hair and are easily brushed away from the hair shaft.

4. White oval particles attached to hair are not indicative of scabies. Scabies is a communicable skin disease caused by an itch mite (*Sarcoptes scabiei*) and is characterized by skin lesions (e.g., small papules, pustules, excoriations, and burrows ending in a vesicle) with intense itching.

7. 1. Microorganisms or endotoxins (lipopolysaccharides that are a component of the cell wall of gram-negative bacteria) stimulate phagocytic cells, which release pyrogens that stimulate the hypothalamic thermoregulatory center, causing fever.

2. Leukocyte migration does not precipitate the inflammatory response, but it is a phase of the inflammatory response. White blood cells reach a wound within a few hours after the injury to ingest bacteria and clean a wound of debris through the process of phagocytosis.

3. Erythema does not increase the flow of blood throughout the body. Increased blood flow to a localized area causes diffuse redness (erythema).

4. Pain does not cause an increase in body temperature directly.

8. 1. A respiratory infection contracted from a visitor is not an example of an infection that directly resulted from a diagnostic or therapeutic procedure.

2. A vaginal infection in a postmenopausal woman is not an example of an infection that directly resulted from a diagnostic or therapeutic procedure.

3. A urinary tract infection in a client who is sedentary is not an example of an infection that directly resulted from a diagnostic or therapeutic procedure.

4. A health-care–associated infection (iatrogenic) directly results from a diagnostic or therapeutic procedure. When a caregiver does not wash his/her hands, thereby transmitting a pathogen that causes a wound infection, the result is an iatrogenic infection.

9. 1. Radiation is not related to heat loss via a cooling (hypothermia) blanket. Radiation is heat loss from one surface to another surface without direct contact.

2. Convection is not related to heat loss via a cooling (hypothermia) blanket. Convection is the loss of heat as a result of the motion of cool air flowing over a warm body. The heat is carried away by air currents that are cooler than the warm body.

3. Conduction is the transfer of heat from a warm object (skin) to a cooler object (hypothermia blanket) during direct contact.

4. Evaporation is unrelated to heat loss via a cooling (hypothermia) blanket. Evaporation is the conversion of a liquid to a vapor, which occurs when perspiration on the skin is vaporized. For each gram of water that evaporates from the skin, approximately 0.6 of a calorie of heat is lost.

10. 1. Catabolism, the destructive phase of metabolism with its resultant release of energy, is related to infection.

2. Serum glucose is increased (hyperglycemia) in the presence of an infection because of the release of glucocorticoids associated with the general adaptation syndrome.

3. The presence of ketones in the urine, a sign that the body is using fat as a source of energy, is related to infection because of the associated increased need for calories for fighting the infection.

4. Metabolic activity increases, not decreases, with an infection as the body mounts a defense to fight invading pathogenic microorganisms.

11. 1. Although this is something the nurse may provide to contain soiled tissues, it is not the first action the nurse should implement to prevent infection.
 2. Although this is something the nurse may do to limit airborne or droplet transmission of microorganisms, it is not the first action the nurse should implement to prevent infection.
 3. Antibiotics generally are prescribed for clients who have infections. However, antibiotics occasionally are prescribed prophylactically.
 4. **This is the most important first step in the prevention of infection. A client who is at risk to transmit an infection or at risk to be physiologically unable to protect the self from infection may require the institution of special precautions (e.g., transmission-based precautions, protective isolation).**

12. 1. Although normal saline is appropriate for cleansing a wound, removal of a gauze dressing that is dry will pull recently granulated tissue off of the wound bed, impeding wound healing.
 2. **Cleaning with normal saline will not damage fibroblasts. Wet-to-damp dressings allow epidermal cells to migrate more rapidly across the wound surface than dry dressings, thereby facilitating wound healing.**
 3. Povidone-iodine is cytotoxic and should not be used on clean granulating wounds. Removal of a dressing that is dry will pull recently granulated tissue off of the wound bed, impeding wound healing.
 4. Hydrogen peroxide is cytotoxic and should not be used on clean granulating wounds. Removal of a dressing that has dried on a wound will pull recently granulated tissue off of the wound bed.

13. 1. Surgery is conducted using sterile technique. In addition, preoperative preparation of the bowel helps to reduce the presence of organisms that have the potential to cause infection.
 2. There is no break in the skin in a first-degree burn; therefore, there is less of a risk for a wound infection than an example in another option.
 3. **Of all the options presented, puncture of the foot by a nail has the greatest risk for a wound infection. A nail is a soiled object that has the potential of introducing pathogens into a deep**

wound that can trap them under the surface of the skin, a favorable environment for multiplication.
 4. Paper generally is not heavily soiled, and the wound edges are approximated. This is less of a risk than an example in another option.

14. 1. **Epithelial cells of the skin are regularly shed, along with potentially dangerous microorganisms that adhere to the skin's outer layers, thereby reducing the risk of infection.**
 2. Epithelial cells on the skin are closely, not loosely, compacted, providing a barrier against pathogens.
 3. Moisture on the skin surface facilitates, not prevents, colonization of pathogens.
 4. Acidity, not alkalinity, of the skin limits the growth of pathogens.

15. 1. Droplet precautions are used for clients who have an illness transmitted by particle droplets larger than 5 μm (micrometers), such as mumps, rubella, pharyngeal diphtheria, *Mycoplasma* pneumonia, pertussis, streptococcal pharyngitis, and pneumonic plague.
 2. **Contact precautions are used for clients who have an illness transmitted by direct contact or with items contaminated by the client. Examples include gastrointestinal, respiratory, skin, or wound infections or colonization with drug-resistant bacteria (including *Clostridium difficile, Escherichia coli, and Shigella*). Contact precautions also are used for other infections/ infestations, such as hepatitis A, herpes simplex virus, impetigo, pediculosis, scabies, syncytial virus, and parainfluenza.**
 3. Reverse precautions, also known as neutropenic precautions or protective isolation, are used for clients who are immunocompromised. Isolation practices are employed, and personal protective equipment is worn by the caregiver to protect the client from the caregiver.
 4. Airborne precautions are used for clients who have an illness transmitted by airborne droplet nuclei smaller than 5 μm (micrometers), such as varicella, rubeola, and tuberculosis.

16. 1. **This is an example of controlling the mode of transmission. Direct transmission of microorganisms from one person to another is interrupted**

when microorganisms are removed from the skin surface by hand washing. Hand washing is part of hand hygiene, which also includes nail care, skin lubrication, and wearing of minimal jewelry in a health-care environment. Hand hygiene should be performed before and after client care and whenever contamination has occurred.

2. The use of a commode is an example of controlling the portal of exit link in the chain of infection.

3. Ingesting a balanced diet is an example of reducing the susceptibility of the host link in the chain of infection.

4. Changing a soiled dressing is an example of controlling the portal of exit link in the chain of infection.

17. 1. Inserting stuffing immediately before putting the turkey in the oven is safe practice. Letting a stuffed turkey stand at room temperature is not advisable because it promotes the multiplication of microorganisms.

2. Hamburger meat should be thoroughly cooked so that disease-producing microorganisms within the meat are destroyed.

3. This statement is about the client's preference about food. The statement does not indicate a lack of knowledge about the use or storage of mayonnaise.

4. This statement does not indicate a lack of knowledge about what to do when it is determined that something does not taste right.

5. This is the correct way to defrost frozen food. Food should not be defrosted in an environment between 45°F and 140°F because bacteria will rapidly grow in this temperature range.

18. **1. Medical aseptic techniques must be instituted to protect others from being exposed to the infestation.**

3. The primary health-care provider must be notified because the surgery must be canceled and treatment instituted.

4. Treatment with a pediculicidal shampoo requires a prescription; it is a dependent function of the nurse.

5. The client's hair should be washed as soon as possible with a medicated shampoo (e.g., permethrin, crotamiton).

2. After the hair is washed with a pediculicidal shampoo, it should be combed

with a fine-toothed comb to remove the nits (eggs).

19. **1. Tears flush the eyes of microorganisms and debris and are a primary defense that protects the body from infection.**

2. Healthy, intact skin prevents entry of many pathogens. In addition, the normal flora of the skin hinder growth of disease-causing microorganisms that settle on the skin.

3. Cilia line the nasal passages, sinuses, trachea, and larger bronchi and are tiny hairlike cells that sweep microorganisms up from the lower airways. These microorganisms are then expelled from the body by coughing and sneezing.

4. Acidity of gastric secretions is a primary defense mechanism that protects the body from infection.

5. A dry epidermis is a primary defense mechanism that protects the body from infection. The exposure to moisture can cause softening and breakdown of skin (masceration), causing skin to become more easily infected with bacteria or fungi.

20. **1. A cut in the skin caused by a sharp instrument with minimal tissue loss can heal by primary intention when the wound edges are lightly pulled together (approximated).**

2. Excoriation heals by secondary, not primary, intention. Excoriation is an injury to the surface of the skin. It can be caused by friction, scratching, and chemical or thermal burns.

3. An abrasion heals by secondary, not primary, intention. With an abrasion, friction scrapes away the epithelial layer, exposing the underlying tissue.

4. A surgical incision is caused by a scalpel, which is a sharp instrument. This type of wound can heal by primary intention when the wound edges are lightly pulled together (approximated) with sutures, staples, or adhesive.

5. A pressure ulcer heals by secondary, not primary, intention. Secondary intention healing occurs when wound edges are not approximated because of full-thickness tissue loss; the wound is left open until it fills with new tissue.

21. **The reservoir link in the chain of infection is where infectious agents live,**

reproduce, and multiply. Reservoirs can be animate (e.g., people, animals, insects) or inanimate (e.g., water, soil, medical devices). Eliminating standing water limits the favorable environment where mosquitoes like to lay their eggs and multiply.

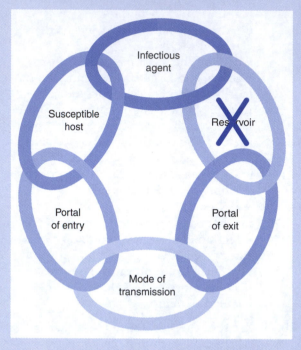

22. 1. An increase in white blood cells (leucocytosis) is a systemic, not local, response to an infection.
   2. Discomfort, uneasiness, or indisposition (malaise) is a systemic, not local, response to infection.
   3. **Chemical mediators increase the permeability of small blood vessels, thereby causing fluid to move into the interstitial compartment, with resulting local edema.**
   4. Fever is a systemic, not local, response to a wound infection. Microorganisms, or endotoxins, stimulate phagocytic cells that release pyrogens, which stimulate the hypothalamic thermoregulatory center to produce an increased temperature (fever, pyrexia).
   5. **Pain is caused by localized edema that puts pressure on the surrounding nerves; this is associated with the local adaptation syndrome.**

23. 1. This is an example of controlling the mode of transmission, not the susceptible host, link in the chain of infection.
   2. **This is an example of an action designed to interrupt the susceptible host link in the chain of infection by increasing the**

resistance of the host to an infectious agent.
   3. Discarding uncapped, used syringes in a sharps container disrupts the chain of infection at the transmission link in the chain of infection. The nurse should never recap a used needle because of the risk of a needle-stick injury.
   4. **Immunoglobulins are a group of related proteins able to act as antibodies. Immunoglobulin therapy helps defend a susceptible host against infection.**
   5. This is an example of controlling the mode of transmission, not the susceptible host, link in the chain of infection.

24. 1. An N95 respirator mask is not necessary when caring for a client receiving contact precautions. Clients receiving contact precautions have infections that are transmitted by contact with wounds, dressings, contaminated supplies, or clients' secretions or excretions. A regular mask with an eye shield is necessary when providing care when splashing of blood, body fluids, or secretions is likely, such as when irrigating a wound.
   2. **This mask is an N95 respirator mask, which should be worn when entering the room of a client receiving airborne precautions. The National Institute for Occupational Safety and Health tests and certifies special fitted masks such as the N95 respirator mask for use when maintaining airborne precautions. Infections such as tuberculosis, severe acute respiratory syndrome (SARS), rubeola (measles), and varicella (chickenpox) are considered airborne infections whereby microorganisms are transmitted via air currents. Clients with these infections receive airborne precautions.**
   3. An N95 respirator mask is not necessary when implementing standard precautions. Standard precautions are actions implemented by the nurse in the care of all persons regardless of their diagnosis.
   4. An N95 respirator mask is not necessary when implementing protective precautions. Protective precautions (reverse isolation, neutropenic precautions) include actions designed to protect the immunocompromised client from infection. The nurse wears a procedural face mask so as not to introduce microorganisms into the air, thereby protecting the client from the nurse. Additional actions include such

actions as restricting fresh fruit, vegetables, and flowers. Depending on the degree of immunosuppression, the client may be placed in a room with positive airflow, have water purity monitored, and have air conduits in the room checked for the presence of microorganisms.

25. 1. Throbbing pain is subjective, not objective, information because pain cannot be observed; it is felt and described only by the client.
    2. **Purulent drainage from the ear is objective information because it can be observed and measured.**
    3. Feeling of pressure is a response to inflammation that causes displacement of tissue. This is subjective information because it cannot be measured or verified other than that which is reported by the client.
    4. Dizziness is subjective, not objective, information because it cannot be measured; dizziness is experienced and described only by the client.
    5. Hearing a buzzing sound (tinnitus) is subjective, not objective, information because it cannot be observed; a buzzing sound is perceived and described only by the client.

26. 1. Antibiotic therapy is the use of chemotherapeutic agents to control or eliminate bacterial infections. It is not a primary defense that protects the body from infection. The inappropriate use of antibiotics destroys the usual flora of the body and can predispose an individual to additional infections.
    2. **Lysozymes in saliva help wash microorganisms from the teeth and gums.**
    3. **The low pH of the skin is caused by phospholipids that help prevent the development of bacterial infections.**
    4. **The acidic environment of the vagina protects it from the growth of pathogens.**
    5. **Mucus produced by epithelial cells in the genitourinary tract adheres to pathogens to facilitate their elimination through urination.**

27. 3. **Using sterile forceps maintains sterility of the drain.**
    2. **Gentle, steady pulling on the drain avoids accidental withdrawal of the drain farther than intended.**
    4. **Removing and reattaching the pin to the drain closer to the surface of the wound prevents the drain from sliding**

back into the wound, where it could become inaccessible. If this were to occur, a surgical procedure would be required to access the drain.
    5. **Cutting off the excess drain by using sterile scissors maintains sterility of the drain. Leaving 2 inches to the length of the drain allows an adequate length of drain to grasp when shortening or removing the drain in the future.**
    1. **Completing the dressing protects the wound and provides an environment conducive for wound healing.**

28. 1. **This is an action designed to interrupt the portal of entry link in the chain of infection. By keeping the collection bag below the level of the client's pelvis, backflow is prevented, which reduces the risk of introducing pathogens into the bladder.**
    2. **Using sterile technique when administering medication parenterally helps to reduce the risk of introducing a pathogen into the body.**
    3. Using a biohazardous transport bag is an example of controlling the mode of transmission link in the chain of infection.
    4. Wearing clean gloves is an example of controlling the mode of transmission link in the chain of infection.
    5. Hand washing is an example of controlling the mode of transmission link in the chain of infection.
    6. **A dressing over a surgical incision provides a barrier between the healing incision and the environment. The dressing protects the client from potential invading microorganisms at the portal of entry portion of the chain of infection.**

29. 1. Although a temperature of 103°F is higher than the expected range of 97.5°F to 99.5°F, it is not as critical as data in another option.
    2. Although abdominal cramping is an important piece of data, it is not as critical as data in another option.
    3. **A white blood cell count of 30,000 cells/mcL or higher is a critical finding indicating a potential life-threatening health situation. The clinical indicators support a medical diagnosis of urosepsis—septicemia from bacteria entering the bloodstream from a urinary cause.**

4. A blood pressure of 110/86 mm Hg is low for an older adult man and probably is low because of dehydration associated with "high" fevers of a few days' duration. Although the blood pressure indicates a need for fluid replacement, it is not as critical as data in another option.

30. 1. A fever is a systemic, not local, response to inflammation.
2. **Chemical mediators released at the site of an injury increase capillary permeability, causing excessive interstitial fluid that results in swelling (edema).**
3. **Local trauma or infection stimulates the release of kinins, which increase capillary permeability and blood flow to the local area. The increase of blood flow to the area causes erythema (redness).**
4. Bradypnea is a regular but excessively slow rate of breathing (less than 12 breaths per minute) and is not a response associated with the local adaptation syndrome.
5. Tachycardia is an elevated heart rate of more than 100 beats per minute and is unrelated to the local adaptation syndrome.

31. 1. **Stool for occult blood does not have to be sterile because test results for the presence of blood are not altered if the specimen is contaminated with exogenous organisms.**
2. **Stool for ova and parasites does not have to be sterile because test results for the presence of parasitic eggs and parasites are not altered if the specimen is contaminated with exogenous microorganisms.**
3. Sterile technique is used to collect a throat culture to avoid contaminating the specimen with exogenous organisms that may alter the accuracy of test results.
4. The bladder is a sterile cavity, and the nurse must use sterile technique to collect urine from the port of a retention catheter (Foley) so as not to introduce any pathogens. In addition, it is important not to introduce exogenous organisms that may contaminate the specimen and alter the accuracy of test results.
5. Sterile technique is used to collect exudate from a wound to avoid contaminating the specimen with exogenous organisms that may alter the accuracy of test results.

32. 1. **Clean gloves protect the nurse from the client's blood and body fluids.**

6. **Loosening the edges of the tape around the entire dressing prepares the tape to be removed by the nurse. Moving from the edge toward the center of the wound avoids pulling on the wound.**
2. **Pulling the tape away from the skin gently reduces discomfort and skin trauma during tape removal.**
5. **Gently lifting the dressing upward and toward the center of the wound avoids dragging the edges of the dressing into the center of the wound and thus contaminating the wound.**
3. **Assessing the status of the exudate provides data for evaluating the progress of wound healing.**
4. **Placing soiled dressings and contaminated gloves in an appropriate waste receptacle breaks the chain of infection at the transmission link.**

33. 1. **Fever is a common systemic response to infection. Microorganisms or endotoxins stimulate phagocytic cells that release pyrogens, which stimulate the hypothalamic thermoregulatory center, resulting in fever.**
2. **An increased heart rate (tachycardia) occurs in response to the increase in the metabolic rate associated with an infection. In addition, blood volume increases as peripheral and visceral vasoconstriction enhances blood flow to the heart and lungs as the body prepares to fight the infection.**
3. **The number of white blood cells increases above the expected range (leukocytosis) to help fight the infection.**
4. **Fatigue or lack of energy are systemic responses to a wound infection. Systemic responses to infection increase the metabolic rate and vital signs, which in turn cause an increase in energy expenditure. In addition, a wound may be painful and require multiple daily dressing changes, which are physiologically demanding. All these factors can contribute to fatigue.**
5. **Chills are caused by rapid muscle contraction and relaxation associated with the onset (cold or chill) phase of a fever. With infection, the brain increases the body's temperature set-point, and contraction and relaxation of muscles (chills) generates heat in an attempt to achieve the new set-point.**

34. **1.** The black foam is cut to the exact size of the cavity of the wound so that suction is applied to the full surface of the wound cavity.

4. Avoiding overlapping surrounding intact skin with the foam allows negative pressure to be exerted only on the wound. Also, it prevents skin from becoming macerated as the foam becomes wet during therapy.

6. The transparent film creates a seal so that negative pressure can be created by the device. Avoiding stretching the film during application prevents excess tension when negative pressure is established, which can cause tissue injury.

2. Creating a 2-cm hole in the transparent film provides a port over which the suction device is applied.

5. The suction device pad placed over the 2-cm hole in the transparent film, once connected to the pump, draws excess exudate away from the wound, through the hole, and into the tubing. Gentle pressure on the suction device pad promotes adherence of the suction device pad to the transparent film.

3. Connecting the suction device tubing to the collection canister and pump establishes negative pressure, which draws excess exudate from the wound. Suctioned exudate exits the wound via the suction device that is secured to the transparent film, is drawn into the tubing, and is collected in the collection canister.

35. **1.** Azithromycin (Zithromax) should be taken 1 hour before or 2 hours after meals because food can decrease the amount of medication absorbed by as much as 50%.

2. The entire regimen of azithromycin (Zithromax) should be completed; the medication should not be discontinued once the client feels better. Taking the entire regimen of an antibiotic eradicates the pathogens that have invaded the body. Stopping an antibiotic early promotes the development of resistant bacteria and a return of the infection.

3. This is the dose and administration regimen for azithromycin (Zithromax).

4. The first dose of azithromycin (Zithromax) can be administered once the specimen for culture and sensitivity is collected. The client does not have to wait for the results of the culture and sensitivity test to initiate therapy. Waiting will only prolong the infection.

5. Antacids may decrease the peak level of azithromycin (Zithromax) and decrease its effectiveness.

Safety

KEYWORDS

The following words include nursing/medical terminology, concepts, principles, and information relevant to content specifically addressed in the chapter or usually associated with topics presented in it. English dictionaries, nursing textbooks, and medical dictionaries, such as *Taber's Cyclopedic Medical Dictionary,* are resources that can be used to expand your knowledge and understanding of these words and related information.

Abdominal thrust (Heimlich maneuver)

Allergies:
  Food
  Latex
  Medication

Aspiration

Call bell

Cardiopulmonary resuscitation (CPR)

Child-proof devices

Dysphagia

Electrical:
  Grounding
  Hazards
  Surge

Falls

Fire safety:
  Fire extinguishers—A, B, C
  RACE model (**R**escue, **A**larm, **C**onfine,
    Extinguish)

Functional alignment

Incident report

Knots:
  Clove hitch
  Half bow
  Slip

Restraints:
  Belt
  Elbow
  Jacket
  Mitt
  Mummy
  Poncho
  Vest

Side rails

SAFETY: QUESTIONS

1. A client brings several electronic devices to a nursing home. One of the devices has a two-pronged plug. Which rationale should the nurse provide when explaining why an electrical device must have a three-pronged plug?
   1. Controls stray electrical currents
   2. Promotes efficient use of electricity
   3. Shuts off the appliance if there is an electrical surge
   4. Divides the electricity among the appliances in the room

2. A nurse is caring for a client with Parkinson's disease who is experiencing difficulty swallowing. For which major potential problem associated with dysphagia should the nurse assess the client?
   1. Anorexia
   2. Aspiration
   3. Self-care deficit
   4. Inadequate intake

3. A nurse is caring for a confused client. Which should the nurse do to prevent this client from falling?
   1. Encourage the client to use the corridor handrails.
   2. Place the client in a room near the nurses' station.
   3. Reinforce how to use the call bell.
   4. Maintain close supervision.

4. A school nurse is teaching children about fire safety procedures. Which is the **first** thing they should be taught to do if their clothes catch on fire?
   1. Yell for help.
   2. Roll on the ground.
   3. Take their clothes off.
   4. Pour water on their clothes.

5. A primary health-care provider prescribes a vest restraint for a client. Which should the nurse do **first** when applying this restraint?
   1. Perform an inspection of the client's skin where the restraint is to be placed.
   2. Ensure that the back of the vest is positioned on the client's back.
   3. Permit four fingers to slide between the client and the restraint.
   4. Secure the restraint to the bed frame using a slipknot.

6. An unconscious client begins vomiting. In which position should the nurse place the client?
   1. Supine
   2. Side-lying
   3. Orthopneic
   4. Low-Fowler

7. A toaster is on fire in the pantry of a hospital unit. Which should the nurse do **first**?
   1. Activate the fire alarm.
   2. Unplug the toaster from the wall.
   3. Put out the fire with an extinguisher.
   4. Evacuate the clients from the room next to the kitchen.

8. The risk management coordinator is preparing a program on the factors that contribute to falls in a hospital setting. Which factor that **most** often contributes to falls should be included in this program?
   1. Wet floors
   2. Frequent seizures
   3. Advanced age of clients
   4. Misuse of equipment by nurses

9. A nurse is assessing a client who is being admitted to the hospital. Which is the **most** important information that indicates whether the client is at risk for physical injury?
   1. Weakness experienced during a prior admission
   2. Medication that increases intestinal motility
   3. Two recent falls that occurred at home
   4. The need for corrective eyeglasses

10. Which should the nurse do to **best** prevent a client from falling?
    1. Provide a cane.
    2. Keep walkways clear of obstacles.
    3. Assist the client with ambulation.
    4. Encourage the client to use hallway handrails.

11. Which is the last step in making an occupied bed that the nurse should teach a nursing assistant?
    1. Elevating the head of the bed to a semi-Fowler position
    2. Ensuring that the client is in a comfortable position
    3. Lowering the height of the bed toward the floor
    4. Raising both the upper side rails on the bed

12. A nurse is caring for a client with a nasogastric tube for gastric decompression. Which nursing action takes **priority**?
    1. Discontinuing the wall suction when providing nursing care
    2. Positioning the client in the semi-Fowler position
    3. Instilling the tube with 30 mL of air every 2 hours
    4. Caring for the nares at least every 8 hours

13. A family member brings an electric radio to a client in a long-term care facility. The client tells the nurse that an electric shock was felt while turning on the radio. Which should the nurse do **first**?
1. Arrange for the maintenance department to examine the radio.
2. Disconnect the radio from the source of energy.
3. Check the client's skin for electrical burns.
4. Take the client's apical pulse.

14. A nurse educator is teaching a group of newly hired nursing assistants. Which hospitalized client should they be taught is at the **highest** risk for injury?
1. School-age child
2. Comatose teenager
3. Postmenopausal woman
4. Confused middle-age man

15. A nurse in the nursing education department of a community hospital is planning an inservice education class about injury prevention. Which factor that **most** commonly causes physical injuries in hospitalized clients should be included in the teaching plan?
1. Malfunctioning equipment
2. Failure to use restraints
3. Visitors
4. Falls

16. Which is the **priority** nursing intervention to prevent client problems associated with latex allergies?
1. Use nonlatex gloves.
2. Identify persons at risk.
3. Keep a latex-safe supply cart available.
4. Administer an antihistamine prophylactically.

17. Which nursing intervention enhances an older adult's sensory perception and thereby helps prevent injury when walking from the bed to the bathroom?
1. Providing adequate lighting
2. Raising the pitch of the voice
3. Holding onto the client's arm
4. Removing environmental hazards

18. A nurse is preparing a client for a physical examination. Which is **most** important for the nurse to do in this situation?
1. Identify the positions contraindicated for the client during the examination.
2. Explore the client's attitude toward health-care providers.
3. Inquire about other professionals caring for the client.
4. Ask when the client last had a physical examination.

19. A client has dysphagia. Which nursing action takes **priority** when feeding this client?
1. Ensuring that dentures are in place
2. Medicating for pain before providing meals
3. Providing verbal cueing to swallow each bite
4. Checking the mouth for emptying between every bite

20. A 3-year-old child is admitted to the pediatric unit. Which should the nurse do to maintain the safety of this preschool-age child?
1. Teach the child how to use the call bell.
2. Put the child in a crib with high side rails.
3. Ensure the child is under continuous supervision.
4. Have the child stay in the playroom most of the day.

21. A nurse is caring for a client with dementia. Which time of day is of **most** concern for the nurse when trying to protect this client from injury?
1. Afternoon
2. Morning
3. Evening
4. Night

22. A nurse is orienting a newly admitted client to the hospital. Which is **most** important for the nurse to teach the client how to do?
    1. Notify the nurse when help is needed.
    2. Get out of the bed to use the bathroom.
    3. Raise and lower the head and foot of the bed.
    4. Use the telephone system to call family members.

23. Profuse smoke is coming out of the heating unit in a client's room. Which should the nurse do **first**?
    1. Open the window.
    2. Activate the fire alarm.
    3. Move the client out of the room.
    4. Close the door to the client's room.

24. A nurse must apply a hospital gown that does not have snaps on the shoulders to a client receiving an IV infusion in the forearm. Which should the nurse do?
    1. Put the gown on the client's arm without the IV, drape the gown over the other shoulder, and adjust the closure behind the neck.
    2. Close the clamp on the IV tubing for no more than 15 seconds while putting the gown on the client.
    3. Disconnect the client's IV at the insertion site, apply the gown, and then reconnect the IV.
    4. Insert the client's IV bag and tubing through the sleeve from inside of the gown first.

25. A nurse is planning care for a client with a wrist restraint. How often should a restraint be removed, the area massaged, and the joints moved through their full range?
    1. Once a shift
    2. Once an hour
    3. Every 2 hours
    4. Every 4 hours

26. A home-care nurse is assigned to care for an older adult living at home. Which is the **first** action the home-care nurse should employ to prevent falls by this older adult?
    1. Conduct a comprehensive risk assessment.
    2. Encourage the client to remove throw rugs in the home.
    3. Suggest installation of adequate lighting throughout the home.
    4. Discuss with the client the expected changes of aging that place one at risk.

27. A nurse is preparing a bed to receive a newly admitted client to the hospital. Which action is **most** important?
    1. Placing the client's name on the end of the bed
    2. Ensuring that the bed wheels are locked
    3. Positioning the call bell in reach
    4. Raising one side rail

28. Which is an appropriately worded goal for a client who is at risk for falling? **Select all that apply.**
    1. _____ "The client will be able to walk from a bed to a chair safely while hospitalized."
    2. _____ "The client will be taught how to call for help to ambulate."
    3. _____ "The client will be kept on bedrest when dizzy."
    4. _____ "The client will be restrained when agitated."
    5. _____ "The client will be free from trauma."

29. A nurse is caring for a client who has a prescription for a mitt restraint. Place an X where the mitt restraint strap should be secured with a quick-release knot.

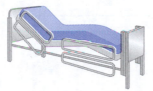

30. Which intervention should a nurse implement when assisting a client to use a bedpan? **Select all that apply.**
   1. _____ Ensure that the bed rails are raised after the client is on the bedpan.
   2. _____ Position the rounded rim of the bedpan under the client's buttocks.
   3. _____ Encourage the client to help as much as possible when using the bedpan.
   4. _____ Raise the head of the bed to the semi-Fowler position once the client is placed on the bedpan.
   5. _____ Dust talcum powder on the rim of the bedpan before placing the bedpan under the client.

31. A nurse identifies the presence of smoke exiting the door to the dirty utility room. Place the nurse's actions in order of priority using the RACE model.
   1. Pull the fire alarm.
   2. Close unit doors and windows.
   3. Shut the door to the utility room.
   4. Provide emotional support to agitated clients.

   Answer: _____

32. Which clinical manifestation indicates that a further nursing assessment is necessary to determine if the client is having difficulty swallowing? **Select all that apply.**
   1. _____ Debris in the buccal cavity
   2. _____ Coughing episodes
   3. _____ Noisy breathing
   4. _____ Slurred speech
   5. _____ Drooling

33. A male client is admitted to ambulatory care for a bilateral herniorrhaphy. A nurse on the unit interviews the client, obtains the client's vital signs, and reviews the primary health-care provider's prescriptions. Which should the nurse do **first**?
   1. Contact the operating suite and inform them of the client's latex allergy.
   2. Ensure the client's allergy band includes the client's identified allergies.
   3. Notify the primary health-care provider of the client's elevated vital signs.
   4. Share the information about the client's anxiety with health team members.

CLIENT'S CLINICAL RECORD

Primary Health-Care Provider's Prescriptions
Nothing by mouth
IVF: 0.9% sodium chloride at 125 mL/hour
Midazolam 5 mg, IM on call to preoperative suite

Vital Signs
Temperature: 99.2°F, orally
Pulse: 96 beats per minute
Respirations: 22 breaths per minute
Blood pressure: 124/82 mm Hg

Client Interview
Client states, "I am a little nervous because I have never had surgery before." During preoperative testing, the client indicated an allergy to oxycodone/acetaminophen but forgot to include allergies to latex and peanuts.

34. A nurse is planning care for a client who requires bilateral arm restraints because the client is delirious and attempting to pull out a urinary retention catheter. Which information is important to consider when planning care for this client? **Select all that apply.**
1. _____ Use of restraints adequately prevents injuries.
2. _____ Reasons for use of restraints must be clearly documented.
3. _____ Most clients recognize that restraints contribute to their safety.
4. _____ Restraints need a health-care provider's prescription before application.
5. _____ Laws permit the use of restraints when specific guidelines are followed.

35. A nurse is implementing the action demonstrated in the illustration. Which is the nurse doing?
1. Transferring a client into a wheelchair
2. Teaching abdominal breathing to a client
3. Dislodging an object from a client's airway
4. Holding a client up after the client became dizzy when walking

36. An adult client consistently tries to pull out a nasogastric tube. As a last resort to maintain integrity of the tube and client safety, the nurse obtains a prescription for a restraint. Which type of restraint is appropriate in this situation? **Select all that apply.**
1. _____ Mummy restraint
2. _____ Elbow restraint
3. _____ Jacket restraint
4. _____ Wrist restraint
5. _____ Mitt restraint

37. A nurse uses the *Get Up and Go* test to assess a client for weakness, poor balance, and decreased flexibility. Place the following actions in the order in which they should be implemented when employing the *Get Up and Go* test.
1. Ask the client to walk 10 feet and then to return to the chair.
2. Ask the client to close the eyes.
3. Ask the client to open the eyes.
4. Ask the client to sit in a chair.
5. Ask the client to stand.

Answer: _____

38. Which action is important when the nurse uses a stretcher? **Select all that apply.**
1. _____ Raising the bed above the level of the stretcher when transferring a client from the stretcher to a bed
2. _____ Guiding the stretcher around a turn by leading with the end with the client's head
3. _____ Ensuring that the client's head is at the end with the swivel wheels
4. _____ Pulling the stretcher on the elevator with the client's feet first
5. _____ Pushing the stretcher from the end with the client's head

39. Which human response to illness alerts the nurse that a client is at risk for aspiration during meals? **Select all that apply.**
1. _____ Bulimia
2. _____ Lethargy
3. _____ Anorexia
4. _____ Stomatitis
5. _____ Dysphagia

40. A nurse is caring for a client with a moderate problem with balance. Place an X over the cane that is most appropriate for this client.

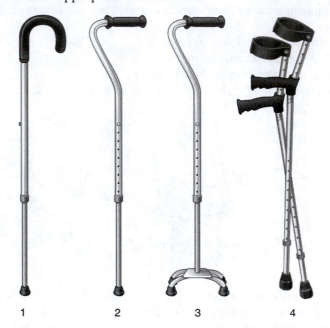

      1   2   3   4

1. 1. **A three-pronged plug functions as a ground to dissipate stray electrical currents.**
   2. The purpose of a three-pronged plug is not to promote efficient use of electricity.
   3. A surge protector shuts off the appliance.
   4. A multiple-outlet plug divides the electricity among appliances in the room.

2. 1. Although lack of an appetite (anorexia) can occur with dysphagia, it is not the most serious associated risk.
   2. **When a person has difficulty with swallowing (dysphagia), food or fluid can pass into the trachea and be inhaled into the lungs (aspiration), rather than swallowed down the esophagus. This can result in choking, partial or total airway obstruction, or aspiration pneumonia.**
   3. Dysphagia is unrelated to self-care deficit. Feeding self-care deficit occurs when a person is unable to cut food, open food packages, or bring food to the mouth.
   4. Inadequate intake of food and fluid can result with dysphagia because of fear of choking. However, it is not the most serious associated risk.

3. 1. A confused client may not be able to follow directions or understand how to use corridor handrails.
   2. Moving the client near the nurses' station may be impossible and impractical.
   3. A confused client may not be able to follow directions or understand how to use a call bell.
   4. **Maintaining safety of the confused client is best accomplished through close or direct supervision. Confused clients cannot be left on their own because they may not have the cognitive ability to understand cause and effect, and therefore their actions can result in harm.**

4. 1. This eventually may be done, but the child must do something immediately before waiting for help to arrive.
   2. **Rolling on the ground will smother the flames and put the fire out. Children should be taught to "Stop, drop, and roll."**
   3. Taking off their clothes may be impossible. In addition, it will take time, and the clothing and skin will continue to burn. Some fabrics may adhere to the skin when they burn, and attempting to remove clothing may cause more damage to the skin.
   4. Finding and obtaining water will take too much time, and the clothing and skin will continue to burn. Something must be done immediately.

5. 1. **Even when applied correctly, restraints can cause pressure and friction. A baseline assessment of the skin under the restraint should be made. In addition, the presence of a dressing, pacemaker, subcutaneous infusion port, or subclavian catheter may influence the type of restraint to use.**
   2. Although the back of the vest should be positioned on the client's back, it is not the first intervention.
   3. The jacket may be too loose if four fingers are used. The jacket should be applied so that two, not four, fingers can slide between the client and the restraint.
   4. Securing the restraint to the bed frame using a slipknot should be done; however, it is the last, not the first, intervention associated with the application of a vest restraint.

6. 1. The supine position will promote aspiration and should be avoided in this situation.
   2. **The side-lying position prevents the tongue from falling to the back of the oropharynx, thus allowing the vomitus to flow out of the mouth by gravity and preventing aspiration.**
   3. The orthopneic position is an unsafe, impossible position in which to maintain an unconscious client.
   4. The low-Fowler position will allow the tongue to fall to the back of the oropharynx, promoting aspiration. This position should be avoided in this situation.

7. 1. **Because no client is in jeopardy, the nurse's initial action should be to activate the fire alarm. The sooner the alarm is set, the sooner professional firefighters will reach the scene of the fire.**
   2. Unplugging the toaster is unsafe because it places the nurse in jeopardy. The nurse may be exposed to an electrical charge or become burned.
   3. This is an inappropriate intervention because the nurse may not be capable of containing or fighting the fire, and this action may place the nurse in jeopardy.
   4. Evacuating clients is premature at this time, but it may become necessary eventually.

8. 1. Although wet floors can contribute to falls, they are not the most common factor that contributes to falls in the hospital setting.
   2. Although seizures can contribute to falls, most clients do not experience seizures.
   3. Older adults who are hospitalized frequently have multiple health problems, are frail, and lack stamina. All of these factors contribute to the inability to maintain balance and ambulate safely.
   4. Although this occasionally happens and is negligence, it is not the most common factor that contributes to falls in the hospital setting.

9. 1. Although this is important information, it is not the most important factor of the options presented in this question. In addition, the prior admission may have been too long ago to have any current relevance.
   2. A client with increased intestinal motility may experience diarrhea, which may place the client at risk for a fluid and electrolyte imbalance, not a physical injury. Although a person with diarrhea may need to use the toilet more frequently, a bedside commode or bedpan can be used to reduce the risk of falls.
   3. This is significant information that must be considered because if falls occurred before, then they are likely to occur again. When a risk is identified, additional injury prevention precautions can be implemented.
   4. Although this is important information, it is not the most important factor of the options presented in this question.

10. 1. The client may or may not need a cane. An unnecessary cane may actually increase the risk of a fall.
    2. Although this should be done, it is not the best intervention of the options presented.
    3. This widens the client's base of support, which improves balance and decreases the risk of a fall.
    4. Although this should be done, it is not the best intervention of the options presented.

11. 1. Elevating the head of the bed may not be necessary. This action should be based on the individual needs of the client.
    2. Assisting the client to a comfortable position should be done while the bed is at an effective working height for the caregiver.
    3. It is safer if the bed is in the lowest position because a higher risk for injury
    to a client occurs when the mattress of the bed is farther from the floor.
    4. Raising the upper side rails on the bed may not be necessary. This action should be based on the individual needs of the client.

12. 1. Discontinuing the wall suction is unnecessary and can result in vomiting and aspiration.
    2. A nasogastric (NG) tube for gastric decompression passes down the esophagus, through the cardiac sphincter, and into the stomach. The cardiac sphincter remains slightly open because of the presence of the NG tube. The semi-Fowler position keeps gastric secretions in the stomach via gravity (preventing reflux and aspiration) and allows the gastric contents to be suctioned out by the NG tube.
    3. Instilling the NG tube with air is not done routinely every 2 hours. This may be done to help reestablish patency of the tube when it is clogged.
    4. Caring for the nares should be done more frequently than every 8 hours to prevent irritation and pressure.

13. 1. Having the radio examined may be done eventually; it is not the priority at this time.
    2. Disconnecting the radio is contraindicated because it may place the nurse in jeopardy.
    3. Inspecting the client's skin is not the priority, and electrical burns may or may not be evident.
    4. An electrical shock can interfere with the electrical conduction system within the heart and result in dysrhythmias. An electrical shock can be transmitted through the body because body fluids (consisting of sodium chloride) are an excellent conductor of electricity.

14. 1. Although a school-age child is at risk for injury in a hospital setting, age-related precautions always are instituted. More nurses generally are assigned to pediatric units, and family members are frequently at the bedside.
    2. A client in a coma is not at as high a risk for injury as a client in another option. A client in a coma demonstrates less response to painful stimuli, generally has an absence of muscle tone and reflexes in the extremities, and appears to be in a deep sleep.
    3. A woman after menopause is not at a high risk for injury.

4. A confused client is at an increased risk for injury because of the inability to comprehend cause and effect; therefore, such a client lacks the ability to make safe decisions.

15. 1. Malfunctioning equipment is not a common cause of injuries in a hospital.
 2. The use of restraints has declined dramatically, and now they are used only when clients may harm themselves or others.
 3. Visitors are not the main cause of injuries in a hospital.
 4. **Research demonstrates that most physical injuries experienced by hospitalized clients occur from falls. Failing to call for assistance, inadequate lighting, and the altered health status of clients all contribute to falls.**

16. 1. Although using nonlatex gloves may be done, it is not the priority.
 2. **Client allergies must be identified (e.g., latex, food, and medication) before any care is provided, be documented in the client's clinical record, and appear on an allergy-alert wristband. After a risk is identified, additional safety precautions can be implemented to prevent exposure to the offending allergen. Assessment is the first step of the nursing process.**
 3. Although keeping a latex-safe supply cart available may be done, it is not the priority.
 4. Administering an antihistamine is unnecessary. A person with a latex allergy should not be exposed to products with latex.

17. 1. **Adequate lighting provides for the safety of clients, staff, and visitors within a hospital. Inadequate lighting causes shadows, a dark environment, and the potential for misinterpreting stimuli (illusions) and is a contributing cause of accidents in the hospital setting. This intervention maximizes a client's sense of sight.**
 2. When talking with older adults, it is better to lower, not raise, the pitch of the voice. As people age, they are more likely to have impaired hearing with higher-pitched sounds.
 3. Holding the client's arm does not enhance a client's sensory perception. Holding a client's arm is not always necessary and therefore could be degrading or promote regression.

4. Although this should be done, removing environmental hazards will not enhance a client's sensory perception.

18. 1. **A physical examination requires a client to assume a variety of positions, such as supine, side-lying, sitting, and standing. To prevent complications, the nurse should inquire about any positions that are uncomfortable or contraindicated because of past or current medical conditions.**
 2. Although the client's attitude toward health-care providers may be obtained before a physical examination, it is not the priority.
 3. Inquiring about other professionals caring for the client is not the priority before a physical examination. This might be done later to ensure continuity of care and prevent fragmentation of care.
 4. Although identifying when the last physical examination was performed may be done, it is not a priority before a physical examination.

19. 1. Although this should be done if a client has dentures, it is not the priority.
 2. Although an analgesic may be administered, it can cause drowsiness that may increase the potential for aspiration in a client with dysphagia.
 3. Although this should be done, the client may be physically incapable of following this direction.
 4. **This is the safest way to ensure that a bolus of food is not left in the mouth, where it can be aspirated and cause an airway obstruction.**

20. 1. A preschool-age child does not have the cognitive and emotional maturity to use a call bell.
 2. A preschool-age child might attempt to climb over the side rails. A crib with high side rails is more appropriate for an infant.
 3. **Constant supervision ensures that an adult can monitor the preschool-age child's activity and environment so that safety needs are met. Preschool-age children are active, curious, and fearless and have immature musculoskeletal and neurological systems, narrow life experiences, and a limited ability to understand cause and effect. All of these factors place preschool-age children at risk for injury unless supervised.**

4. This is inappropriate because most preschoolers still take one or two naps daily, the child may be on bedrest, and periods of activity and rest should be alternated to conserve the child's energy.

21. 1. The sunlight and usual afternoon activities generally help keep clients with dementia more oriented and safe.
2. The sunlight and the routine morning activities of hygiene, grooming, dressing, and eating generally help keep clients with dementia more oriented and safe.
3. As the day progresses and the sun sets, the concern for safety increases because of altered cognition (sundowner syndrome). However, in the evening there are activities of daily living and available caregivers to distract the client and provide for safety.
4. **At night, clients with dementia often continue to experience confusion and agitation. At night there is less light, less activity, and fewer caregivers, so there are fewer orienting stimuli. Clients who are confused or agitated are at an increased risk for injury because they may not comprehend cause and effect and therefore lack the ability to make safe judgments.**

22. 1. **Explaining how to use a call bell meets safety and security needs. It reinforces that help is immediately available at a time when the client may feel physically or emotionally vulnerable in an unfamiliar environment.**
2. Clients generally do not need teaching about how to get out of bed to go to the bathroom. This instruction depends on the individual needs of a client.
3. How to manipulate the bed is part of orienting a client to the hospital environment; however, it is not the most important point to emphasize with a client.
4. Use of the telephone is part of orienting a client to the hospital environment; however, it is not the most important point to emphasize with a client.

23. 1. Opening a window is contraindicated because environmental air will feed the fire and cause it to increase in severity.
2. Although activating the alarm will be done, it is not the priority at this point in time.
3. **The client's physical safety is the priority. The client must be removed**

from direct danger before the alarm is activated and the fire contained.
4. Although closing the door will be done eventually, it is not the priority at this point in time.

24. 1. Draping the gown over the shoulder leaves the client exposed unnecessarily. It interferes with privacy, and the client may feel cold.
2. Stopping the flow of the IV solution can result in blood coagulating at the end of the catheter in the vein, compromising the patency of the IV tubing.
3. Disconnecting the IV tubing at the catheter insertion site is unnecessary. This increases the risk of contaminating the equipment and the potential for infection.
4. **Inserting the IV bag and tubing through the sleeve from inside of the gown first ensures that the IV bag and tubing are safely passed through the armhole of the gown before the client puts the arm with the insertion site through the gown. This prevents tension on the tubing and insertion site, which limits the possibility of the catheter dislodging from the vein.**

25. 1. Once a shift is too long a period; it promotes the development of injuries (e.g., contractures, pressure ulcers).
2. Once an hour generally is too often and unnecessary.
3. **Restraints should be removed every 2 hours. The extremities must be moved through their full range of motion to prevent muscle shortening and contractures. The area must be massaged to promote circulation and prevent pressure injuries.**
4. Four hours is too long a period between activities and promotes the development of injuries.

26. 1. **Assessment is the first step of the nursing process. The best way to prevent falls is by identifying those at risk and instituting multiple interventions that prevent falls.**
2. This is inadequate. Removing throw rugs is just one strategy.
3. This is inadequate. Ensuring adequate lighting is just one strategy.
4. This is inadequate. Exploring the issues of aging with a client is just one strategy.

27. 1. Placing clients' names on the end of their beds violates the client's right to privacy.

An identification wristband must be worn for client identification.

2. **Locked bed wheels are an important safety precaution. The bed must be an immovable object because the client may touch the bed for support, lean against it when getting in or out of bed, or move around when in bed. If bed wheels are unlocked during these maneuvers, the bed may move and the client can fall.**

3. The call bell cord may become an obstacle when moving the client into the bed. This should be done after the client is in the bed.

4. The side rail may become an obstacle when moving the client into the bed. This should be done after the client is in the bed.

28. 1. **This is an appropriate goal. It is realistic, specific, measurable, and has a time frame. It is realistic to expect that all clients be safe. It is specific and measurable because safety from trauma can be compared with standards of care within the profession of nursing. It has a time frame because the words "while hospitalized" reflect the time frame of "continuously" while directly under the care of a health team.**

2. Being taught how to call for help is a planned intervention, not a goal.

3. Maintaining a client on bedrest is a planned intervention, not a goal.

4. This is a planned intervention, not a goal. In addition, it is inappropriate to restrain a person automatically for agitation. A restraint should be used as a last resort to prevent the client from self-injury or injuring others.

5. **This is an appropriate goal. It is realistic, specific, and measurable and has a time frame. It is realistic to expect that all clients be safe. It is specific and measurable because safety from trauma can be compared with standards of care within the profession of nursing. It has a time frame because the words "free from" reflect the time frame of "continuously."**

29. **A restraint strap should always be tied with a quick-release knot to the frame of the bed. Tying a restraint strap to the side rail is contraindicated because when the side rail is lowered, it may become too tight, causing an injury.**

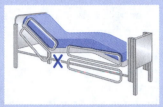

30. 1. Client safety is a priority. A bedpan is not a stable base of support, and the effort of elimination may require movements that alter balance. Side rails provide a solid object to hold while balancing on the bedpan and supply a barrier to prevent falling out of bed.

2. **The rounded rim of a bedpan should be placed under the client's buttocks because the rounded rim supports the client's weight when sitting on the bedpan.**

3. **Encouraging the client to help promotes the client's independence and limits strain on the nurse.**

4. **The semi-Fowler position is comfortable and provides a more normal position for defecation that helps prevent straining.**

5. The use of talcum powder should be avoided because it is a respiratory irritant.

31. 1. **Pulling the fire alarm ensures that appropriate hospital personnel and the fire department are notified of the fire. Trained individuals will arrive to contain and extinguish the fire and help move clients if necessary. The RACE model should be followed in a fire emergency: rescue, alarm, confine, and extinguish. The fire is in the dirty utility room, and no clients at this time need to be rescued.**

3. **Closing the door to the dirty utility room protects the clients and staff**

members in the immediate vicinity of the fire.

2. Closing unit doors and windows provides a barrier between the clients and the fire and limits drafts that could exacerbate the fire.

4. Clients should be supported emotionally during a crisis because anxiety can be contagious.

32. 1. **Retention of food in the oral cavity indicates that the client is not swallowing ingested food completely. Food collects in the buccal cavity because the area between the teeth and cheek forms a pocket that traps food.**

2. **When a person has difficulty swallowing, coughing episodes may occur in an effort to clear aspirated material from the respiratory tract.**

3. **When a person has difficulty swallowing, noisy breathing may occur as secretions, food, or liquid is aspirated into the respiratory tract.**

4. **Slurred speech reflects an inability of the tongue and muscles of the face to form words. Dysfunction of the muscles of the face and tongue will interfere with the ability to chew and swallow food.**

5. **Drooling indicates that oral secretions are accumulating in the mouth. This may occur when a person has difficulty swallowing.**

33. 1. This intervention should be performed immediately after the priority intervention. Clients with latex allergies require special precautions to be taken in the operating suite. The use of latex products can be life-threatening for the client if appropriate precautions are not taken. All equipment, such as gloves and tubes, must be latex free to protect the client from experiencing an allergy that can progress to anaphylaxis.

2. **Protecting the client is the priority, and a red allergy band is the first line of defense. In addition, the client's allergies must be included on other designated places on the client's medical record.**

3. Although the client's vital signs are on the high side of normal or slightly elevated, their elevations probably are related to the client's anxiety. These elevations should be documented and reported, but they are not the priority at this time. Normal ranges for vital signs are temperature, 97.5°F to 99.5°F; pulse, 60 to 100 beats per minute; respirations, 12 to 20 breaths per minute; and blood pressure: systolic pressure, less than 120 mm Hg; and diastolic pressure, less than 80 mm Hg.

4. Although this should be done, this is not the priority at this time. Mild to moderate anxiety is a common response when anticipating surgery, especially when surgery is being experienced for the first time. The client's anxiety should be documented and communicated to other members of the health team, but it is not the priority at this time. However, when a client has a sense of impending doom, the surgeon should be notified immediately because the client may not be in the right frame of mind for surgery; if surgery is performed, it can be a self-fulfilling prophesy.

34. 1. This statement is not true. Injuries and falls can occur if restraints are not applied appropriately. In addition, research indicates that clients incur less severe injuries if they are left unrestrained.

2. **The reason for the use of restraints must adhere to standards of care and be documented on the client's clinical record to create a legal document that protects the client as well as health-care providers.**

3. The opposite is true. Clients resist the use of restraints and usually are mentally or emotionally incompetent to understand their necessity or benefits.

4. Restraints can be applied by nurses in emergencies without a primary health-care provider's prescription to protect clients from harming themselves or others. Restraints can be used for nonviolent clients who are at risk for harming themselves (level 1 restraint) or violent clients who are at risk for harming themselves or others (level 2 restraint). A primary health-care provider must assess the client and document the need for the original application of the restraint and its continued use within specified time frames. For example, for a level 1 restraint, a primary health-care provider's prescription must be obtained within 12 hours after its application and daily thereafter, whereas for a level 2 restraint, a primary health-care provider must evaluate the client within 1 hour after its application and every 4 hours thereafter.

5. Federal and state laws provide specific guidelines regarding clients' rights and responsibilities of caregivers associated with the use of restraints. In addition, The Joint Commission has specific guidelines that require documentation of the following: previous restraint-free interventions that have failed to protect the client; a description of the situation indicating a need for the restraint; the least restrictive restraint that has been selected; and assessments and prescriptions by a primary health-care provider within specified time frames.

35. 1. A nurse stands in front of a client when transferring the client from a bed to a wheelchair.

2. Abdominal breathing is best taught when the nurse demonstrates placement of the hands on one's own abdomen. The nurse teaches the client to contract and relax the diaphragm when inhaling and exhaling. With the client's hands resting on his or her own abdomen, the abdomen will rise on inspiration and relax on exhalation when abdominal breathing is implemented correctly.

3. This is an illustration of the abdominal thrust maneuver (Heimlich maneuver) used to dislodge a foreign object from a person's airway. An abdominal thrust applies pressure up against the diaphragm that forces air out from the lungs, exerting pressure behind the obstruction, thus dislodging the foreign object from the airway.

4. When a client becomes dizzy and begins to fall, the nurse should not try to keep the client in the standing position because this can cause injury to the client and/or nurse. The nurse should project one hip forward and with a wide base of support guide the client down along that leg until the client reaches the floor. Once the client is on the floor, the nurse protects the client's head to prevent a head injury.

36. 1. A mummy restraint usually is used to immobilize an infant or a very young child during a procedure.

2. A soft limb splint that extends from the mid-forearm to the mid-upper arm can be applied to inhibit flexion of the elbow, which can prevent the pulling out of a nasogastric tube.

3. A jacket restraint usually is used to keep a person from falling out of bed while not immobilizing the extremities.

4. A wrist restraint encircles the wrist and has ties that are secured with a slipknot to the bed frame so that a client is unable to reach tubes.

5. A mitt restraint covers the hand to prevent the fingers from grasping and pulling out tubes.

37. 4. The first step involves asking the client to sit in a chair. This allows the nurse time to observe the client's posture while sitting in a straight-backed chair before any other activity.

5. The second step involves asking the client to stand. This allows the nurse to observe the client's use of the leg muscles to stand or whether the client has to push up and off the seat with the hands to stand. This helps to assess leg strength when moving to a standing position.

2. The third step involves asking the client to close the eyes. This allows the nurse to observe if the client sways to maintain balance when the eyes are closed.

3. The fourth step involves asking the client to open the eyes. This prepares the client for the next step in the procedure.

1. The fifth step involves asking the client to walk 10 feet, turn around, and return to the chair. This allows the nurse to observe the client's gait, posture, stability, pace, and balance when ambulating.

38. 1. Keeping a bed lower, not higher, than a stretcher when transferring a client from the stretcher to a bed uses gravity, which places less stress and strain on both the client and nurses.

2. It is too difficult and unsafe to maneuver a stretcher with the nonswivel wheels on the leading end of the stretcher. The end of the stretcher with the client's head does not have swivel wheels.

3. The swivel-wheeled end of the stretcher should be the leading end of the stretcher, and it is unsafe to lead with the client's head. In addition, the end of the stretcher with the swivel wheels moves through greater arcs; this can cause dizziness. The swivel wheels of a stretcher should be at the end under the client's feet, not the head.

4. This is unsafe and places the client in physical jeopardy. The elevator doors may inadvertently close by the client's head while the nurse is pulling the feet end of the stretcher into the elevator. The client should be moved into an elevator head, not feet, first.

5. **A stretcher should always be pushed from the end of the stretcher with the client's head so that the client's head is protected. The swivel wheels must be under the client's feet on the leading end of the stretcher for safe maneuverability.**

39. 1. The risk for aspiration in a client with bulimia occurs after, not during, meals. Bulimia is characterized by episodes of binge eating followed by purging, depression, and self-deprecation.

2. **When a person is sleepy, sluggish, or stuporous (lethargic), there may be a reduced level of consciousness and diminished reflexes, including the gag and swallowing reflexes. This condition can result in aspiration of food or fluids that can compromise the person's airway and respiratory status.**

3. A lack of appetite (anorexia) is unrelated to aspiration. The less food or fluid that is placed in the mouth, the less the risk is for aspiration.

4. **An inflammation of the mucous membranes of the mouth (stomatitis) may result in dysphagia and increase the risk of aspiration.**

5. **Dysphasia (difficulty swallowing) places a client at risk for aspiration generally because of impaired innervation of the tongue and muscles used for swallowing.**

40. 1. This is a single-ended cane with a half-circle handle. It is used by clients who can navigate stairs and need minimal support.

2. This is a single-ended cane with a straight handle. It is used by clients who need minimal support but have hand weakness.

3. **This is a quad cane and is the most appropriate cane to meet this client's needs. It has four prongs that provide a wide base of support, and it has a straight handle. It is used by clients with moderate balance problems.**

4. This is a Lofstrand (forearm support) crutch, not a cane. It is used by clients who need to limit or eliminate weight-bearing on a lower extremity. The client relies on the strength in the arms and shoulders when walking. The Lofstrand crutch supports the wrist, thus making walking safer.

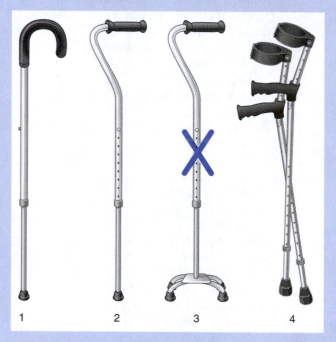

Medication Administration

The following words include nursing/medical terminology, concepts, principles, and information relevant to content specifically addressed in the chapter or associated with topics presented in it. English dictionaries, nursing textbooks, and medical dictionaries, such as *Taber's Cyclopedic Medical Dictionary,* are resources that can be used to expand your knowledge and understanding of these words and related information.

Air-lock (air-bubble) technique

Bevel

Bolus

Canthus, inner/outer

Diluent

Drug levels:
  Peak
  Therapeutic
  Toxic
  Trough

Filtered needle

Five Rights:
  Right client
  Right dose
  Right frequency
  Right medication
  Right route

Gauge

Injection sites:
  Abdomen
  Deltoid
  Dorsogluteal
  "Love handles"
  Rectus femoris
  Vastus lateralis
  Ventrogluteal

Instillation

Interaction:
  Drug
  Food

Medication-dispensing systems

Medication prescriptions:
  prn prescriptions
  Single prescriptions
  Standing prescriptions

STAT prescriptions
  Stop prescriptions
  Telephone prescriptions

Metered-dose inhaler

Over-the-counter drugs (OTCs)

Parenteral

Reconstitution

Routes of administration:
  Buccal
  Ear (otic)
  Epidural
  Eye (ophthalmic)
  Intradermal
  Intramuscular
  Intrathecal
  Intravenous:
      Intravenous piggyback infusion
        (IVPB), intermittent infusion
      IV push
  Nasal cavity
  Rectal
  Subcutaneous
  Sublingual
  Topical
  Transdermal
  Urinary bladder
  Vaginal

Substance misuse

Systemic/local effects

Titrate

Troche

Tuberculin syringe

Unit-dose system

Z-track

MEDICATION ADMINISTRATION: QUESTIONS

1. A nurse instructs a client to close the eyes gently after the administration of eyedrops. Which rationale for this instruction should the nurse explain to the client?
   1. Limits corneal irritation
   2. Forces excess medication from the eyes
   3. Disperses the medication over the eyeballs
   4. Prevents medication from entering the lacrimal duct

2. How often should "docusate sodium 100 mg PO bid" be given?
   1. Three times a day
   2. Two times a day
   3. Every other day
   4. At bedtime

3. A nurse is preparing to reconstitute a medication in a multiple-dose vial. Which is the **most** essential step in the preparation of this medication?
   1. Instilling an accurate amount of diluent into the vial
   2. Using a filtered needle when drawing up the medication from the vial
   3. Instilling air into the vial before withdrawing the reconstituted solution
   4. Wiping the rubber seal of the vial with alcohol before and after each needle insertion

4. Which characteristic is associated with a subcutaneous injection of 5,000 units of heparin?
   1. 3-mL syringe
   2. 22-gauge needle
   3. 1½-inch needle length
   4. 90-degree angle of insertion

5. A home-care nurse observes the spouse of a client inserting a rectal suppository into the client. Which behavior indicates that the nurse must provide further teaching about suppository administration?
   1. Lubricates the tip of the suppository
   2. Inserts the suppository while wearing a glove
   3. Inserts the suppository while the client bears down
   4. Places the suppository a finger length into the rectum

6. A primary health-care provider prescribes a medication that must be administered via the intramuscular route. Which site should the nurse eliminate from consideration because it has the **highest** potential for injury when administering an intramuscular injection?
   1. Vastus lateralis
   2. Rectus femoris
   3. Ventrogluteal
   4. Dorsogluteal

7. Which information about a parenteral medication indicates that the nurse should use a filtered needle when preparing the medication?
   1. Has to be reconstituted
   2. Is supplied in an ampule
   3. Appears cloudy in the vial
   4. Is to be mixed with another medication

8. Which should the nurse use when administering a subcutaneous injection?
   1. 5-mL syringe
   2. 25-gauge needle
   3. Tuberculin syringe
   4. 1½-inch-long needle

9. When the nurse brings a pill to a client, the client is unable to hold the paper cup with the medication. Which should the nurse do?
   1. Use the cup to introduce the pill into the client's mouth.
   2. Crush the pill and mix it with a small amount of applesauce.
   3. Have the primary health-care provider prescribe the liquid form of the drug.
   4. Put the pill into the client's hand and have the client self-administer the pill.

10. Which route is inappropriate for a topical medication?
    1. Intradermal
    2. Bladder
    3. Rectum
    4. Vagina

11. A nurse holds a bottle with the label next to the palm of the hand when pouring a liquid medication. Which is the rationale for this action?
    1. Prevent soiling of the label by spilled liquid
    2. Conceal the label from the curiosity of others
    3. Ensure accuracy of the measurement of the dose
    4. Guarantee the label is read before pouring the liquid

12. A primary health-care provider prescribes a medicated powder to be applied to a client's lower leg. Which is **most** essential for the nurse to do when applying the medicated powder?
    1. Apply a thin layer in the direction of hair growth.
    2. Protect the client's face with a small towel.
    3. Dress the area with dry sterile gauze.
    4. Ensure that the skin surface is dry.

13. A nurse must administer a medication that is supplied in an ampule. Which should the nurse do **first** to access the ampule?
    1. Break the constricted neck using a barrier.
    2. Wipe the constricted neck with an alcohol swab.
    3. Insert the needle into the center of the rubber seal.
    4. Inject the same amount of air as the fluid to be removed.

14. A nurse must administer a medication into the ear of an adult. Which should the nurse do to limit client discomfort when administering the eardrops?
    1. Warm the solution to body temperature.
    2. Place the client in a comfortable position.
    3. Pull the pinna of the ear upward and backward.
    4. Instill the fluid in the center of the auditory canal.

15. A nurse instructs a client to inhale deeply and hold each breath for a second when using a hand-held nebulizer. The client asks, "Why do I have to hold my breath?" Which information should the nurse include in the response to the client's question?
    1. "It prolongs treatment."
    2. "It limits hyperventilation."
    3. "It disperses the medication."
    4. "It prevents bronchial spasms."

16. Which abbreviation indicates that the primary health-care provider wants a medication administered before meals?
    1. pc
    2. ac
    3. PO
    4. OD

17. A home-care nurse is helping a client with short-term memory loss with how to remember to take multiple drugs throughout the day. Which should the nurse do when teaching this client?
    1. Suggest that the client wear a watch with an alarm.
    2. Ask a family member to call the client when medications are to be taken.
    3. Design a chart of the medications the client takes each day during the week.
    4. Instruct the client to put medications in a weekly organizational pill container.

18. Which action should be implemented by the nurse when a medication is delivered by the Z-track method?
    1. Use a special syringe designed for Z-track injections.
    2. Pull the skin laterally away from the injection site before inserting the needle.
    3. Administer the injection in the muscle on the anterolateral aspect of the thigh.
    4. Insert the needle in a separate spot for each dose on a Z-shaped grid on the abdomen.

19. A nurse must reconstitute a powdered medication. Which action should the nurse implement?
    1. Keep the needle below the initial fluid level as the rest of the fluid is injected.
    2. Instill the solvent that is consistent with the manufacturer's directions.
    3. Score the neck of the ampule before breaking it.
    4. Shake the vial to dissolve the powder.

20. A nurse is preparing to administer a tablet to a client. When should the nurse remove the medication from its unit dose package?
    1. Outside the door to the client's room
    2. When next to the client's bed
    3. In the medication room
    4. At the medication cart

21. A client has a prescription for an analgesic. Which nursing action is appropriate when administering this medication?
    1. Reassess drug effectiveness every 8 hours.
    2. Follow the prescription exactly for the first 24 hours.
    3. Seek a new prescription after two doses that do not achieve a tolerable level of relief.
    4. Ask the primary health-care provider to prescribe another medication for breakthrough pain.

22. The primary health-care provider prescribes a troche. In which part of the body should the nurse administer the troche?
    1. Ear
    2. Eye
    3. Mouth
    4. Rectum

23. A nurse teaches a client about taking a sublingual nitroglycerin tablet. Which part of the body identified by the client indicates that the client understands the teaching?
    1. "On my skin."
    2. "Inside my cheek."
    3. "Under my tongue."
    4. "In my eye on the lower lid."

24. A nurse plans to administer a bolus dose of a medication via a currently running IV infusion. Which should the nurse do **first**?
    1. Use a volume-control infusion set with microdrip tubing.
    2. Ensure that it is compatible with the IV solution being infused.
    3. Pinch the tubing above the infusion port while instilling the bolus.
    4. Instill it into a 50-mL bag of normal saline and infuse it via a secondary line.

25. A nurse is administering an intradermal injection. At which angle should the nurse insert the needle?
    1. 90-degree angle
    2. 45-degree angle
    3. 30-degree angle
    4. 15-degree angle

26. A nurse plans to administer a 3-mL intramuscular injection. Which muscle is the **least** desirable to use for the administration of this medication?
    1. Deltoid
    2. Dorsogluteal
    3. Ventrogluteal
    4. Vastus lateralis

27. A nurse is preparing to administer a subcutaneous injection of insulin. Which site should the nurse use to **best** promote its absorption?
    1. Upper lateral arms
    2. Anterior thighs
    3. Love handles
    4. Upper chest

28. A client has a prescription for a vaginal cream. Which should the nurse use when placing the cream into the client's vaginal canal?
    1. A finger
    2. A gauze pad
    3. An applicator
    4. An irrigation kit

29. A primary health-care provider prescribes a medication that must be administered transdermally. Which information about the route of administration does the nurse understand is related to a drug prescribed to be administered transdermally?
    1. Inhaled into the respiratory tract
    2. Dissolved under the tongue
    3. Absorbed through the skin
    4. Inserted into the rectum

30. Which should the nurse do to limit discomfort when administering an injection to an adult?
    1. Pull back on the plunger before injecting the medication.
    2. Apply ice to the area before the injection.
    3. Pinch the area while inserting the needle.
    4. Inject the medication slowly.

31. A nurse is preparing to draw up medication from a vial. Which action should the nurse implement **first**?
    1. Ensure that the needle is firmly attached to the syringe.
    2. Rub vigorously back and forth over the rubber cap with an alcohol swab.
    3. Inject air into the vial with the needle bevel below the surface of the medication.
    4. Instill slightly more air than the volume of medication to be withdrawn from the vial.

32. A primary health-care provider prescribes 18 units of regular insulin and 26 units of NPH insulin to be given at 0730 a.m. in the same syringe. Indicate on the syringe, by shading in the appropriate area, how many total units of regular and NPH insulin are to be drawn into the syringe.

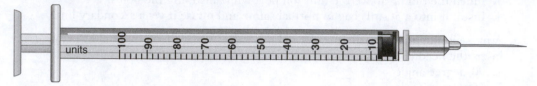

33. A primary health-care provider prescribes a medicated cream for a client to be administered topically to an area of excoriated skin. Place the following steps in the order in which they should be implemented.
1. Don clean gloves.
2. Evaluate the results of the cream on the skin.
3. Warm the tube of medication before application.
4. Cleanse the skin gently with soap and water and pat dry.
5. Don sterile gloves and apply a thin layer of cream to the desired area.

Answer: _____

34. The instructions with a medication state to use the Z-track method of administration. Which action should the nurse implement that is specific to this procedure? **Select all that apply.**
1. _____ Pinch the site throughout the procedure.
2. _____ Massage the site after the needle is removed.
3. _____ Add 0.1 to 0.3 mL of air after drawing up the correct dosage.
4. _____ Remove the needle immediately after the medication is injected.
5. _____ Inject the medication quickly, at a rate of 1 second per mL of solution.

35. A primary health-care provider prescribes benztropine (Cogentin)1.5 mg PO STAT. Benztropine is available in 0.5-mg scored tablets. How many tablets should the nurse administer? **Record your answer using a whole number.**

Answer: _____ tablets.

36. Which routes are unrelated to the parenteral administration of medications? **Select all that apply.**
1. _____ Buccal
2. _____ Z-track
3. _____ Sublingual
4. _____ Intravenous
5. _____ Intradermal

37. Which intervention is uniquely related to the administration of an intradermal injection? **Select all that apply.**
1. _____ Using the air-bubble technique
2. _____ Circling the injection site with a pen
3. _____ Pinching the skin during needle insertion
4. _____ Inserting the needle with the bevel upward
5. _____ Massaging the area after the fluid is instilled

38. A primary health-care provider prescribes an IV antibiotic to be administered four times a day. The client has a primary infusion of 0.9% sodium chloride. The medication is compatible with the sodium chloride. Place an X over the port that should be used when administering this drug as an IV piggyback infusion.

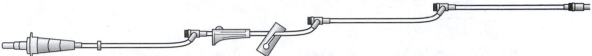

39. A nurse is assessing a client to determine if it is appropriate to administer a prescribed medication via the oral route. Which information indicates that the nurse should ask the primary health-care provider for a change in route? **Select all that apply.**
1. _____ Nausea
2. _____ Unconsciousness
3. _____ Gastric suctioning
4. _____ Emergency situation
5. _____ Difficulty swallowing

40. A primary health-care provider prescribes a medication via a transdermal patch. Place the following steps in the order in which they should be implemented when administering this medication.
1. Remove the previous patch.
2. Contain and dispose of the used patch.
3. Wear clean gloves throughout the procedure.
4. Write the date, time, and your initials on the patch.
5. Apply a new patch to a different section of the skin.
6. Wash and dry the skin after removal of the used patch.

Answer: _____

41. A primary health-care provider prescribes an oral medication for a client. The nurse identifies that the client is having some difficulty swallowing. What should the nurse plan to do? **Select all that apply.**
1. _____ Crush tablets that are crushable and mix with a small amount of applesauce.
2. _____ Have the client hyperextend the neck slightly when swallowing.
3. _____ Give water before, during, and after medication administration.
4. _____ Stroke under the chin over the larynx.
5. _____ Have the client use a straw.

42. The primary health-care provider prescribes 500 mL of D_5W with 10 mEq of KCl to be administered over 10 hours. The IV tubing states that each mL delivers 60 gtts. To what rate per minute should the nurse adjust the flow rate of the intravenous solution? **Record your answer using a whole number.**

Answer: _____ gtts/min.

43. A primary health-care provider prescribes nose drops to be administered twice a day. Which should the nurse do when instilling the nose drops? **Select all that apply.**
1. _____ Tell the client not to sniff the medication once administered.
2. _____ Place the client in the supine position with the head tilted backward.
3. _____ Pinch the nares of the nose together briefly after the drops are instilled.
4. _____ Instruct the client to blow the nose 5 minutes after the drops are instilled.
5. _____ Insert the drop applicator ½ inch into the nose toward the base of the nasal cavity.

44. Which route is associated with the administration of a suppository? **Select all that apply.**
    1. _____ Ear
    2. _____ Nose
    3. _____ Mouth
    4. _____ Vagina
    5. _____ Rectum

45. A primary health-care provider prescribes a monthly intramuscular injection of fluphenazine decanoate 37.5 mg. The medication is available as 25 mg/mL. How much solution of fluphenazine should the nurse administer? **Record your answer using one decimal place.**

    Answer: _____ mL.

46. A nurse is to administer an eye irrigation to a client's right eye. Which should the nurse do? **Select all that apply.**
    1. _____ Direct the flow of solution from the inner to the outer canthus.
    2. _____ Irrigate with a bulb syringe held several inches above the eye.
    3. _____ Expose the conjunctival sac and hold open the upper lid.
    4. _____ Don sterile gloves before beginning the procedure.
    5. _____ Position the client in a right lateral position.

47. A primary health-care provider prescribes medicated eardrops for a client. Place the following steps in the order in which they should be implemented after cleaning the client's ear.
    1. Release the pinna and gently press on the tragus several times.
    2. Pull up and back on the cartilaginous part of the pinna gently.
    3. Place the drops on the side of the ear canal without touching the canal with the dropper.
    4. Position the client in the side-lying position with the affected ear facing toward the ceiling.
    5. Warm the refrigerated eardrops to room temperature by holding the container in the palm of a hand for several minutes.

    Answer: _____

48. A primary health-care provider prescribes a rectal suppository for an adult client. Which action should the nurse implement when administering the rectal suppository? **Select all that apply.**
    1. _____ Lubricate the medication before insertion.
    2. _____ Warm the medication equal to body temperature.
    3. _____ Instruct the client to take deep breaths through the mouth.
    4. _____ Insert the medication just inside the rectum's external sphincter.
    5. _____ Place the client in the prone position to administer the medication.

49. A primary health-care provider prescribes an IV infusion of 1,000 mL 0.9% sodium chloride to be followed by 1,000 mL D_5W with 20 mEq of potassium chloride. The infusion is to be administered at 125 mL/hr. The drop factor of the IV tubing states 10 drops/mL. To how many drops per minute should the nurse set the IV infusion? **Record your answer using a whole number.**

    Answer: _____ gtts/min.

50. A primary health-care provider prescribes a liquid medication that has an unpleasant taste for a school-age child. What should the nurse do to facilitate administration of this medication? **Select all that apply.**
    1. _____ Mix it with the child's favorite food.
    2. _____ Teach that the taste only lasts a short time.
    3. _____ Give an ice pop just before giving the medication.
    4. _____ Have a parent administer the medication if present.
    5. _____ Offer the child the choice of a spoon, needleless syringe, or dropper.

51. A primary health-care provider prescribes acetaminophen 320 mg PO every 6 hours prn for pain for a 12-year-old child. The child has difficulty swallowing pills, and the nurse obtains a liquid form of the drug. The bottle of acetaminophen states that there are 160 mg/5 mL. Put an X at the point on the graduated medicine cup that indicates how much solution of acetaminophen should be administered.

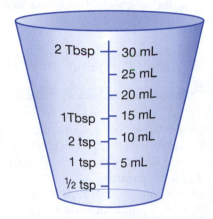

52. A nurse is interviewing a newly admitted client in the process of completing a nursing admission history and physical assessment. Which information should be included in a medication reconciliation form? **Select all that apply.**
    1. _____ Vitamins
    2. _____ Drug allergies
    3. _____ Food supplements
    4. _____ Over-the-counter herbs
    5. _____ Prescribed medications

53. Which action should the nurse implement when administering an intramuscular injection into the ventrogluteal site? **Select all that apply.**
    1. _____ Use a 1-inch needle.
    2. _____ Use a 25-gauge needle.
    3. _____ Insert the needle at a 45-degree angle.
    4. _____ Aspirate before instilling the medication.
    5. _____ Massage the insertion site after needle removal.

54. A primary health-care provider prescribes a vaginal suppository for a client. The nurse obtains the suppository, pulls the curtain around the client's bed, encourages the client to void, provides perineal care, and then dons a new pair of clean gloves. Place the following steps in the order in which they should now progress to complete the administration of the vaginal suppository.
    1. Drape the client, exposing only the vaginal area.
    2. Position the client in the dorsal recumbent position.
    3. Encourage the client to remain in the supine position for 10 to 20 minutes.
    4. Lubricate the suppository and the nurse's index finger with a water-soluble jelly.
    5. Insert the suppository downward and backward using the full length of the index finger.

    Answer: _____

55. A primary health-care provider prescribes a liquid oral medication for a client. Which action should the nurse implement when administering this medication? **Select all that apply**.

1. _____ Vigorously shake the liquid before pouring a dose.
2. _____ Measure oral liquids in a calibrated medication cup at eye level.
3. _____ Pour liquids with the label facing away from the palm of the hand.
4. _____ Place an opened top of a container on a surface with the inside lid facing up.
5. _____ Use a needleless syringe to measure an oral liquid less than 5 mL and transfer it to a medication cup.

56. A client in the emergency department becomes agitated, and limit setting by the nurse is ineffective. The client's behavior escalates, and the client attempts to punch the nurse. The primary health-care provider prescribes a STAT dose of haloperidol (Haldol) 2.5 mg IM. The haloperidol available states that there is 5 mg/mL. Indicate on the syringe, by shading in the appropriate area, how much solution of haloperidol should be administered.

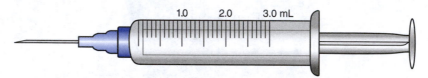

57. A primary health-care provider prescribes two oral medications for a client with a nasogastric tube on low continuous suction. Which action should the nurse implement when administering this medication? **Select all that apply.**

1. _____ Give each medication separately.
2. _____ Follow medication administration with 100 mL of free water.
3. _____ Crush crushable tablets into a fine powder and mix with 30 mL of warm water.
4. _____ Shut off nasogastric tube suctioning for 30 minutes after medication administration.
5. _____ Ensure nasogastric tube placement by instilling 30 mL of air while auscultating over the epigastric area for a "whooshing" sound.

58. An older adult is transported via ambulance to the emergency department of the hospital after being found unconscious on the living room floor by a family member. The client regains consciousness and tells the nurse that everything went blank after the client stood up abruptly from a lounge chair. The client is diagnosed with dehydration and is admitted for observation and rehydration therapy. The nurse performs a routine client assessment 18 hours after initiation of the IV therapy. What should the nurse do **first** after reviewing the client's clinical record and assessing the client?
    1. Administer oxygen via a nasal cannula.
    2. Slow the rate of the intravenous infusion.
    3. Elevate the head of the bed to the semi-Fowler position.
    4. Notify the primary health-care provider of the client's status.

CLIENT'S CLINICAL RECORD

Vital Signs on Admission
Temperature: 99.6°F
Pulse: 96 beats per minute
Respirations: 22 breaths per minute, regular rhythm
Blood pressure: 100/60 mm Hg

Primary Health-Care Provider Prescriptions
IVF: 0.9% sodium chloride at 125 mL/hr for 24 hours
Docusate sodium 100 mg PO once a day

Nurse's Physical Assessment of the Client
Temperature: 99.8°F
Pulse: 112 beats per minute
Respirations: 26 breaths per minute, labored
Blood pressure: 150/98 mm Hg
Breath sounds: Fine rales at base of lungs

---

59. A primary health-care provider prescribes a unit of packed red blood cells for a client with a low hemoglobin level. Which action should be implemented by the nurse when administering this transfusion? **Select all that apply.**
    1. _____ Adjust the flow rate to 20 drops per minute for the first 15 minutes.
    2. _____ After 15 minutes, vital signs should be taken every 15 to 30 minutes.
    3. _____ Ensure that an 18-gauge needle is used for administering the blood transfusion.
    4. _____ Discontinue the blood transfusion if it extends beyond 4 hours after its initiation.
    5. _____ Stay with the client for 15 minutes after initiating the blood transfusion while taking vital signs every 5 minutes.

60. A primary health-care provider prescribes NPH and regular insulin to be administered to a client with diabetes. Place the following illustrations in the order in which they should be implemented when mixing NPH and regular insulin in the same syringe.

Answer: _____

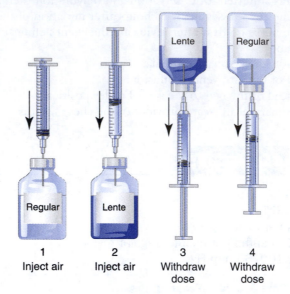

1	2	3	4
Inject air	Inject air	Withdraw dose	Withdraw dose

1. 1. Instilling medication into the conjunctival sac prevents the trauma of drops falling on the cornea.
2. Closing the eyes gently, rather than squeezing the lids shut, prevents the loss of medication from the conjunctival sac.
3. **Closing the eyes moves the medication over the conjunctiva and the eyeball and helps ensure an even distribution of medication.**
4. Gentle pressure over the inner canthus for 1 minute after administration prevents medication from entering the lacrimal duct.

2. 1. The abbreviation for three times a day is tid (ter in die).
2. **The abbreviation bid (bis in die) represents twice a day.**
3. Bid does not mean every other day. Every other day must be written out. The Joint Commission disallows the use of the abbreviation for every other day QOD (quaque altera die) because of the frequency of errors with its use.
4. Bid (bis in die) represents twice a day, not at bedtime. Formerly, the abbreviation for bedtime (hour of sleep) was hs (hora somni); however, The Joint Commission disallows the use of the abbreviation of hs because of the frequency of errors with its use.

3. 1. **The required amount of diluent must be followed exactly in a multiple-dose formulation to ensure accurate dosage preparation. The diluent for a single-dose formulation also must be measured exactly so that the medication is diluted enough not to injure body tissues.**
2. A filtered needle should be used when drawing up fluid from an ampule, not a vial. A filter prevents shards of glass from entering the syringe.
3. Although this is an advisable practice, it is not as important as administering an accurate dose.
4. The rubber seal must be wiped with alcohol before, not after, needle insertion.

4. 1. Most doses of heparin are less than 1 mL. It would be difficult to withdraw an appropriate amount of heparin in a 3-mL syringe because the volume markings on the syringe are widely spaced.
2. A 22-gauge needle is too large and can cause unnecessary trauma and bleeding at the insertion site. A 25- or 26-gauge needle is adequate.
3. A 1½-inch length needle is unnecessarily long and may enter a muscle rather than subcutaneous tissue.
4. **A ½-inch-length needle inserted at a 90-degree angle will ensure that the heparin is inserted into subcutaneous tissue.**

5. 1. Lubrication is required to limit tissue trauma and ease insertion.
2. Standard precautions should be employed when there is exposure to clients' body fluids.
3. **Bearing down increases intra-abdominal pressure, which impedes the insertion of the suppository. The client should be instructed to relax and breathe deeply and slowly while the suppository is inserted.**
4. In an adult, a suppository should be inserted 4 inches to ensure it is beyond the internal sphincter.

6. 1. The vastus lateralis site is not near large nerves or blood vessels, and the muscle does not lie over a joint. It is a preferred site for infants 7 months of age and younger.
2. The rectus femoris site is not near major nerves, blood vessels, or bones. It is an appropriate site for adults.
3. The ventrogluteal site is not near large nerves or blood vessels. It is a preferred site in adults and children.
4. **The dorsogluteal site has the highest risk for injury because of the close proximity of the sciatic nerve, blood vessels, and bone.**

7. 1. Reconstitution occurs within a closed vial and does not require a filtered needle.
2. **The top of an ampule must be snapped off at its neck to access the fluid. A filtered needle prevents glass particles from being drawn into the syringe.**
3. The majority of medications in vials are clear solutions. Cloudy fluid usually indicates contamination. Additional information from a drug guide or a pharmacist is necessary to determine if the cloudiness is an expected characteristic of the drug or it indicates contamination.
4. It is not necessary to use a filtered needle when mixing medications.

8. 1. A subcutaneous injection should not exceed 1 mL. A 3-mL, not a 5-mL, syringe is acceptable for a subcutaneous injection.
   2. **A subcutaneous injection should use a 25- to 29-gauge needle, which minimizes tissue trauma. The diameter of a needle is referred to as its gauge, which ranges from 28 (small) to 14 (large).**
   3. The volume of a tuberculin syringe is only 1 mL. For most subcutaneous injections, a syringe that can accommodate up to 3 mL is preferred to facilitate handling of the syringe.
   4. A 1½-inch length is appropriate for an intramuscular, not a subcutaneous, injection.

9. 1. **The client needs assistance. Keeping medication in the cup, rather than touching it with the hands, maintains medical asepsis.**
   2. Mixing medication with applesauce is done if the client has dysphagia.
   3. It is not necessary to obtain a prescription for the liquid form of the medication. A prescription is required if a route other than oral is necessary.
   4. This action is unrealistic and unsafe. The client requires assistance.

10. 1. **An intradermal injection is inserted below, not on top of, the epidermis.**
    2. Medications in the form of solutions can be instilled into the bladder. They are designed to work locally and are considered topical medications.
    3. Medications in the form of a suppository can be inserted into the rectum and are considered topical medications. Most are designed to work locally, although some are absorbed systemically.
    4. Medications in the form of a suppository, tablet, cream, foam, or jelly can be instilled into the vagina. They are designed to work locally and are considered topical medications.

11. 1. **Liquid medication may drip down the side of the bottle and soil the label, which may interfere with the ability to read the label accurately.**
    2. Although client confidentiality should always be maintained, this is not the reason for holding the label toward the palm of the hand.
    3. Accuracy of the dose is ensured by using a calibrated cup and measuring the liquid at the base of the meniscus while positioning the cup at eye level.

4. The label should be read before holding it against the palm of the hand.

12. 1. This action is done with lotions, creams, or ointments.
    2. It is unnecessary to protect the client's face. When the powder is sprinkled gently on the site, the powder should not become aerosolized.
    3. A dressing is not a universal requirement. When necessary, a dressing is applied with a primary health-care provider's prescription.
    4. **Moisture harbors microorganisms, and when mixed with a powder it will result in a pastelike substance. The site should be clean and dry to ensure effective action of the drug.**

13. 1. **A barrier, such as a commercially manufactured ampule opener, gauze, or an alcohol swab, should be used to protect the nurse's hands from broken glass.**
    2. The rubber seal of a vial, not the neck of an ampule, should be wiped with alcohol.
    3. Piercing a rubber seal is done with a vial, not an ampule.
    4. Injecting air is done with a vial, not an ampule.

14. 1. **Instilling cold medication into the ear canal is uncomfortable and can cause vertigo and nausea. Holding the bottle of medication in the hand for several minutes warms the solution to body temperature.**
    2. A comfortable position may not be the side-lying position, which is required for administration of an ear drop. The side-lying position with the involved ear upward must be maintained for 2 to 3 minutes while the instilled medication disperses throughout the ear canal.
    3. These actions straighten the ear canal and facilitate the flow of medication toward the eardrum in an adult; they do not limit discomfort.
    4. This action is contraindicated because the force of the fluid may injure the eardrum. The drops should be directed along the side of the ear canal.

15. 1. There is no advantage in prolonging the treatment.
    2. Slow, deep breathing will limit hyperventilation.
    3. **A pause at the height of inspiration will promote distribution and absorption of the medication before exhalation begins.**

4. Slow inhalations and exhalations with pursed lips help prevent bronchial spasms.

16. 1. The abbreviation for after meals is pc (post cibum).
    2. **The abbreviation for before meals is ac (ante cibum).**
    3. The abbreviation for by mouth is PO (per os).
    4. The abbreviation for right eye is OD. However, this abbreviation should be spelled out because there is confusion among the following abbreviations: right eye—OD (oculus dexter), left eye—OS (oculus sinister), and both eyes—OU (oculus utro).

17. 1. This suggestion is unrealistic. When the alarm goes off, the client may not remember why it is ringing.
    2. This suggestion is unrealistic and puts an excessive burden on family members.
    3. A chart is unrealistic. The chart may be complex, confusing, and require repeated cognitive decisions throughout the day that may be beyond the client's ability.
    4. **Pill distribution can be set up once a week. After the medication is taken, the empty section reminds the client that the medication was taken, which prevents excessive doses. This is a major issue for clients with short-term memory loss.**

18. 1. A special syringe is not needed for administering a medication via Z-track. The barrel of the syringe must be large enough to accommodate the volume of solution to be injected (usually 1 to 3 mL) and the needle long enough to enter a muscle (usually 1½ inches).
    2. **This action creates a zigzag track through the various tissue layers. The track prevents backflow of medication up the needle track when simultaneously removing the needle and releasing the traction on the skin after the medication is injected.**
    3. The use of the vastus lateralis muscle for a Z-track injection may cause discomfort for the client. Z-track injections are tolerated more when the well-developed gluteal muscles are used.
    4. The needle is inserted into the muscle once for a Z-track injection. The Z represents the zigzag pattern of the needle track that results when the skin traction and the needle are simultaneously removed.

19. 1. This will create excessive bubbles that can interfere with complete reconstitution or result in bubbles being drawn into the syringe. Both occurrences can result in an inaccurate dose.
    2. **Compatibility is necessary so that a compound or precipitate that is harmful to a client does not result.**
    3. Reconstitution occurs in a vial (a closed system), not an ampule (an open system).
    4. Shaking the vial will create excessive bubbles. The vial should be rotated between the hands to facilitate reconstitution.

20. 1. Opening the package outside the room exposes the medication to the environment, where it may become contaminated or grouped with other medications being administered to the client, thus interfering with safe administration of one or more of the medications.
    2. **The medication should be opened at the bedside and administered immediately to the client, thereby limiting the potential for contamination. Reading the label immediately before opening the package is an additional safety check. Immediate administration prevents accidental disarrangement of medications that may result in a medication error.**
    3. Opening the package in the medication room exposes the medication to the environment because it requires the nurse to carry the medication through the unit to the client's room. In addition, it can become confused with the medications for other clients.
    4. Opening the package at the medication cart exposes the medication unnecessarily to the environment, and it can be inadvertently confused with the medications for other clients.

21. 1. The client should be assessed every 1 to 2 hours to ensure effectiveness of the drug.
    2. The prescription should be followed exactly if it is a safe dose; however, if the medication is not effective, 24 hours is too long a period not to intervene.
    3. **Two doses provide enough time to evaluate the effectiveness of a medication for pain. Clients should not have to endure intolerable levels of pain.**
    4. Requesting additional medication is unnecessary if the drug is the appropriate dose.

22. 1. Medications in the form of a solution are instilled into the ear.
2. Ophthalmic medications in the form of a solution or an ointment are administered in the eye.
3. **A troche, a lozengelike tablet, dissolves slowly in the mouth in the buccal cavity to provide a localized effect.**
4. Medications in the form of suppositories are inserted through the anus into the rectum.

23. 1. Topical medications are applied on the skin.
2. A troche or lozenge given by the buccal route is placed between the cheek and gums.
3. **A sublingual medication is placed under the tongue. It is absorbed quickly through the mucous membranes into the systemic circulation.**
4. A medication placed in the lower conjunctival sac of the eye is administered for its local effect and is considered a topical medication.

24. 1. The volume of fluid of a bolus dose is too small to necessitate a volume-control infusion set.
2. **An incompatible solution can increase, decrease, or neutralize the effects of the medication. In addition, an incompatibility may result in a compound or cause a precipitate that is harmful to the client.**
3. Pinching the tubing is not done first. Pinching is done immediately before and while instilling the medication to ensure that the medication flows toward the client, rather than in the opposite direction up the tubing.
4. Instilling a bolus dose of medication into a 50-mL bag of normal saline and infusing it via a secondary line is done for a medication administered via an intermittent IV infusion over a 30- to 90-minute period rather than for an IV bolus (IV push) dose that is administered over 1 to 5 minutes.

25. 1. A 90-degree angle is appropriate for an intramuscular, not an intradermal, injection.
2. A 45-degree angle is appropriate for a subcutaneous injection when using a needle that is 1 inch long, not for an intradermal injection.
3. A 30-degree angle is too steep an angle for an intradermal injection, and a wheal will not form.

4. **An intradermal injection is administered by inserting a needle at a 10- to 15-degree angle through the skin with the bevel of the needle facing upward toward the skin. The small volume of medication instilled just below the epidermis causes the formation of a wheal (a localized area of swelling that appears like a small bubble).**

26. 1. **The deltoid muscle, on the lateral aspect of the upper arm, is a small muscle that is incapable of absorbing a large medication volume. This site is more appropriate for 1 mL of solution.**
2. The dorsogluteal site uses the gluteus maximus muscles in the buttocks, which can absorb larger medication volumes.
3. The ventrogluteal site uses the gluteus medius and minimus muscles in the area of the hip, which can absorb larger medication volumes.
4. The vastus lateralis muscles are located on the anterolateral aspect of the thighs, which can absorb larger medication volumes.

27. 1. Although insulin can be administered at the deltoid site, it is a small area that is not conducive to injection rotation within the site. The rate of absorption at this site is slower than at the preferred site for insulin administration.
2. Although insulin can be administered in this site, tissues of the thighs and buttocks have the slowest absorption rate.
3. **The areas around the waist lateral to the abdomen are the preferred sites for the administration of insulin. These areas have abundant subcutaneous tissue that has a fast rate of absorption, and they promote a systematic rotation of injections.**
4. The chest is not an acceptable site for the administration of insulin because of the lack of adequate subcutaneous tissue.

28. 1. Either a gloved finger or an applicator is used to insert a vaginal suppository, not a cream.
2. It is impossible to insert a cream into the vaginal canal with a gauze pad. If attempted, it will traumatize the mucous membranes of the vagina.
3. **The consistency of a cream requires that an applicator be used to ensure that the medication is deposited along the full length of the vaginal canal.**

4. The consistency of a cream is too thick to be inserted into the vagina with an irrigating kit.

29. 1. A medication that is aerosolized is inhaled.
2. A tablet, such as nitroglycerin, is dissolved under the tongue.
3. **A medicated patch or disk can be applied directly to the skin, where the medication is released and absorbed over time. This method ensures a continuous therapeutic drug level and reduces fluctuations in circulating drug levels.**
4. Medications in the form of a suppository are inserted into the rectum.

30. 1. Testing for a blood return prevents injecting medication directly into the circulatory system, rather than limiting the discomfort of an injection.
2. Applying ice is contraindicated because it causes vasoconstriction, which limits absorption of the medication.
3. Pinching the skin aids in needle insertion when administering a subcutaneous injection. It does not limit the discomfort of an injection.
4. **Injecting slowly allows the fluid to be dispersed gradually, which limits tissue trauma and discomfort.**

31. 1. **This will ensure a tight seal and a closed system. If not firmly connected, the hub of the needle may disengage from the barrel of the syringe during preparation or administration of the medication when internal and external pressures are exerted on the needle and syringe.**
2. The top just needs to be swiped. Rubbing back and forth is a violation of surgical asepsis because it reintroduces microorganisms to the area being cleaned.
3. Injecting air below the surface of the solution should be avoided because it causes bubbles that may interfere with the drawing up of an accurate volume of solution.
4. Excess air in the closed system raises pressure in the vial that may cause bubbles when withdrawing the fluid and result in an inaccurate volume of solution.

32. **Answer: 44 units total.**
A total of 44 units of insulin should be drawn into the syringe. Eighteen units of regular insulin are drawn into the syringe first, and then the 26 units of NPH insulin are drawn into the syringe. It is done in this order to ensure that the NPH insulin, which is longer acting, does not dilute the regular insulin in the vial, which is fast acting.

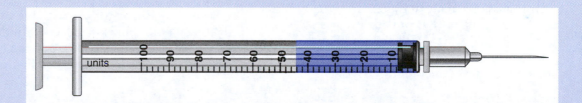

33. 1. **Using clean gloves conforms to standard precautions; they protect the nurse from the client's body fluids.**
4. **Cleansing the area removes debris and previously applied topical medication; doing so allows the skin to be accessible to the cream. Patting the skin dry is less irritating to the skin than rubbing, and the dry surface facilitates adherence of the cream.**
3. **Warming the medication promotes comfort for the client when it is applied.**
5. **Sterile gloves maintain sterility of the procedure and prevent the nurse from contacting and absorbing the medication. Excessive cream can irritate the skin.**
2. **Evaluating the results of the cream on the skin ensures that therapeutic and nontherapeutic responses to the medication are identified. These responses must be documented and communicated to other members of the healthcare team.**

34. 1. When the Z-track method is used during an intramuscular injection, the skin and the subcutaneous tissue are pulled laterally 1 to 1½ inches away from the injection site, not pinched.
2. Massage is contraindicated because it will force medication back up the needle track, which may result in tissue irritation or staining.

3. The injection of a small amount of air after the medication is administered instills air into the Z track, and this helps to keep the medication deeply seated in the muscle.

4. Removal of the needle should be delayed 10 seconds to allow the medication to begin to be dispersed and absorbed.

5. The medication should be injected slowly, at a rate of 10 seconds per mL of solution. This allows time for the medication to become dispersed in the tissue, reducing back pressure on the line of needle insertion.

35. Answer: 3 tablets.
Solve the problem using the "Desire Over Have" formula.

$$\frac{\text{Desired}}{\text{Have}} \quad \frac{1.5 \text{ mg}}{0.5 \text{ mg}} = \frac{x \text{ tablets}}{1 \text{ tablet}}$$
$$0.5x = 1 \times 1.5$$
$$x = 1.5 \div 0.5$$
$$x = 3 \text{ tablets}$$

36. 1. A parenteral route is outside the gastrointestinal tract. A medication administered by the buccal route dissolves between the cheeks and gums, where it acts on the oral mucous membranes or is swallowed with saliva. Most troches are used for their local effect.

2. Z-track is a method of administering an intramuscular injection. The intramuscular route is a parenteral route.

3. A parenteral route is outside the gastrointestinal tract. With the sublingual route, medication dissolves under the tongue, where it is rapidly absorbed.

4. The IV route, a parenteral route, instills medication directly into the venous circulation.

5. The intradermal route, a parenteral route, injects medication just under the epidermis.

37. 1. The air-bubble or air-lock technique can be used with intramuscular, not intradermal, injections.

2. Circling the injection site with a pen indicates the area that must be evaluated; generally, the site is assessed 72 hours after the intradermal injection.

3. Pinching or bunching up tissue is appropriate with subcutaneous, not intradermal, injections.

4. When medication is injected with the bevel up, a small wheal will form under the skin. This technique is used only with intradermal injections.

5. Massaging the site of an intradermal injection will disperse the medication beyond the intended injection site and is contraindicated.

38. This port is accessible to the short length of a secondary administration set tubing. The port is above the roller clamp on the primary tubing. When the bag of medication is hung higher than the primary solution bag, the back check valve on the primary tubing will shut off the flow of the primary infusion until the IV piggyback (secondary intermittent infusion) is almost complete. See figure.

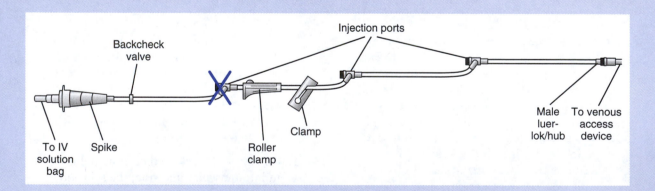

39. 1. Vomiting, not nausea, is a contraindication for oral medications.
2. **Nothing that requires swallowing should ever be placed into the mouth of an unconscious client because of the risk for aspiration.**
3. Gastric suctioning can be interrupted for 20 to 30 minutes after medication has been instilled via a nasogastric tube.
4. **In an emergency, a drug is best administered IV, rather than orally, because it is faster acting.**
5. Nursing interventions, such as positioning, mixing a crushed medication in applesauce, and dissolving a medication in a small amount of fluid, can be employed to facilitate the ingestion of medication.

40. 3. **Wearing clean gloves protects the nurse from contact with the medication.**
1. **Removing the previous patch reduces the risk of an overdose of the medication.**
2. **Containing and disposing of the used patch protects others from contact with active matter on the patch.**
6. **Washing and drying the skin after removing a used patch eliminates lingering medication from the skin and minimizes the risk of overdose.**
5. **Applying a patch to a different surface of the skin avoids irritation to a surface that is used excessively.**
4. **Writing the date, time, and your initials on the patch allows for accountability and helps minimize the risk of a medication error.**

41. 1. **Reducing the size of a tablet and mixing it with a food the consistency of applesauce facilitate ingestion and minimize the risk of aspiration. The thickness of applesauce is easier to control in the mouth than water for a person who has difficulty swallowing.**
2. Hyperextending the neck when swallowing facilitates entry of the substance ingested into the trachea; this action is unsafe. Slightly flexing, not hyperextending, the neck helps to open the esophagus and bypass the trachea when swallowing.
3. **Giving a small amount of fluid before, during, and after medication administration lubricates the oral cavity and facilitates movement of medication toward the esophagus and stomach.**

4. **Stroking under the chin over the larynx encourages laryngeal elevation, which facilitates swallowing.**
5. A straw deposits fluid in the back of the mouth and does not allow time for a coordinated approach to swallowing. The use of a straw increases the risk of aspiration.

42. **Answer: 50 gtts/min.**
Solve the problem by using the following formula.

$$\frac{\text{Total volume to be infused} \times \text{drop factor}}{\text{Total time in minutes}}$$

$$\frac{500 \text{ (total volume to be infused)} \times 60 \text{ (drop factor of the IV tubing)}}{60 \text{ (minutes within an hour)} \times 10 \text{ (number of hours prescribed)}}$$

$$\frac{500 \times 60 = 30{,}000}{60 \times 10 = 600}$$

$$30{,}000 \div 600 = 50 \text{ drops per minute (gtts/min)}$$

43. 1. **Avoiding sniffing the nose drops after administration allows the medication to reach desired areas (ethmoid and sphenoid sinuses) via gravity.**
2. **This position ensures that gravity will promote the flow of medication to the nasopharynx. Five minutes is the length of time the client should remain in the supine position with the head tilted backward.**
3. Pinching the nose is unnecessary and can frighten the client, who already may be having difficulty breathing.
4. Blowing the nose should be avoided because it may remove medication from the nose.
5. Nose drops should be directed toward the midline of the ethmoid bone, with the dropper held ½ inch above the nares. Holding the dropper ½ inch above the nares prevents contamination of the dropper.

44. 1. Medicated solutions are administered via drops in the ear.
2. Medicated solutions are dropped or sprayed in the nose.
3. Tablets, lozenges, and troches are administered in the mouth.
4. **Semisolid cone-shaped or oval suppositories that melt at body temperature can be inserted into the vagina.**
5. **Semisolid cone-shaped or oval suppositories that melt at body temperature are inserted rectally.**

45. Answer: 1.5 mL.
Solve the problem using the "Desire Over Have" formula.

$$\frac{\text{Desired}}{\text{Have}} \quad \frac{37.5 \text{ mg}}{25 \text{ mg}} = \frac{x \text{ mL}}{1 \text{ mL}}$$

$$25x = 37.5$$
$$x = 37.5 \div 25$$
$$x = 1.5 \text{ mL}$$

46. 1. **This action prevents secretions and fluid from entering and irritating the lacrimal ducts.**
2. A bulb syringe produces a flow of fluid that is forceful and difficult to control. An IV bag of solution is preferred to provide a flow of fluid by gravity that is gentle and controllable.
3. **These actions provide access to the eye.**
4. Medical, not surgical, asepsis is required for this procedure.
5. The client should be placed in a sitting or back-lying position with the head tilted toward the affected eye.

47. 5. **Warming the medication to room temperature minimizes discomfort when the medication enters the external ear canal.**
4. **The side-lying position helps to retain the drops in the external ear canal via gravity.**
2. **Gently pulling up and back on the pinna for an adult helps to straighten the ear canal, and this promotes the flow of drops toward the tympanic membrane.**
3. **Placing the drops on the side of the ear canal allows the fluid to flow down the wall of the external ear canal and avoid injury to the tympanic membrane.**
1. **Pressing gently on the tragus several times moves the medication along the external ear canal toward the tympanic membrane.**

48. 1. **Lubrication eases insertion by reducing friction, which limits tissue trauma and discomfort.**
2. Warming the medication causes it to melt, making it impossible to insert. Most rectal suppositories are kept refrigerated until used.
3. **Taking deep breaths relaxes the rectal sphincters.**
4. Rectal suppositories should be inserted 3 inches into the rectal canal past the rectum's internal sphincter of an adult. This can be accomplished by using the full length of a lubricated, gloved index finger to place the suppository.
5. The client should be placed in the left-lateral or left-Sims position to take advantage of the anatomical curve of the rectum and sigmoid colon.

49. Answer: 21 gtts/min.
Solve the problem by using the following formula.

$$\frac{\text{Total volume to be infused} \times \text{drop factor}}{\text{Total time in minutes}}$$

$$\frac{125 \text{ (volume to be infused in 1 hour)} \times 10 \text{ (drop factor of the IV tubing)}}{60 \text{ (number of minutes in 1 hour)}}$$

$$125 \times 10 = 1{,}250$$
$$1{,}250 \div 60 = 20.8$$

Because 0.8 is greater than 0.5, round the answer up to 21 gtts/min.

50. 1. Using a favorite food or liquid to mask the taste of a medication may promote a negative association with and subsequent refusal of the favorite food or liquid. This practice should be avoided.
2. Although this may be a true statement, it denies the child's dislike of the medication's unpleasant taste.
3. **An ice pop just before administration may numb the taste buds and minimize the unpleasant taste of the medication.**
4. A parent should not be asked to administer unpleasant-tasting medication, to avoid the child associating the parent with the unpleasant medication.
5. **Offering the child a choice supports a sense of control. Involvement in decisions limits resistance.**

51. Answer: 10 mL.
Solve the problem using the "Desire Over Have" formula.

$$\frac{\text{Desire}}{\text{Have}} \quad \frac{320 \text{ mg}}{160 \text{ mg}} = \frac{\text{x mL}}{5 \text{ mL}}$$

$$160x = 320 \times 5$$
$$160x = 1,600$$
$$x = 1,600 \div 160$$
$$x = 10 \text{ mL}$$

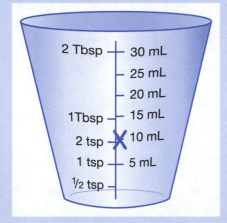

52. 1. Vitamins are a medication and should be included on a medication reconciliation form. An accurate list of all the drugs that a client is taking (e.g., name, dose, route, and frequency) should be reconciled on admission and during transitions (e.g., transfer between units, shift reports, when new medication administration records are implemented, and at discharge). This list should be compared with new medications prescribed and education provided to the client about each medication.

2. Generally, drug allergies are documented on a health history, not on the drug reconciliation form.

3. **Food supplements are considered medications because they often contain ingredients that may interact with medicinal products.**

4. **Over-the-counter herbs are considered medications because they contain ingredients that may unfavorably interact with medicinal products.**

5. **Prescribed medications should be included on a medication reconciliation form.**

53. 1. A 1½-inch needle is required to reach muscular tissue.

2. A 22-gauge needle usually is used for an intramuscular injection; a 25-gauge needle usually is used for a subcutaneous injection.

3. The needle should be inserted at a 90-degree angle; a 45-degree angle is used for a subcutaneous injection when using a 1-inch needle.

4. Research indicates that aspiration before instilling an intramuscular injection is not necessary when using the ventrogluteal, vastus lateralis, and rectus femoris sites. There are no major blood vessels at these sites. Aspiration is recommended before instilling the medication in the gluteus maximus site because of the close proximity of blood vessels. A blood return indicates that the needle is in a blood vessel and the procedure should be discontinued.

5. **Massage promotes dispersement of the medication.**

54. 2. **Positioning the client in the dorsal recumbent position provides access to the vaginal area and is a comfortable position for the client during the procedure.**

1. **Exposing only the vaginal area provides for privacy and supports dignity.**

4. **Lubricating the suppository and the nurse's gloved index finger facilitates insertion and limits tissue trauma. A water-soluble jelly is gentle and soothing to the mucous membranes of the vagina.**

5. **Directing insertion downward and backward using the full length of the nurse's index finger follows the contour of the vaginal anatomy and ensures that the medication is inserted deep in the vaginal canal.**

3. **Encouraging the client to remain in the supine position for 10 to 20 minutes after insertion allows time for the suppository to melt and to keep it in contact with vaginal tissue, which facilitates absorption.**

55. 1. Not all liquids should be vigorously shaken. Only liquids that contain constituents that must be evenly distributed need to be vigorously shaken; the nurse should follow the manufacturer's directions.

2. **Measuring oral liquids in a calibrated medication cup at eye level ensures accuracy of the dose.**

3. Liquids should be poured with the label against the palm of the hand to prevent the liquid from dripping on and obscuring the label.

4. **Placing an opened top of a container on a surface with the inside lid facing**

up prevents contamination of the inside of the lid and subsequent contamination of the bottle when the lid is returned and closed.

5. Using a needleless syringe to measure an oral liquid volume less than 5 mL and transferring it to a medication cup are acceptable practices because they ensure accuracy of the dose.

56. Answer: 0.5 mL.
Solve the problem using the "Desire Over Have" formula.

$$\frac{Desire}{Have} \quad \frac{2.5 \text{ mg}}{5 \text{ mg}} = \frac{x \text{ mL}}{1 \text{ mL}}$$
$$5x = 2.5$$
$$x = 2.5 \div 5$$
$$x = 0.5 \text{ mL}$$

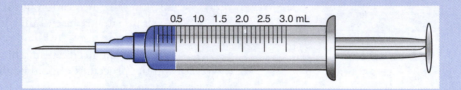

57. 1. If the tube used to administer a medication via a nasogastric tube becomes accidentally disconnected during administration, the nurse can identify the approximate volume of the one medication that was lost when reporting the event to the primary health-care provider.
2. Oral medication via a nasogastric tube should be followed by 30 mL, not 100 mL, of tap water to ensure tube patency. Free water refers to larger volumes of water administered at routine intervals as per a prescription by a primary health-care provider.
3. Crushing crushable tablets into a fine powder and mixing the powder with 30 mL of warm water dissolves the medication and prevents clogging the enteral tube.
4. Shutting off nasogastric tube suctioning for 30 minutes after medication administration enhances medication absorption in the stomach.
5. This method is the most unreliable method of assessing placement of a nasogastric tube. Measuring the pH of gastric aspirate is more accurate. A low pH (1 to 5; acidic) indicates the tube probably is in the stomach; a high pH (more than 6; alkaline) indicates the tube probably is in the intestine or the respiratory tract.

58. 1. Although this should be done to increase the amount of oxygen reaching body cells, it is not the priority.
2. The client is exhibiting signs of fluid volume overload and pulmonary edema. The IV infusion rate should be slowed to 15 to 30 mL per hour.

This action will decrease the amount of fluid entering the client's intravenous compartment while maintaining the integrity of the IV access site until the rapid response team is notified and arrives.
3. Although elevating the head of the bed should be done because it will promote respirations and reduce the amount of blood returning from the lower extremities, it is not the priority.
4. Notifying the primary health-care provider should be done eventually. However, the client requires immediate intervention.

59. 1. This is the recommended initial flow rate. It delivers a small amount of blood that allows the nurse to evaluate the client's response to the blood. If the client does not experience a reaction within the first 15 minutes, then the remainder of the packed red blood cells can be administered over 2 to 4 hours.
2. Vital signs should be taken every 15 to 30 minutes depending on the agency's policy; this supports early detection of a transfusion reaction or fluid overload, which enables early intervention.
3. The standard practice is to use an 18-gauge needle when performing a blood transfusion. The width of the lumen of an 18-gauge needle allows red blood cells to infuse without hemolysis of cells.
4. Blood transfusions that extend to 4 hours are discontinued because bacterial growth may occur in the product.

5. The majority of severe transfusion reactions occur during the first 15 minutes of the procedure. Identifying a reaction early minimizes consequences. Clinical indicators of a transfusion reaction include back pain, chills, itching, or shortness of breath.

60. 2. First: The nurse should use an insulin syringe to draw up environmental air equal to the combined volume of both insulins. While keeping the NPH vial right-side up, the nurse should inject air equal to the prescribed amount of NPH into the air pocket at the top of the vial. This air prevents negative pressure inside the NPH vial when the NPH solution is withdrawn later in the procedure. Injecting air into the air pocket at the top of the vial avoids needle exposure to the NPH insulin and prevents bubbles that later can cause an inaccurate dose when the NPH insulin is withdrawn.

1. Second: The nurse should inject the remaining air into the air pocket of the regular insulin vial while the vial is right-side up. Keeping the needle in the air pocket avoids causing bubbles in the solution. Bubbles displace solution, increasing the risk of an incorrect dose. Also, the injected air prevents negative pressure inside the regular insulin vial later when withdrawing the regular insulin.

4. Third: The nurse should invert the regular insulin vial and draw up the prescribed amount of regular insulin. By drawing up the regular insulin first, it prevents contamination of the regular insulin vial with NPH insulin, which is slower acting.

3. Fourth: The nurse should reinsert the needle into the NPH vial, invert the vial, and withdraw the prescribed amount of NPH insulin. The mixed insulin is now ready to be administered.

Pharmacology

The following words include nursing/medical terminology, concepts, principles, and information relevant to content specifically addressed in the chapter or associated with topics presented in it. English dictionaries, nursing textbooks, and medical dictionaries, such as *Taber's Cyclopedic Medical Dictionary,* are resources that can be used to expand your knowledge and understanding of these words and related information.

Adverse effect
Allergic/allergy
Blood level
Controlled substance
Dependence
Drug effect:
  Adverse
  Anaphylaxis, anaphylactic
  Idiosyncratic
  Local
  Side
  Synergistic
  Systemic
  Therapeutic
  Topical
  Toxic, toxicity
Drug levels, terms related to:
  Duration
  Peak
  Onset
  Therapeutic range
  Trough
Drug names:
  Generic
  Trade
Food and Drug Administration (FDA)
Half-life
Hypersensitivity
Interaction
Prophylactic
Teratogenic
Tolerance/threshold

CLASSIFICATIONS OF DRUGS

Analgesic
Antacid
Antianxiety agent
Antiarrhythmic, antidysrhythmic
Antibacterial
Antibiotic
Anticholinergic
Anticoagulant
Anticonvulsant/antiepileptic

Antidepressant
Antidiabetic
Antidiarrheal
Antiemetic
Antifungal
Antihistamine
Antihypertensive
Anti-inflammatory
Antineoplastic
Antiparkinson
Antipsychotic
Antipyretic
Antiretroviral
Antitussive
Antiulcer
Bronchodilator
Cathartic
Diuretic
Emetic
Expectorant
Hypnotic
Laxative
Lipid-lowering agent
Mucolytic
Narcotic
Opioid
Skeletal muscle relaxant
Thyroid agent
Vasodilator
Vitamins and minerals

DRUG FORMS

Caplet
Capsule
Cream
Elixir
Emulsion
Enteric-coated
Extract
Liniment
Lotion
Metered-dose inhaler (MDI)
Ointment

Paste	Syrup
Pill	Tablet
Powder	Tincture
Solution	Transdermal
Suppository	Troche, lozenge
Suspension	

PHARMACOLOGY: QUESTIONS

1. Which effect on the body does the nurse understand is the reason for the need to discontinue a medication when a client's liver function tests become elevated as a result of the medication?
   1. Side effect
   2. Toxic effect
   3. Adverse effect
   4. Synergistic effect

2. Which nursing action is important in relation to the administration of most antibiotics?
   1. Assessing for constipation
   2. Administering between meals
   3. Encouraging foods high in vitamin K
   4. Monitoring the volume of urinary output

3. A nurse is preparing to administer an injection of heparin. Which is the preferred site for this injection?
   1. Leg
   2. Arm
   3. Buttock
   4. Abdomen

4. Which concept associated with drug therapy and quality of sleep is important for a nurse to consider when planning nursing care?
   1. Aggressive pain management will reduce pain but increase insomnia.
   2. Abrupt discontinuation of hypnotic drugs can lead to withdrawal.
   3. Sedatives support restful sleep for people experiencing hypoxia.
   4. Barbiturates are the drugs of choice for insomnia.

5. A primary health-care provider prescribes a medication that is known to cause nephrotoxicity. Which element of pharmacokinetics does the nurse understand is critical when assessing this client's response to this medication?
   1. Excretion
   2. Absorption
   3. Distribution
   4. Biotransformation

6. After administering a drug, the nurse monitors the client for reactions. Which reaction has the **highest** potential to be life-threatening?
   1. Toxicity
   2. Habituation
   3. Anaphylaxis
   4. Idiosyncratic

7. A nurse is assessing clients' responses to medications received. Which must the nurse know about these drugs to **best** evaluate whether the expected outcomes of the drug therapy have been achieved?
   1. Side effects
   2. Therapeutic effect
   3. Mechanism of action
   4. Chemical composition

8. A nurse is to administer a variety of analgesics. For which medication is it **most** important that the nurse know its daily dose limit?
   1. Meperidine
   2. Ibuprofen
   3. Morphine
   4. Codeine

9. A client in pain requests the prescribed pain medication, which is an opioid. Which nursing assessment is **essential** before administering the opioid?
   1. Blood pressure
   2. Respirations
   3. Temperature
   4. Pulse

10. A primary health-care provider prescribes an antihypertensive medication to be administered twice a day. Which is **essential** for the nurse to assess before administering the antihypertensive agent to the client?
    1. Level of consciousness
    2. Apical heart rate
    3. Blood pressure
    4. Respirations

11. Which is a common concern of the nurse when caring for clients taking drugs that depress the immune system?
    1. Inability to follow the therapeutic regimen
    2. Sensory perceptual alterations
    3. Constipation
    4. Infection

12. After the nurse administers an opioid, the client becomes excitable. Which response should the nurse identify as being experienced by the client?
    1. Toxic
    2. Allergic
    3. Synergistic
    4. Idiosyncratic

13. A client experiences unrelenting neuropathic pain. Which classification of drug should the nurse anticipate will be prescribed for this client?
    1. Anticonvulsant
    2. Antidepressant
    3. Antihistamine
    4. Anesthetic

14. A nurse is administering 10 a.m. medications to several clients on a hospital unit. Which condition should the nurse anticipate places a client at the **highest** risk for toxicity associated with most drugs?
    1. Liver disease
    2. Kidney insufficiency
    3. Respiratory difficulty
    4. Malabsorption syndrome

15. A nurse is discussing with a client the variety of routes that medications can be administered. Which route should the nurse explain allows medications to be absorbed most efficiently?
    1. Orally
    2. Rectally
    3. Intravenously
    4. Intramuscularly

16. A client who has 4+ dependent edema is receiving a diuretic. Which is the **best** way for the nurse to evaluate the effectiveness of the diuretic therapy?
    1. Weigh daily.
    2. Assess skin turgor.
    3. Measure calf girth.
    4. Monitor urine specific gravity.

17. A client has a prescription for an antiemetic as an adjunct to antineoplastic therapy. Which dosing schedule should the nurse anticipate that the primary health-care provider will prescribe?
    1. After the client vomits
    2. 30 minutes before meals
    3. When the client reports nausea
    4. 4 and 8 hours after the initial chemotherapeutic dose

18. After the ingestion of a new medication, the client develops a rash, urticaria, and pruritus. Which should the nurse conclude that the client is experiencing?
    1. Allergic response
    2. Idiosyncratic effect
    3. Anaphylactic reaction
    4. Synergistic interaction

19. A client is taking hydrochlorothiazide (HCTZ) once a day. Which fruit should the nurse encourage the client to eat because it contains the **highest** amount of potassium?
    1. Plum
    2. Orange
    3. Banana
    4. Tangerine

20. A nurse must administer a medication that is a digitalis derivative. Which nursing assessment is **essential** before administering this medication?
    1. Pulse rate
    2. Blood pressure
    3. Respiratory rate
    4. Level of consciousness

21. A nurse teaches a client to use a metered-dose inhaler (MDI). The client asks, "Why do I need this instead of just taking a pill?" Which response should the nurse use regarding the primary purpose of a MDI?
    1. "It provides you with a sense of control."
    2. "It directs the medication into your upper respiratory tract."
    3. "It delivers medication via positive pressure into your lungs."
    4. "It releases the medication in small particles that you can inhale deeply."

22. A client with multiple health problems goes to a variety of medical specialists. Which response to medication should the nurse monitor in the client?
    1. Interactions
    2. Habituation
    3. Tolerance
    4. Allergies

23. A nurse is responsible for administering medications via various routes to a group of clients. Which route of administration is the **most** effective way to achieve and maintain a drug's therapeutic level?
    1. IV push
    2. Sublingual route
    3. Oral administration
    4. Large-volume infusion

24. A nurse is administering a variety of medications via the following routes. Which of these routes is the **fastest** acting?
    1. Buccal
    2. Transdermal
    3. Subcutaneous
    4. Intramuscular

25. A client asks the nurse why a lipid-lowering drug was prescribed. Before formulating a response, which should the nurse consider is the reason why primary health-care providers generally prescribe a hyperlipidemic drug?
    1. After failure of diet therapy
    2. For those who are unable to exercise
    3. For clients older than 60 years of age
    4. After 2 consecutive months of elevated serum lipid levels

26. A nurse administers a prescribed antiemetic. Which clinical manifestation, when reduced, indicates that the client is experiencing a therapeutic response?
    1. Fever
    2. Anxiety
    3. Vomiting
    4. Coughing

27. A nurse is contrasting prefilled, disposable unit-dose intramuscular drug cartridges with multidose vials. Which does the nurse conclude is the **primary** purpose of unit-dose cartridges?
    1. Ensure that the appropriate-length needle is attached
    2. Reduce the incidence of drug interactions
    3. Limit preparation time in emergencies
    4. Ensure purity of the drugs

28. Which human response does the nurse understand is prevented by weaning a client from a long-term prescribed corticosteroid rather than suddenly discontinuing the corticosteroid?
    1. Shock
    2. Seizures
    3. Bleeding
    4. Hypothermia

29. The nurse is administering an antihypertensive medication to a client. Which clinical manifestation should the nurse identify as an excessive response to the antihypertensive agent?
    1. Respirations of 24 breaths per minute
    2. Heart rate of 60 beats per minute
    3. Blood pressure of 80/60 mm Hg
    4. Oral temperature of 98°F

30. A client has a prescription for sertraline, an antidepressant. Which is **most** important for the nurse to do?
    1. Monitor the client for suicidal tendencies.
    2. Advise the client to engage in psychotherapy.
    3. Teach the client to limit alcohol intake to one drink per day.
    4. Encourage the client to diet because weight gain is common with this drug.

31. A client is receiving an antipyretic agent. Which client assessment should be performed to determine if the medication has achieved a therapeutic response?
   1. Urine output
   2. Pain tolerance
   3. Respiratory rate
   4. Body temperature

32. Which is the **most** important action by the nurse before instituting client-controlled analgesia via a continuous IV route for the relief of pain?
   1. Identify the client's pain tolerance.
   2. Assess the client's respiratory status.
   3. Determine the client's pain threshold.
   4. Monitor the client's analgesic blood levels.

33. Identify the drug classification that is correctly associated with its expected therapeutic outcomes. **Select all that apply.**
   1. _____ Bronchodilators: relieve dyspnea
   2. _____ Diuretics: increase urinary output
   3. _____ Antitussives: prevent or relieve coughing
   4. _____ Expectorants: decrease mucus production
   5. _____ Antiemetics: prevent or treat nausea and vomiting

34. A primary health-care provider prescribes aluminum hydroxide/magnesium hydroxide tablets, an antacid agent, for a client with symptoms of indigestion. Which is the important thing the nurse should teach this client to do? **Select all that apply.**
   1. _____ Document the characteristics of gastric discomfort in a log.
   2. _____ Notify the health team if coffee-ground vomitus occurs.
   3. _____ Monitor for the presence of diarrhea.
   4. _____ Take the drug an hour before meals.
   5. _____ Swallow the tablets whole.

35. A nurse in the hospital is evaluating client responses to medications. Which classification of drugs commonly precipitates diarrhea? **Select all that apply.**
   1. _____ Sedatives
   2. _____ Narcotics
   3. _____ Laxatives
   4. _____ Antibiotics
   5. _____ Antiemetics

36. A public health nurse is planning a health class about herbal remedies for a group of older adults at the community center. Which information about herbal remedies should the nurse include in the class? **Select all that apply.**
   1. _____ Herbal remedies are capable of causing serious herbal-to-prescription drug interactions.
   2. _____ Herbal remedies are required to be labeled with information about their structure.
   3. _____ Herbal remedies are approved by the Food and Drug Administration.
   4. _____ Herbal remedies are natural because they are botanical in origin.
   5. _____ Herbal remedies are safe because they are organic.

37. A primary health-care provider tells a client who is receiving an antibiotic that several blood specimens will be taken to evaluate the effectiveness of the antibiotic therapy. The client asks the nurse, "Why do these tests have to be done?" Which information included in a response by the nurse answers this client's question? **Select all that apply.**
   1. _____ Test results help maintain constant drug levels in the body.
   2. _____ Test results will determine the half-life of a drug in the body.
   3. _____ Test results identify whether the dose is adequate for the body.
   4. _____ Test results establish where biotransformation occurs in the body.
   5. _____ Test results help monitor the rate of absorption of the drug in the body.

38. The primary health-care provider prescribes 1.5 grams of an antibiotic to be administered IV piggyback 30 minutes before surgery to prevent infection. The medication is supplied in a 10-g vial that states that after reconstitution there will be 500 mg/mL. How much solution should the nurse administer? **Record your answer using a whole number.**

    Answer: _____ mL.

39. A client with a severe upper respiratory tract infection is being treated with a bronchodilator. Which client response indicates that the therapeutic effect has been achieved? **Select all that apply.**
    1. _____ Oxygen saturation of 95%
    2. _____ Presence of viscous secretions
    3. _____ Experiencing no difficulty breathing
    4. _____ Exhibiting a decrease in respiratory excursion
    5. _____ Decrease in bronchovesicular breath sounds on auscultation

40. A client admits to taking magnesium hydroxide for its laxative effect several times a week. Which information should the nurse teach the client about this medication? **Select all that apply.**
    1. _____ It can cause dependence and dehydration if taken for more than 2 weeks.
    2. _____ It can cause an accumulation of sodium and potassium ions in the body.
    3. _____ It should be discontinued if you experience watery diarrhea.
    4. _____ It should be accompanied by 2 to 3 glasses of fluid.
    5. _____ It should be taken at bedtime.

41. While the nurse is applying a transdermal patch, the client asks the nurse, "Why can't I just take a pill?" Which should the nurse explain is the advantage of administering a medication via a transdermal patch? **Select all that apply.**
    1. _____ "It limits allergic responses."
    2. _____ "It prevents drug interactions."
    3. _____ "It delivers the drug over a period of time."
    4. _____ "It bypasses the harsh, acidic digestive system."
    5. _____ "It provides a local rather than a systemic effect."

42. A client has a prescription for diphenoxylate/atropine, an antidiarrheal agent. Which should the nurse teach the client about this medication? **Select all that apply.**
    1. _____ Report the occurrence of decreased urination, muscle cramps, weakness, or fainting.
    2. _____ Inform the primary health-care provider if diarrhea persists for more than 2 days.
    3. _____ Be aware that the medication may cause hyperactivity.
    4. _____ Limit fluid intake to 2,000 mL/day.
    5. _____ Avoid crushing the tablets.

43. A primary health-care provider prescribes famotidine 20 mg PO bid to inhibit gastric acid secretion for a client reporting epigastric discomfort. What should the nurse do when caring for this client? **Select all that apply.**
    1. _____ Assess for constipation.
    2. _____ Evaluate the oral cavity for stomatitis.
    3. _____ Check for a decreased serum creatinine.
    4. _____ Monitor a complete blood count with differential.
    5. _____ Encourage the intake of the full course of therapy as prescribed.

44. A primary health-care provider prescribes zolpidem, an extended-release tablet, 12.5 mg PO at hour of sleep, for a client experiencing insomnia. What is important for the nurse to teach the client about this medication? **Select all that apply.**
    1. _____ Avoid drinking alcohol.
    2. _____ Swallow the tablet whole.
    3. _____ Take it with food for best results.
    4. _____ Repeat the dose if you are not asleep in 3 hours.
    5. _____ Take it when you are able to stay in bed for at least 6 hours.

45. Place the elements of pharmacokinetics in order from the first step to the last step as a medication moves from its entry to its exit from the body.
    1. Excretion
    2. Absorption
    3. Distribution
    4. Biotransformation

    Answer: _____

46. A client at the outpatient clinic reports increasing joint pain caused by arthritis associated with the aging process. The primary health-care provider prescribes ibuprofen 600 mg PO qid for joint pain. What should the nurse teach the client about this medication? **Select all that apply.**
    1. _____ Take it with a few sips of water.
    2. _____ Do not exceed 4,000 mg of this drug daily.
    3. _____ Double a dose if a previous dose is forgotten.
    4. _____ Report the intake of the drug if dental treatment or surgery is necessary.
    5. _____ Use an oatmeal bath for a mild skin rash because it is a common side effect.

47. A primary health-care provider prescribes nitrofurantoin 100 mg oral suspension PO every 6 hours for a client who reports clinical manifestations of a urinary tract infection. What should the nurse teach the client to do when taking nitrofurantoin? **Select all that apply.**
    1. _____ Take this drug on an empty stomach.
    2. _____ Use a straw to take the medication, and rinse the mouth afterward.
    3. _____ Note that urine will be reddish/orange in color, but do not be alarmed.
    4. _____ Report diarrhea, abdominal cramping, fever, and bloody stools if they occur.
    5. _____ Inform the primary health-care provider if clinical manifestations do not resolve within a week of therapy.

48. An active older adult female client reports episodes of urinary urgency and frequency, urge incontinence, and bladder spasms. The primary health-care provider diagnoses an overactive bladder and prescribes oxybutynin, an extended-release tablet, 5 mg PO tid. What should the nurse teach this client? **Select all that apply.**
    1. _____ Crush the tablet thoroughly, mix with a little water, and take it on an empty stomach.
    2. _____ Sedation and weakness may occur when taking this medication.
    3. _____ Avoid requiring alertness when drowsiness occurs.
    4. _____ Report an inability to pass urine if it should occur.
    5. _____ Avoid strenuous activity in a warm environment.

49. A nurse is caring for a client who is receiving two types of analgesics concurrently. Which effect does the nurse understand occurs when these medications are administered together? **Select all that apply.**
    1. _____ Curative
    2. _____ Palliative
    3. _____ Synergistic
    4. _____ Potentiation
    5. _____ Antagonistic

50. A primary health-care provider prescribes the corticosteroid budesonide 180 mcg, 2 inhalations, bid, along with a bronchodilator. What should the nurse teach the client about these medications? **Select all that apply.**

1. _____ "Let the health team know if you develop a skin rash during therapy."
2. _____ "Use your budesonide inhaler and the bronchodilator 5 minutes later."
3. _____ "It will take 2 weeks for you to see an improvement in your symptoms."
4. _____ "Use tap water to rinse and spit after each time you use your budesonide inhaler."
5. _____ "If you experience an acute bronchospasm between doses, you can take an additional dose of budesonide."

51. A tablet containing dextromethorphan 30 mg and guaifenesin 600 mg PO every 4 hours prn is prescribed for a client with a cough and a respiratory tract infection. What should the nurse teach the client who is taking this medication? **Select all that apply.**

1. _____ "Increase your fluid intake to a minimum of 2 quarts of fluid daily."
2. _____ "Report if clinical manifestations do not improve after 2 weeks of therapy."
3. _____ "Obtain medical advice before taking another over-the-counter cold remedy."
4. _____ "Avoid taking alcohol or other central nervous system depressants concurrently with this medication."
5. _____ "Tell your primary health-care provider if severe dizziness, anxiety, confusion, or slow or shallow breathing occur.

52. Which information documented in the clinical record of an adult male client should the nurse consider problematic?

1. Calcium: 5.4 mEq/L
2. Temperature: 97.8°F
3. Docusate sodium: 1,000 mg, PO, daily
4. Respirations: 14 breaths per minute, unlabored

CLIENT'S CLINICAL RECORD

Laboratory Results
Calcium: 5.4 mEq/L
Sodium: 137 mEq/L
Potassium: 4.2 mEq/L

Physical Assessment
Temperature (oral): 97.8°F
Pulse: 62 beats per minute
Respirations: 14 breaths per minute, unlabored
Blood pressure: 128/84 mm Hg

Medication Reconciliation Form
Aspirin 81 mg, PO, daily
Docusate sodium 1,000 mg, PO, daily
Alprazolam 0.5 mg, PO, tid

53. A primary health-care provider prescribes simvastatin 20 mg PO daily, a lipid-lowering agent, for a client with an elevated cholesterol level. What should the nurse teach the client receiving this medication? **Select all that apply.**
1. _____ Exchange vegetable oils containing monounsaturated fatty acids with vegetable oils containing polyunsaturated fatty acids.
2. _____ Report the presence of muscle aches, pains, stiffness, or weakness to the primary health-care provider immediately.
3. _____ Consume 2 to 3 servings of fish high in omega-3 fatty acids weekly.
4. _____ Monitor for cola-colored urine or if output is reduced or absent.
5. _____ Take the medication in the morning.

54. A primary health-care provider prescribes esomeprazole 20 mg PO daily for a client reporting gastroesophageal reflux at night. What should the nurse teach the client receiving this medication? **Select all that apply.**
1. _____ Take the drug one hour before meals.
2. _____ Do not crush or chew the medication.
3. _____ Taking antacids and esomeprazole concurrently is acceptable.
4. _____ Avoid nonsteroidal anti-inflammatory drugs while on this medication.
5. _____ Mix the capsule contents with applesauce if it is difficult to swallow.
6. _____ Painful swallowing, nausea, and chest pain should be reported immediately.

55. A primary health-care provider prescribes acetylsalicylic acid for a client experiencing body aches and fever associated with an upper respiratory tract infection. Which nontherapeutic response related to acetylsalicylic acid should the nurse teach the client to report to the primary health-care provider? **Select all that apply.**
1. _____ Rash
2. _____ Tinnitus
3. _____ Bleeding
4. _____ Dizziness
5. _____ Constipation

56. A nurse is caring for a client receiving morphine for intractable pain associated with cancer. For what nontherapeutic effect should the nurse monitor the client? **Select all that apply.**
1. _____ Sedation
2. _____ Confusion
3. _____ Tachypnea
4. _____ Constipation
5. _____ Hypertension

57. Which word is associated with the medication levothyroxine? **Select all that apply.**
1. _____ Trade
2. _____ Generic
3. _____ Curative
4. _____ Antidote
5. _____ Substitutive

58. A primary health-care provider prescribes a medication that must maintain effective blood concentrations of the drug to be effective. Which information is **essential** for the nurse to know about this medication to ensure its effectiveness? **Select all that apply.**
1. _____ Therapeutic range
2. _____ Trough level
3. _____ Peak level
4. _____ Half-life
5. _____ Onset

59. A primary health-care provider prescribes medication for a hospitalized older adult client with a diagnosis of the flu, an oral *Candida* infection, and a history of hypothyroidism, hyperlipidemia, and moderate dementia. Which prescription should the nurse discuss with the primary health-care provider before administering medications? **Select all that apply.**

1. _____ Clotrimazole 1 lozenge 10 mg, via buccal cavity, 5 times a day for 14 days
2. _____ Acetaminophen 325 mg, PO, every 4 hours prn for headache
3. _____ Levothyroxine 100 mcg PO once a day
4. _____ Simvastatin 20 mg PO hour of sleep
5. _____ Docusate sodium 100 mg PO bid

60. Which type of insulin is reflected by the illustration regarding its length of action?

1. Glargine
2. Regular
3. Lispro
4. NPH

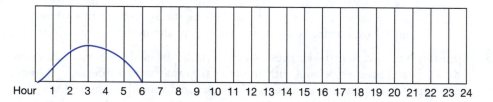

Hour 1 2 3 4 5 6 7 8 9 10 11 12 13 14 15 16 17 18 19 20 21 22 23 24

1. 1. A side effect is an unintended response that generally is predictable and well tolerated. Usually, it does not require discontinuation of the drug because the drug's benefit outweighs the discomfort. Dry mouth and nausea are examples of side effects that do not require discontinuation of the drug, and usually they respond to palliative interventions.
   2. **Liver impairment is an example of a toxic effect that requires discontinuation of a medication. Toxic effects are dangerous and harmful responses to a medication that often are predictable. When a client exhibits a toxic effect to a medication, the nurse should hold the medication and notify the primary health-care provider immediately. The only time holding a dose would not apply is if the drug dose must be tapered to discontinue the drug safely.**
   3. An adverse effect is an unintended, usually unpredictable response to a medication that is more severe than a side effect. When an adverse effect occurs, the medication may or may not be discontinued, depending on the severity of the adverse effect.
   4. A synergistic effect does not apply in this situation. A synergistic effect occurs when the combined effect of two medications is greater than when the effects of each are just added together.

2. 1. Most antibiotics tend to cause diarrhea, not constipation.
   2. **Food often interferes with the dissolution and absorption of antibiotics and delays their action. Also, food can combine with molecules of certain drugs, and it can change their molecular structure and ultimately inhibit or prevent their absorption.**
   3. Yogurt, not foods high in vitamin K, is encouraged for a client receiving antibiotics. Yogurt helps to recolonize the endogenous flora of the gastrointestinal tract that can be eradicated by antibiotics.
   4. Antibiotics do not affect the volume of urinary output.

3. 1. The tissues in the legs are not preferred for the administration of heparin (Hep-Lock) because muscle activity associated with walking increases the risk of hematoma formation.
   2. The tissues in the arms are not preferred for the administration of heparin because muscle activity associated with movement of the arms increases the risk of hematoma formation.
   3. The tissues associated with walking are not preferred for the administration of heparin because muscle activity increases the risk of hematoma formation.
   4. **The abdomen, from among the options presented, is the preferred site for the administration of heparin because it lacks major muscles and muscle activity. This site has the least risk for hematoma formation.**

4. 1. Effective pain management will facilitate rest and sleep, not promote insomnia.
   2. **Barbiturate sedative-hypnotics depress the central nervous system and, when withdrawn abruptly, can cause withdrawal symptoms such as restlessness, tremors, weakness, and insomnia. Long-term use should be tapered by 25% to 30% weekly.**
   3. Sedatives, central nervous system depressants, are not advocated for clients with hypoxia because they depress respirations, which may exacerbate the hypoxia.
   4. Barbiturates depress the central nervous system, alter rapid eye movement and non-rapid eye movement sleep, result in daytime drowsiness, and cause rebound insomnia. For this reason, antianxiety drugs or tranquilizers, rather than barbiturates, are preferred.

5. 1. **Medication elimination occurs primarily via urine produced by the nephrons of the kidneys (*excretion*). If a medication is toxic to nephrons, damage to nephrons can result. A drug that can cause damage to nephrons is known as nephrotoxic. A nurse must assess the client for a decrease in urine production and identify laboratory results that indicate impairment of the kidneys, such as elevated creatinine and blood urea nitrogen levels.**
   2. Nephrotoxicity is unrelated to the process of movement of a medication into the bloodstream (*absorption*).
   3. Nephrotoxicity is unrelated to the transport of a medication from the site of absorption to the site of medication action (*distribution*).
   4. Nephrotoxicity is unrelated to the process of biotransformation. Biotransformation is

the conversion of a medication to a less active form (*detoxification*) in preparation for excretion.

6. 1. Medication toxicity results from excessive amounts of the drug in the body because of overdosage or impaired metabolism or excretion. Most drug toxicity that occurs immediately after administration is preventable through accurate prescribing and administering of the medication. Toxicity that occurs through the cumulative effect occurs over time and, if recognized early, is not life-threatening.
   2. Drug habituation is a mild form of psychological dependence that occurs over time and is not life-threatening.
   3. **Anaphylaxis, a severe allergic reaction, requires immediate intervention (e.g., epinephrine, IV fluids, corticosteroids, and antihistamines) because it can be fatal.**
   4. An idiosyncratic effect is an unexpected, individualized response to a drug. The response can be an underresponse or an overresponse, or it can cause unpredictable, unexplainable symptoms. Usually, it is not life-threatening.

7. 1. Side effects are unintended effects and are not as important as another aspect of a medication when evaluating whether expected outcomes of medication therapy have been achieved.
   2. **Therapeutic effects are the desired, intended effects of the drug. They are the reason for which the drug is prescribed.**
   3. Although it is important to know the mechanism of action of a drug (pharmacodynamics), this knowledge is not as important as another aspect of a medication when evaluating whether expected outcomes of medication therapy have been achieved.
   4. Although it is important to know the chemical composition of a drug, it is not as significant as knowing another aspect of a medication when evaluating whether expected outcomes of medication therapy have been achieved.

8. 1. When administered to an adult under the supervision of a primary health-care provider, meperidine may exceed the recommended oral dosage of 1,200 mg/day or the IV dose of 15 to 35 mg/hr.
   2. **In adults, ibuprofen should not exceed 3,600 mg/day when used as an anti-inflammatory agent or 1,200 mg/day**

when used as an analgesic or antipyretic. Higher doses do not increase effectiveness and may cause major gastrointestinal and central nervous system adverse effects. Ibuprofen is an over-the-counter medication that increases the risk for an overdose as a result of self-medication by an uninformed consumer.
   3. Recommended daily doses for morphine vary based on weight of the client and route of administration. Recommended dosages routinely are exceeded in pain management of clients with chronic, intractable (malignant) pain when prescribed by a primary health-care provider.
   4. When administered to an adult under the supervision of a primary health-care provider, codeine may exceed the recommended daily dosage of 120 mg.

9. 1. An opioid can cause the side effect of hypotension. However, assessment of blood pressure is not as essential as another vital sign.
   2. **An opioid depresses the respiratory center in the medulla, which results in a decrease in the rate and depth of respirations. When a client's respiratory rate is less than 10 breaths per minute, the drug should be withheld and the primary health-care provider notified.**
   3. The side effects and adverse reactions to opioids do not include alterations in temperature.
   4. An opioid analgesic can cause the side effect of bradycardia, so the pulse should be assessed before administration. However, assessment of heart rate is not as essential as another vital sign.

10. 1. This is unnecessary because antihypertensives do not alter the level of consciousness.
    2. The apical heart rate should be assessed before administering cardiac glycosides and antidysrhythmics, not antihypertensives.
    3. **Antihypertensives, such as beta-adrenergic blockers, calcium channel blockers, vasodilators, and angiotensin-converting enzyme (ACE) inhibitors, all act to reduce blood pressure; therefore, the blood pressure should be obtained before and monitored after administration.**
    4. Respirations and breath sounds should be assessed before administering bronchodilators and expectorants, not antihypertensive agents.

11. 1. Although this is a concern for any client who must follow a pharmacological regimen, it is not the most common risk associated with drugs that suppress the immune system.
    2. Medications that depress the immune system usually do not cause sensory problems. Although some antineoplastic drugs can cause peripheral neuropathy, this response is not as common as gastrointestinal, hematological, integumentary, and immune system adverse effects.
    3. Medications that depress the immune system are more likely to cause gastrointestinal disturbances such as anorexia, nausea, vomiting, and diarrhea, not constipation.
    4. **Medications that suppress the immune system, such as antineoplastics (destroy stem cells that are precursors to white blood cells), corticosteroids (suppress function and numbers of eosinophils and monocytes), and antibiotics (destroy body flora), lower the body's ability to fight microorganisms that can cause infection.**

12. 1. Toxicity is manifested by sedation, respiratory depression, and coma. The antidote naloxone may be necessary.
    2. Allergic responses frequently manifest as a rash, urticaria, and pruritus.
    3. A synergistic response associated with an opioid is reflected by a lowered level of consciousness and sedation.
    4. **Excitability is an unexpected, unexplainable response to an opioid. Opioids are central nervous system depressants that relieve pain and promote sedation; they do not cause excitability.**

13. 1. Anticonvulsants do not relieve pain. Anticonvulsants depress abnormal neuronal discharges in the central nervous system and limit or prevent seizures.
    2. **Antidepressants, particularly amitriptyline, potentiate the effects of opioids and have innate analgesic properties.**
    3. Antihistamines do not relieve pain. Antihistamines block the effects of histamine at H_1 receptors.
    4. Although anesthetics do block pain, usually they are not used to relieve neuropathic pain. General anesthetics depress the central nervous system sufficiently to allow pain-free invasive procedures (e.g., surgery), and local anesthetics produce brief episodes of decreased nerve transmission when general anesthesia is not warranted.

14. 1. **Drug-metabolizing enzymes in the liver detoxify drugs to a less active form (biotransformation). With liver dysfunction, biotransformation is impaired and drugs accumulate, ultimately reaching toxic levels.**
    2. Although decreased kidney function will adversely affect drug excretion, which can contribute to toxicity, it does not pose the highest risk for toxicity, as does information in another option.
    3. Most drugs are degraded in an organ other than the lungs and then are excreted through the kidneys.
    4. Most drugs are degraded in a body system other than the gastrointestinal tract and are excreted through the kidneys.

15. 1. Food, fluid, and gastric acidity can influence the dissolution and absorption of oral medications.
    2. The absorption of rectal medications is influenced by the presence of fecal material and is unpredictable.
    3. **IV medications enter the bloodstream directly by way of a vein. IV administration offers the quickest rate of absorption, and it is within the circulatory system for easy distribution.**
    4. The intramuscular route is not the most efficient route for absorption of medication. Factors such as local edema and inadequate blood supply to the area will limit drug absorption.

16. 1. **To obtain the most accurate comparable data, clients should be weighed at the same time every day (preferably first thing in the morning), after toileting, before breakfast, wearing the same clothing, and using the same scale. This controls as many variables as possible to make the daily measurements an objective, accurate reflection of the client's weight. Approximately 1 kilogram (2.2 lb) of weight gained or lost is equivalent to 1 liter of fluid.**
    2. Although skin turgor is assessed, it is a less accurate assessment than others because it is based on the nurse's perception and interpretation. Assessing skin turgor is less desirable than a measurement that is objective.
    3. Measuring calf girth assesses the progression or resolution of edema in only a small area of the body, which does not reflect total body fluid losses or gains. Edema generally is not observable until 2.5 to 3 liters of fluid have been retained.

4. Monitoring urine specific gravity is not an accurate method of assessing the effectiveness of diuretic therapy because it should be considered in relation to other variables, such as urine volume and serum osmolality.

17. 1. Administering an antiemetic after a client vomits is too late. When an antiemetic is administered as an adjunctive to chemotherapy, it is given so that vomiting should not occur.
    2. Administering an antiemetic 30 minutes before meals is inappropriate when an antiemetic is prescribed as a component of a chemotherapeutic regimen. It is administered in relation to when the chemotherapeutic agent is given, not meals.
    3. Administering an antiemetic after a client reports nausea is too late. When an antiemetic is administered as an adjunctive to chemotherapy, it is given so that nausea should not occur.
    4. **Antiemetics should be administered 30 minutes before initiation of chemotherapy and then 4 and 8 hours after the initial dose of the antiemetic.**

18. 1. **A drug allergy is an immunological response to a drug. In addition to integumentary responses, the client may develop angioedema, rhinitis, lacrimal tearing, nausea, vomiting, wheezing, dyspnea, and diarrhea.**
    2. An idiosyncratic effect is an unexpected, individualized response to a drug. The response can be an underresponse or an overresponse, or it may cause unpredictable, unexplainable signs or symptoms.
    3. The early signs of anaphylaxis are shortness of breath, acute hypotension, and tachycardia.
    4. When a drug interaction occurs where the action of one or both drugs is potentiated, it is called a synergistic effect.

19. 1. One medium-size plum contains approximately 114 mg of potassium.
    2. One medium-size orange contains approximately 237 mg of potassium.
    3. **One medium-size banana contains approximately 450 mg of potassium. Hydrochlorothiazide (HCTZ), by its action in the distal convoluted tubule, promotes the excretion of potassium. Potassium must be replenished because of its vital role in the sodium-potassium pump.**

4. One medium-size tangerine contains approximately 132 mg of potassium.

20. 1. **A medication that is a digitalis derivative, such as digoxin, decreases conduction through the sinoatrial (SA) and atrioventricular (AV) nodes and prolongs the refractory period of the AV node, resulting in a slowing of the heart rate (negative chronotropic effect). When the heart rate is less than preset parameters (e.g., 60 beats per minute) or higher than preset parameters (e.g., 100 beats per minute), the medication should be held and a serum digoxin level assessed for exceeding its therapeutic range of 0.5 to 2 ng/mL. It is important to remember that the heart rate may exceed a rate of 100 beats per minute with toxicity.**
    2. Dysrhythmias, not alterations in blood pressure, are cardiovascular signs of toxicity.
    3. An assessment of the respiratory rate is unnecessary because a change in respiratory status is not a symptom of toxicity.
    4. Toxicity may cause confusion and disorientation, not an altered level of consciousness. Level of consciousness refers to level of arousability and responsiveness to the environment.

21. 1. Although this may be a secondary benefit for some clients, it is not the reason for using a metered-dose inhaler (MDI).
    2. The medication from an MDI is delivered to the lungs, which comprise the lower, not upper, respiratory tract.
    3. Although an MDI delivers the medication via pressure to the client's mouth, it is the act of the client's inhalation that delivers the medication to its site of action.
    4. **An MDI aerosolizes the medication so that the suspension of microscopic liquid droplets can be inhaled deep into the lung.**

22. 1. **A drug interaction occurs when one drug affects the action of another drug. The effect of one or both drugs increases, decreases, or is negated. The risk for drug interactions increases when multiple drugs are prescribed by several primary health-care providers with inadequate communication among the providers.**
    2. Drug habituation is a mild form of psychological dependence and is

unrelated to the concern presented in the question.

3. Tolerance occurs when a client develops a decreased response to a medication and therefore requires an increased dose to achieve the therapeutic response; it is unrelated to the concern presented in the question.

4. An allergic reaction results from an immunological response to a medication to which the client has been sensitized; it is unrelated to the concern presented in the question.

23. 1. An IV push (bolus) is the administration of a drug directly into the systemic circulation. Usually, it is administered as a single dose in an emergency. It achieves the desired level quickly but does not maintain it.

2. The sublingual route is used intermittently and only when necessary. It is not used to maintain constant therapeutic drug levels.

3. Although the oral route is the safest, easiest, and most desirable way to administer medications, there are fluctuations in serum blood levels because the medication is administered intermittently one or more times throughout the day.

4. **With a large-volume infusion, a drug is added to an IV container (usually 250 mL, 500 mL, or 1,000 mL), and the resulting solution is administered over time. This approach maintains a constant serum drug level.**

24. 1. Medications administered via the buccal route dissolve between the teeth and gums, mix with saliva, and are swallowed. This route has a slow onset of action.

2. The transdermal route is noted for its ability to sustain the absorption of medication, not because it produces a rapid response. The absorption of medications administered via the transdermal route is influenced by the condition of the skin, the presence of interstitial fluid, and the adequacy of circulation to the area.

3. The subcutaneous route is faster-acting than some routes because it is a parenteral route but slower-acting than other parenteral routes because subcutaneous tissue does not have a large blood supply.

4. **Of the options presented, the intramuscular route is the fastest-acting route because muscles have a large vascular network that ensures rapid absorption into the bloodstream.**

25. 1. **Generally, conservative management of hyperlipidemia through dietary modifications and exercise is attempted before resorting to a medication. Lipid-lowering agents have side effects and adverse effects and may interact with other drugs.**

2. Exercise is only one factor that influences the client's lipid status. Factors such as diet, cigarette smoking, stress, concurrent diseases, and family history are additional factors that must be considered when a pharmacological regimen is prescribed.

3. Lipid-lowering agents are prescribed for clients who are older than 60 years old only when necessary, not because they are older than 60 years of age.

4. Only people with chronically elevated lipid levels receive antilipidemics because of their significant side effects. Lifestyle modifications are attempted first.

26. 1. Antipyretics, not antiemetics, reduce fever.

2. Anxiolytics, not antiemetics, reduce anxiety.

3. **Antiemetics block the emetogenic receptors to prevent or treat nausea or vomiting.**

4. Antitussives, not antiemetics, reduce the frequency and intensity of coughing.

27. 1. Although generally this is true, sometimes the attached needle is inappropriate for a particular client and the nurse must change the needle or transfer the medication into a standard syringe.

2. Drug interactions can still occur with prefilled, disposable cartridges because the drug within the cartridge may alter or be altered by the concurrent presence of another medication in the client's body.

3. Although prefilled cartridges are convenient in an emergency, it is not the primary purpose of having prefilled cartridges.

4. **Single-dose cartridges prepared by a medication manufacturer or pharmacy ensure the purity of the drug. Multiple-dose vials can be contaminated by rubber debris and microorganisms.**

28. 1. **Exogenous glucocorticoids cause adrenal suppression. When exogenous corticosteroids are withdrawn abruptly, the adrenal glands are unable to produce adequate amounts of**

glucocorticoids, thus causing acute adrenal insufficiency and shock.
2. Acute adrenal insufficiency may cause dizziness and syncope, not seizures.
3. Acute adrenal insufficiency is unrelated to hemorrhage.
4. Acute adrenal insufficiency may cause hyperthermia, not hypothermia.

29. 1. Antihypertensive agents do not directly affect respirations. Respirations may return to the expected range of 12 to 20 breaths per minute when cardiac output improves.
2. This heart rate is within the expected range of 60 to 100 beats per minute.
3. **The acceptable range for the systolic pressure is 90 to less than 120 mm Hg. This client's systolic reading is outside the expected range, which is an excessive decrease when receiving an antihypertensive agent.**
4. Antihypertensive agents do not influence body temperature. Expected adult oral temperatures range between 97.5°F and 99.5°F.

30. 1. **When depression lifts during the early stages of antidepressant therapy, the individual has renewed energy that may support the implementation of suicidal ideation. Client safety is the priority.**
2. Although encouraging psychotherapy should be done, it is not the priority.
3. Alcohol should be avoided because it potentiates the central nervous system depressive effects of sertraline (Zoloft).
4. A person will more likely lose, not gain, weight when taking sertraline (Zoloft) because its side effects include anorexia, nausea, and vomiting.

31. 1. Intake and output are monitored when a client is taking a diuretic, not an antipyretic.
2. Pain tolerance is monitored when a client is taking an analgesic, not an antipyretic.
3. Respirations are monitored when a client is taking a central nervous system depressant or bronchodilator, not an antipyretic.
4. **Antipyretics lower fever by affecting thermoregulation in the central nervous system, inhibiting the action of prostaglandins peripherally, or both.**

32. 1. Although this may be done, it is not the priority. Pain tolerance is the highest intensity of pain that the person is willing to endure.

2. **Analgesics depress the central nervous system; therefore, the respiratory status must be monitored before and routinely throughout administration for signs of respiratory depression.**
3. Although this may be done, it is not the priority. Pain threshold is the amount of pain stimulation a person requires before pain is felt.
4. Monitoring analgesic blood levels is unnecessary.

33. 1. **Bronchodilators relax smooth muscles of the bronchi and bronchioles, thus increasing the diameter of their lumens (bronchodilation) and resulting in a decrease in airway resistance.**
2. **Diuretics increase the urinary excretion of water and electrolytes such as sodium, potassium, calcium, and chloride.**
3. **Antitussives prevent or relieve coughing by depressing the cough center in the medulla.**
4. Expectorants increase, not decrease, the flow of respiratory secretions; they decrease the viscosity of secretions and promote the coughing up and removal of mucus from the lungs.
5. **Antiemetics, depending on the agent (e.g., antihistamines, anticholinergics, neuroleptic agents, prokinetic agents, serotonin antagonists, and substance P neurokinin-1 receptor antagonists), act in a variety of ways to prevent, limit, or treat nausea and vomiting.**

34. 1. **A log will help evaluate the client's response to the aluminum and magnesium hydroxide (Mylanta) regimen. Characteristics include location, duration, intensity, and description of the discomfort.**
2. **These are symptoms of gastric bleeding, and the primary health-care provider should be notified immediately. Enzymes act on blood to produce coffee-ground emesis and tarry stools.**
3. **The magnesium in the aluminum and magnesium hydroxide can cause diarrhea in some people.**
4. This medication should be taken 1 to 3 hours after a meal and at bedtime to neutralize gastric acid.
5. This medication should be thoroughly chewed and taken with at least a half glass of water to prevent the tablet from entering the intestine undissolved.

35. 1. Sedatives, used to promote sleep, depress the central nervous system, which may cause constipation, not diarrhea.
2. Narcotics, opium derivatives used to relieve pain, depress the central nervous system, which may cause constipation, not diarrhea.
3. **Diarrhea is an adverse reaction to a laxative. Laxatives are agents that increase evacuation of the bowel via various mechanisms. An excessive dose or taking a laxative when it is not necessary can cause diarrhea.**
4. **Antibiotics can alter the flora of the body, with resulting superinfections. Opportunistic fungal infections of the gastrointestinal system may cause a black, furred tongue, nausea, and diarrhea.**
5. Antiemetics, used to prevent or alleviate nausea and vomiting, may cause constipation, not diarrhea.

36. 1. **Some herbal supplements can cause dangerous herbal-to-drug interactions or nontherapeutic responses when taken concurrently with over-the-counter or prescribed medication.**
2. **The Dietary Supplement Health and Education Act of 1994 stipulated that herbs must be labeled with information about their effects on the structure and function of the body. Herbal substances officially are considered food supplements.**
3. The Food and Drug Administration (FDA), a division of the U.S. Department of Health and Human Services, regulates the manufacture, sale, and effectiveness of prescription and nonprescription medications, not herbal remedies.
4. Herbs, considered by some to be "natural," are plants that are valued for their medicinal properties. As medicinal substances, they should be viewed by the consumer as drugs.
5. Just because herbs are organic does not ensure that they are safe. Many herbs, even though organic, can be toxic if ingested in unsafe amounts.

37. 1. **Drug levels are maintained within a therapeutic range that is less than the peak level and more than the trough level. The peak serum level of a drug is the maximum concentration of a drug in the blood (occurs when the elimination rate equals the absorption rate). Trough levels indicate the serum level**

of a drug just before the next dose is to be administered. The results of these two values determine the dose of the drug and the time a drug should be administered to maintain a serum level of the drug within its therapeutic range.
2. Although a drug's half-life, the usual amount of time needed by the body to reduce the concentration of the drug by one-half, is helpful in determining how frequently a drug should be given initially, it does not reflect an individual client's response to the drug.
3. **On the basis of peak and trough levels of a drug, the dosage is adjusted to ensure that the concentration of the drug in the blood remains in the therapeutic range over a 24-hour period.**
4. Biotransformation, the process of inactivating and breaking down a drug, takes place primarily in the liver. Peak and trough levels may indirectly reflect the rate of biotransformation, not the place where it occurs.
5. This is not the purpose of peak and trough levels, although peak and trough levels indirectly measure both the absorption and the inactivation and elimination of a drug from the body.

38.   Answer: 3 mL.
Use ratio and proportion to convert grams to milligrams first, and then perform a calculation to determine the dose.

$$\frac{\text{Desired}}{\text{Have}} \quad \frac{1.5 \text{ g}}{1 \text{ g}} = \frac{\text{x mg}}{1,000 \text{ mg}}$$

$$1x = 1.5 \times 1,000$$
$$x = 1,500 \text{ mg; therefore,}$$
$$1,500 \text{ mg is equal to } 1.5 \text{ g}$$

Now perform a calculation to determine how many mL to administer.

$$\frac{\text{Desired}}{\text{Have}} \quad \frac{1,500 \text{ mg}}{500 \text{ mg}} = \frac{\text{x mL}}{1 \text{ mL}}$$

$$500x = 1,500$$
$$x = 1,500 \div 500$$
$$x = 3 \text{ mL}$$

39. 1. Oxygen saturation measures the ratio of oxyhemoglobin to the total concentration of hemoglobin in the blood. It indicates how much a person is being oxygenated. An oxygen saturation level of 95% or higher indicates an acceptable range.
2. Mucolytic agents, not bronchodilators, liquefy thick, sticky (viscous) secretions.

3. **Bronchodilators expand the airways of the respiratory tract, and this promotes air exchange and easier respirations.**
4. The ability of the chest to expand (respiratory excursion) increases, not decreases.
5. Bronchovesicular breath sounds will increase, not decrease, after the administration of a bronchodilator. Bronchovesicular sounds are expected blowing sounds heard over the mainstem bronchi. They are blowing sounds that are moderate in pitch and intensity and equal in length on inspiration and expiration.

40. 1. **Prolonged laxative use weakens the bowel's natural responses to fecal distention and results in chronic constipation. The osmotic action of magnesium salts in magnesium hydroxide (Milk of Magnesia) draws water into the intestine, which can cause dehydration and electrolyte imbalances.**
2. Magnesium hydroxide (Milk of Magnesia) causes sodium and potassium to be lost from, rather than accumulate in, the body. The magnesium in magnesium hydroxide may be absorbed and result in hypermagnesemia.
3. **Watery diarrhea is a sign of an overdose of magnesium hydroxide (Milk of Magnesia). The drug should be discontinued because watery diarrhea can lead to a serious imbalance in fluid and electrolytes.**
4. Each dose of magnesium hydroxide (Milk of Magnesia) should be followed by 8 ounces of water to promote a faster effect and help replenish lost fluid. Daily fluid intake should be 2,000 to 3,000 mL.
5. This will interrupt sleep. Magnesium hydroxide (Milk of Magnesia) causes bowel elimination 3 to 6 hours after its administration.

41. 1. The composition of the drug and the client's response to the drug, not the route by which it is administered, determine if an allergic response occurs.
2. The composition of a drug and its molecular reaction with another drug that is concurrently present determine if a drug interaction will occur.
3. **A transdermal patch placed on the skin gradually releases a predictable amount of medication that is absorbed into the bloodstream for a prescribed period. This approach maintains therapeutic**
blood levels and reduces fluctuations in circulating drug levels.
4. **A drug administered via a transdermal patch cannot be inactivated by gastric acidity. Drugs taken orally can cause gastric irritation, which can be avoided if the drugs are administered via a transdermal patch.**
5. Transdermal patches are used for their systemic, not local, effects.

42. 1. **These are clinical indicators of dehydration and should be reported to the primary health-care provider because rehydration therapy may be necessary.**
2. **Diphenoxylate/atropine (Lomotil) depresses intestinal motility and effectively controls diarrhea within 24 to 36 hours. If diarrhea persists beyond 48 hours, the primary health-care provider should be notified.**
3. Diphenoxylate/atropine (Lomotil) may depress the central nervous system, which causes drowsiness and sedation, not hyperactivity.
4. When a client is experiencing diarrhea, fluid should be encouraged, not restricted, to prevent dehydration and electrolyte imbalances.
5. The tablets for this medication are not enteric coated and do not have extended-release properties; therefore, they may be crushed if necessary.

43. 1. **Constipation and diarrhea are both side effects of famotidine (Pepcid) for which the nurse should assess the client.**
2. Although administered by mouth, famotidine (Pepcid) is not known to cause stomatitis.
3. An increase, not a decrease, in serum creatinine is a side effect associated with famotidine (Pepcid). Seventy percent of famotidine is excreted unchanged via the kidneys, and the drug may cause kidney damage.
4. **The nurse should monitor a client's complete blood count with differential periodically during famotidine (Pepcid) therapy to identify hematological adverse reactions. Serious hematological adverse reactions include agranulocytosis, aplastic anemia, anemia, neutropenia, and thrombocytopenia.**
5. **Completing the full course of famotidine (Pepcid) therapy and not discontinuing the famotidine when feeling**

better support the achievement of the maximum therapeutic effect.

44. 1. **Mixing alcohol and zolpidem (Ambien CR) can intensify the effects of both and can precipitate dangerous side effects such as dizziness, shallow breathing, and impaired motor control, judgment, and thinking; it can even cause loss of consciousness or coma.**

2. **Controlled-release (CR) medications should never be chewed, crushed, divided, or dissolved. A damaged tablet alters the process by which the medication is released. Too much medication may be released into the system at once, causing an excessive dose. Zolpidem (Ambien CR) is a dual-layer tablet: 10.5 mg is released immediately and another 2.5 mg later. The first layer dissolves rapidly to help a person get to sleep, and the second layer dissolves gradually to help a person stay asleep.**

3. Zolpidem (Ambien CR) is better absorbed and therefore more effective when taken when the stomach is empty.

4. Zolpidem (Ambien CR) is a central nervous system depressant that has a habit-forming potential if taken in higher doses than prescribed. Excessive doses can lead to tolerance and misuse. Also, a second dose so close to a previous dose can dramatically increase the risk of adverse reactions associated with the central nervous system, such as irregular heart rate, impaired breathing, and memory loss.

5. **Zolpidem (Ambien CR) is a central nervous system depressant that has a duration of action of approximately 7 to 8 hours. If the person is active before the medication is metabolized, drowsiness, dizziness, light-headedness, and impaired balance may occur, increasing the risk for injury.**

45. 2. **The process of movement of a medication into the bloodstream *(absorption)* is the first element of pharmacokinetics as medication moves from its entry to its exit from the body.**

3. **The transport of a medication from the site of absorption to the site of medication action *(distribution)* is the second element of pharmacokinetics as medication moves from its entry to its exit from the body.**

4. **Conversion of a medication to a less active form *(biotransformation)* in preparation for excretion is the third element of pharmacokinetics as medication moves from its entry to its exit from the body.**

1. **Elimination of a medication by the body *(excretion)* is the fourth element of pharmacokinetics as medication moves from its entry to its exit from the body.**

46. 1. Taking ibuprofen with a full glass of water and maintaining adequate fluid intake help to prevent renal adverse reactions.

2. The client should not exceed 1,200 mg of ibuprofen for over-the-counter use daily and not exceed 3,200-mg prescription strength daily to avoid stomach or intestinal damage.

3. The client should avoid taking a double dose. However, if a forgotten dose is remembered, it can be taken as long as it not too close to the next scheduled dose.

4. **Research demonstrates that bleeding time is increased when taking ibuprofen; therefore, ibuprofen should be discontinued if dental treatment or surgery is scheduled.**

5. If a skin rash occurs, the client should discontinue taking ibuprofen immediately. A rash may indicate toxic epidermal necrolysis or Stevens-Johnson syndrome, which can be life-threatening.

47. 1. Nitrofurantoin (Macrodantin) oral suspension should be administered with food, not on an empty stomach, to minimize gastric irritation and to improve drug absorption.

2. **This helps to prevent staining of the teeth associated with nitrofurantoin (Macrodantin).**

3. The urine is brown or rust colored, not reddish/orange, with nitrofurantoin (Macrodantin). Reddish/orange urine is associated with the drug phenazopyridine, a urinary tract analgesic that contains a type of azo dye.

4. **The client should monitor for these clinical manifestations because they are indicative of pseudomembranous colitis, a serious adverse reaction to nitrofurantoin (Macrodantin).**

5. A week is too long to wait to report lack of improvement in clinical manifestations of the urinary tract infection. The client should be instructed to notify the primary

health-care provider if clinical manifestations do not resolve within several days.

48. 1. Oxybutynin (Ditropan XL) is a tablet designed to release the drug over a certain period and should not be crushed, broken, or chewed. Oxybutynin (Ditropan XL) can be administered with or without food. Drugs that are CD-controlled delivery, CR-controlled release, LA-long acting, SR-sustained release, TR-timed release, XL-extended release, and XR-extended release are all designed to release medication over time to maintain a consistent level of the drug in the bloodstream. If the integrity of these types of tablets is altered by crushing, chewing, or breaking them in half, the entire dose will be given at once, causing an overdose of the medication.

2. **Sedation and weakness may result from the anticholinergic effects of oxybutynin (Ditropan XL), especially in older adults.**

3. **Drowsiness is a side effect of oxybutynin (Ditropan XL) because of its anticholinergic effects. The client should avoid activities such as driving when the level of alertness is diminished.**

4. **Urinary retention requires immediate medical attention to avoid permanent bladder damage resulting from overstretching of the bladder and kidney damage caused by a backup of urine into the kidneys. Oxybutynin (Ditropan XL) exerts an antispasmodic effect on smooth muscle by inhibiting the action of acetylcholine and also relaxes the bladder's detrusor muscle. These actions can lead to urinary retention in some people.**

5. **Oxybutynin (Ditropan XL) decreases the ability to perspire because of its anticholinergic effect, which may cause fever and heatstroke if a person engages in strenuous activity in a warm environment.**

49. 1. Analgesics do not have a curative action.

2. **Analgesics decrease the intensity of pain (palliative treatment). Palliative treatments minimize clinical manifestations or promote comfort; palliative treatments do not produce a cure.**

3. **When two analgesics are administered together, they exert a synergistic effect. A synergistic effect occurs when the combined effect of two medications is greater than when the effects of each are added together.**

4. **When two analgesics are given together, they potentiate the action of each other. Potentiation occurs when drugs administered together increase the action of one or both drugs.**

5. Two analgesics will increase, not decrease (antagonize), the action of each other.

50. 1. **Budesonide (Pulmicort Flexhaler), an inhaled corticosteroid, may cause a rash, which may indicate Stevens-Johnson syndrome (a life-threatening condition), or toxic epidermal necrolysis.**

2. The opposite should be done. The bronchodilator reduces airway resistance, and then the budesonide can be aspirated deeper into the lungs for maximal effect.

3. Improvement in asthma control can occur within 24 hours of starting treatment. Maximum benefit from an inhaled corticosteroid may take 1 to 2 weeks of treatment.

4. **Rinsing the mouth with water and avoiding swallowing after use of budesonide (Pulmicort Flexhaler) will help to reduce the risk of an oral fungal (*Candida*) infection.**

5. Budesonide (Pulmicort Flexhaler), a corticosteroid, is not indicated for the immediate relief of bronchospasms. A short-acting beta$_2$-agonist medication is indicated in the event of a sudden asthma attack or in the presence of breathing problems.

51. 1. **Increased fluid intake will help to decrease the viscosity of respiratory secretions and moisten the throat. At least 2,000 mL or more of fluid is suggested when taking dextromethorphan and guaifenesin (Mucinex DM).**

2. One week, not 2 weeks, is long enough to wait before informing the primary health-care provider of a lack of improvement. Another intervention may be required.

3. **Dextromethorphan, a cough suppressant, and guaifenesin, an expectorant, are contained in many over-the-counter cough remedies. Taking multiple drugs with the same or similar properties can cause an overdose of these elements.**

4. **Taking alcohol or other central nervous system depressants concurrently with this medication has caused fatalities.**

5. **These are serious side effects of dextromethorphan and guaifenesin (Mucinex DM); these medications should be discontinued with medical supervision.**

52. 1. A calcium level of 5.4 mEq/L is within the expected range of 4.5 to 5.5 mEq/L and is not a cause for concern.
2. A temperature of 97.8°F is within the expected range of 97.5°F to 99.5°F for an adult and is not a cause for concern.
3. **One thousand milligrams of docusate sodium (Colace) daily exceeds the recommended daily dose of 50 to 500 mg and is a cause for concern.**
4. A respiratory rate of 14 breaths per minute is within the expected range of 12 to 20 breaths per minute for an adult and is not a cause for concern.

53. 1. The opposite should be encouraged. Vegetable oils with polyunsaturated fatty acids should be exchanged for vegetable oils with monounsaturated fatty acids.
2. **These human responses may indicate a serious adverse reaction to simvastatin (Zocor) and must be evaluated. In addition to reducing the liver's production of cholesterol, simvastatin affects several enzymes in muscle cells that are responsible for muscle growth; this may be the cause of muscle symptoms. However, these symptoms may indicate the presence of rhabdomyolysis. Rhabdomyolysis is a condition that breaks down skeletal muscle fibers and myocyte cell membranes, which leads to muscle necrosis. Because rhabdomyolysis can be fatal, muscle symptoms must be evaluated immediately.**
3. **Research demonstrates that omega-3 fatty acids help limit triglycerides, inflammation, hypertension, and cardiovascular and autoimmune diseases.**
4. **Cola-colored urine indicates the presence of myoglobin, which is a skeletal muscle protein involved in metabolism. When skeletal muscles are damaged, they release myoglobin into the bloodstream. The blood is then filtered by the kidneys, thus causing urine to be cola- or tea-colored. Reduced urine output or absence of urine may indicate kidney damage caused by rhabdomyolysis, necessitating immediate medical attention.**
5. Simvastatin (Zocor) should be taken at bedtime or during the evening meal, not in the morning. Research demonstrates that the body makes cholesterol at night and that cholesterol levels are lower when simvastatin is taken in the evening rather than in the morning.

54. 1. **Food activates the proton pump mechanism, which releases gastric acid in the stomach. When esomeprazole (Nexium), a proton pump inhibitor, is taken 30 minutes to 1 hour before a meal, it allows time for esomeprazole to be absorbed into the bloodstream, which then prevents the final transport of hydrogen ions into the gastric lumen.**
2. **Not chewing or crushing this medication prevents damage to the delayed-release pellets within the esomeprazole (Nexium) capsule.**
3. **Antacids may be used when taking esomeprazole (Nexium).**
4. **Nonsteroidal anti-inflammatory drugs may cause an increase in gastrointestinal irritation and should be avoided when taking esomeprazole (Nexium).**
5. **Opening the esomeprazole (Nexium) capsule can be done as long as the pellets are not crushed or chewed.**
6. **These are clinical indicators of esophageal ulcers. Gastroesophageal reflux disease is the main cause of ulcers or sores in the lining of the esophagus.**

55. 1. **One type of rash is a hypersensitivity (allergic) reaction to a chemical element in a drug. Hypersensitivity reactions can be mild if localized, but if the exposure is systemic, the reaction is on a larger scale and may even be life-threatening.**
2. **Tinnitus is caused by damage to the eighth cranial nerve, which is a toxic effect of acetylsalicylic acid.**
3. **Acetylsalicylic acid has antiplatelet agglutination properties that cause an increase in clotting time.**
4. Dizziness is indicative of hypotension, which is not a common nontherapeutic response to acetylsalicylic acid.
5. Diarrhea, rather than constipation, is more likely to occur with the intake of acetylsalicylic acid. Aspirin inhibits the COX-1 enzyme and causes a thinning of the stomach lining that increases the prospect of gastrointestinal irritation from digestive juices and contributes to diarrhea, heartburn, abdominal pain, bloating, and bleeding.

56. 1. Morphine, an opioid analgesic, is a central nervous system depressant. A central nervous system depressant reduces the activity and slows down the normal functions of the brain, thus leading to a decreased level of alertness.
2. Morphine, an opioid analgesic, is a central nervous system depressant. A central nervous system depressant has a sedating effect on brain function that can lead to confusion.
3. Morphine, an opioid analgesic, is a central nervous system depressant. A central nervous system depressant decreases the respiratory center of the brain, thus causing bradypnea, not tachypnea.
4. Morphine, an opioid analgesic, is a central nervous system depressant. A central nervous system depressant decreases gastrointestinal motility and contributes to constipation.
5. Morphine, an opioid analgesic, is a central nervous system depressant. A central nervous system depressant relaxes the neurovascular system and contributes to hypotension, not hypertension.

57. 1. Synthroid is a proprietary brand (trade) name for levothyroxine. Trade names of drugs are patented by drug companies. They begin with a capital letter and usually are short and easy to recall.
2. Levothyroxine is the generic (nonproprietary, official) name for the synthetic thyroid hormone that is chemically identical to thyroxine (T4). It is used to treat thyroid hormone deficiency.
3. Levothyroxine does not have a curative action. It is a synthetic hormone used to treat a thyroid deficiency.
4. Levothyroxine does not have an antidotal action. An antidote is used to reverse the toxic effect of another medication. An example of a medication that is an antidote is naloxone; it limits central nervous system depression resulting from opioids.
5. Levothyroxine is a supportive (substitutive) medication because it maintains health by providing an essential hormone that is deficient in the body.

58. 1. Knowing a drug's therapeutic range is essential. It indicates the lowest blood concentration level that is effective and the highest blood concentration level that is effective without causing toxicity.

2. A trough level reflects the lowest plasma concentration of a drug in the client's body. The nurse must determine if a trough level is within the drug's therapeutic range. A trough plasma level is determined by a blood test that assesses the level of the drug in the client's body just before the administration of a prescribed dose of the medication.
3. A peak level reflects the highest plasma concentration of a drug in the client's body. The nurse must determine if a peak level is high enough to be within the therapeutic range yet not too high to be toxic. A peak plasma level is determined by a blood test that assesses the level of the drug in the client's body 30 minutes to 1 hour after administration of the medication.
4. Knowing the time needed by the body to metabolize or inactivate one-half the amount of a medication (half-life) will not help the nurse determine if an effective blood concentration level of the drug is being maintained.
5. Knowing the length of time it takes the body to respond to a medication (onset) will not help the nurse determine if an effective blood concentration level of the drug is being maintained.

59. 1. The prescription for the clotrimazole (Mycelex) 1 lozenge 10 mg, via buccal cavity, 5 times a day for 14 days, should be discussed with the primary health-care provider. It is unlikely that a client with moderate dementia will be able to follow directions to keep a lozenge in the mouth for the length of time necessary for it to dissolve (15 to 30 minutes) without swallowing. Also, it places the client at risk for aspiration.
2. Acetaminophen 325 mg administered every 4 hours will deliver 1,950, mg of acetaminophen daily. This dose is within the maximum daily intake of 3,000 mg recommended by Johnson & Johnson, the manufacturer. The latest guidelines allow clients to take up to nine 325-mg doses per 24 hours.
3. It is not necessary to discuss the prescription for levothyroxine (Synthroid) 100 mcg PO once a day. It is within the appropriate range of dosage for this medication, and it will not interact with any of the other prescribed medications.

4. It is not necessary to discuss the prescription for simvastatin (Zocor) 20 mg PO hour of sleep with the primary health-care provider. There are no concerns associated with administering simvastatin concurrently with the other prescribed medications, and the dose is within the acceptable dosage range for an adult.

5. It is not necessary to discuss the prescription for docusate sodium (Colace) 100 mg PO bid with the primary health-care provider. There are no concerns associated with administering docusate sodium concurrently with the other prescribed medications, and the dose is within the acceptable dosage range for an adult.

60. 1. Glargine is a long-acting insulin with an onset of 1 to 2 hours. It has no pronounced peak, and it has a duration of 24 hours or more.

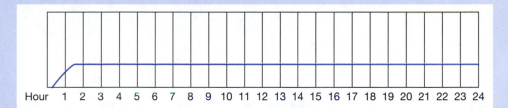

2. **The graphic illustrates that regular insulin is short-acting, with an onset of 30 minutes to 1 hour. It has a peak of 2 to 3 hours and a duration of 3 to 6 hours.**

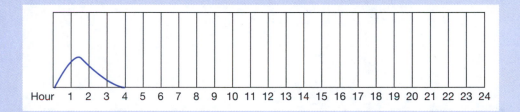

3. Lispro is a rapid-acting insulin with an onset of 15 minutes, a peak of 60 to 90 minutes, and a duration of 3 to 4 hours.

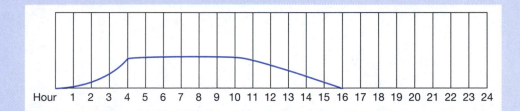

4. NPH is an intermediate-acting insulin with an onset of 2 to 4 hours, a peak of 4 to 10 hours, and a duration of 10 to 16 hours.

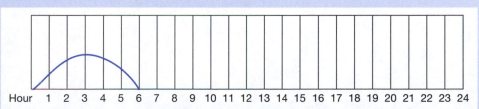

Basic Human Needs and Related Nursing Care

5

Hygiene

KEYWORDS

The following words include nursing/medical terminology, concepts, principles, and information relevant to content specifically addressed in the chapter or associated with topics presented in it. English dictionaries, nursing textbooks, and medical dictionaries, such as *Taber's Cyclopedic Medical Dictionary,* are resources that can be used to expand your knowledge and understanding of these words and related information.

Activities of daily living
Asepsis
Back massage
Baths:
  Bag bath (towel bath)
  Bed bath (partial, complete)
  Shower (standup, shower chair)
  Sitz bath
  Tub bath
Canthus, outer and inner
Cerumen
Circumcised, uncircumcised
Cuticles
Dental caries
Dentures
Distal
Effleurage
Flossing
Halitosis
Heat loss, mechanisms of:
  Conduction
  Convection

Evaporation
  Radiation
Hirsutism
Integumentary
Labia, majora and minora
Mucous membrane
Oral hygiene
Orange stick
Pediculosis
Perianal area
Perineal care
Peripheral neuropathy
Plaque
Proximal
Sebaceous glands
Skin, dermis and epidermis
Smegma
Sordes
Toe pleat

HYGIENE: QUESTIONS

1. A nurse is bathing a client who has a fever. Why should the nurse use tepid bath water for this procedure?
   1. Increases heat loss
   2. Removes surface debris
   3. Reduces surface tension of skin
   4. Stimulates peripheral circulation

2. A nurse must make the decision to give a client a full or partial bed bath. Which criterion is **most** important for the basis of this decision?
   1. Primary health-care provider's prescription for the client's activity
   2. Immediate need of the client
   3. Time of client's last bath
   4. Client preference

3. A client has had a nasogastric tube to decompress the stomach for 3 days and is scheduled for intestinal surgery in the morning. For which of the following is the client at the **highest** risk?
   1. Physical injury
   2. Ineffective social interaction
   3. Decreased nutritional intake
   4. Altered oral mucous membranes

4. A client is incontinent of urine and stool. For which client response should the nurse be **most** concerned?
   1. Impaired skin integrity
   2. Altered sexuality
   3. Dehydration
   4. Confusion

5. A nurse is giving a client a bed bath. Which nursing action is **most** important?
   1. Lower the 2 side rails on the working side of the bed.
   2. Ensure that the bathwater is at least 110°F.
   3. Fold the washcloth like a mitt on the hand.
   4. Raise the bed to the highest position.

6. A nurse plans to give a client a back rub. Which product should the nurse use for this intervention?
   1. Baby powder
   2. Rubbing alcohol
   3. Moisturizing lotion
   4. Antimicrobial cream

7. A nurse changes the sheets and pillowcase of a bed while the client sits in a chair. Of the options presented, which is the **most** important nursing action when changing bed linens?
   1. Ensuring the hem of the bottom sheet is facing the mattress
   2. Arranging the linen in the order in which it is to be used
   3. Shifting the mattress up to the headboard of the bed
   4. Checking the soiled bed linens for personal items

8. A nurse is responsible for providing hair care for a client. Which should the nurse do to distribute oil evenly along hair shafts?
   1. Brush the hair from the scalp toward the hair ends.
   2. Lift opened fingers through the length of the hair.
   3. Apply a hydrating conditioner to wet hair.
   4. Comb hair with a fine-toothed comb.

9. Which condition identified by the nurse places a client at the **highest** risk for impaired self-care when toileting?
   1. Amputation of a foot
   2. Early dementia
   3. Fractured hip
   4. Pregnancy

10. A client asks the nurse, "Why do I have to use mouthwash if I brush my teeth?" Which rationale about the use of all mouthwashes should the nurse include when responding to this question?
1. Reduces offensive mouth odors
2. Minimizes the formation of cavities
3. Softens debris that accumulates in the mouth
4. Destroys pathogens that are found in the oral cavity

11. A nurse is planning to shampoo the hair of a client who has a prescription for bedrest. Which should the nurse do **first**?
1. Wet hair thoroughly before applying shampoo.
2. Encourage the use of dry shampoo.
3. Brush the hair to remove tangles.
4. Tape eye shields over both eyes.

12. A client just had perineal surgery. Which type of bath should the nurse expect to be prescribed for this client?
1. Sponge bath
2. Sitz bath
3. Tub bath
4. Bed bath

13. A nurse plans to assist a client who has impaired vision with a bed bath. Which is the **most** appropriate nursing intervention to facilitate bathing for this client?
1. Providing the client with a liquid bath gel rather than a bar of soap
2. Giving the client an adapted toothbrush to use when brushing the teeth
3. Checking the client's ability to give self-care through a crack in the curtain
4. Ensuring the client can locate bathing supplies placed on the over-bed table

14. A nurse plans to meet the hygiene needs of a hospitalized client who is experiencing hemiparesis because of a brain attack (cerebrovascular accident). Which is an appropriate nursing intervention?
1. Assisting the client to bathe as needed
2. Giving total assistance with a complete bath
3. Providing minimal supervision during the bath
4. Encouraging a family member to bathe the client

15. A nurse is making an occupied bed. Which nursing action is **most** important?
1. Securing top linens under the foot of the mattress and mitering the corners
2. Ensuring that the client's head is supported and is in functional alignment
3. Fan-folding soiled linens as close to the client's body as possible
4. Placing the bed in the horizontal position

16. A nurse must bathe the feet of a client with diabetes. Which should the nurse do before bathing this client's feet?
1. File the nails straight across with an emery board.
2. Teach that daily foot care is essential for adequate hygiene.
3. Ensure a provider's prescription for hygienic foot care is obtained.
4. Assess for additional risk factors that may contribute to localized problems.

17. Which should be the nurse's **first** intervention after removing a bedpan from under a debilitated client who has just had a bowel movement?
1. Document results.
2. Provide perineal care.
3. Reposition the client.
4. Cover the client with the top linens.

18. Which common problem with the hair should the nurse anticipate when clients are on complete bedrest?
1. Dry hair
2. Oily hair
3. Split hair
4. Matted hair

19. A nurse is helping a client who has right hemiparesis to get dressed. Which action should the nurse implement?
1. Put the gown's right sleeve on first.
2. Keep the client in an open-backed gown.
3. Encourage the client to dress independently.
4. Leave the right sleeve off while adjusting the tie at the neck.

20. A cognitively impaired client is incontinent of loose stools. Which action should the nurse implement to help the client prevent skin breakdown?
1. Wash the buttocks with strong soap and water.
2. Bathe immediately after a bowel movement.
3. Apply Talcum powder after the bath.
4. Put a pad under the buttocks.

21. A nurse covers the client with a cotton blanket during a bath. Which of the following mechanisms of heat loss is prevented by the nurse's action?
1. Vasodilation
2. Conduction
3. Convection
4. Diffusion

22. A client who has a fever experienced significant diaphoresis during the night. The client states, "I am tired, and I just want to sleep this morning." Which should the nurse do regarding bathing the client?
1. Wait until the client feels better.
2. Postpone bathing until the afternoon.
3. Give a bed bath with complete assistance.
4. Consult with the primary health-care provider before providing care.

23. A nurse gives a bedbound client a bed bath. Which is the **primary** reason why the nurse provides hygiene care to this client?
1. Support a sense of well-being by increasing self-esteem.
2. Promote circulation by stimulating peripheral nerve endings.
3. Remove excess oil, perspiration, and bacteria by mechanical cleansing.
4. Exercise muscles by contraction and relaxation of muscles when bathing.

24. Which human response, identified by the nurse, **best** supports the concern that a client has a reduced capacity to provide for activities of daily living?
1. Presence of joint contractures
2. Inability to wash body parts
3. Postoperative lethargy
4. Visual disorders

25. When giving a client a bed bath, a nurse washes the client's extremities from distal to proximal. Which is the rationale for this nursing action?
1. Decreases the chance of infection
2. Facilitates removal of dry skin
3. Stimulates venous return
4. Minimizes skin tears

26. During oral care, the nurse identifies a patch of dried food and debris adhered to the hard palate of the client's mouth. Which word should the nurse use when documenting this condition?
    1. Sordes
    2. Plaque
    3. Glossitis
    4. Stomatitis

27. A nurse is teaching a client about how many times a day it is necessary to brush the teeth to achieve effective dental hygiene. According to the American Dental Association, how many times a day should the nurse teach the client to brush the teeth?
    1. 6
    2. 4
    3. 3
    4. 2

28. A nurse is providing hygiene to a client with peripheral neuropathy. Which action should the nurse implement?
    1. Seek a prescription for foot care.
    2. File the toenails straight across the nail.
    3. Wash the feet with lukewarm water and dry well.
    4. Apply moisturizing lotion to the feet, especially between the toes.

29. Which nursing intervention **most** requires the nurse to consider the concept of intimate space?
    1. Providing a bed bath
    2. Obtaining the vital signs
    3. Performing a health history
    4. Ambulating the client down the hall

30. Which nursing action is common to both a bed bath and a tub bath? **Select all that apply.**
    1. _____ Obtaining a prescription from the primary health-care provider
    2. _____ Helping the client wash body parts that cannot be reached
    3. _____ Exposing just the part of the body being washed
    4. _____ Providing for privacy throughout the bath
    5. _____ Ensuring that the call bell is in reach

31. A nurse plans to provide a client with a partial bath. Place the following steps in the order in which the nurse should proceed.
    1. Back
    2. Face
    3. Axilla
    4. Both hands
    5. Genital area
    6. Change water

    Answer: _____

32. Which should the nurse implement when caring for a client who wears eyeglasses? **Select all that apply.**
    1. _____ Encourage use of artificial tears while hospitalized.
    2. _____ Store eyeglasses in a safe place when not being worn.
    3. _____ Dry the lenses with a paper towel after they are washed.
    4. _____ Limit the time that eyeglasses are worn in an effort to rest the eyes.
    5. _____ Use warm water to clean the lenses of eyeglasses at least once a day.

33. When providing morning care for a client, the nurse identifies crusty debris around the client's eyes. Which of the following should the nurse implement when cleaning the client's eyes? **Select all that apply.**
    1. _____ Wear sterile gloves.
    2. _____ Use a tear-free baby soap.
    3. _____ Position the client on the same side as the eye to be cleaned.
    4. _____ Wash the eyes with cotton balls from the inner to outer canthus.
    5. _____ Use a separate cotton ball for each stroke when washing the eyes.

34. A nurse must make an unoccupied bed. Which nursing action is **essential**? **Select all that apply.**
    1. _____ Position the call bell in reach.
    2. _____ Place a pull sheet on top of the draw sheet.
    3. _____ Ensure that the bottom sheet is free of wrinkles.
    4. _____ Ensure that there is a toe pleat at the foot of the bed.
    5. _____ Complete one side of the bed before completing the other side.

35. A nurse plans to administer a foot bath to a client who is sitting in a chair and has no contraindications for this intervention. Place the following steps in the order in which they should be implemented.
    1. Soak each foot individually for 5 to 20 minutes, subject to the client's tolerance, condition of the skin, and absence of a history of diabetes or peripheral vascular disease.
    2. Don clean gloves and assist the client to position one foot in the water, verifying with the client that the water temperature is comfortable.
    3. Position a waterproof pad on the floor on which to place a basin half-filled with warm water (approximately 105°F to 110°F).
    4. Wash each foot with rinse-free soap and clean under the nails with an orange stick.
    5. Apply lotion to each foot, avoiding between the toes.
    6. Dry each foot gently, especially between the toes.

    Answer: _____

36. A nurse teaches a client effective oral hygiene practices. Which of the following indicates that the teaching about preventing and removing dental plaque was understood by the client? **Select all that apply.**
    1. _____ Uses a nonabrasive toothpaste
    2. _____ Brushes the teeth with a toothbrush
    3. _____ Gargles with antiplaque mouthwash
    4. _____ Flosses the teeth with unwaxed floss
    5. _____ Has teeth cleaned regularly by a dental hygienist

37. A nurse is providing for the hygiene and grooming needs of an obese client who easily becomes short of breath when moving about. Which nursing intervention is important? **Select all that apply.**
    1. _____ Administering oxygen during provision of care
    2. _____ Maintaining the bed in a high-Fowler position
    3. _____ Assessing the client's response to the activity
    4. _____ Bathing areas that the client cannot reach
    5. _____ Providing rest periods every ten minutes

38. A nurse plans to shave a male client's facial hair with a safety razor. Which of the following should the nurse implement? **Select all that apply.**
    1. _____ Hold the razor perpendicular to the skin.
    2. _____ Use long, downward strokes with the razor.
    3. _____ Shave in the opposite direction of hair growth.
    4. _____ Ensure that the client is not receiving an anticoagulant.
    5. _____ Use a hot, wet washcloth to wrap the face before shaving.

39. A nurse is caring for a client who was newly admitted to a rehabilitation facility. After reviewing the client's clinical record, the nurse chooses which of the following bathing plans to meet the client's hygiene needs?
   1. Complete bath with partial assistance
   2. Towel bath with total assistance
   3. Shower with partial assistance
   4. Tub bath with total assistance

CLIENT'S CLINICAL RECORD

History
A 74-year-old woman admitted for rehabilitation after a total hip replacement 6 days ago due to chronic pain from osteoarthritis. Postoperative status was uneventful; suture line intact and free of signs or symptoms of complications. Ingesting a regular diet; fluid and electrolytes in balance. Vital signs stable, although the respiratory rate is slightly elevated and labored due to a history of emphysema.

Nursing Admission Assessment
Resting in the semi-Fowler position with an abduction pillow in place. Oriented to person but not time and place. Client keeps saying, "This does not look like my home. I want to go home." Surgical site is dry and intact, wound edges approximated, and is free of any signs or symptoms of complications. Client is pulling on the linen, appears agitated, and is attempting to turn from side to side. Incontinent of urine.

Vital Signs
Temperature: 99.4°F, temporal
Pulse: 98 beats per minute, regular
Respirations: 28 breaths per minute, pursed-lip breathing
Blood pressure: 150/90 mm Hg

40. A nurse is caring for a client with an excessively dry mouth. Which nursing action is important when providing mouth care for this client? **Select all that apply.**
   1. _____ Wearing clean gloves
   2. _____ Providing oral care every 2 hours
   3. _____ Rinsing frequently with mouthwash
   4. _____ Cleansing 4 times a day with a water pick
   5. _____ Swabbing with a sponge-tipped applicator of lemon and glycerin

41. A nurse is providing perineal care to a male client. Which should the nurse do? **Select all that apply.**
   1. _____ Wash the genital area with hot, sudsy water.
   2. _____ Wash the scrotum before washing the glans penis.
   3. _____ Wash the shaft of the penis while moving toward the urinary meatus.
   4. _____ Wash the penis with one hand while holding it firmly with the other hand.
   5. _____ Wash the glans with a circular motion, starting at the tip and then proceeding down the shaft.

42. A school nurse teaches an adolescent who has dry skin and acne about skin care. Which statement by the adolescent indicates that the information is understood? **Select all that apply.**
   1. _____ "I will scrub my face every day with a strong soap."
   2. _____ "I will break pustules carefully after washing my face."
   3. _____ "I will apply an oil-based emollient after washing my face."
   4. _____ "I will bathe my face with cool water when I shower in the morning."
   5. _____ "I will use mild soap to gently cleanse my face thoroughly twice a day."

43. A nurse is observing a nursing assistant in a home-care setting administering a bed bath. Which issue apparent in the photograph indicates that the nursing assistant has violated the standards of care for a bed bath? **Select all that apply.**

1. _____ The pillows behind the client's body should be removed before the bath.
2. _____ The nursing assistant's uniform is in contact with the client's linens.
3. _____ The nursing assistant should be making eye contact with the client.
4. _____ The client's left leg should be covered with the bath blanket.
5. _____ The nursing assistant is not wearing clean gloves.

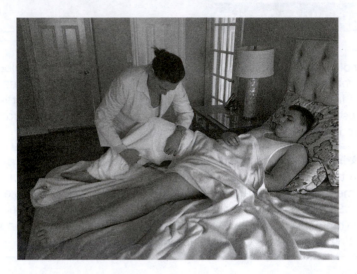

44. Which statement made by an older adult indicates to the nurse that additional teaching about skin care is necessary? **Select all that apply.**

1. _____ "I limit my baths to twice a week."
2. _____ "I humidify my home in the winter."
3. _____ "I apply moisturizing lotion to my body daily."
4. _____ "I use a bubble-bath product when I take a bath."
5. _____ "I love to relax in a hot bath before going to bed."

45. Which of the following should the nurse implement when providing fingernail care during a client's bath? **Select all that apply.**

1. _____ Push cuticles back with a section of a soft washcloth.
2. _____ File nails straight across, rounding corners slightly.
3. _____ Apply a moisturizing lotion around cuticles.
4. _____ Clean under nails with an orange stick.
5. _____ Soak hands in warm water first.

1. 1. **Heat is transferred from the warm surface of the skin to the water that is in direct contact with the body, and evaporation of the water promotes cooling. Tepid water is slightly below body temperature, and a person with a fever has an elevated body temperature (febrile).**
2. Friction, not the temperature of the bathwater, helps to remove surface debris.
3. Soap, not the temperature of bathwater, reduces the surface tension of water, not the surface tension of skin.
4. Peripheral circulation is increased by warm water and by rubbing the skin with a washcloth.

2. 1. Full or partial bed baths can be administered regardless of the activity prescription written by the primary health-care provider because this task is an independent function of the nurse.
2. **A total client assessment with an analysis of the data identifies the needs of the client and the appropriate intervention to meet those needs.**
3. Time has no relevance in relation to identifying what type of bed bath to administer to a client.
4. Although client preference is a consideration, client teaching should convince a client what should be done to meet physical needs.

3. 1. This client is not at risk for physical injury. A person at risk for physical injury is in jeopardy for harm because of a perceptual or physiological deficit, a lack of awareness of hazards, or maturational age.
2. This client is not at risk for ineffective social interaction. A person at risk for ineffective social interaction is in jeopardy of experiencing negative, insufficient, or unsatisfactory interactions with others.
3. Inadequate nutritional intake generally is not a concern when it exists for just several days. Most postoperative clients usually progress from a clear liquid to a regular diet in 2 to 3 days once bowel function returns. This is too short a time frame to be concerned about decreased nutritional intake.
4. **Not drinking anything by mouth and having a tube through the nose and posterior pharynx can result in drying of the oral mucous membranes and a coated, furrowed tongue.**

4. 1. **Fecal material contains enzymes that erode the skin, and urine is an acidic fluid that macerates the skin. As a result, altered skin integrity is a serious concern.**
2. Although incontinence may contribute to low self-esteem, which may have an impact on a person's sexual patterns, it is not the priority.
3. Incontinence is unrelated to dehydration.
4. Although confusion may contribute to a client experiencing incontinence, confusion is not a reaction to incontinence.

5. 1. Although lowering the two side rails on the working side of the bed might be done to promote safe body mechanics of the nurse, it is not a necessity.
2. **The temperature of bathwater should be between 110°F and 115°F to promote comfort, dilate blood vessels, and prevent chilling. A lower temperature can cause chilling, and a higher temperature can cause skin trauma.**
3. Although a mitt retains water and heat and prevents loose ends from irritating the skin, it is not as essential as other factors that relate to client safety.
4. Although the height of the bed should be adjusted to promote the nurse's body mechanics, it is not as essential as other factors that relate to client safety.

6. 1. Baby powder mixed with secretions of the skin forms a pastelike substance that supports antimicrobial growth and irritates the skin, promoting skin breakdown. Also, baby powder should be avoided because it is a respiratory irritant.
2. Rubbing alcohol causes drying of the skin and should not be used.
3. **Moisturizing lotion lubricates the skin and reduces friction between the nurse's hands and the client's back. Lotion facilitates smooth movement of the hands across the client's skin, which is relaxing and prevents trauma to the skin. The use of a moisturizing lotion for a back rub does not require a primary health-care provider's prescription.**
4. An antimicrobial cream is inappropriate for a back rub. It can dry the skin and eliminate the integument's natural flora. Use of an antimicrobial cream requires a primary health-care provider's prescription.

7. 1. Although it is important to provide a smooth surface by placing the seam of a hem facing the mattress, it is not the priority.
2. Arranging linen in the order in which it is to be used is an efficient approach that permits each item to be accessible when needed; however, it is not a priority.
3. Although shifting the mattress up to the headboard of the bed is important to ensure that the client is well supported when the head of the bed is elevated or the knee gatch employed, it is not the priority.
4. **A nurse must take reasonable precautions to ensure that a client's personal belongings, especially eyeglasses, dentures, and prosthetic devices, are kept safe. Checking for personal belongings before placing soiled linen into a linen hamper is a reasonable, prudent nursing action.**

8. 1. **Brushing the hair from the scalp to the ends of the hair massages the scalp and distributes oils secreted by the scalp down along the length of the hair shaft.**
2. Lifting opened fingers through the hair to distribute oil evenly along hair shafts is inadequate hair care. It might be done at the completion of hair care to style the hair.
3. Although a hydrating conditioner will make hair more supple, it will not facilitate distribution of oil along the hair shaft.
4. A fine-toothed comb has pointed ends and should not be used for daily grooming because it can injure the scalp, damage the hair shaft, and split the ends of hair.

9. 1. A client with an amputation of a foot can still transfer to a bedside commode or ambulate with crutches to a bathroom.
2. When a person has early dementia, frequent reminders to perform self-toileting activities or declarative directions about toileting usually are adequate.
3. **Discomfort resulting from the proximity of the fracture to the pelvic area and the limitations placed on the positioning of, or weight-bearing on, the affected leg influence a client's ability to use a bedpan or transfer to a commode.**
4. Although the enlarging uterus exerts pressure on the bladder, causing urinary frequency and alteration of the person's center of gravity, self-toileting usually is not impaired.

10. 1. **An offensive odor to the breath (halitosis) can be caused by inadequate oral hygiene, periodontal disease, or systemic disease. Rinsing the mouth with mouthwash will flush the oral cavity of debris and microorganisms, which will reduce halitosis if it is caused by a localized problem.**
2. Dental caries is caused by plaque. Therefore, brushing and flossing, not the use of mouthwash, are the most efficient ways to prevent dental caries.
3. Mouthwash flushes debris away from the teeth; it does not soften debris.
4. Only bactericidal mouthwashes can limit the amount of bacterial flora in the mouth; prolonged or excessive use can result in oral fungal infections.

11. 1. Although wetting the hair thoroughly before applying shampoo is done, it is not the first intervention.
2. Dry powder shampoos can irritate the scalp and dry the hair.
3. **It is easier and causes less trauma to the hair to brush out tangles when the hair is dry rather than wet.**
4. Taping eye shields over both eyes is unnecessary. Appropriate positioning will let the water flow by gravity away from the face, and a washcloth can be placed over the eyes.

12. 1. A sponge bath is given to reduce a client's fever through heat loss via conduction and vaporization. Giving a sponge bath is an independent function of the nurse and does not require a primary health-care provider's prescription.
2. **A sitz bath immerses a client from the mid-thighs to the iliac crests, or umbilicus, in a special tub, or the client sits in a basin that fits onto the toilet seat, so the legs and feet remain out of the water. The moist heat to the genital area increases local circulation, cleans the skin, reduces soreness, and promotes relaxation, voiding, drainage, and healing. A sitz bath requires a primary health-care provider's prescription because it is a method of applying local heat to the perineal area.**
3. Tubs generally are used for therapeutic baths when medications are added to the water to soothe irritated skin.
4. A bed bath is indicated for clients with restricted mobility or decreased energy. Giving a bed bath is an independent

function of the nurse and does not require a primary health-care provider's prescription.

13. 1. Manipulating a bottle of bath gel may be more difficult than using a bar of soap for a client who is vision impaired.
    2. Adapted toothbrushes are intended for people who have neuromuscular problems that interfere with grasping and manipulating a toothbrush, not for people with impaired vision.
    3. Monitoring a client through a crack in the bedside curtain is a violation of client privacy. Clients have a right to know when they are being assessed.
    4. **Identifying the placement of supplies on the over-bed table facilitates the use of equipment by a person with impaired vision and encourages self-care.**

14. 1. **Hemiparesis is a weakness on one side of the body that can interfere with the performance of activities of daily living. Encouraging the client to do as much as possible will support self-esteem, and assisting when necessary will ensure that hygiene needs are met.**
    2. Providing total assistance is unnecessary and may lower the client's self-esteem, precipitate regression, or promote dependence.
    3. Minimal supervision may result in the completion of an inadequate bath.
    4. It is not the responsibility of the family to meet the physical needs of a hospitalized relative.

15. 1. These actions will promote plantar flexion and should not be done without a toe pleat.
    2. **Maintaining functional alignment of a client's head when making an occupied bed promotes comfort and minimizes stress to the respiratory passages and vital anatomy in the neck.**
    3. Although fan-folding soiled linens as close to the client's body as possible is done, it is not the priority.
    4. Although placing the bed in the horizontal position may be done to facilitate tight sheets with minimal wrinkles, it is not the priority. In addition, many clients cannot assume this position.

16. 1. A podiatrist should file or cut the toenails of a client with diabetes. The toenails usually are thickened and hardened, and

an accidental injury can take a long time to heal, become infected, and, if gangrene occurs, can even lead to an amputation.
    2. Although client teaching about daily foot care is important, it is not the priority.
    3. A primary health-care provider's prescription is unnecessary. Foot care in relation to hygiene is within the scope of independent nursing practice.
    4. **A thorough assessment of the client is the first step of the nursing process. People with diabetes frequently have thick, hardened toenails, peripheral neuropathy, impaired arterial and venous circulation in the feet, and foot or leg ulcers.**

17. 1. Documenting results is done after the client's immediate needs are met.
    2. **When rolling a debilitated client off a bedpan, the perianal area is exposed, which permits the nurse to provide immediate perineal hygiene. A bed-bound, debilitated client is incapable of providing self-hygiene after having a bowel movement on a bedpan.**
    3. Repositioning the client is not the priority after removing a debilitated client from a bedpan.
    4. The top linens should not have been removed during this procedure because they provide privacy and maintain dignity.

18. 1. Bedrest does not cause dry hair. Malnutrition, aging, and excessive shampooing cause dry hair.
    2. Bedrest does not cause oily hair. Infrequent shampooing results in oily hair.
    3. Bedrest does not cause hair to split. Excessive brushing, blow drying, and coloring the hair can cause hair to split.
    4. **Bedrest causes matted, tangled hair because of friction and pressure related to the movement of the head on a pillow.**

19. 1. **Putting the right sleeve of the gown on the weak extremity first puts less stress on affected muscles; the stronger side can stretch more easily to dress.**
    2. Although dressing the client in an open-backed gown is helpful, the nurse still needs to put the gown on without stressing the joints, tendons, muscles, and nerves of the weak arm.
    3. Encouraging the client to dress independently may be frustrating and tiring and may cause further damage to the weak arm.

4. Leaving the right sleeve off while adjusting the tie at the neck is unnecessary. The client should be dressed appropriately.

20. 1. Strong soap may further irritate the skin.
    2. **Loose stool contains digestive enzymes that are irritating to the skin and should be cleaned from the skin as soon as possible after soiling.**
    3. The use of Talcum powder is unsafe because it is a respiratory irritant.
    4. Placing a pad under the buttocks will not keep stool off the skin.

21. 1. Vasodilation increases blood flow to the surface of the skin, which promotes, not prevents, heat loss.
    2. Conduction is the transfer of heat between two objects in physical contact.
    3. **Convection is the transfer of heat by movement of air along a surface. Using a bath blanket limits the amount of air flowing across the client, which prevents heat loss.**
    4. Diffusion is the movement of molecules from a solution of higher concentration to a solution of lower concentration.

22. 1. Waiting until the client feels better is inappropriate because the client may never feel better. Physical needs can be met while addressing the client's concerns.
    2. Postponing the bath until the afternoon is unsafe. With significant diaphoresis, there is moisture on the client's skin that can contribute to skin breakdown and cause chilling.
    3. **After explaining the need for the bath, the nurse should administer a bath with complete assistance. This will meet the client's immediate hygiene needs while conserving the client's energy.**
    4. Consulting with the primary health-care provider is unnecessary. Bathing a client is within the scope of independent nursing practice.

23. 1. Although a bath is refreshing and relaxing and may support self-esteem, this is not the primary reason for bathing.
    2. Although friction from rubbing the skin increases surface temperature, which increases circulation to the area, this is not the primary purpose of a bed bath.
    3. **The removal of accumulated oil, perspiration, dead cells, and bacteria from the skin limits the environment conducive**

to the growth of bacteria and skin breakdown. Intact, healthy skin is one of the body's first lines of defense.
    4. Although range-of-motion exercises may be performed while a client is being bathed, this is not the purpose of the bath.

24. 1. Although someone may have contractures, that person may still be able to provide self-care.
    2. **Being unable to wash body parts is a human response indicating that a client is unable to provide for one's own activities of daily living, such as meeting hygiene and grooming needs.**
    3. People who are lethargic or listless generally are still able to provide for their own basic self-care needs. However, they may require frequent rest periods or more time to complete the task.
    4. People who are legally blind are still able to provide for their own self-care needs.

25. 1. Friction, regardless of the direction of the washing strokes, in conjunction with soap and water, mechanically removes secretions, dirt, and microorganisms that decrease the potential for infection.
    2. Friction, regardless of the direction of the washing strokes, mechanically removes dry, dead skin cells.
    3. **The pressure exerted on the skin surface by long, smooth strokes moving from distal to proximal areas also presses on the veins, which promotes venous return.**
    4. Long, smooth washing strokes that avoid a shearing force minimize skin tears.

26. 1. **The accumulation of matter, such as food, epithelial elements, dried secretions, and microorganisms (sordes) eventually can lead to dental caries and periodontal disease and therefore must be removed during oral hygiene.**
    2. Plaque is an invisible film composed of secretions, epithelial cells, leukocytes, and bacteria that adheres to the enamel surface of teeth.
    3. Glossitis is an inflammation of the tongue.
    4. Stomatitis is an inflammation of the oral mucosa.

27. 1. Brushing the teeth six times a day is more than the number of times a day recommended by the American Dental Association. Brushing the teeth six times a day is unnecessary for effective dental hygiene. It

may cause gum recession, which can
lead to dentine hypersensitivity or cause
damage to the neck of the teeth.

2. Brushing the teeth four times a day is
more than the number of times a day
recommended by the American Dental
Association. It is important to know that
excessive brushing with a soft brush using
minimal pressure will not wear away
enamel in the absence of an acidic environment. However, brushing the teeth
four or more times a day may cause problems such as gum recession, which can
lead to dentine hypersensitivity or cause
damage to the neck of the teeth.

3. Brushing the teeth three times a day is
more than the number of times a day
recommended by the American Dental
Association. However, some reputable
Web sites recommend brushing the teeth
after each meal. Some sites recommend
brushing the teeth upon awakening to
facilitate removal of bacteria from the
mouth.

**4. The American Dental Association
recommends brushing the teeth for
2 minutes two times a day, and it
should be done at least 30 minutes
after consuming acidic food or drinks.**

28. 1. A primary health-care provider's prescription is unnecessary because providing
foot care is within the scope of nursing
practice.

2. When the client has peripheral neuropathy, cutting or filing toenails should be
provided by a podiatrist.

**3. Lukewarm water is comfortable and
limits the potential for burns. Drying
the feet limits moisture that promotes
bacterial growth.**

4. Lotion between the toes in the dark,
warm environment of shoes promotes the
growth of bacteria and the development of
an infection.

29. **1. Touching a client during a bed bath
invades the person's intimate space
(physical contact to 1½ feet) because of
the need to expose and touch personal
body parts.**

2. Although the nurse enters a client's intimate space when obtaining vital signs, this
task does not involve touching the intimate parts of a client's body and is therefore less intrusive than other procedures.

3. Performing a health history can be
accomplished by remaining in a person's

personal space (1½ to 4 feet) or social
space (4 to 12 feet).

4. Although touching a client while ambulating invades the person's intimate space,
it does not involve touching the intimate
parts of a client's body and is therefore
less intrusive than other procedures.

30. 1. Providing a bed bath is within the scope of
nursing practice, so a primary health-care
provider's prescription is unnecessary. A
prescription is necessary for a tub bath or
a shower because it requires an activity
prescription and is therefore a dependent
function of the nurse.

**2. Clients should provide self-care within
their abilities. When they have limitations, such as an inability to reach a
body area, an activity intolerance, a
decreased level of consciousness, or
cognitive impairment, it is the nurse's
responsibility to assist the client
regardless of the type of bath.**

3. It is impossible to expose just the body
parts being washed during a tub bath or a
shower. During a tub bath or a shower,
the entire body is exposed.

**4. Bathing is a private matter and an inva-
sion of personal space. The nurse
provides privacy by pulling a curtain,
closing a door, and keeping the client
covered as much as possible. These interventions maintain the client's dignity.**

5. There is no need for a call bell when a
client is taking a tub bath or a shower because it is unsafe to leave a client alone.

31. **2. The bath should follow a cephalocaudal progression and be based on the
principle of from "clean to dirty."
The face is washed first, before soap
is placed in the bathwater.**

**3. The axillae are less soiled than the
hands but are more soiled than the
face.**

**4. The hands are more soiled than the
axilla.**

**6. The water is changed after washing the
soiled hands so as not to contaminate
other areas of the body.**

**1. The back is less soiled than the genital
area.**

**5. The genital area is considered more
soiled than the back and should be
washed last.**

32. 1. Encouraging the use of artificial tears is
unnecessary. Not everyone who wears

eyeglasses has dry eyes. Also, this intervention requires a health-care provider's prescription.

2. **Storing eyeglasses in a safe place when not being worn protects them from loss or damage.**

3. A paper towel is coarse and may scratch the lenses of eyeglasses. A soft, nonabrasive cloth or chamois should be used.

4. Client preference determines how long eyeglasses can be worn.

5. **Eyeglasses should be cleaned at least once a day because dirty lenses impair vision. Warm, not hot, water is used to prevent distortion of the lens or frame, particularly if it is made of a plastic compound.**

33. 1. Medical, not surgical, asepsis is necessary. Clean gloves are adequate.

2. Soap is never used around the eyes. The eyes should be washed only with water.

3. **Tilting the head or turning the client toward the same side as the eye to be washed facilitates the flow of water from the inner to the outer canthus. This limits secretions from entering the lacrimal ducts.**

4. **Washing the eyes from the inner canthus to the outer canthus moves debris away from the lacrimal duct.**

5. **Using a new cotton ball for each stroke prevents reintroducing debris removed during the previous stroke.**

34. 1. The call bell does not have to be positioned until there is a client occupying the bed.

2. A pull sheet is not included in the procedure for an unoccupied bed. In addition, this creates too many layers of linens that may wrinkle under a client. A draw sheet can be used as a pull sheet. A draw sheet may not be used when using a fitted bottom sheet.

3. **Wrinkles create ridges that exert additional pressure on the skin, promoting discomfort, skin irritation, and the development of pressure ulcers.**

4. **A toe pleat is essential because it allows room for movement of the feet and helps to prevent plantar flexion as a result of top sheets that are too tight.**

5. Although completing one side of the bed before the other side is advisable to conserve the nurse's time and energy, it is not a priority.

35. 3. The first step involves positioning a waterproof pad on the floor on which to place the foot basin. Warm water promotes circulation. Avoiding hot water protects the client from sustaining a burn injury.

2. The second step involves donning clean gloves to protect the nurse from the client's body fluids. The heel of a foot is a common place for skin cracks and skin breakdown. Ensuring that the water temperature is comfortable helps to prevent a burn injury.

1. The third step involves soaking a foot for the appropriate length of time considering the client's condition. A foot bath for a client with diabetes or peripheral vascular disease may dry the skin, placing the client at risk for cracks in the skin, and should be conducted over 5 minutes or less.

4. **The fourth step involves washing each foot with rinse-free soap because this avoids the drying effect of soap residue. Cleaning under the nails with an orange stick removes debris and minimizes the risk of injury that could occur when using a sharp instrument.**

6. **The fifth step involves drying each foot, especially between the toes, because moisture can cause maceration and support the growth of fungal infections.**

5. **The sixth step involves applying lotion to each foot while avoiding between the toes. Lotion hydrates the skin and keeps skin supple, reducing the risk of cracks in the skin. Lotion between the toes should be avoided because it can cause skin maceration and support the growth of fungal infections.**

36. 1. **A nonabrasive toothpaste and a soft toothbrush should be used to clean the teeth. An abrasive toothpaste can harm the enamel of teeth.**

2. Brushing the teeth involves several techniques: brushing back-and-forth strokes across the biting surface of teeth; brushing from the gum line to the crown of each tooth; and, with the bristles at a 45-degree angle at the gum line, vibrating the bristles while moving from under the gingival margin to the crown of each tooth. Brushing removes plaque, which is a soft, thin film of food debris, mucin, and dead

epithelial cells that provides a medium for bacterial growth. Plaque plays an etiological role in the development of periodontal and gingival disease as well as dental caries.

3. **Mouthwash with anti-plaque properties can help prevent plaque buildup.**

4. **Unwaxed floss is thin, slides between the teeth easily, and is more effective than waxed floss. This removes debris that contributes to plaque formation.**

5. **A dental hygienist is a licensed oral health-care professional educated to provide such services as dental education, dental radiographs, oral prophylaxis, and removal of calcified plaque.**

37. 1. Administration of oxygen is a dependent function of the nurse and requires a primary health-care provider's prescription unless it is needed in an emergency situation. The situation in this question is not an emergency.

2. When an obese client is in the high-Fowler position, the abdominal organs press against the diaphragm, which limits respiratory excursion. The semi-Fowler position is preferred.

3. **Evaluation of a client's response to care allows the nurse to alter care to meet the client's individual needs.**

4. **Bathing body parts that the client cannot reach ensures that the client receives adequate hygiene care.**

5. A rest period every 10 minutes may be inadequate or may unnecessarily prolong the bath. This intervention is not individualized to the client's needs.

38. 1. A safety razor should be held at a 45-, not 90-, degree angle to the skin.

2. Short, gentle strokes should be used when shaving a client.

3. Shaving in the opposite direction of hair growth irritates the skin and promotes the development of ingrown hairs.

4. **Ensuring that the client is not receiving an anticoagulant is essential. A client receiving an anticoagulant should use an electric razor to avoid the risk of blood loss associated with an accidental cut made by using a safety razor.**

5. A hot washcloth may cause a burn injury. A warm, not hot, washcloth applied to the face for several minutes before shaving helps to soften the beard.

39. 1. The client is too confused to provide self-care, even with partial assistance.

2. **A towel bath is the most appropriate bathing plan for this client. It is quick and easy to administer and is the intervention that is least taxing physically, considering the client's recent surgery, confusion, and respiratory status.**

3. The client is too confused and physically dependent to participate in a shower, even with partial assistance.

4. It is too soon after surgery to submerse the client's body in a tub bath. Generally, a tub bath is contraindicated until a surgical wound is fully healed.

40. 1. **Wearing clean gloves protects the nurse from the blood and body fluids of the client. This interrupts the chain of infection.**

2. **Mouth breathing, oxygen use, unconsciousness, and debilitation, among other conditions, can lead to dry oral mucous membranes. The nurse should provide oral hygiene with saline rinses frequently to keep the oral mucosa moist.**

3. Mouthwash contains astringents that can injure sensitive, delicate, dry mucous membranes.

4. Oral hygiene four times a day is inadequate for a client with a dry mouth, and a water pick is contraindicated because the force of the water can injure delicate, dry mucous membranes.

5. Lemon and glycerin swabs are counterproductive because their use can lead to further dryness of the mucosa and an alteration in tooth enamel.

41. 1. Warm, not hot, water is used to clean the perineal area because the skin and mucous membranes of the genital area are sensitive, and hot water may cause harm.

2. The glans penis, foreskin, and shaft of the penis are cleaned before the scrotum. The scrotum is considered more soiled than the penis because of its proximity to the rectum.

3. When cleaning the shaft of the penis, bathing should start at the glans penis and then proceed down the shaft toward the scrotum.

4. **Stabilizing the penis and holding it firmly facilitates the bathing procedure and usually prevents an erection.**

5. **Washing from the tip of the penis in a circular motion and then down the**

shaft of the penis follows the principle of "clean to dirty," with the meatus being the cleanest area.

42. 1. Strong soap may irritate fragile skin.
     2. Breaking pustules should be avoided because it can spread infection and cause skin damage and scarring. Acne with pustules requires the intervention of a dermatologist because topical or oral medications may be necessary to treat the acne.
     3. An oil-based emollient can block sebaceous gland ducts and hair follicles, which will aggravate the acne. A water-based emollient should be used.
     4. Washing once a day is inadequate to cleanse the skin. Warm, not cool, water is necessary to remove the oily accumulation on the face.
     5. **Washing the face with mild soap and water twice a day will remove dirt and oil, which helps prevent secondary infection. Washing the face more than twice a day can irritate the skin and make acne worse.**

43. 1. The pillows can remain under the client's head throughout the bath as long as this position is not contraindicated by the client's condition. A client does not have to remain in the supine position to receive a bed bath.
     2. **When a nursing care provider's uniform touches a client's linens, the uniform is considered contaminated. Microorganisms from the client can be carried on the uniform to other clients. This is a violation of medical asepsis.**
     3. The nursing assistant should not be making eye contact with the client. The nursing assistant should be concentrating on looking at the action being implemented.
     4. **Body parts should be covered when not being bathed to prevent heat loss and chilling. The left leg should be covered to promote comfort, prevent heat loss, and provide for privacy.**
     5. Clean gloves should be worn to provide a barrier between the nursing assistant's hands and the client's body

fluids. **This is an important medical aseptic practice associated with standard precautions.**

44. 1. Limiting baths to twice a week is an acceptable practice. Excessive exposure to warm water and soap exacerbates dry skin associated with aging.
     2. A humidified environment limits the amount of insensible loss of moisture through the skin, which helps the skin retain fluid and remain supple.
     3. Applying moisturizing lotion to the body daily is an acceptable practice. Older adults experience less sebum produced by sebaceous glands, causing dry and scaly skin. Moisturizing lotion helps to keep skin supple and less dry.
     4. **Bubble-bath preparations cause irritation and dryness of the skin because they remove essential skin surface oils. Showers are preferable to baths because baths require submersion in warm water, which is detrimental to skin hydration and resiliency.**
     5. **Hot bathwater removes essential skin surface oils, causing skin to be dry and scaly, and should be avoided. A short shower with warm water should be encouraged instead.**

45. 1. **Using a soft washcloth is a gentle way of moving cuticles toward the base of the nails. An orange stick also can be used. Metal instruments should be avoided.**
     2. Filing nails straight across helps to avoid ingrown nails. Rounding corners slightly reduces sharp edges that may scratch the skin.
     3. **Applying a moisturizing lotion around cuticles helps to soften cuticles.**
     4. **An orange stick is an implement that is shaped to facilitate removal of debris from under the nails without causing tissue injury. Removal of dirt and debris decreases the risk of infection.**
     5. **Warm water helps to remove debris and soften the cuticles in preparation for further nail care.**

Mobility

KEYWORDS

The following words include nursing/medical terminology, concepts, principles, and information relevant to content specifically addressed in the chapter or associated with topics presented in it. English dictionaries, nursing textbooks, and medical dictionaries, such as *Taber's Cyclopedic Medical Dictionary,* are resources that can be used to expand your knowledge and understanding of these words and related information.

Ambulation
Atrophy
Blanchable erythema
Body mechanics
Bony prominence
Contracture
Exercises:
  Aerobic
  Anaerobic
  Isometric
  Isotonic
Flaccidity
Footdrop
Functional alignment
Gait
Hemiparesis
Hemiplegia
Joints:
  Ball and socket
  Condyloid
  Hinge
  Pivot
  Saddle
Mechanical lift, Hoyer lift
Paraplegia
Paresis
Popliteal
Positioning devices:
  Bed cradle
  Hand roll
  Hand-wrist splint
  Heel and elbow protectors
  Pillow
  Side rail
  Trapeze bar
  Trochanter roll
  Turning and pull sheet
Positions:
  Contour
  Dorsal recumbent
  Fowler (low-, semi-, high-)
  Knee-chest

Lateral
Lithotomy
Orthopneic
Prone
Sims
Supine
Trendelenburg
Posture
Pressure relief, reduction devices:
  Air cushion/mattress
  Dense foam cushion/mattress
  Egg-crate cushion/mattress
  Gel cushion/mattress
  Sheepskin cushion, heel/elbow
    protectors
Pressure ulcer, stages I, II, III, IV
Quadriplegia
Range-of-motion exercises:
  Active
  Active-assistive
  Passive
Range-of-motion movements:
  Abduction
  Adduction
  Circumduction
  Eversion
  Extension
  Flexion:
    Dorsal flexion
    Lateral flexion
    Plantar flexion
    Radial flexion
    Ulnar flexion
  Hyperextension
  Inversion
  Opposition of thumb
  Pronation
  Rotation:
    External
    Internal
    Supination
Reactive hyperemia

Restraints:
  Belt
  Chest
  Elbow
  Four-point

Mitt
Poncho
Vest
Wrist
Shearing force

MOBILITY: QUESTIONS

1. A nurse turns a client's ankle so that the sole of the foot moves medially toward the midline. Which word should the nurse use when documenting exactly what was done during range-of-motion exercises?
   1. Inversion
   2. Adduction
   3. Plantar flexion
   4. Internal rotation

2. A nurse is transferring a client from a bed to a wheelchair. Which should the nurse do to quickly assess this client's tolerance to this activity?
   1. Obtain a blood pressure.
   2. Monitor for bradycardia.
   3. Determine if the client feels dizzy.
   4. Allow the client time to adjust to the change in position.

3. A nurse is transferring a client from the bed to a wheelchair using a mechanical lift. Which is a basic nursing intervention associated with this procedure?
   1. Lock the base lever in the open position when moving the mechanical lift.
   2. Raise the mechanical lift so that the client is six inches off the mattress.
   3. Keep the wheels of the mechanical lift locked throughout the procedure.
   4. Ensure the client's feet are guarded when sitting on the mechanical lift.

4. A client has hemiplegia as a result of a brain attack (cerebrovascular accident). Which complication of immobility that may be associated with this client is a concern for the nurse?
   1. Dehydration
   2. Contractures
   3. Incontinence
   4. Hypertension

5. Which stage pressure ulcer requires the nurse to measure the extent of undermining?
   1. Stage 0
   2. Stage I
   3. Stage II
   4. Stage III

6. A client has a cast from the hand to above the elbow because of a fractured ulna and radius. After the cast is removed, the nurse teaches the client active range-of-motion exercises. Which client action indicates that further teaching is necessary?
   1. Moves the elbow to the point of resistance
   2. Keeps 90° elbow flexion after the procedure
   3. Assesses the elbow's response after this procedure
   4. Puts the elbow through its full range at least 3 times

7. Which word is **most** closely associated with nursing care strategies to maintain functional alignment when clients are bedbound?
   1. Endurance
   2. Strength
   3. Support
   4. Balance

8. A client with impaired mobility is to be discharged from the hospital within a week. Which is an example of a discharge goal for this client?
   1. The client will understand range-of-motion exercises before they are initiated.
   2. The client will be taught range-of-motion exercises after they are prescribed.
   3. The client will transfer independently to a chair by discharge.
   4. The client will be kept clean and dry at all times.

9. A nurse is performing passive range-of-motion exercises for a client who is in the supine position. Which motion occurs when the nurse bends the client's ankle so that the toes are pointed toward the ceiling?
   1. Adduction
   2. Supination
   3. Dorsal flexion
   4. Plantar extension

10. A nurse is caring for a client with impaired mobility. Which position contributes **most** to the formation of a hip flexion contracture?
    1. Low-Fowler
    2. Orthopneic
    3. Supine
    4. Sims

11. A client is diagnosed with a stage IV pressure ulcer with eschar. Which medical treatment should the nurse anticipate the primary health-care provider will prescribe for this client?
    1. Heat lamp treatment three times a day
    2. Application of a topical antibiotic
    3. Cleansing irrigations twice daily
    4. Débridement of the wound

12. A nurse raises a client's arm forward and upward over the head during range-of-motion exercises. Which word should the nurse use when documenting exactly what was done during this range-of-motion exercise?
    1. Flexion
    2. Supination
    3. Opposition
    4. Hyperextension

13. A client with a history of thrombophlebitis should not have pressure exerted on the popliteal space. In which position should the nurse **avoid** placing this client?
    1. Prone
    2. Supine
    3. Contour
    4. Trendelenburg

14. A nurse is caring for a variety of clients, each experiencing one of the following problems. Which health problem places a client at the **highest** risk for complications associated with immobility?
    1. Incontinence
    2. Quadriplegia
    3. Hemiparesis
    4. Confusion

15. A nurse in a community center is conversing with a group of older adults who voiced fears about falling. Which is the **most** common consequence associated with older adults' fear of falling that the nurse should discuss with them?
    1. Impaired skin integrity
    2. Occurrence of panic attacks
    3. Self-imposed social isolation
    4. Decreased physical conditioning

16. A nurse is evaluating an ambulating client's balance. Which factor about the client is **most** important for the nurse to assess?
    1. Posture
    2. Strength
    3. Energy level
    4. Respiratory rate

17. A client with a prescription for bedrest has diaphoresis. Which should the nurse use to **best** limit the negative effects of perspiration on dependent skin surfaces of this client?
    1. Ventilated heel protectors
    2. Air-filled rings
    3. Air mattress
    4. Sheepskin

18. A nurse is teaching a class to nursing assistants about how to care for clients who are immobile. Which should the nurse include about why immobilized people develop contractures?
    1. Muscles that flex, adduct, and internally rotate are stronger than weaker opposing muscles.
    2. Muscular contractures occur because of excessive muscle flaccidity.
    3. Muscle mass and strength decline at a progressive rate weekly.
    4. Muscle catabolism exceeds muscle anabolism.

19. A nurse turns the palm of a client's hand downward when performing range-of-motion exercises. Which word should the nurse use when documenting exactly what was done?
    1. Pronation
    2. Lateral flexion
    3. Circumduction
    4. External rotation

20. Which nursing action is **most** effective in relation to the concept *Immobility can lead to occlusion of blood vessels in areas where bony prominences rest on a mattress*?
    1. Encouraging the client to breathe deeply 10 times per hour
    2. Performing range-of-motion exercises twice a day
    3. Placing a sheepskin pad under the sacrum
    4. Repositioning the client every 2 hours

21. A nurse plans to use a trochanter roll when repositioning a client. Where should the nurse place the trochanter roll?
    1. Under the small of the back
    2. Behind the knees when supine
    3. Alongside the ilium to mid-thigh
    4. In the palm of the hand with the fingers flexed

22. Which is the earliest nursing assessment that indicates damage to tissue because of compression of soft tissue between a bony prominence and a mattress?
    1. Nonblanchable erythema
    2. Circumoral cyanosis
    3. Tissue necrosis
    4. Skin abrasion

23. An emaciated client is at risk for developing a pressure ulcer. In which position should the nurse **avoid** placing the client?
    1. Thirty-degree lateral position
    2. Side-lying position
    3. Supine position
    4. Prone position

24. A nurse is making an occupied bed. Which is the easiest way for the nurse to prevent plantar flexion?
    1. Tuck in the top linens on just the sides of the bed.
    2. Place a toe pleat in the top linens over the feet.
    3. Let the top linens hang off the end of the bed.
    4. Position the top linens over a bed cradle.

25. A nurse identifies that a client's pressure ulcer has just partial-thickness skin loss involving the epidermis and dermis. Which stage pressure ulcer should the nurse document based on this assessment?
    1. Stage I
    2. Stage II
    3. Stage III
    4. Stage IV

26. Which nursing action should be implemented when assisting a client to move from a bed to a wheelchair?
    1. Lowering the height of the bed to 2 inches below the height of the client's wheelchair
    2. Applying pressure under the client's axillae areas when assisting the client to stand
    3. Letting the client help as much as possible when transferring to the wheelchair
    4. Keeping the client's feet within 6 inches of each other

27. A nurse places a client in the orthopneic position. Which is the **primary** reason for the use of this position?
    1. Facilitates breathing
    2. Supports hip extension
    3. Prevents pressure ulcers
    4. Promotes urinary elimination

28. An immobilized bedbound client is placed on a 2-hour turning and positioning program. Which should the nurse explain to the client is the **primary** reason why this program is important?
    1. Supports comfort
    2. Promotes elimination
    3. Maintains skin integrity
    4. Facilitates respiratory function

29. Which do nurses sometimes do that increases their risk for injury when moving clients?
    1. Use longer, rather than shorter, muscles when moving clients
    2. Place their feet wide apart when transferring clients
    3. Pull rather than push when turning clients
    4. Rotate their backs when moving clients

30. Which systemic response in immobilized clients should nurses monitor for? **Select all that apply.**
    1. _____ Pressure ulcer
    2. _____ Dependent edema
    3. _____ Hypostatic pneumonia
    4. _____ Plantar flexion contracture
    5. _____ Increased cardiac workload

31. A nurse moves a client's leg through the range of motion demonstrated in the figure. Which word should the nurse use when documenting exactly what was done during the range-of-motion exercise?
1. Eversion
2. Circumduction
3. Plantar flexion
4. External rotation

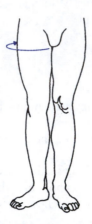

32. A nurse is placing a client in the left-lateral position. Which of the following should the nurse implement when positioning this client? **Select all that apply.**
1. _____ Maintain the left knee flexed at ninety degrees.
2. _____ Rest the right leg on top of the left leg.
3. _____ Place the ankles in plantar flexion.
4. _____ Align the shoulders with the hips.
5. _____ Protract the left shoulder.

33. A nurse places a client with a sacral pressure ulcer in the left-Sims position. How should the nurse position the client's right arm? **Select all that apply.**
1. _____ On a pillow
2. _____ Behind the back
3. _____ With the palm up
4. _____ In internal rotation
5. _____ With the elbow extended

34. A nurse concludes that a client has the potential for impaired mobility. Which of the following reflect risk factors that **support** this conclusion? **Select all that apply.**
1. _____ Joint pain
2. _____ Exertional fatigue
3. _____ Sedentary lifestyle
4. _____ Limited range of motion
5. _____ Increased respiratory rate

35. A nurse enters the room of the client in the photograph. The client has right-sided weakness and is attempting to transfer out of bed without the nurse's knowledge. What should the nurse do **first**?
1. Lower the height of the bed to its lowest position to the floor.
2. Reposition the client back to the semi-Fowler position.
3. Move the wheelchair parallel to the foot of the bed.
4. Put on the client's slippers.

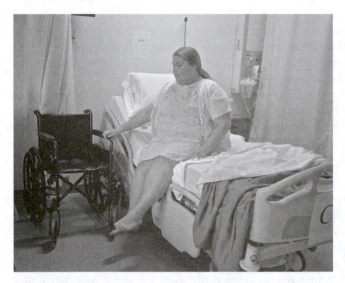

36. A nurse plans to teach a client with hemiparesis to use a cane. Which should the nurse teach the client to do? **Select all that apply.**
1. _____ Move forward 1 step with the weak leg first, followed by the strong leg and cane.
2. _____ Adjust the cane height 12 inches lower than the waist.
3. _____ Hold the cane in the strong hand when walking.
4. _____ Look at the feet when walking with the cane.
5. _____ Lean over onto the cane when walking.

37. A nurse is planning to help move a client up in bed. Which of the following can the nurse implement to reduce the risk of self-strain when performing this action? **Select all that apply.**
1. _____ Use the force of gravity to facilitate the move.
2. _____ Keep the upper and lower body in alignment.
3. _____ Use the large muscles of the legs.
4. _____ Keep the knees slightly bent.
5. _____ Raise the bed to waist level.

38. A primary health-care provider prescribes crutches for a person who has a left lower leg injury. The nurse is teaching the person how to move from a standing to a sitting position in a chair. Place the following steps in the order in which they should be implemented.
1. While standing, back up so that the unaffected leg is against the edge of the center of the chair seat.
2. Hold the hand bars of both crutches with the left hand.
3. Lean forward slightly and flex the knees and hips.
4. Grasp the arm of the chair with the right hand.
5. Lower the body slowly into the chair.

Answer: _____

39. A client sits for excessive lengths of time in a wheelchair. Which site should the nurse assess for skin breakdown in this client? **Select all that apply.**
1. _____ Ischial tuberosities
2. _____ Bilateral scapulae
3. _____ Trochanters
4. _____ Malleolus
5. _____ Sacrum

40. A client with limited mobility has a prescription to be out of bed to a chair for 1 hour daily. The nurse plans to transfer the client using a mechanical lift. Which of the following should the nurse implement? **Select all that apply.**
1. _____ Apply gentle pressure against the client's knees while lowering the client into the chair.
2. _____ Ensure that there is a prescription to use this device to transfer the client out of bed.
3. _____ Hook the longer straps on the end of the sling closest to the client's feet.
4. _____ Place a sheepskin inside the sling so that it is under the client.
5. _____ Lead with the client's feet when exiting the bed.

41. A primary health-care provider prescribes a standard walker for a client who has left-sided weakness and requires some assistance with balance but can bear weight on both legs. Which should the nurse teach the client about how to use the walker safely? **Select all that apply.**
1. _____ Advance the strong leg last by itself.
2. _____ Lift the walker before moving it forward twelve inches.
3. _____ Advance the walker and the weak leg ahead together first.
4. _____ Adjust the height of the walker so that it is equal with the hip joint.
5. _____ Roll the walker a comfortable distance ahead before stepping forward.

42. A nurse is to transfer a client from a bed to a chair. After washing the hands, providing privacy, and explaining the transfer to the client, the nurse ensures that the wheels on the bed are locked and moves the bed to the lowest position. Place the following steps in the order in which they should be implemented.
1. Verify if the client feels dizzy.
2. Assess the client's vital signs and strength while in the supine position.
3. Assist the client to a sitting position on the side of the bed, with the feet on the floor.
4. Elevate the head of the bed to the high-Fowler position and put footwear on the client's feet.
5. Support the client sitting on the side of the bed for several minutes before transferring to a chair.

Answer: _____

43. Which action employed by the nurse indicates acceptable body mechanics to avoid self-injury? **Select all that apply.**
1. _____ Keep back, neck, pelvis, and feet aligned.
2. _____ Position oneself close to the client.
3. _____ Keep knees and hips slightly flexed.
4. _____ Arrange for adequate help.
5. _____ Keep feet close together.

44. A nurse is assessing a client's risk for thrombus formation associated with impaired mobility. Which of the following constitute Virchow's triad? **Select all that apply.**
1. _____ Compression of small vessels in the legs
2. _____ Orthostatic hypotension
3. _____ Coagulation activation
4. _____ Hypostatic pneumonia
5. _____ Venous stasis

45. A nurse is caring for a male client who is at risk for a pressure ulcer. After reviewing the client's clinical record, which area of the body should the nurse identify is **most** at risk for a pressure ulcer?
1. Greater trochanters
2. Ischial tuberosities
3. Medial malleolus
4. Spinal processes

CLIENT'S CLINICAL RECORD

Primary Health-Care Provider Prescriptions
Oxygen via simple face mask, humidified, 8 L flow rate
Levofloxacin 500 mg, PO, daily for 14 days
Prednisone 30 mg, PO, daily for 2 days; 20 mg, PO, daily for 2 days; 10 mg, PO, daily for 2 days; and 5 mg, PO, daily for 2 days
Position for comfort
OOB to bathroom
Fluid intake, at least 3,000 mL daily, soft diet

Nurse's Progress Note
Client sitting in an upright position leaning on a pillow on the over-bed table, oxygen face mask in place and set at a flow rate of 8 L, client has a productive cough, expectorating clear-colored mucous. Respirations are 34 and labored, with mild retractions and flaring of nares. Assisted with activities of daily living, shortness of breath on activity.

Client Interview
Client states that he was fine until he caught his 5-year-old granddaughter's cold. He developed a fever, nasal stuffiness, and a "heavy cough" that got progressively worse. The primary health-care provider admitted him to the hospital with the diagnosis of pneumonia and an oxygen saturation rate of 88%. He said that since he is in the hospital he "feels much better." He stated that he is able to breathe best leaning over the over-bed table, that his cough is improved, and his fever is resolving.

1. 1. **Inversion, a gliding movement of the foot, occurs by turning the sole of the foot medially toward the midline of the body.**
   2. Adduction occurs when an arm or leg moves toward or beyond the midline of the body (or both).
   3. Plantar flexion occurs when the joint of the ankle is in extension by pointing the toes of the foot downward and away from the anterior portion of the lower leg.
   4. Internal rotation of a leg occurs by turning the foot and leg inward so that the toes point toward the other leg.

2. 1. Although a blood pressure reading may indicate the presence of hypotension, the blood pressure should be obtained before and after a transfer to allow a comparison to conclude that the hypotension is orthostatic hypotension.
   2. If the client is experiencing orthostatic hypotension, the heart rate will increase, not decrease.
   3. **Feeling dizzy is a subjective response to orthostatic hypotension. Obtaining feedback from the client provides a quick evaluation of the client's tolerance of the transfer.**
   4. Allowing the client time to adjust to the change in position is not an assessment. This is a safe intervention for a client who is experiencing orthostatic hypotension.

3. 1. The width of the base depends on the configuration of the bed, objects in the room, and the ultimate destination. The base usually is locked open when lifting or lowering the client and locked closed when moving the lift.
   2. Raising the mechanical lift so that the client is 6 inches off the mattress is unsafe. The lift should raise the client only high enough to clear the surface of the bed.
   3. The wheels must be unlocked to move the lift from under the bed to its ultimate destination.
   4. **The legs dangle from the sling and therefore may drag across the linens or hit other objects if not protected.**

4. 1. Dehydration is not a response to immobility.
   2. **Contractures can result from permanent shortening of muscles, tendons, and ligaments and are a complication associated with a brain attack if routine** range-of-motion exercises and maintaining the body in functional alignment are not provided.
   3. The decreased tone of the urinary bladder and the inability to assume the usual voiding position in bed promote urinary retention, rather than urinary incontinence.
   4. With immobility, the increased heart rate reduces the diastolic pressure. In addition, there is a decrease in blood pressure related to postural changes from lying to sitting or standing (orthostatic hypotension). This situation is manageable with a priority on maintaining client safety.

5. 1. There is no stage 0 in the classification system for staging pressure ulcers.
   2. The skin is still intact and there is no undermining in a stage I pressure ulcer.
   3. Tissue damage is superficial and there is no undermining in a stage II pressure ulcer.
   4. **In a stage III pressure ulcer, there is full-thickness skin loss involving damage to subcutaneous tissue that may extend to the fascia, and there may or may not be undermining, which is tissue destruction underneath intact skin along wound margins.**

6. 1. Moving the elbow to the point of resistance is desirable. Performing range-of-motion exercises beyond resistance may injure muscles and joints and should be avoided.
   2. **Keeping the elbow flexed after the procedure is undesirable because it contributes to a flexion contracture. Slight flexion to maintain functional alignment is preferred because it minimizes stress and strain on muscles, tendons, ligaments, and joints.**
   3. Responses to range-of-motion exercises must be evaluated and compared with the assessment performed before the procedure.
   4. Sequential flexion and extension of a hinge joint are efficient in facilitating full range of motion of the joint.

7. 1. Endurance relates to aerobic exercise that improves the body's capacity to consume oxygen for producing energy at the cellular level.
   2. Strength relates to isometric and isotonic exercises, which contract muscles and promote their development.
   3. **The line of gravity passes through the center of gravity when the body is**

correctly aligned; this results in the least amount of stress on the muscles, joints, and soft tissues. Bedbound clients often need assistive devices such as pillows, sandbags, bed cradles, wedges, rolls, and splints to support and maintain the vertebral column and extremities in functional alignment.

4. Balance relates to body mechanics and is achieved through a wide base of support and a lowered center of gravity.

8. 1. This goal is not measurable as stated. Understanding is not measurable unless parameters are identified.
2. This statement is a nursing intervention, not a client goal.
3. **This is a client-centered goal that is specific and measurable and has a time frame.**
4. This statement is a nursing goal, not a client goal.

9. 1. Adduction occurs when an arm or leg moves toward or beyond the midline of the body (or both).
2. Supination occurs when the hand and forearm rotate so that the palm of the hand is facing upward.
3. **Dorsal flexion (dorsiflexion) of the joint of the ankle occurs when the toes of the foot point upward and backward toward the anterior portion of the lower leg.**
4. There is no range of motion called plantar extension. Plantar flexion occurs when the joint of the ankle is in extension by pointing the toes of the foot downward and away from the anterior portion of the lower leg.

10. 1. In the low-Fowler position, the hips are slightly flexed.
2. **While in the high-Fowler position, the client is then positioned leaning forward with the arms resting on an over-bed table (orthopneic position). In the orthopneic position, the hips are extensively flexed, creating an angle of less than 90 degrees.**
3. In the supine position, the hips are extended (180 degrees), not flexed.
4. In the Sims position, the hip and the knee of the upper leg are just slightly flexed.

11. 1. Heat lamp treatments will further dry out the wound and can cause burns.
2. Topical antibiotics are used only when the ulcer is infected, not to treat eschar.

3. Cleansing irrigations are ineffective in removing the thick, fibrin-containing cells of eschar covering the surface of the wound.
4. **Thick, leatherlike, necrotic, devitalized tissue (eschar) must be removed surgically or enzymatically before wound healing can occur.**

12. 1. **The shoulder, a ball-and-socket joint, flexes by raising the arm from a position by the side of the body forward and upward to a position beside the head.**
2. Supination occurs when the hand and forearm rotate so that the palm of the hand is facing upward.
3. Opposition is the touching of the thumb of the hand to each fingertip of the same hand.
4. Hyperextension of the arm occurs by moving an arm from a resting position at the side of the body to a position behind the body.

13. 1. In the prone position, there is pressure in front of, not behind, the knees.
2. In the supine position, the hips and legs are extended, which does not exert pressure on the popliteal spaces.
3. **In the contour position, the head of the bed and the knee gatch are slightly elevated. The elevated knee gatch puts pressure on the popliteal spaces.**
4. In the Trendelenburg position, the hips and knees are extended, which does not exert pressure on the popliteal spaces.

14. 1. Clients who are incontinent are not necessarily immobile.
2. **Quadriplegia, paralysis of all four extremities, places the client at highest risk for pressure ulcers because the client has no ability to shift body weight off of bony prominences or change position without total assistance.**
3. Hemiparesis, muscle weakness on one side of the body, does not prevent a person from shifting or changing position to relieve pressure on the skin.
4. Confused clients can move independently when uncomfortable or when encouraged and assisted to move by the nurse.

15. 1. A person who chooses not to ambulate still has the ability to assume many different sitting or lying-down positions.
2. The occurrence of panic attacks is not the most common consequence. Anxiety and

ultimately panic that is precipitated by a situation can be prevented by avoiding the situation.

3. A person who chooses not to ambulate because of a fear of falling still can socialize.

4. Most falls occur when ambulating. Fear of falling results in the conscious choice not to place oneself in a position where a fall can occur. Disuse and muscle wasting cause a reduction of muscle strength at the rate of 5% to 10% per week, so that within 2 months of immobility more than 50% of a muscle's strength can be lost. In addition, there is a decreased cardiac reserve. These responses result in decreased physical conditioning.

16. **1. Assessing posture will identify whether the client's center of gravity is in the midline from the middle of the forehead to a midpoint between the feet and therefore balanced within the client's base of support.**

2. Strength has more to do with the exertion of power, not balance.

3. Energy has more to do with endurance, not balance.

4. Assessing the respiratory rate before activity establishes a baseline against which to compare the respiratory rate after activity to determine tolerance for activity, not balance.

17. 1. Ventilated heel protectors protect only the heels, not the other dependent areas of the body.

2. Air-filled rings usually are made of plastic, which tends to promote sweating. Air rings rarely are used because they are designed for just the sacral area, and often they increase, not decrease, pressure.

3. Air mattresses usually are made of plastic, which tends to promote sweating.

4. The soft tuffs of sheepskin allow air to circulate, thereby promoting the evaporation of moisture that can precipitate skin breakdown.

18. **1. The state of balance between muscles that serve to contract in opposite directions is impaired with immobility. The fibers of the stronger muscles contract for longer periods than do those of the weaker, opposing muscles. This results in a change in the loose connective tissue to a denser**

connective tissue and to fibrotic changes that limit range of motion.

2. Contractures occur because of muscle spasticity and shortening, not muscle flaccidity.

3. Disuse and muscle wasting cause a reduction in muscle strength at the rate of 5% to 10% a week, so that within 2 months more than 50% of a muscle's strength can be lost. This results in muscle atrophy, not contractures.

4. Muscle catabolism exceeding muscle anabolism is unrelated to contractures. In unused muscles, catabolism exceeds anabolism, and the muscles decrease in size (disuse atrophy).

19. **1. Pronation of the hand occurs by rotating the hand and arm so that the palm of the hand is facing down toward the floor.**

2. Lateral flexion of the hand occurs with both abduction (radial flexion) and adduction (ulnar flexion). With the hand supinated, radial flexion occurs by bending the wrist laterally toward the thumb, and ulnar flexion occurs by bending the wrist laterally toward the fifth finger.

3. Circumduction, associated with a ball-and-socket joint, occurs when an extended extremity moves forward, up, back, and down in a full circle.

4. External rotation is associated with ball-and-socket joints. External rotation of a shoulder occurs when the upper arm is held parallel to the floor, the elbow is at a 90-degree angle, the fingers are pointing toward the floor, and the person moves the arm upward so that the fingers point toward the ceiling. External rotation of the hip occurs when a leg in extension is turned so that the foot points outward from the midline of the body.

20. 1. Deep breathing prevents atelectasis and hypostatic pneumonia, not pressure ulcers, which this question is about.

2. Range-of-motion exercises help prevent contractures, not pressure ulcers.

3. Although sheepskin reduces friction and limits pressure, its main purpose is to allow air to circulate under the client to minimize moisture and maceration of skin.

4. Turning a client relieves pressure on the capillary beds of the dependent areas of the body, particularly the skin overlying bony prominences, which

reestablishes blood flow to the area. When pressure on a capillary exceeds 15 to 32 mm Hg, its lumen is occluded, depriving oxygen from local body cells.

21. 1. Placing a trochanter roll under the small of the back is unsafe. A trochanter roll placed in the small of the back is uncomfortable and produces an excessive lumbar curvature.
    2. Placing a trochanter roll behind the knees when supine is contraindicated because it places unnecessary pressure on the popliteal area.
    3. **A trochanter roll is a rolled wedge, pillow, or sandbag placed by the lateral aspect of the leg extending from the iliac crest to the knee to prevent external hip rotation.**
    4. The diameter of a trochanter roll is too wide to maintain the hand in functional alignment.

22. 1. **Nonblanchable erythema refers to redness of intact skin that persists when finger pressure is applied. This is the classic sign of a stage I pressure ulcer.**
    2. Circumoral cyanosis (slightly bluish, grayish, slatelike, or dark purple discoloration of the skin around the mouth) is an indication of hypoxia, not pressure ulcers.
    3. With necrosis, death of cells has occurred. Necrosis occurs in stage III and stage IV pressure ulcers.
    4. With an abrasion, the superficial layers of the skin are scraped away. This stage II, not stage I, pressure ulcer appears reddened and may exhibit localized serous weeping or bleeding.

23. 1. The 30-degree lateral position is the preferred position to prevent pressure ulcers because it limits body weight directly over bony prominences, versus other positions.
    2. **In the side-lying position, the majority of the body weight is borne by the greater trochanter. The bone is close to the surface of the skin, with minimal overlying protective tissue.**
    3. In the supine position, the occiput, scapulae, spine, elbows, sacrum, and heels are at risk for pressure; however, the body weight is distributed more evenly than in some other positions.
    4. In the prone position, the ears, cheeks, acromion process, anterior-superior spinous process, knees, toes, male genitalia, and female breasts are at risk for pressure;

however, the body weight is distributed more evenly than in some other positions.

24. 1. Top sheets tucked in along the sides of the bed still exert pressure on the upper surface of the feet, which may promote plantar flexion. The sides of top sheets, mitered at the foot of the bed, hang freely off the side of the bed.
    2. **Making a vertical or horizontal toe pleat in the linen at the foot of the bed over the client's feet leaves room for the feet to move freely and avoids exerting pressure on the upper surface of the feet, thus minimizing plantar flexion.**
    3. The weight of the top sheets still exerts pressure on the upper surface of the feet, promoting plantar flexion.
    4. Although the use of a bed cradle will hold the linen off the legs and feet of the client, it is not the easiest way for the nurse to prevent plantar flexion of the options presented.

25. 1. In a stage I pressure ulcer, the skin is still intact and manifests clinically as reactive hyperemia.
    2. **In a stage II pressure ulcer, the partial-thickness skin loss manifests clinically as an abrasion, blister, or shallow crater.**
    3. In a stage III pressure ulcer, there is full-thickness skin loss involving the subcutaneous tissue that may extend to the underlying fascia. The ulcer manifests clinically as a deep crater with or without undermining.
    4. In a stage IV pressure ulcer, there is full-thickness skin loss with extensive destruction, tissue necrosis, or damage to muscle, bone, or supporting structures.

26. 1. The bed should be higher, not lower, than the wheelchair so that gravity can facilitate the transfer.
    2. Applying pressure under the client's axillae areas when standing up should be avoided because it can injure local nerves and blood vessels.
    3. **Encouraging the client to be as self-sufficient as possible ensures that the transfer is conducted at the client's pace, promotes self-esteem, and decreases the physical effort expended by the nurse.**
    4. Keeping the client's feet within 6 inches of each other will provide a narrow base of support and is unsafe.

27. 1. Sitting in the high-Fowler position and leaning forward (orthopneic position) allow the abdominal organs to drop by gravity, which promotes contraction of the diaphragm. The arms resting on an over-bed table increase thoracic excursion. This position promotes breathing.
2. The hips will be in extreme flexion, not extension.
3. Pressure ulcers can still occur on the ischial tuberosities.
4. Standing (for men) and sitting on a toilet/commode (for women) are superior to any position for promoting urinary elimination.

28. 1. Although turning the client to a new position every 2 hours provides variety and increased comfort, these are not the primary reasons for this intervention.
2. Although turning frequently promotes elimination, the upright positions, such as high-Fowler and sitting, have a greater influence on elimination because of the effect of gravity.
3. **Compression of soft tissue greater than 15 to 32 mm Hg interferes with capillary circulation and compromises tissue oxygenation in the compressed area. Turning the client relieves the compression of tissue in dependent areas, particularly those tissues overlying bony prominences.**
4. Although turning and positioning promote respiratory functioning, other interventions, such as sitting, deep breathing, coughing, and incentive spirometry, have a greater influence on respiratory status.

29. 1. Nurses should use the longer, stronger muscles of the thighs and buttocks when moving clients to protect their weaker back and arm muscles.
2. Nurses should have a wide base of support when moving clients to provide better stability.
3. Nurses should use a pulling motion to turn clients because the muscles that flex, rather than extend, the arm are stronger, and pulling, rather than pushing, creates less friction and therefore less effort.
4. **Twisting (rotation) of the thoracolumbar spine and flexion of the back place the line of gravity outside the base of support, which can cause muscle strain and disabling injuries. Misaligning the back when moving clients**

occurs most often when not facing the direction of the move.

30. 1. Prolonged pressure on skin over a bony prominence interferes with capillary blood flow to the skin, which ultimately can result in a pressure ulcer. A pressure ulcer is a localized, not systemic, response to immobility.
2. **Decreased calf muscle activity and pressure of the bed on the legs allow blood to accumulate in the distal veins. The resulting increased hydrostatic pressure moves fluid out of the intravascular compartment and into the interstitial compartment, causing edema. Dependent edema is a systemic response to immobility.**
3. **Static respiratory secretions provide an excellent media for bacterial growth that can result in hypostatic pneumonia, which is a systemic response to immobility.**
4. Plantar flexion contracture (footdrop) is a localized response to prolonged extension of the ankle.
5. **An increased cardiac workload results from a decrease in vessel resistance and redistribution of blood in the body, with blood pooling in the lower extremities. These are systemic responses to immobility.**

31. 1. Eversion, a gliding movement of the foot, occurs by turning the sole of the foot away from the midline of the body.
2. Circumduction is a range of motion that is performed with a ball-and-socket joint. It occurs when an extended extremity moves forward, up, back, and down in a full circle.
3. Plantar flexion occurs when the joint of the ankle is in extension by pointing the toes of the foot downward and away from the anterior portion of the lower leg.
4. **External rotation occurs when the entire leg is rolled outward from the body so that the toes point away from the opposite leg.**

32. 1. This excessive flexion can result in contractures of the hip and knee. The left leg should be slightly flexed or extended.
2. The right leg should be supported on a pillow in front of the left leg.
3. The ankles should be maintained at 90 degrees.

4. **Maintaining alignment of the shoulders and hips avoids stress and strain on the bones, muscles, and joints.**

5. **In the left-lateral (side-lying) position, the left arm is positioned in front of the body with the shoulder pulled forward (protracted). This position reduces pressure on the joint in the shoulder and acromial process.**

33. 1. **In the left-Sims position, the client's right arm and leg are supported on pillows to prevent internal rotation of the shoulder and hip.**

    2. The right arm is positioned in front of, not behind, the back.

    3. The right hand is positioned in pronation, not supination.

    4. The right arm is positioned to maintain the shoulder in functional alignment, not internal rotation.

    5. The right arm should be flexed slightly at the elbow; this supports comfort and functional alignment.

34. 1. **Joint pain may prevent the client from moving about, leading to contractures that result in impaired mobility.**

    2. Exertional fatigue is associated with activity intolerance. People who are fatigued are still able to move.

    3. People who are sedentary are still able to move.

    4. **Limited range of motion is associated with contracture formation and impaired mobility.**

    5. An increased respiratory rate is a response to activity, not impaired mobility.

35. 1. The client may fall if the bed is lowered while the client is sitting on the side of the bed. Although lowering the height of the bed closer to the floor should be done, it is not the first thing that the nurse should do in this scenario.

    2. **The client should be repositioned back in bed. The height of the bed from the floor is in the highest position and must be lowered before the client can be transferred out of bed. It is unsafe to lower the height of the bed while the client is sitting on the side of the bed. The client should exit from the left side of the bed, leading with the strong left arm and leg.**

    3. Repositioning the wheelchair is not the first thing that the nurse should do. Also,

the wheelchair should be positioned at the head of the left side of the bed.

    4. Putting on the client's slippers is not the first thing the nurse should do in this scenario. Once the client is returned to bed, slippers can be placed on the client's feet, and then the client can be transferred.

36. 1. The unaffected leg should be advanced first because the weight of the body is supported by the leg with the greatest strength.

    2. With the tip of the cane placed 6 inches lateral to the foot, the handle should be at the level of the client's greater trochanter to ensure that the elbow will be flexed 15 to 30 degrees when using the cane.

    3. **A cane is a hand-gripped assistive device; therefore, the hand opposite the hemiparesis should hold the cane. Exercises can strengthen the flexor and extensor muscles of the arms and the muscles that dorsiflex the wrist.**

    4. This action will cause flexion of the neck, hips, or waist that will move the center of gravity outside the base of support. Body alignment is essential for balance, stability, and safe ambulation.

    5. Leaning over onto the cane should be avoided. The client should distribute weight between the feet and the cane while standing in an upright posture. This is the most stable position when using a cane.

37. 1. **Muscle strain is reduced when clients are moved by using gravity, not with the added effort needed to move clients against gravity.**

    2. **Keeping the upper and lower body in alignment decreases strain on the sacrospinal muscles and intervertebral disks.**

    3. **To exert an upward lift, the gluteal and leg muscles should be used, rather than the sacrospinal muscles of the back. The gluteal and leg muscles are larger than the sacrospinal muscles and therefore fatigue less quickly, and their use protects the intervertebral disks.**

    4. **The muscles of the legs are most efficient when the knees and hips are slightly bent. This reduces strain on the muscles being used.**

    5. **Positioning the bed at waist height avoids the need to reach and stretch,**

which may strain a caregiver's muscles, bones, joints, tendons, or ligaments.

38. 1. **Being as close as possible to the chair allows a person to use the chair for support when sitting. Also, it supports sitting deeper into the seat of the chair, which is safer than sitting on the edge of the seat.**
    2. **Holding the hand bars of both crutches with the left hand frees the right hand for the next step in the procedure.**
    4. **Grasping the arm of the chair with the right hand allows the person to support body weight partially on the right arm and the right leg.**
    3. **Leaning forward slightly and flexing the knees and hips partially lowers the body and prepares it for the next step in the procedure.**
    5. **Lowering the body slowly into the chair protects the body from injury.**

39. 1. **When in the sitting position, the hips and knees are flexed at 90 degrees and the body's weight is borne by the pelvis, particularly the ischial tuberosities, which are bony protuberances of the lower portion of the ischium. Using a wheelchair results in prolonged sitting unless interventions are implemented to promote local circulation.**
    2. **Pressure to the scapulae occurs when in a sitting position as well as when in the supine and Fowler positions.**
    3. Pressure to a trochanter occurs in a side-lying, not the sitting, position.
    4. Pressure to the lateral malleolus of an ankle occurs in a side-lying, not a sitting, position.
    5. **Pressure to the sacrum occurs when in a sitting position, as well as when in the supine and Fowler positions.**

40. 1. **Applying gentle pressure against the client's knees while lowering the client into the chair facilitates an upright sitting position in a chair.**
    2. Moving clients with a mechanical lift is within the scope of nursing practice, and a primary health-care provider's prescription is unnecessary.
    3. **The longer straps/chains go in the holes for the seat support, which keep the legs and pelvis below the upper body. Appropriate placement of the upper and lower straps/chains creates a**

bucket seat in which a client is moved safely.
    4. Placing a sheepskin inside the sling so that it is under the client may result in the client's sliding down and out of the sling during the transfer. Nylon, net, or canvas slings are available.
    5. It does not matter whether the feet or the head exit the bed first as long as functional alignment and safety are maintained.

41. 1. **Advancing the unaffected leg last by itself allows weight to be borne by the affected leg while both arms are supported on the walker.**
    2. Six, not 12, inches is the proper distance to advance a walker. Twelve inches will require the client to reach too far forward, moving beyond a stable center of gravity.
    3. **Advancing the walker and the affected leg together ensures that weight is borne by the unaffected leg.**
    4. Adjusting the height of the walker so that it is equal with the hip joint is too low and will require the client to stoop to reach the hand bar. The hand bar should be at a height just below the client's waist, allowing the elbows to be slightly flexed. A walker that is the correct height allows a client to assume a more functional posture.
    5. A standard walker does not have wheels. Directing a person to advance a walker a comfortable distance is unsafe. The word "comfortable" is subjective and unclear. Walkers should be advanced 6 inches at a time to ensure that a person's weight does not extend beyond the center of gravity.

42. 2. **Assessing vital signs is the first step in the procedure because results provide baseline data against which to compare outcomes when evaluating activity tolerance.**
    4. **Elevating the head of the bed is the second step in the procedure. It minimizes the effort required by the client to move to a sitting position in the bed as well as minimizes lifting by the nurse. Footwear protects the client's feet from physical injury and contamination from pathogens that may be on the floor.**
    3. **Assisting the client to a sitting position on the side of the bed, with the client's feet on the floor, facilitates pivoting of the trunk of the body perpendicular to the length of the bed. This prepares**

the body eventually to assume a wide base of support, with the greatest mass between the feet.

1. **Verifying if the client feels dizzy evaluates tolerance to the activity and is the fourth step in the transfer procedure. Dizziness indicates orthostatic hypotension. If dizziness occurs, the nurse should support the client in the sitting position for a few minutes. If dizziness does not resolve, then return the client to a semi-Fowler position to provide for the safety of the client.**

5. **Supporting the client in the sitting position for several minutes before transferring to a chair is the fifth step in the transfer procedure. This reduces the possibility of orthostatic hypotension and allows more time for an evaluation of the client's response to the change in position.**

43. 1. **Alignment reduces the risk of lumbar vertebrae and muscle group injury resulting from torquing (twisting).**
    2. **Positioning oneself close to the client keeps the client closer to your center of gravity. Increased stability reduces strain on back muscles.**
    3. **Keeping knees and hips slightly flexed facilitates using the large muscles of the legs, rather than the back, to move the client.**
    4. **Multiple caregivers share the load of moving a client safely.**
    5. Feet should be positioned wide apart, not close together, to provide a wide base of support, which increases stability.

44. 1. **Compression of small vessels in the legs is one of the three factors that make up Virchow's triad. Immobility leads to vessel compression, which can cause injury to small vessels.**
    2. Orthostatic hypotension is not one of the three factors that make up Virchow's

triad. Orthostatic hypotension occurs when prolonged inactivity deactivates the baroreceptors associated with constriction and distention of blood vessels. When one is changing position, there is a decrease in venous return, followed by a decrease in cardiac output and a decline in blood pressure. It may take several seconds to several minutes for the blood pressure to respond to the change in position.

3. **Coagulation activation is one of the three factors that make up Virchow's triad. As a result of venous pooling, there is a decreased clearance of coagulation factors, resulting in activation of clotting (i.e., the blood clots faster).**

4. Hypostatic pneumonia is not one of the three factors that make up Virchow's triad. Hypostatic pneumonia is an inflammation of the lung as a result of stasis of respiratory secretions.

5. **Venous stasis is one of the three factors that make up Virchow's triad. Inactive skeletal muscles of the legs do not adequately compress the peripheral vessels in the legs and therefore do not assist with the return of blood back to the heart; this results in stasis of blood in the lower extremities.**

45. 1. Greater trochanters are at risk when a client is in the side-lying position.
    2. **Ischial tuberosities are at greatest risk when a client is in the orthopneic or mid- to high-Fowler positions because the greatest weight of the body is exerted against the genital, perianal, and sacral areas of the body.**
    3. A lateral malleolus is at risk when a client is in a side-lying position.
    4. Spinal processes are at risk when a client is in the supine position or a Fowler position.

Nutrition

KEYWORDS

The following words include nursing/medical terminology, concepts, principles, and information relevant to content specifically addressed in the chapter or associated with topics presented in it. English dictionaries, nursing textbooks, and medical dictionaries, such as *Taber's Cyclopedic Medical Dictionary*, are resources that can be used to expand your knowledge and understanding of these words and related information.

Amino acids:
  Essential
  Nonessential
Basal metabolic rate
Calorie, kilocalorie
Calorie count
Cellular metabolism:
  Anabolism
  Catabolism
Fiber:
  Insoluble
  Soluble
Food consistency:
  Chopped
  Liquid
  Pureed
  Regular
  Soft
Ideal body weight
Laboratory values:
  Blood urea nitrogen
  Serum albumin
  Total cholesterol
  Transferrin level
  Triglycerides
Malnutrition
MyPlate
Nausea
Nutrients:
  Carbohydrates
  Fats
  Minerals:
    Fluoride
    Iodine
    Iron
    Potassium
    Sodium
  Protein:
    Complete
    Incomplete
  Water

Obesity
Recommended dietary allowances
Stomatitis
Therapeutic diets:
  2-g sodium
  Clear liquid
  Full liquid
  Low residue
  Mechanical soft
  Protein restricted
Tube feedings:
  Continuous
  Gastrostomy
  Intermittent
  Jejunostomy
  Nasogastric
Underweight
Vegetarian:
  Flexitarian
  Lactovegetarian
  Ovolactovegetarian
  Vegan
Vitamins:
  Fat soluble:
    A
    D
    E
    K
  Water soluble:
    B_1 (thiamine)
    B_2 (riboflavin)
    B_3 (niacin)
    B_6 (pyridoxine)
    B_{12} (cobalamin)
    Biotin
    C (ascorbic acid)
    Folic acid
    Pantothenic acid
Vomiting

NUTRITION: QUESTIONS

1. A client is admitted to the hospital with a history of liver dysfunction associated with hepatitis. With which metabolic problem does the nurse anticipate that this client may have a problem?
1. Emulsifying fats
2. Digesting carbohydrates
3. Manufacturing red blood cells
4. Reabsorbing water in the intestines

2. A nurse is assessing a client who is admitted to the hospital with withdrawal from alcohol. Which effect of alcohol on the body will influence the client's plan of care?
1. Interferes with the absorption of glucose
2. Accelerates the absorption of medications
3. Decreases the absorption of many important nutrients
4. Lengthens passage time of stool through the intestinal tract

3. An obese client of a nursing home who is receiving a 1,500-calorie weight reduction diet has not lost weight in the past 2 weeks. Which should the nurse do **first**?
1. Inform the primary health-care provider of the client's lack of progress.
2. Instruct the client to limit intake to 1,000 calories per day.
3. Schedule a multidisciplinary team conference.
4. Keep a log of the oral intake for 3 days.

4. A nurse is screening clients who are in various age groups for clinical manifestation of eating disorders. In which age group should the nurse expect more problems to become evident?
1. Toddlerhood
2. Adolescence
3. Senescence
4. Infancy

5. A client is diagnosed with a vitamin A deficiency. The client loves pie for dessert. Which type of pie should the nurse encourage the client to ingest?
1. Blueberry
2. Pumpkin
3. Cherry
4. Pecan

6. A client is anorexic because of stomatitis related to chemotherapy. Which should the nurse be **most** concerned about when planning care for this client?
1. Aspiration
2. Dehydration
3. Malnutrition
4. Constipation

7. A nurse is counseling a client with the diagnosis of osteoporosis. In addition to calcium, which vitamin supplement should the nurse anticipate that the primary health-care provider will prescribe for this client?
1. B
2. K
3. D
4. E

8. An older adult is admitted to the hospital for multiple health problems. Assessment reveals that the client has no teeth and is having difficulty eating. Which diet should the nurse encourage the primary health-care provider to prescribe for this client?
   1. Liquid supplements
   2. Mechanical soft
   3. Pureed
   4. Soft

9. A nurse is caring for clients with a variety of nutrition-related problems. Which problem should the nurse anticipate eventually may require a client to have a feeding tube inserted?
   1. Malabsorption syndrome
   2. Difficulty swallowing
   3. Stomatitis
   4. Vomiting

10. A nurse is caring for a client who is confused and disoriented. Which type of food containing chicken is **most** appropriate for this client?
    1. Soup
    2. Salad
    3. Fingers
    4. Casserole

11. An older adult tends to bruise easily, and the primary health-care provider recommends that the client eat foods high in vitamin K. In addition to teaching the client about food sources of vitamin K, the nurse should include nutrients that must be ingested for vitamin K to be absorbed. Which foods that increase the absorption of vitamin K should be included in the teaching plan?
    1. Carbohydrates
    2. Starches
    3. Proteins
    4. Fats

12. A school nurse is preparing a health class about vitamins. Which information about vitamins that is based on a scientific principle should the nurse include?
    1. Eating a variety of foods prevents the need for supplements.
    2. Megadoses of vitamins have proved to be most effective in preventing illness.
    3. Taking a prescribed vitamin supplement is the best way to ensure adequate intake.
    4. Vitamins that are more expensive are purer than those that are less expensive.

13. A client without any identified current health problems is having a yearly physical examination. The laboratory results indicate the presence of ketosis. Which rationale explains the presence of ketosis in this otherwise healthy adult?
    1. Inadequate intake of carbohydrates
    2. Increased intake of protein
    3. Excessive intake of starch
    4. Decreased intake of fiber

14. Which vitamin that does not require fat in the diet to be absorbed should a nurse teach a client about?
    1. Vitamin C
    2. Vitamin A
    3. Vitamin E
    4. Vitamin D

15. An occupational nurse is facilitating a group discussion on weight reduction. Which should the nurse explain is the **most** common contributing factor to obesity?
    1. Sedentary lifestyle
    2. Low metabolic rate
    3. Hormonal imbalance
    4. Excessive caloric intake

16. A nurse is evaluating the effectiveness of a nutritional program for a client with anemia. For which clinical finding should the nurse monitor the client because it is a short-term indicator of an improved nutritional status?
1. Weight gain of two pounds daily
2. Increasing transferrin level
3. Decreasing serum albumin
4. Appropriate skin turgor

17. A client is diagnosed with iron-deficiency anemia. Which major cause of iron deficiency will influence a focused assessment by the nurse?
1. Metabolic problems
2. Inadequate diets
3. Malabsorption
4. Hemorrhage

18. A primary health-care provider identifies that a client may have a fluoride deficiency. Which physical characteristic identified by the nurse **supports** this conclusion?
1. Stomatitis
2. Dental caries
3. Bleeding gums
4. Mottling of the teeth

19. A nurse identifies that a vegetarian understands the importance of eating kidney beans when the client indicates that they are essential because they contain which nutrient?
1. Carbohydrates
2. Minerals
3. Protein
4. Fat

20. Which is the **most** common independent nursing intervention to help a debilitated older adult maintain body weight while in the hospital?
1. Making mealtime a social activity
2. Taking a thorough nutritional history
3. Providing assistance with the intake of meals
4. Encouraging dietary supplements between meals

21. Which total cholesterol level in a healthy adult female client necessitates that the client receives health teaching about a low-cholesterol diet?
1. 210 mg/dL
2. 190 mg/dL
3. 150 mg/dL
4. 120 mg/dL

22. A nurse is caring for a client who is expending energy that is greater than the client's caloric intake. For which human response should the nurse monitor the client?
1. Fever
2. Anorexia
3. Malnutrition
4. Hypertension

23. A nurse is reviewing the laboratory findings of a client to assess the client's nutritional status. Which laboratory result from among the following tests is an indicator of inadequate protein intake?
1. High hemoglobin
2. Low serum albumin
3. Low specific gravity
4. High blood urea nitrogen

24. A woman who is advised to follow a low-fat diet frequently eats in Chinese restaurants. Which of the following foods should the nurse teach the woman is lowest in fat?
    1. Egg rolls
    2. Spareribs
    3. Crispy noodles
    4. Hot and sour soup

25. A nurse is teaching a client about the importance of balancing protein, carbohydrates, and fats in the diet. The nurse identifies that the teaching was successful. Which of the following did the client indicate is provided by carbohydrates?
    1. Electrolytes
    2. Vitamins
    3. Minerals
    4. Energy

26. A client has been blind in one eye for several years because of the complications associated with diabetes mellitus. The client is admitted to the hospital with a detached retina and resulting loss of sight in the other eye. Which should the nurse do to assist this client with meals?
    1. Explain to the client where items are located on the plate according to the hours of a clock.
    2. Encourage eating one food at a time according to the preference of the client.
    3. Order finger foods that are permitted on the client's diet.
    4. Feed the client the prescribed meals.

27. Which is unrelated to the balance of calcium in the body?
    1. Osteoporosis
    2. Vitamin D
    3. Tetany
    4. Iron

28. A nurse is caring for a client receiving bolus enteral feedings several times daily. Which nursing intervention is **most** important to help prevent diarrhea?
    1. Flush the tube after every feeding.
    2. Check the residual before each feeding.
    3. Elevate the head of the bed 30 degrees continuously.
    4. Discard the refrigerated opened cans of formula after 24 hours.

29. A nurse teaches a client about the prescribed low-fat diet. Which food selected by the client indicates that the teaching was understood? **Select all that apply.**
    1. _____ Eggs
    2. _____ Liver
    3. _____ Cheese
    4. _____ Turkey
    5. _____ Scallops
    6. _____ Flounder

30. A client has a high serum cholesterol level. Which of the following should the nurse teach the client to **avoid**? **Select all that apply.**
    1. _____ Liver
    2. _____ Shrimp
    3. _____ Skim milk
    4. _____ Turkey burger
    5. _____ Sliced bologna

31. A primary health-care provider prescribes folic acid 0.8 mg PO once daily for a client with anemia. Unit-dose tablets of 0.4 mg/tablet are available. How many tablets should the nurse administer? **Record your answer using a whole number.**

    Answer: _____ tablets.

32. A client has a decreased hemoglobin level because of a low intake of dietary iron. Which food that is an excellent source of iron should the nurse include when teaching the client? **Select all that apply.**
    1. _____ Eggs
    2. _____ Fruit
    3. _____ Meat
    4. _____ Bread
    5. _____ Spinach

33. A primary health-care provider prescribes a low-residue diet for a client with inflammatory bowel disease. Which of the following should the nurse teach the client to include in the diet? **Select all that apply.**
    1. _____ Scrambled eggs
    2. _____ Cooked oatmeal
    3. _____ Orange juice
    4. _____ Green beans
    5. _____ Rye bread

34. A client is admitted to the hospital with a diagnosis of alcoholism. The primary health-care provider prescribes thiamine hydrochloride (vitamin B_1) 50 mg IM three times a day. The drug is supplied 100 mg/mL. Indicate on the syringe the line to which the nurse should fill the syringe to administer the prescribed dose.

35. A client has multiple fractures from a skiing accident. To **best** facilitate bone growth, the nurse should encourage the client to eat more foods high in calcium. Which food selected by the client indicates an understanding of those that are high in calcium? **Select all that apply.**
    1. _____ Orange juice
    2. _____ Peanut butter
    3. _____ Cottage cheese
    4. _____ Baked flounder
    5. _____ Low-fat yogurt
    6. _____ Cooked spinach

36. A nurse is obtaining a health history from a client. Which of the following reflects healthy behaviors? **Select all that apply.**
    1. _____ Increasing fruits and vegetables to 50% of food intake
    2. _____ Substituting fish for meat in the diet
    3. _____ Wanting to lose 20 pounds
    4. _____ Consuming 4 eggs a week
    5. _____ Eating foods low in fat

37. A nurse is caring for a postoperative client. The nurse reviews the client's concurrent health problems, checks the medications prescribed by the primary health-care provider, and performs a focused assessment. Which should the nurse do at 12 p.m.?
    1. Administer 5 units of regular insulin subcutaneously to the client.
    2. Notify the primary health-care provider of the client's status.
    3. Give the oral solution of 15 mg of oxycodone.
    4. Provide an additional dose of ipratropium.

CLIENT'S CLINICAL RECORD

Concurrent Health Problems
Diabetes mellitus for 10 years
Obstructive lung disease (COPD) for 6 years

Prescribed Medications
Ipratropium 17 mcg aerosol inhaler, 2 inhalations four times a day
Oxycodone oral solution 15 mg PO every 6 hours whenever necessary
NPH insulin 20 units subcutaneously 8 a.m.
Regular insulin 8 units subcutaneously 8 a.m.
Regular insulin coverage subcutaneously before meals and at hour of sleep
   <150 mg/dL to 0 units
   151–200 mg/dL to 3 units
   201–250 mg/dL to 5 units
   251–300 mg/dL to 7 units
   301–350 mg/dL to 9 units
   >351: Call provider

Physical Assessment
11:50 a.m.: Breath sounds indicate slight wheezing over right sternal border
Respirations: 22 breaths per minute, unlabored
Serum glucose finger stick: 235 mg/dL
Incisional pain of 3 on pain scale of 0 to 10v

---

38. A primary health-care provider prescribes a clear liquid diet for a client. Which of the following should the nurse teach the client to **avoid** when following this diet? **Select all that apply.**
    1. _____ Strawberry gelatin
    2. _____ Decaffeinated tea
    3. _____ Strong coffee
    4. _____ Pureed soup
    5. _____ Ice cream

39. A nurse teaches a postoperative client about foods high in protein that will promote wound healing. Which food selection by the client indicates that the teaching was effective? **Select all that apply.**
    1. _____ Milk
    2. _____ Meat
    3. _____ Fruit
    4. _____ Bread
    5. _____ Vegetables

40. A nurse must obtain the serum glucose level of a client with diabetes mellitus. The nurse completes all the initial preparations for the procedure, including verifying the prescription, identifying the client, and washing the hands. Place the following steps in the order in which they should be performed.

1. Don clean gloves.
2. Wipe away the first drop with sterile gauze.
3. Hold the client's finger in a dependent position.
4. Drop the second drop of blood on the reagent strip.
5. Puncture the side of the end of a finger with a sterile lancet.
6. Wipe the intended puncture site with an approved antiseptic.

Answer: _____

41. A client is scheduled for surgery, and the nurse is teaching the client about the importance of vitamin C in wound healing. Which source of vitamin C should the nurse include in the teaching plan? **Select all that apply.**

1. _____ Potatoes
2. _____ Papayas
3. _____ Yogurt
4. _____ Beans
5. _____ Milk

42. A nurse is administering enteral nutrition via the method depicted in the photograph. Which of the following steps should be implemented when administering enteral nutrition via this method? **Select all that apply.**

1. _____ Administer water after the feeding.
2. _____ Administer the bolus over 60 minutes.
3. _____ Ensure that the formula is at room temperature.
4. _____ Elevate the head of the bed 15° above horizontal.
5. _____ Add formula continuously to the syringe just before it empties.

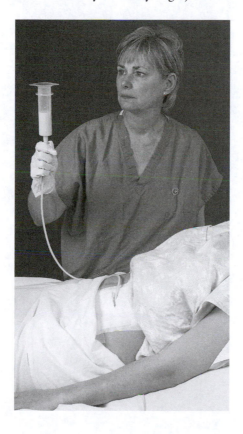

43. A young adult woman tells the nurse that she has been taking St. John's wort for several weeks for depression. Which should the nurse teach the client that is important to know about taking St. John's wort? **Select all that apply.**
    1. _____ It should not be taken without an evaluation by a primary health-care provider.
    2. _____ Use a different method of birth control if taking an oral contraceptive.
    3. _____ Discontinue it if there is no change in symptoms within 3 months.
    4. _____ Stop taking it 2 weeks before surgery with general anesthesia.
    5. _____ Apply sunscreen to skin exposed to the sun.

44. An older adult states that he is experiencing all the signs and symptoms of an enlarged prostate and is interested in taking the herbal supplement saw palmetto. Which is important for the nurse to teach the client about treatment with saw palmetto? **Select all that apply.**
    1. _____ Saw palmetto should be avoided until after an evaluation by a urologist.
    2. _____ Taking saw palmetto generally is considered safe as a dietary supplement.
    3. _____ Saw palmetto interferes with the measurement of prostate-specific antigen.
    4. _____ Some clients report an improvement in erectile dysfunction after taking saw palmetto.
    5. _____ The most recent research by reputable institutions indicates that saw palmetto is more effective than a placebo in reducing the symptoms of an enlarged prostate.

45. A nurse is providing for the nutritional needs of several clients. Which problem increases clients' caloric requirements? **Select all that apply.**
    1. _____ Burns
    2. _____ Nausea
    3. _____ Dysphagia
    4. _____ Pneumonia
    5. _____ Depression

NUTRITION: ANSWERS AND RATIONALES

1. 1. **Bile is produced and concentrated in the liver and stored in the gallbladder. As fat enters the duodenum, it precipitates the release of cholecystokinin, which stimulates the gallbladder to release bile. Bile, an emulsifier, enlarges the surface area of fat particles so that enzymes can digest the fat.**
   2. The liver is not involved with carbohydrate digestion. Ptyalin (secreted by the parotid glands), amylase (secreted by the pancreas), and sucrase, lactase, and maltase (secreted by the walls of the small intestine) digest carbohydrates.
   3. The liver is not involved with red blood cell production. People who are deficient in iron and protein have difficulty with red blood cell production.
   4. The large intestine, not the liver, is involved with reabsorbing water. The majority of the water in chyme is reabsorbed in the first half of the colon, leaving the remainder (approximately 100 mL) to form and eliminate feces.

2. 1. Alcohol interferes with the absorption of thiamine, which is essential to oxidize, not absorb, glucose.
   2. The damaging effects of alcohol decrease, not increase, the efficiency of the process of absorption of medications in the stomach and intestines. However, alcohol can potentiate the action of drugs, such as central nervous system depressants.
   3. **Alcohol interferes with vitamin intake, absorption, metabolism, and excretion. It specifically interferes with the absorption of vitamins A, D, K, thiamine, folic acid, pyridoxine, and B_{12}.**
   4. Alcohol increases intestinal motility so that it decreases, not increases, the length of time it takes intestinal contents to pass through the body.

3. 1. Informing the primary health-care provider of the client's status is premature. The nurse is abdicating the responsibility to help the client.
   2. A change in diet requires a primary health-care provider's prescription. Generally, calories should not be restricted below 1,200 calories/day for women or 1,500 calories/day for men so that they receive adequate amounts of essential nutrients.

   3. Conducting a multidisciplinary team conference may eventually be done, but it is premature at this time.
   4. **When the expected outcome of an intervention is not attained, the situation must be reassessed to determine the problem and the plan changed appropriately. A record of a dietary intake provides objective information about the amounts and types of food consumed. This information provides data about nutrient deficiencies or excesses, eating patterns, behaviors associated with eating, and potential problems and needs.**

4. 1. Although toddlers may experience an eating disorder called failure to thrive, in which they fail to ingest enough nutrients to be adequately nourished, it is not as common as eating disorders in an age group in another option.
   2. **Studies report that 2% to 5% of young women in the United States between 12 and 25 years of age experience either anorexia nervosa (self-imposed dieting leading to starvation) or bulimia (destructive episodic binge eating followed by purging/self-induced vomiting to prevent weight gain). Thirty percent of adolescents in the United States are obese (weight 20% greater than ideal body weight).**
   3. Although older adults have many stressors in relation to nutrition, such as decline in metabolism; difficulty with procuring, cooking, and chewing food; and physiological changes affecting absorption and utilization of nutrients, they are not at as high a risk for eating disorders as members in another age group.
   4. Although infants may experience an eating disorder called failure to thrive, in which they fail to ingest enough nutrients to be adequately nourished, it is not as common as eating disorders as in another age group.

5. 1. One piece of blueberry pie contains only 14 mcg retinol equivalents (RE) of vitamin.
   2. **Pumpkin is an excellent source of vitamin A. One piece (one-sixth of a 9-inch-diameter pie) contains 3,750 mcg RE of vitamin A.**
   3. One piece of cherry pie contains only 70 mcg RE of vitamin A.

4. One piece of pecan pie contains only 115 mcg RE of vitamin A.

6. 1. Although in some clients stomatitis may cause difficulty with swallowing (dysphagia), which may contribute to aspiration, a bland diet soft in consistency will help to minimize dysphagia.
2. Ingesting adequate amounts of fluid generally is not a problem as long as acidic fluids are avoided because they irritate the lesions of the mucous membranes.
3. **Stomatitis, inflammation of the mucous membranes of the oral cavity, can be painful. Clients with stomatitis frequently avoid eating to limit discomfort, which can lead to inadequate nutritional intake and malnutrition.**
4. Although a loss of appetite may contribute to constipation, an increase in fluid intake and activity can help prevent constipation.

7. 1. The B-complex vitamins are related to protein synthesis and cross-linking of collagen fibers, which are essential for integrity of the integumentary system, not strong bones.
2. Vitamin K promotes blood clotting by increasing the synthesis of prothrombin by the liver; it does not promote strong bones.
3. **Vitamin D (also regarded as a hormone) promotes bone mineralization by producing transport proteins that bind calcium and phosphorus, which increases intestinal absorption, stimulates the kidneys to return calcium to the bloodstream, and stimulates bone cells to use calcium and phosphorus to build and maintain bone tissue.**
4. Vitamin E prevents the oxidation of unsaturated fatty acids and thereby prevents cell damage; it does not promote strong bones.

8. 1. A person with few or no teeth should be able to meet all daily nutrient requirements without liquid supplements.
2. **A mechanical soft diet is modified only in texture. It includes moist foods that require minimal chewing and eliminates most raw fruits and vegetables and foods containing seeds, nuts, and dried fruit.**
3. A person with few or no teeth can handle a diet with a more solid consistency than pureed foods. A pureed diet is a soft diet processed to a semisolid consistency.
4. A person with few or no teeth can handle a diet with a more solid consistency than a

soft diet. A soft diet is moderately low in fiber and lightly seasoned. A soft diet usually is prescribed as a transition between liquids and a regular diet for clients who are unable to tolerate a regular diet after surgery.

9. 1. A nasogastric feeding (enteral feeding) enters the stomach and is not an appropriate therapy for a client with malabsorption syndrome. The formula would still have to be absorbed by the gastrointestinal tract.
2. **If a client with difficulty swallowing (dysphagia) does not respond to a dysphagia diet (mechanical soft, soft, blended, or pureed liquids), there may be a need for the insertion of a gastrostomy tube. Gastrostomy feedings can be administered to meet nutritional needs and minimize the risk of aspiration.**
3. Nasogastric feedings are a drastic measure for stomatitis. Stomatitis, an inflammation of the mouth, usually is a temporary problem that responds to pharmacological therapy and frequent, appropriate oral hygiene.
4. Nasogastric feedings are contraindicated in the presence of vomiting because of the potential for aspiration. The cause of the vomiting should be identified and treated.

10. 1. A confused and disoriented client may not know how to manipulate a spoon to eat soup. This may result in spilling and frustration.
2. Eating chicken salad requires the use of a utensil, which may be beyond the cognitive ability of a client who is confused and disoriented.
3. **Chicken fingers are a single food item that usually is familiar to most people in the United States. A single familiar food is an easier symbol to decode cognitively than food mixed together in one dish. Food that can be held with the fingers, rather than using a utensil, promotes independence for a client who is confused and disoriented.**
4. Eating a casserole requires the use of a utensil, which may be beyond the client's cognitive ability. In addition, for a client who is confused and disoriented, food mixed together is more confusing than food that is presented individually.

11. 1. Carbohydrates are not necessary for the absorption of vitamin K.

2. Starches are not necessary for the absorption of vitamin K.

3. Proteins are not necessary for the absorption of vitamin K.

4. **Vitamin K is one of the fat-soluble vitamins (A, D, E, and K) that require the presence of fat to be absorbed. Vitamin K plays an essential role in the production of the clotting factors II (prothrombin), VII, IX, and X.**

12. 1. **A balanced diet with choices in moderation from a variety of foods will provide the recommended daily allowances of essential nutrients without the need for supplements.**

2. Megadoses of vitamins no longer operate as nutritional agents, and excesses are detrimental to the body, particularly to the liver and the brain.

3. Vitamins by themselves will not ensure an adequate intake. Their action contributes to chemical reactions (i.e., they act as catalysts), and they must have their substrate materials to work on, which are carbohydrates, protein, and fats and their metabolites.

4. It may or may not be true that expensive vitamins are more pure than inexpensive vitamins.

13. 1. **When the amount of carbohydrates ingested does not meet the energy requirements of an individual, the body will break down stored fat to meet its energy needs. Ketone bodies are produced during the oxidation of fatty acids.**

2. The presence of ketosis in an otherwise healthy adult is not caused by an increased intake of protein. An increased intake of protein helps meet energy demands because when the energy from carbohydrates is depleted, the body converts protein and fatty acids to glucose (gluconeogenesis).

3. The presence of ketosis in an otherwise healthy adult is not caused by an increased intake of starch. Starch is the major source of carbohydrates in the diet, and it yields simple sugars on digestion. Adequate serum glucose levels provide for energy needs, thus negating the need to break down body fat, resulting in ketosis.

4. The presence of ketosis in an otherwise healthy adult is not caused by an increased intake of fiber. An increase in fiber intake

supplies roughage or bulk to the diet, which assists the gastrointestinal tract to function effectively and facilitates elimination of intestinal waste.

14. 1. **Vitamin C (ascorbic acid) is a water-soluble vitamin. The presence of fat or bile salts is unnecessary for its absorption.**

2. Vitamin A is a fat-soluble vitamin that requires fat and bile salts to promote its absorption.

3. Vitamin E is a fat-soluble vitamin that requires fat and bile salts to promote its absorption.

4. Vitamin D is a fat-soluble vitamin that requires fat and bile salts to promote its absorption.

15. 1. A sedentary lifestyle is only one theory associated with the cause of obesity.

2. A low metabolic rate is only one theory associated with the cause of obesity.

3. A hormonal imbalance is only one theory associated with the cause of obesity.

4. **An excessive caloric intake is the basis of all weight gain, regardless of the etiology. Excess ingested nutrients are stored in adipose tissue (fat) and muscle, which increases body weight. Obesity is body weight 20% or greater than ideal body weight. Glucose is stored as glycogen in the liver and muscle, with surplus amounts being converted to fat. Glycerol and fatty acids are stored as triglycerides in adipose tissue. Excess amino acids are used for glucose formation or are stored as fat.**

16. 1. A rapid weight gain indicates fluid retention, not an improved nutritional status. One liter of fluid weighs 2.2 pounds.

2. **Transferrin is a glycoprotein formed in the liver. Serum transferrin is a marker for iron metabolism and protein status. Because serum transferrin's half-life is 8 days (compared with a half-life of 20 days for albumin), serum transferrin levels will provide earlier objective information concerning a person's increasing or decreasing nutritional status. Serum transferrin levels range from 215 to 380 mg/dL in adults, depending on gender.**

3. A decreasing serum albumin level indicates a deteriorating, not improving, nutritional status. A serum albumin

level should range from 3.5 to 5 g/dL. Mild depletion values range from 2.8 to 3.4 g/dL. Moderate depletion values range from 2.1 to 2.7 g/dL. In severe depletion, values are less than 2.1 g/dL.

4. Appropriate skin turgor, fullness, and elasticity that allow the skin to spring back to its previous state after being pinched reflect an adequate fluid, not nutritional, balance.

17. 1. Although the inability to form hemoglobin in the absence of other necessary factors, such as vitamin B_{12} (in pernicious anemia), can result in iron deficiency, it is not the major cause of iron deficiency.

2. The most common nutrient deficiency in the United States is iron, which results from an inadequate supply of dietary iron. The major condition indicating iron deficiency is anemia because iron is a key component of red blood cells.

3. Malabsorption of iron is not the major cause of iron deficiency. However, the malabsorption of iron can be caused by a lack of gastric hydrochloric acid, which is necessary to help liberate iron for absorption, and the presence of phosphate or phytate, inhibitors of iron absorption.

4. Although hemorrhage can precipitate iron deficiency, it is not the major etiological factor.

18. 1. Stomatitis, inflammation of the mucous membranes of the mouth, is most often caused by infectious sources (e.g., herpes simplex virus, *Candida albicans*, and hemolytic streptococci) or chemotherapy, not fluoride deficiency.

2. Fluoride strengthens the ability of the tooth structure to withstand the erosive effects of bacterial acids on the teeth. The recommended daily intake of fluoride for adults is 1.5 to 4.0 mg.

3. Bleeding gums is caused by inflammation of the gums (gingivitis), not fluoride deficiency.

4. Mottling of the teeth is related to a fluoride excess, not a fluoride deficiency. Yellow, brown, or black discoloration of teeth may indicate other problems, such as staining, a partial or total nonviable nerve, or tetracycline administration during the prenatal period or early childhood.

19. 1. Although kidney beans are an excellent source of carbohydrates, a vegetarian diet has many other foods that can be selected to provide carbohydrates.

2. Although kidney beans are an excellent source of minerals, especially sodium, potassium, and phosphorus, a vegetarian diet has many other foods that can be selected to provide minerals.

3. Kidney beans are high in protein. One cup of kidney beans contains 15 g of protein. Complete proteins come from animal sources, such as meat, poultry, and fish, but these foods are not included on a vegetarian diet. Kidney beans combined with a grain are a substitute for a complete protein.

4. One cup of kidney beans contains only 1 g of fat.

20. 1. Although making mealtime a social activity is desirable, it may be impractical or impossible in an acute care facility. Client rooms may be private or semiprivate, which limits exposure to other clients, and clients often are too sick to socialize.

2. Although obtaining a nutritional history is done, the information will not necessarily improve intake.

3. Sick older adults often are debilitated, lack energy, and do not feel well. Assistance with meals conserves the client's energy and demonstrates a caring concern, which may increase the intake of food.

4. Dietary supplements require a primary health-care provider's prescription. Providing dietary supplements is a dependent function of the nurse.

21. **1. A total cholesterol level of 210 mg/dL in a woman is 11 mg more than the acceptable limit of less than 200 mg/dL. To prevent excessive cholesterol levels, clients should be taught which foods are high in cholesterol and should thus be avoided.**

2. 190 mg/dL is an acceptable level of total cholesterol for a healthy adult woman.

3. 150 mg/dL is an acceptable level of total cholesterol for a healthy adult woman.

4. 120 mg/dL is in the low normal range of 120 to 140 mg/dL, which is an acceptable level of cholesterol for a healthy adult woman.

22. 1. During the states of malnutrition and starvation, the basal metabolic rate (BMR) decreases because the lean body mass

decreases. Fever is associated with an increased, not decreased, BMR.

2. When energy expended is greater than the caloric intake, an individual will experience hunger, not anorexia. Hunger is a dull or acute pain felt around the epigastric area that is caused by a lack of food. Anorexia is the loss or lack of appetite.

3. **When energy expenditure exceeds caloric intake, eventually body fat and muscle mass break down to supply the fuel needed for metabolism. Malnutrition results when the body's cells have a deficiency or excess of one or more nutrients.**

4. When a person is malnourished, eventually the serum protein will be low, which may result in decreased colloid osmotic pressure and then movement of fluid from the intravascular compartment into the peritoneal cavity. When the circulating blood volume decreases, the blood pressure decreases, not increases.

23. 1. Hemoglobin concentration of the blood correlates closely with the red blood cell count. Elevated hemoglobin suggests hemoconcentration from increased numbers of red blood cells (polycythemia) or dehydration.

2. **Serum proteins, particularly albumin, reflect a person's skeletal muscle and visceral protein status. An expected serum albumin level ranges between 3.5 and 5.0 g/dL. Mild depletion ranges between 2.8 and 3.4 g/dL. Moderate depletion ranges between 2.1 and 2.7 g/dL. Severe depletion is less than 2.1 g/dL.**

3. Specific gravity is a urine test that measures the kidney's ability to concentrate urine. A low specific gravity reflects dilute urine that suggests a high urine volume, diabetes insipidus, kidney infection, or severe renal damage with disturbances in concentrating and diluting abilities.

4. Blood urea nitrogen (BUN) measures the nitrogen fraction of urea, a product of protein metabolism. An elevated BUN suggests renal disease, reduced renal perfusion, urinary tract obstruction, and increased protein metabolism.

24. 1. Egg rolls are a fried food. Frying involves cooking food in a solution consisting of saturated or unsaturated fat, which is composed mostly of fatty acids. Fatty

acids combine with glycerol to form triglycerides.

2. Spareribs are high in saturated fat and cooked with sauces that are high in saturated or unsaturated fat.

3. Crispy noodles are a fried food that should be avoided. Frying involves cooking food with a saturated or unsaturated fat solution, which is composed mostly of fatty acids.

4. **Hot and sour soup contains less fat than the other food choices listed.**

25. 1. An electrolyte is a chemical substance that, in solution, dissociates into electrically charged particles. Electrolytes maintain the chemical balance between cations and anions in the body, which is essential for acid-base balance.

2. Vitamins are organic compounds that do not provide energy but are needed for the metabolism of energy.

3. Minerals are inorganic elements or compounds essential for regulating body functions. The major minerals of the body are calcium, phosphorus, sodium, potassium, magnesium, chloride, and sulfur.

4. **Carbohydrates, a group of organic compounds, such as saccharides, starch, cellulose, and gum, are the main fuel sources for energy. Athletes competing in endurance events often adhere to a diet that increases carbohydrates to 70% of the diet for 3 days before a race (carbohydrate loading) to maximize muscle glycogen storage.**

26. 1. **The clock system, which identifies where certain foods are on a plate in relation to where numbers are located on a clock, allows the client to be independent when eating. Independence with activities of daily living supports self-esteem.**

2. Eating one food at a time is unnecessary and may decrease the client's appetite.

3. Ordering finger foods is unnecessary and limits the client's food choices.

4. Feeding the client does not promote independence and may precipitate feelings of low self-esteem.

27. 1. Osteoporosis is a disease characterized by a decrease in total bone mass and deterioration of bone tissue that leads to bone fragility and the risk of fractures. Adequate calcium is necessary for building and strengthening bones and preventing osteoporosis.

2. Vitamin D promotes bone mineralization by producing transport proteins that bind calcium and phosphorus. This increases intestinal absorption, stimulates the kidneys to return calcium to the bloodstream, and stimulates bone cells to use calcium and phosphorus to build and maintain bone tissue.

3. A decrease in calcium in the blood (hypocalcemia) can eventually lead to tetany, which is characterized by muscle spasms, paresthesias, and convulsions.

4. Iron is unrelated to calcium balance. Iron is essential for hemoglobin formation.

28. 1. Flushing the tube after every feeding moves the formula into the stomach and helps maintain tube patency; it does not reduce the risk of diarrhea.

2. Checking residual volume informs the nurse about the absorption of the last feeding. This step prevents the addition of more feeding than the client can digest; it does not prevent diarrhea. Generally, feedings are withheld when a certain residual volume is identified. Protocols may include withholding the next feeding when a residual of half the volume of the last feeding is removed just before the next feeding, or the primary health-care provider may give specific instructions if there is a residual volume.

3. Elevating the head of the bed 30 degrees at all times helps to keep the formula in the stomach via the principle of gravity and helps to prevent aspiration; it does not prevent diarrhea.

4. Contaminated formula can cause diarrhea. Opened cans of formula support bacterial growth and must be discarded after 24 hours, even when refrigerated.

29. 1. Eggs should be avoided on a low-fat diet. One egg contains 1.7 g of saturated fat.

2. Liver should be avoided on a low-fat diet. Three ounces of liver contains 2.5 g of saturated fat.

3. Cheese should be avoided on a low-fat diet. Depending on the cheese, 1 ounce contains 4.4 to 6.2 g of saturated fat.

4. Turkey is permitted on a low-fat diet. Three ounces of turkey contains 0.9 g of saturated fat. A low-fat food should contain less than 1.0 g of saturated fat per serving.

5. Scallops are permitted on a low-fat diet. Three ounces of scallops contains 0.1 g of saturated fat.

6. Flounder is permitted on a low-fat diet. Three ounces of flounder contains 0.3 g of saturated fat.

30. 1. Liver is high in cholesterol. Three ounces of beef, calf, and chicken liver contains 331, 477, and 537 mg of cholesterol, respectively.

2. Shrimp is high in cholesterol. Three ounces of shrimp contains 166 mg of cholesterol.

3. One cup of skim milk contains only 18 mg of cholesterol.

4. Three ounces of turkey contains only 59 mg of cholesterol.

5. Two slices of bologna contain only 31 mg of cholesterol.

31.   **Answer: 2 tablets.**
       Solve the problem by using ratio and proportion.

$$\frac{\text{Desired}}{\text{Have}} \quad \frac{0.8 \text{ mg}}{0.4 \text{ mg}} = \frac{\text{x tab}}{1 \text{ tab}}$$
$$0.4 \text{ x} = 0.8$$
$$\text{x} = 0.8 \div 0.4$$
$$\text{x} = 2 \text{ tablets}$$

32. 1. One egg contains only 1.0 mg of iron.

2. One serving of fruit contains less than 1.0 mg of iron.

3. Meat, especially liver, is an excellent source of iron. Three ounces of meat contains 1.6 to 5.3 mg of iron, depending on the type of meat and whether it is a regular or lean cut.

4. One slice of bread contains 0.7 to 1.4 mg of iron, depending on the type of bread.

5. Spinach is an excellent source of iron. A half cup of boiled spinach contains 3.2 mg of iron.

33. **1. All eggs, except fried, are permitted on a low-residue (low-fiber) diet. A low-residue diet is easily digested and absorbed and limits bulk in the intestines after digestion.**

2. Cooked oatmeal is not permitted on a low-residue diet. One cup of cooked oatmeal contains 4 g of fiber.

3. Orange juice contains pulp, a soluble fiber, which is not permitted on a low-residue diet.

4. Green beans contain polysaccharides that provide structure to plants and result in a

residual after digestion that is not permitted on a low-residue diet. One cup of green beans contains 4.19 g of dietary fiber.

5. Whole-grain breads, breads with seeds or nuts, and breads made with bran consist of insoluble fibers that are not permitted on a low-residue diet. Two slices of whole-wheat bread contain 4 g of fiber.

34. **Solve the problem by using ratio and proportion.**

$$\frac{\text{Desired}}{\text{Have}} \quad \frac{50 \text{ mg}}{100 \text{ mg}} = \frac{\text{x mL}}{1 \text{ mL}}$$
$$100 \text{ x} = 50$$
$$\text{x} = 50 \div 100$$
$$\text{x} = 0.5 \text{ mL}$$

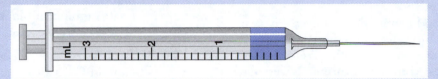

35. 1. One cup of orange juice contains only 27 mg of calcium.
2. One tablespoon of peanut butter contains only 5 mg of calcium.
3. **Cottage cheese is an excellent source of calcium, which is essential for bone growth. One cup of cottage cheese contains 155 mg of calcium. The NIH Consensus Conference—Optimal Calcium Intake recommends an average intake of 1,000 to 1,500 mg of calcium daily for an adult, depending on various factors.**
4. Three ounces of baked flounder contains only 13 mg of calcium.
5. **Low-fat yogurt is an excellent source of calcium, which is essential for bone growth. One cup of low-fat yogurt contains 345 mg of calcium.**
6. **Cooked spinach is an excellent source of calcium, which is essential for bone growth. One cup of cooked spinach contains 276 mg of calcium.**

36. 1. **The Center for Nutrition Policy and Promotion advocates in the MyPlate diet that vegetables and fruits should be 50% of one's diet, with slightly more vegetables than fruits.**
2. **Fish, such as flounder and haddock, contain extremely low levels of saturated fat compared with meat, which is much higher in saturated fat.**
3. Wanting to lose 20 pounds reflects cognition, not behavior. Desiring something may or may not progress to action.
4. **Although eggs are high in cholesterol, they are low in saturated fats, and they can be eaten in moderation (e.g., 4 to 6 eggs or less a week). Recent studies indicate that even 1 egg a day is not**

associated with an increased risk of coronary heart disease or stroke.
5. **Eating foods low in fat is a healthy behavior because it is an action that promotes a healthy lifestyle. Implementing health-promotion behaviors is based on the perceived benefits of the actions.**

37. 1. **The client's serum glucose level is 235. The primary health-care provider wrote a prescription for regular insulin coverage. When the serum glucose level is between 201 and 250, the client is to receive 5 units of regular insulin subcutaneously.**
2. It is unnecessary to notify the primary health-care provider of the client's status.
3. The client's pain is at level 3 on a scale of 0 to 10. The nurse can delay the administration of oxycodone, a potent analgesic, until the client is experiencing a higher level of pain.
4. The client's respiratory status is stable. There is no prescription to administer an additional dose of ipratropium. The administration of medication is a dependent function of the nurse.

38. 1. Gelatin is a clear liquid that is a solid when refrigerated and a liquid at room temperature. It is permitted in either form on a clear liquid diet.
2. Caffeinated or decaffeinated tea is permitted on a clear liquid diet.
3. Weak or strong coffee and caffeinated or decaffeinated coffee are permitted on a clear liquid diet.
4. Pureed soups are permitted on a full-liquid, not a clear liquid, diet. Pureed

soups have a high-solute load, including fats and proteins, which stimulates the digestive process.

5. Milk and milk products are not included on a clear liquid diet. Ice cream contains a high-solute load, including fat and proteins, which stimulates the digestive process.

39. 1. One cup of milk contains only 8 g of protein.

2. Food from animal sources (e.g., meat, poultry, fish, and eggs) provides complete proteins and therefore is the best source of protein. Three ounces of meat or poultry contains 19 to 25 g of protein, depending on the type of meat or poultry.

3. Fruit does not contain protein. Fruit contains glucose, minerals, and vitamins, depending on the fruit.

4. Although a serving of a grain product contains approximately 2 g of protein, it primarily provides carbohydrates and fiber.

5. The majority of vegetables provide only 1 to 3 g of protein.

40. 1. Wearing clean gloves protects the nurse from the client's blood. This is not a sterile procedure.

3. Holding the finger in a dependent position allows more blood to enter the distal portion of the finger. Avoid squeezing the finger because it increases the likelihood of an inaccurate low reading.

6. Wiping the site with an approved antiseptic will remove some surface microorganisms that could enter the skin when punctured. The antiseptic used should not interfere with the reagent on the strip, and it should dry on the skin before the puncture occurs. The use of alcohol is controversial because it dries the skin, and if it interacts with the reagent, it will give a false low reading.

5. The side of a finger has fewer nerve endings than the pad of a fingertip and, therefore, during and after the procedure the discomfort will be less. Some advocate using just the two last digits of a hand because they are not used as much as the other fingers.

2. The first drop of blood should be wiped away with sterile gauze because

the first drop contains more serous fluid, which can alter test results. Sterile gauze limits microorganisms from entering the puncture site.

4. The finger should hover over the reagent strip, and the drop of blood should make minimal contact with the reagent strip. This provides a full drop of blood for testing. A smeared blood sample will provide an inadequate amount of blood, resulting in an inaccurate reading.

41. 1. Potatoes are an excellent source of vitamin C (ascorbic acid). One medium potato contains approximately 42 mg of vitamin C.

2. Papayas are an excellent source of vitamin C. One cup of papayas contains 87 mg of vitamin C.

3. Eight ounces of yogurt contains only 1 mg of vitamin C.

4. Dried beans (legumes) contain no vitamin C. One cup of green beans contains only 12 mg of vitamin C.

5. One cup of milk contains only 2 mg of vitamin C.

42. 1. This is a photograph of a formula being administered via a gastrostomy tube. Thirty to 60 mL of water should be added to the catheter-tip syringe when the syringe is nearly empty of formula. This will clear the tube of formula at the end of the feeding and will prevent occlusion of the tube.

2. This is a photograph of a formula being administered via a gastrostomy tube. Bolus feedings administered over a 60-minute period generally are controlled by a feeding pump, not administered by gravity, as indicated in the photograph.

3. This is a photograph of a formula being administered via a gastrostomy tube. A formula at room temperature is less likely to cause gastric discomfort.

4. This is a photograph of a formula being administered via a gastrostomy tube. The head of the bed should be elevated 30 to 45 degrees during the feeding and for 1 hour after the feeding to minimize the risk of gastroesophageal reflux and aspiration.

5. This is a photograph of a formula being administered via a gastrostomy tube. Formula is added continuously to the catheter-tip syringe just before

it empties until the entire feeding is administered. Just before the final amount of formula exits the syringe, 30 to 60 mL of water is added to the syringe to clear the tubing of formula.

43. 1. **A primary health-care provider should assess the client's level of depression. St. John's wort is not recommended for moderate to severe depression. Other medications may be of greater benefit.**
    2. **St. John's wort may decrease the effectiveness of oral contraceptives.**
    3. A lifting of depression may be identified as early as 2 to 3 weeks after initiation of St. John's wort. If no improvement is identified in 4 to 6 weeks, discontinue the medication.
    4. **St. John's wort must be discontinued before surgery because clients exposed to general anesthesia may experience cardiovascular collapse.**
    5. **A heightened reaction to the sun (photosensitization) is a response that can occur with exposure to sunlight when taking St. John's wort.**

44. 1. **It is advisable to be evaluated by a urologist because the symptoms that the client is experiencing may be caused by a serious medical condition other than benign enlargement of the prostate.**
    2. **Side effects are not common and generally are mild. Side effects include dizziness, headache, nausea, vomiting, constipation, and diarrhea. Primary health-care providers generally permit a client to take saw palmetto if the client is insistent because it has so few side effects.**
    3. There is no evidence that saw palmetto interferes with the measurement of prostate-specific antigen (PSA), a protein associated with prostate cancer. However, a primary health-care provider may prescribe a PSA test and implement a rectal examination for baseline data before initiating treatment with saw palmetto.

4. Some men do report an enhanced ability to maintain an erection. It is believed that saw palmetto relaxes smooth muscle, allowing blood to flow smoothly and supporting an erection.
5. Research supported by the National Institute of Diabetes and Digestive and Kidney Diseases, the National Center for Complementary and Alternative Health, and the National Institutes of Health Office of Dietary Supplements indicates that saw palmetto has no greater effect on the signs and symptoms of benign prostatic hypertrophy than treatment with a placebo.

45. 1. **Burns interrupt the integrity of the skin and, as a result, a primary defense against infection is disrupted. The body's metabolic rate increases dramatically in an attempt to repair the skin and protect the body from infection. Nutrients are required to provide the building blocks for skin cells and immunoglobulins.**
    2. Nausea does not precipitate a need for an increase in caloric intake above average requirements. However, frequent small, dry feedings and medications to limit nausea may be used.
    3. Difficulty swallowing (dysphagia) does not precipitate a need for an increase in caloric intake above average requirements. However, the texture of foods and the rate of feeding may have to be adjusted.
    4. **An individual with pneumonia requires an increase in caloric requirements because of an increased resting energy expenditure and hypermetabolic state. With an infection, more energy is needed to regulate an elevated body temperature, and extra protein is needed to produce antibodies and white blood cells.**
    5. Depression does not precipitate a need for an increase in caloric intake above average requirements. If a depressed client becomes withdrawn and sedentary, caloric requirements may decrease.

Oxygenation

The following words include English vocabulary, nursing/medical terminology, concepts, principles, and information relevant to content specifically addressed in the chapter or associated with topics presented in it. English dictionaries, nursing textbooks, and medical dictionaries, such as *Taber's Cyclopedic Medical Dictionary,* are resources that can be used to expand your knowledge and understanding of these words and related information.

Abdominal thrust (Heimlich maneuver)
Accessory muscles of respiration
Activity intolerance
Aerosol therapy
Airway clearance
Airway obstruction
Airway resistance
Alveoli
Arterial blood gases
Aspiration
Atelectasis
Auscultation
Breathing, types of:
  Abdominal
  Apnea
  Bradypnea
  Deep
  Diaphragmatic
  Eupnea
  Pursed-lip
  Tachypnea
  Thoracic
Breath sounds:
  Adventitious:
    Crackles (rales)
    Gurgles (rhonchi)
    Pleural friction rub
    Stridor
    Wheezes
  Normal:
    Bronchial
    Bronchovesicular
    Vesicular
Bronchial spasm
Bronchoscopy
Capillary refill
Cardiac output
Cardiac workload
Cardiopulmonary resuscitation
Cardiovascular
Chest physiotherapy
Chest percussion
Chest vibration

Chest radiograph (x-ray)
Chest tube
Choking
Cilia
Circumoral cyanosis
Cough:
  Nonproductive
  Productive
Cyanosis
Diffusion
Dyspnea
Dysrhythmias
Electrocardiogram
Endotracheal tube
Excursion
Exhale, exhalation
Expectorate
Expiration
Extubation
Fatigue
Hemoglobin saturation
Hemoptysis
Hemorrhage
Humidify
Hypercapnia
Hypertension/hypotension
Hyperventilation/hypoventilation
Hypostatic pneumonia
Hypovolemic shock
Hypoxia, hypoxemia
Incentive spirometer
Inhale, inspiration
Intrathoracic pressure
Intubation
Iron-deficiency anemia
Laryngeal spasm
Metered-dose inhaler (MDI)
Mucous membranes
Mucus
Nares
Nebulizer
Oropharynx
Orthopnea

Orthostatic hypotension
Oxygen delivery systems:
  Face mask
  Nasal cannula
  Nonrebreather mask
  Venturi mask
Oxygen liter-flow gauge
Oxygen saturation
Oxygen therapy
Pallor
Palpable
Patency, patent
Peripheral pulses
Pneumothorax
Positive-pressure ventilation
Postural drainage
Postural hypotension
Pulmonary embolus
Pulmonary function tests
Pulse oximetry
Secretions:
  Tenacious
  Viscous

Sedentary
Sputum
Sternum
Suctioning:
  Nasal
  Oropharyngeal
  Tracheal
Thoracentesis
Thoracic
Thoracotomy
Thrombophlebitis
Tidal volume
Tissue perfusion
Tracheostomy
Valsalva maneuver
Vasoconstriction
Vasodilation
Ventilation
Vital capacity
Xiphoid process

OXYGENATION: QUESTIONS

1. A nurse teaches a client how to use an incentive spirometer. Which projected client outcome **supports** the conclusion that the use of the incentive spirometer was effective?
   1. Expiratory volume will be decreased.
   2. Inspiratory volume will be increased.
   3. Sputum will be expectorated.
   4. Coughing will be stimulated.

2. A primary health-care provider prescribes chest physiotherapy with percussion and vibration for a newly admitted client. Which information obtained by the nurse during the health history should alert the nurse to question the provider's prescription?
   1. Emphysema
   2. Osteoporosis
   3. Cystic fibrosis
   4. Chronic bronchitis

3. Which nursing assessment **best** indicates a client's ability to tolerate activity?
   1. Vital signs that take three minutes to return to preactivity level
   2. Absence of adventitious breath sounds on auscultation
   3. Flexibility of both muscles and joints
   4. Reports of weakness after activity

4. Which should the nurse do **first** when an adult who is choking on food becomes unconscious?
   1. Apply upward thrusts over the client's xiphoid process.
   2. Initiate a cardiopulmonary resuscitation protocol.
   3. Strike the middle of the client's back firmly.
   4. Perform a blind finger sweep of the mouth.

5. A client has thick, tenacious respiratory secretions. Which should the nurse do to liquefy the client's respiratory secretions?
   1. Change the client's position every two hours.
   2. Get a prescription for an antitussive agent.
   3. Encourage the client to drink more fluid.
   4. Teach effective deep breathing.

6. Which action is effective in meeting the needs of a client experiencing laryngospasm after extubation?
   1. Ensuring hyperextension of the head
   2. Providing positive-pressure ventilation
   3. Instituting cardiopulmonary resuscitation
   4. Administering oxygen by using a face mask

7. A client's hemoglobin saturation via pulse oximetry indicates inadequate oxygenation. Which should the nurse do **first**?
   1. Notify the primary health-care provider.
   2. Encourage breathing deeply.
   3. Raise the head of the bed.
   4. Administer oxygen.

8. A nurse is reviewing the laboratory results of a client with the preliminary diagnosis of anemia. An abnormal response of which diagnostic test would reflect iron-deficiency anemia?
   1. Hemoglobin
   2. Platelet count
   3. Serum albumin
   4. Blood urea nitrogen

9. A client is admitted with the diagnosis of lower extremity arterial disease. Which is a specific desirable outcome for a client with this diagnosis?
   1. Respirations within the expected range
   2. Oriented to the environment
   3. Palpable peripheral pulses
   4. Prolonged capillary refill

10. A primary health-care provider prescribes bedrest for a client. Which should the nurse explain to the client is the **primary** purpose of bedrest?
    1. Conserve energy.
    2. Maintain strength.
    3. Enhance protein synthesis.
    4. Reduce intestinal peristalsis.

11. A nurse is planning to teach one client pursed-lip breathing and another client diaphragmatic breathing. Which technique associated with diaphragmatic breathing is different from pursed-lip breathing and should be included by the nurse in the teaching plan?
    1. Inhale through the mouth.
    2. Exhale through pursed lips.
    3. Raise both shoulders while inhaling deeply.
    4. Tighten the abdominal muscles while exhaling.

12. A meal tray arrives for a client who is receiving 24% oxygen via a Venturi mask. Which should the nurse do to meet this client's needs?
    1. Discontinue the oxygen when the client is eating meals.
    2. Request a prescription to use a nasal cannula during meals.
    3. Obtain a prescription to change the mask to a nonrebreather mask during meals.
    4. Arrange for liquid supplements that can be administered via a straw through a valve in the mask.

13. A nurse hears a client explain the purpose of pursed-lip breathing to a relative. Which information would indicate to the nurse that the client correctly understood the nurse's teaching about pursed-lip breathing?
    1. Precipitates coughing
    2. Helps maintain open airways
    3. Decreases intrathoracic pressure
    4. Facilitates expectoration of mucus

14. An unconscious client who had oral surgery is admitted to the postanesthesia care unit. In which position should the nurse place the client?
    1. Prone
    2. Supine
    3. Fowler
    4. Lateral

15. A primary health-care provider prescribes chest physiotherapy with percussion and vibration for a client. After the primary health-care provider leaves, the client says, "I still don't understand the purpose of this therapy." Which statement should be included in the nurse's response?
    1. "It eliminates the need to cough."
    2. "It limits the production of bronchial mucus."
    3. "It helps clear the airways of excessive secretions."
    4. "It promotes the flow of secretions to the base of the lungs."

16. A nurse raises the head of the bed for a client who has difficulty breathing. Which science includes the principle that explains how this intervention facilitates respiration?
    1. Physics
    2. Biology
    3. Anatomy
    4. Chemistry

17. Which clinical manifestation is of **most** concern when the nurse assesses a client who has impaired mobility?
    1. Shallow respirations
    2. Increased oxygen saturation
    3. Decreased chest wall expansion
    4. Gurgling sounds when breathing

18. A nurse teaches a client to make a series of short, forceful exhalations (huffing) just before actually coughing. Which information should the nurse include when explaining the purpose of this action?
    1. Conserves energy when coughing
    2. Limits pain precipitated when coughing
    3. Liquefies respiratory secretions when coughing
    4. Raises sputum to a level where it can be expectorated when coughing

19. Which are effective leg exercises the nurse should encourage a client to perform to prevent circulatory complications during the postoperative period?
    1. Knee flexion
    2. Isometric exercises
    3. Dorsiflexion exercises
    4. Passive range of motion

20. Which outcome **best** reflects achievement of the goal, "The client will expectorate lung secretions with no signs of respiratory complications"?
    1. Absence of adventitious breath sounds
    2. Deep breathing and coughing nonproductively
    3. Drinking 3,000 mL of fluid in the last 24 hours
    4. Expectorating sputum three times between 3 p.m. and 11 p.m.

21. Which should the nurse do **first** when caring for a nonverbal client who is restless, agitated, and irritable?
    1. Administer oxygen.
    2. Suction the oropharynx.
    3. Reduce environmental stimuli.
    4. Determine patency of the airway.

22. Which action should the nurse implement to increase both the respiratory and the circulatory functions of a client in a coma?
    1. Encourage the client to cough.
    2. Massage the client's bony areas.
    3. Assist the client with breathing exercises.
    4. Change the client's position every two hours.

23. A client sucking on a hard candy inhales while laughing and develops a total airway obstruction. Which is the nurse attempting to do when implementing an abdominal thrust?
    1. Produce a burp.
    2. Pump the heart.
    3. Push air out of the lungs.
    4. Put pressure on the stomach.

24. A nurse in the postanesthesia care unit is monitoring several clients who received general anesthesia. Which client response causes the **most** concern?
    1. Pain
    2. Stridor
    3. Lethargy
    4. Diaphoresis

25. A primary health-care provider prescribes oxygen for a client to be delivered at a high flow rate. Which additional nursing action is necessary when implementing a high-liter flow as opposed to a low-liter flow?
    1. Attaching a flowmeter to the wall outlet
    2. Providing oral hygiene whenever necessary
    3. Using an oil-based lubricant when caring for the nares
    4. Humidifying oxygen before it is delivered to the client

26. A nurse is teaching a client how to use an incentive spirometer. Which position should the nurse assist the client to assume during this procedure?
    1. Sitting
    2. Side-lying
    3. Orthopneic
    4. Low-Fowler

27. Which is the **most** important action by the nurse after a client has a chest tube inserted to treat a pneumothorax?
    1. Ensure the client's intake is at least 3,000 mL of fluid per 24 hours.
    2. Provide the client with adequate medication for pain relief.
    3. Maintain the integrity of the client's chest tube.
    4. Reposition the client every 2 hours.

28. A nurse is assessing a postoperative client. Which complication has occurred when the client experiences purulent sputum, dyspnea, and chest pain?
    1. Hypostatic pneumonia
    2. Hypovolemic shock
    3. Thrombophlebitis
    4. Pneumothorax

29. An obese client has limited mobility after an open reduction and internal fixation of a fractured hip. For which human response related to increased blood coagulability should the nurse monitor this client?
1. Muscle deterioration
2. Pain in the calf
3. Hypotension
4. Bradypnea

30. For which clinical manifestation should the nurse monitor the client when concerned about a potential for respiratory distress?
1. Productive cough
2. Sore throat
3. Orthopnea
4. Eupnea

31. A nurse, working in the emergency department, identifies that a client's hands are edematous when attempting to apply a pulse oximetry probe for short-term use. Which action should the nurse implement?
1. Attach the probe to one of the client's toes.
2. Connect the probe to one of the client's earlobes.
3. Wash the client's hand before attaching the probe to the finger.
4. Encourage the client to perform active range-of-motion exercises of the hand with the probe.

32. A primary health-care provider's prescription reads, "6 L oxygen via face mask." The client, who has been extremely confused since being in the unfamiliar environment of the hospital, becomes agitated and repeatedly pulls off the mask. Which should the nurse do?
1. Tighten the strap around the head.
2. Reapply the mask every time the client pulls it off.
3. Provide an explanation of why the oxygen is necessary.
4. Request that the prescription for oxygen be changed to a nasal cannula.

33. A nurse is caring for a male client who had several laboratory tests performed. Which of the following increase this client's risk for an impaired ability to tolerate activity? **Select all that apply.**
1. _____ Hct of 45%
2. _____ Hb of 10 g/dL
3. _____ O_2 saturation of 97%
4. _____ WBC count of 7,500 cells/mcL
5. _____ RBC count of 4.8 million cells/mcL

34. A nurse teaches a preoperative client how to use an incentive spirometer. Place the following steps of the use of an incentive spirometer in the order in which they should be performed.
1. Inhale slowly.
2. Hold the incentive spirometer level.
3. Remove the mouthpiece and exhale normally.
4. Keep the visual indicator at the inspiratory goal for several seconds.
5. Maintain a firm seal, with the lips around the mouthpiece during inhalation.

Answer: _____

35. A primary health-care provider prescribes a loading dose of theophylline 6 mg/kg IV over 30 minutes. The client weighs 150 pounds. How many milligrams of theophylline should the nurse administer? **Record your answer using a whole number.**

Answer: _____ mg.

36. A nurse in the operative suite is preparing an older adult for surgery. Which of the following physiological factors place the older adult at **greater** risk of life-threatening complications associated with surgery? **Select all that apply.**
1. _____ Skin elasticity
2. _____ Bladder emptying
3. _____ Tolerance for pain
4. _____ Respiratory excursion
5. _____ Cardiovascular capacity

37. Which of the following should the nurse instruct a client to do when using the apparatus in the illustration?
1. Breathe out normally, seal your mouth around the mouthpiece, breathe in as slowly and deeply as possible, hold your breath at least three seconds, and remove the mouthpiece and exhale.
2. Hold the device, seal your mouth around the mouthpiece, and breathe in and out slowly and deeply.
3. Seal your mouth around the mouthpiece, and breathe in and out normally.
4. Take a deep breath, and forcefully exhale through the mouthpiece.

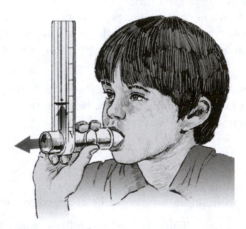

38. A nurse is caring for a client who has a chest tube after thoracic surgery. Which of the following should the nurse implement when caring for this client? **Select all that apply.**
1. _____ Encourage the client to cough and deep breathe at regular intervals.
2. _____ Clamp the tube when providing for activities of daily living.
3. _____ Position the collection device below the level of the chest.
4. _____ Maintain an airtight dressing over the puncture wound.
5. _____ Empty drainage from the device every shift.
6. _____ Avoid using pins to secure tubing.

39. A nurse is caring for a client with thrombophlebitis. For which of the following clinical manifestations of a complication associated with thrombophlebitis should the nurse monitor the client? **Select all that apply.**
1. _____ Postural hypotension
2. _____ Difficulty breathing
3. _____ Blanchable erythema
4. _____ Dependent edema
5. _____ Acute chest pain

40. Which is the nurse preparing to do with the equipment depicted in the photograph?
   1. Perform gastric lavage.
   2. Obtain a sputum specimen.
   3. Institute gastric decompression.
   4. Administer a nebulizer treatment.

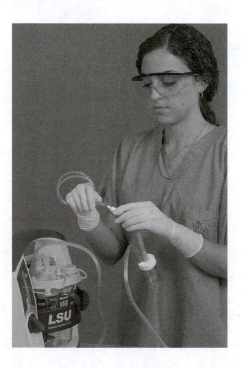

41. A nurse is caring for a client receiving oxygen via a nasal cannula. Which of the following should the nurse implement? **Select all that apply.**
   1. _____ Apply a water-based lubricant to the client's nares.
   2. _____ Adjust the flowmeter to the prescribed oxygen flow rate.
   3. _____ Reassess nares, cheeks, and ears for signs of pressure every 2 hours.
   4. _____ Place the nasal prongs so that they curve downward when in the nares.
   5. _____ Loop the tubing over the client's ears and adjust it gently under the chin.

42. A nurse is assessing a client with a respiratory problem. Which clinical manifestation is reflective of an early response to hypoxia that requires a nursing intervention? **Select all that apply.**
   1. _____ Dysrhythmias
   2. _____ Restlessness
   3. _____ Irritability
   4. _____ Cyanosis
   5. _____ Apnea

43. Which piece of information documented in the clinical record of a male adult should the nurse consider problematic?
   1. Simvastatin 20 mg, PO, in the evening
   2. Pulse 100 beats per minute
   3. Oxygen saturation 85%
   4. WBC 8,000 cells/mcL

CLIENT'S CLINICAL RECORD

Laboratory Results
WBC 8,000 cells/mcL
Hb 17 g/dL
Hct 50%

Physical Assessment
BP: 132/70 mm Hg
Pulse: 100 beats per minute
Respirations: 22 breaths per minute
Temperature: 99°F, oral
Oxygen saturation: 85%

Medication Reconciliation Form
Levothyroxine 100 mcg, PO, daily
Simvastatin 20 mg, PO, hs
Montelukast 10 mg, PO, hs

---

44. A primary health-care provider prescribes oxygen via a simple face mask at a flow rate of six liters for a client. The nurse explains the procedure to the client and maintains standard precautions. Place the following steps in the order in which they should be implemented.
   1. Place the mask on the client's face from the bridge of the nose to under the chin.
   2. Secure the elastic bands around the back of the client's head.
   3. Attach the prefilled humidifier to the flowmeter.
   4. Attach the flowmeter to the wall oxygen source.
   5. Attach the face mask tubing to the humidifier.
   6. Turn the oxygen flowmeter on to six liters.

   Answer: _____

45. A primary health-care provider prescribes zafirlukast 40 mg daily to be divided into two doses, one in the morning and one in the evening. The package insert indicates that each tablet is 10 mg. How many tablets should the nurse administer for each dose? **Record your answer using a whole number.**

   Answer: _____ tablets.

1. 1. The expiratory volume should increase, not decrease, with the use of an incentive spirometer.

2. An incentive spirometer provides a visual goal for and measurement of inspiration. It encourages the client to execute and maintain a sustained inspiration. A sustained inspiration opens airways, increases the inspiratory volume, and reduces the risk of atelectasis.

3. Although sputum may be expectorated after the use of an incentive spirometer, this is not the primary reason for its use.

4. Although the deep breathing associated with the use of an incentive spirometer may stimulate coughing, this is not the primary reason for its use.

2. 1. These are appropriate interventions for a client with emphysema. Emphysema is a chronic obstructive pulmonary disease characterized by an abnormal increase in the size of air spaces distal to the terminal bronchioles with destructive changes in their walls.

2. Implementing the primary health-care provider's prescription may compromise client safety because percussion and vibration in the presence of osteoporosis may cause fractures. Osteoporosis is an abnormal loss of bone mass and strength.

3. These are appropriate interventions for a client with cystic fibrosis. Cystic fibrosis causes widespread dysfunction of the exocrine glands. It is characterized by thick, tenacious secretions in the respiratory system that block the bronchioles, creating breathing difficulties.

4. These are appropriate interventions for a client with chronic bronchitis. Bronchitis is an inflammation of the mucous membranes of the bronchial airways.

3. **1. Vital signs reflect cardiopulmonary functioning of the body. Vital signs obtained before and after activity provide data that can be compared to determine the body's response to the energy demands of ambulation. When the vital signs return to the preactivity level within 3 minutes, it indicates that the client has tolerated the activity.**

2. The absence of abnormal breath sounds (adventitious sounds) indicates the nonexistence of a respiratory problem. Adventitious breath sounds (e.g., wheezes, rhonchi, rales, pleural friction rub, and stridor) indicate narrowed airways, presence of excessive respiratory secretions, pleural inflammation, or diminished ventilation and are not the best signs to use when assessing a person's tolerance to activity.

3. Flexibility relates to mobility, not one's physiological capacity to endure activities that require energy.

4. A report of weakness indicates that the client has not tolerated the activity.

4. 1. Abdominal thrusts should not be performed on people who are unconscious because of a foreign body airway obstruction. Another intervention is more effective.

2. Chest compressions are more effective than abdominal thrusts when attempting to eject a foreign body obstructing the airway of an unconscious adult. Chest compressions more effectively raise intrathoracic pressure.

3. Hitting the middle of the client's back firmly should never be done for an unconscious adult who is choking. The American Red Cross advocates alternating 5 back blows and 5 abdominal thrusts for a conscious adult who is choking.

4. A blind finger sweep should never be performed because it may push the foreign body deeper into the airway.

5. 1. Changing positions will mobilize, not liquefy, respiratory secretions.

2. Mucolytics, not antitussives, liquefy respiratory secretions. Antitussives prevent or relieve coughing.

3. A fluid intake of 2,500 to 3,000 mL is recommended to maintain the moisture of the respiratory mucous membranes. Adequate fluid keeps respiratory secretions thin so that they can be moved by ciliary action or be coughed up and spat out (expectorated).

4. Deep breathing mobilizes, not liquefies, respiratory secretions.

6. 1. Although tilting the head backward (hyperextension of the head) elongates the pharynx, reducing airway resistance, it will do nothing to correct the obstruction at the glottis (opening through the vocal cords). Also, the tongue will block the airway unless there is forward pressure applied on the lower angle of the jaw (jaw thrust maneuver).

2. **Positive pressure will push the vocal cords backward toward the wall of the larynx, opening the glottis (space between the vocal cords), which allows ventilation of the lung.**

3. Instituting cardiopulmonary resuscitation is unnecessary. The client is having a respiratory, not a cardiac, problem.

4. Administering oxygen by using a face mask is useless because the glottis is obstructed and the oxygenated air will not enter the lung.

7. 1. Notifying the primary health-care provider is premature. The client's needs must be met first.

2. Although encouraging deep breathing might be done eventually, it is not the priority at this time. It may or may not help. Inadequate oxygenation can be caused by a variety of problems other than shallow breathing.

3. **A nurse can implement this immediate, independent action. Nurses are permitted to treat human responses. Raising the head of the bed facilitates the dropping of the abdominal organs by gravity away from the diaphragm, which permits the greatest lung expansion.**

4. Obtaining and setting up the equipment take time that can be used for other more appropriate interventions first.

8. 1. **Iron is necessary for hemoglobin synthesis. Therefore, reduced intake of dietary iron results in iron-deficiency anemia. Hemoglobin is the main component of red blood cells and transports oxygen and carbon dioxide through the bloodstream.**

2. Platelets are unrelated to iron-deficiency anemia. Platelets (thrombocytes) are non-nucleated, round or oval, flattened, disk-shaped, formed elements in the blood that are necessary for blood clotting.

3. Albumin is unrelated to iron-deficiency anemia. Albumin is a protein in the blood that helps to maintain blood volume and blood pressure.

4. Blood urea nitrogen (BUN) is unrelated to iron-deficiency anemia. BUN is a test that measures the nitrogen portion of

urea present in the blood. It is an index of glomerular function in the production and excretion of urea.

9. 1. Respirations within the expected range are unrelated to lower extremity arterial disease (LEAD).

2. LEAD does not involve inadequate circulation to the brain.

3. **Palpable peripheral pulses are an appropriate expected outcome for a client with LEAD, which is a decrease in nutrition and respiration at the peripheral cellular level because of a decrease in capillary blood supply. A physiological response associated with LEAD is diminished or absent arterial pulses.**

4. A prolonged capillary refill indicates a continued problem with peripheral tissue perfusion. After compression, blanched tissue should return to its original color within 2 seconds (blanch test).

10. 1. **Bedrest reduces cardiopulmonary demands, muscle contraction, and other bodily functions. All of this reduces the basal metabolic rate, which conserves energy.**

2. Activity, not bedrest, maintains strength.

3. Protein synthesis is enhanced by the intake of amino acids, not bedrest.

4. Although bedrest may limit peristalsis, it is not the most common reason bedrest is prescribed.

11. 1. Inhalation is through the nose for both diaphragmatic and pursed-lip breathing.

2. Exhalation through pursed lips is performed only with pursed-lip breathing.

3. Raising both shoulders while breathing deeply is not part of diaphragmatic or pursed-lip breathing. The use of these accessory muscles of respiration is a compensatory mechanism that helps to increase thoracic excursion when inhaling.

4. **With diaphragmatic breathing, the contraction of abdominal muscles at the end of expiration helps to reduce the amount of air left in the lungs (residual volume).**

12. 1. Discontinuing oxygen when the client is eating is unsafe because it can compromise the client's respiratory status while the oxygen is disconnected.

2. **A Venturi mask interferes with eating because it covers the nose and mouth.**

Using a nasal cannula during meals will help meet both the nutritional and oxygen needs of the client. A nasal cannula delivers oxygen via prongs placed in the client's nares, leaving the mouth unobstructed, which promotes talking and eating. Specific oxygen delivery systems require a prescription, and their use is a dependent function of the nurse, except in emergency situations.

3. A Venturi mask and a nonrebreather mask are both masks that cover the mouth, which interferes with eating.

4. Liquid supplements are unnecessary. The client should eat the diet prescribed by the primary health-care provider.

13. 1. Deep breathing and huff coughing, not pursed-lip breathing, stimulate effective coughing.

2. Pursed-lip breathing involves deep inspiration and prolonged expiration against slightly closed lips. The pursed lips create a resistance to the air flowing out of the lungs, which prolongs exhalation and maintains positive airway pressure, thereby maintaining an open airway and preventing airway collapse.

3. Pursed-lip breathing increases, not decreases, intrathoracic pressure.

4. The huff cough stimulates the natural cough reflex and is effective for clearing the central airways of sputum. Saying the word huff with short, forceful exhalations keeps the glottis open, mobilizes sputum, and stimulates a cough.

14. 1. Although the prone position allows for drainage from the mouth, it is contraindicated because lying on the side of the face compresses oral tissues, impedes assessment, complicates oral suctioning, and may compromise the airway.

2. The supine position is unsafe. In an unconscious client, the gag and swallowing reflexes may be impaired, increasing the risk for aspiration as well as letting the tongue fall to the back of the oropharynx, occluding the airway.

3. The Fowler position is unsafe. An unconscious client is unable to maintain an upright position.

4. The lateral position facilitates the flow of secretions out of the mouth by gravity, keeps the tongue to the side of the mouth, maintaining the airway, and permits effective assessment

of the oropharynx and respiratory status.

15. 1. Chest physiotherapy promotes, not eliminates, the need for coughing.

2. Chest physiotherapy promotes the expectoration of, not limits the production of, bronchial mucus.

3. The striking of the skin over the lung (percussion, clapping) and fine, vigorous, shaking pressure with the hands on the chest wall during exhalation (vibration) mobilize secretions so that they can be coughed up and expectorated.

4. Chest physiotherapy mobilizes secretions, thus facilitating expectoration and interfering with the flow of secretions to the base of the lungs.

16. **1. Raising the head of the bed drops the abdominal organs away from the diaphragm via the principle of gravity, facilitating breathing. Gravity, the tendency of weight to be pulled toward the center of the earth, is a physics principle.**

2. Raising the head of the bed is not related to biology. Biology is the study of living organisms.

3. Raising the head of the bed is not related to anatomy. Anatomy is the study of the form and structure of living organisms.

4. Raising the head of the bed is not related to chemistry. Chemistry is the study of elements, compounds, and atomic relations of matter.

17. 1. Although shallow respirations are a concern, they are not as serious as a clinical manifestation in another option.

2. Oxygen saturation may be decreased, not increased, with immobility.

3. Although decreased chest wall expansion is a concern, it is not as serious as a clinical manifestation in another option.

4. Impaired activity contributes to accumulation of respiratory secretions in lung segments. Activity promotes drainage of secretions from lung segments and aerates lung tissue, thereby reducing the risk of airway obstruction and infection. Respirations that sound gurgling (gurgles, rhonchi) indicate air passing through narrowed air passages because of secretions, swelling, or a tumor. A partial or total obstruction

of the airway can occur, which is
life-threatening.

18. 1. Regardless of the type of cough, coughing
       uses, not conserves, energy. However,
       after the airway is cleared of sputum, the
       client's oxygen demands will be met more
       effectively.
    2. Limiting pain precipitated by coughing
       is not the purpose of huff coughing.
       Coughing usually is not painful unless the
       thoracic muscles are strained or the client
       has had abdominal or pelvic surgery.
    3. An increased fluid intake, not coughing,
       liquefies respiratory secretions.
    **4. The huff cough stimulates the natural
       cough reflex and is effective for clear-
       ing the central airways of sputum.
       Saying the word "huff" with short,
       forceful exhalations keeps the glottis
       open and raises sputum to a level
       where it can be coughed up and
       expectorated.**

19. 1. Flexing the knees exerts pressure on the
       veins in the popliteal space; this reduces
       venous return, which increases, not
       decreases, the risk of postoperative
       circulatory complications.
    2. Isometric exercises strengthen muscles;
       they do not prevent postoperative
       circulatory complications. Isometric
       exercises change the muscle tension but
       do not change the muscle length or move
       joints.
    **3. Alternating dorsiflexion and plantar
       flexion (calf pumping) contracts and
       relaxes the calf muscles, including the
       gastrocnemius muscles. This muscle
       contraction promotes venous return,
       preventing venous stasis that con-
       tributes to the development of
       postoperative thrombophlebitis.**
    4. Passive range-of-motion exercises are
       done by another person moving a client's
       joints through their complete range of
       movement. This does not prevent postop-
       erative circulatory complications because
       the power is supplied by a person other
       than the client. To facilitate circulation, a
       client should contract and relax muscles
       actively.

20. **1. Adventitious breath sounds are abnor-
       mal breath sounds that occur when
       pleural linings are inflamed or when
       air passes through narrowed airways
       or through airways filled with fluid.**

The absence of abnormal sounds is
desirable.
    2. To expectorate secretions, coughing must
       be productive, not nonproductive. A
       nonproductive cough is dry, which means
       that no respiratory secretions are raised
       and spat out (expectorated) because of
       coughing.
    3. Drinking fluid is an intervention that
       will liquefy respiratory secretions, thus
       facilitating their expectoration. However,
       just drinking fluid will not ensure that the
       secretions will be expectorated.
    4. Although spitting out sputum reflects
       achievement of the goal in relation to
       expectorating lung secretions, it does not
       address the absence of respiratory compli-
       cations, which is the ultimate goal of de-
       creasing stasis of respiratory secretions.

21. 1. Administering oxygen may or may not be
       necessary. The need for oxygen adminis-
       tration will depend on the results of other
       interventions that should be done first.
    2. Suctioning the oropharynx is premature.
       Mucus or sputum may not be the cause of
       the problem.
    3. Reducing environmental stimuli will
       serve no purpose at this time and is not
       the priority.
    **4. Early signs of hypoxia are restlessness,
       agitation, and irritability resulting from
       reduced oxygen to brain cells. A partial
       or completely obstructed airway pre-
       vents the passage of gases into and
       out of the lungs. The ABCs (Airway,
       Breathing, Circulation) of emergency
       care identify airway as the priority.**

22. 1. A client in a coma is unable to respond to
       an instruction to cough.
    2. Massage increases circulation only in the
       localized area being massaged. In addition,
       massage should be performed around, not
       over, bony prominences.
    3. A client in a coma is unable to respond
       to an instruction to perform breathing
       exercises.
    **4. Changing the client's position every
       2 hours helps respirations by promot-
       ing drainage of secretions from lung
       segments and aerating lung tissue,
       which helps prevent airway obstruction
       and respiratory infections. Changing
       position helps circulation because
       activity increases blood flow and
       relieves local pressure.**

23. 1. Producing a burp originating from the stomach in this situation is ineffective. Whatever is causing the obstruction is not caught in the esophagus, which leads to the stomach, but in the respiratory system.
2. Pressing on the heart (compression) is used in cardiopulmonary resuscitation (CPR).
3. **When trapped air behind an obstruction is forced out in response to an abdominal thrust, the forced air may push out what is causing the obstruction.**
4. Applying pressure against the stomach is ineffective in this situation. Whatever is causing the obstruction is not lodged in the esophagus, which leads to the stomach, but in the respiratory system.

24. 1. Pain is an expected response to the trauma of surgery and usually can be managed effectively.
2. **Stridor is an obvious audible, shrill, harsh sound caused by laryngeal obstruction. The larynx can become edematous because of the trauma of intubation associated with general anesthesia. Obstruction of the larynx is life-threatening because it prevents the exchange of gases between the lungs and the atmosphere.**
3. Lethargy, which is drowsiness or sluggishness, is an expected response to anesthesia and opioid medications because these medications depress the central nervous system.
4. Although diaphoresis is a cause for concern, it is not as immediately life-threatening as an adaptation in another option. Diaphoresis can be related to a warm environment, impaired thermoregulation, the general adaptation syndrome, or shock.

25. 1. All oxygen systems should have a flowmeter to control and maintain the flow of oxygen.
2. All oxygen is drying to the oral mucosa. Therefore, oral hygiene should be provided frequently to moisten the mucous membranes.
3. The use of an oil-based lubricant is unsafe because it is a volatile, flammable material in the presence of oxygen. A water-based lubricant should be used.
4. **A low-liter flow system administers a volume of oxygen designed to**
supplement the inspired room air to provide airflow equal to the person's minute ventilation (total volume of gas in liters exhaled from the lung per minute). A high-liter flow system administers a volume of oxygen designed to exceed the volume of air required for the person's minute ventilation. **The low-liter flow system is less drying than the high-liter flow system, and humidification is unnecessary. A humidifier is a mechanical device that adds water vapor to air in a particle size that can carry moisture to the small airways.**

26. 1. **An upright sitting position in a bed or a chair facilitates maximum thoracic excursion because it permits the diaphragm to contract without pressure being exerted against it by abdominal viscera.**
2. The side-lying position is not ideal for the use of an incentive spirometer because it limits thoracic expansion. The side-lying position allows abdominal viscera to exert pressure against the diaphragm during inspiration, and the lung on the lower side of the body is compressed by the weight of the body.
3. Although the orthopneic position allows for thoracic expansion, leaning forward with the arms on an over-bed table does not free the hands for holding the spirometer.
4. The low-Fowler position does not maximize the effects of gravity. In the high-Fowler position, gravity moves abdominal viscera away from the diaphragm and thus facilitates the contraction of the diaphragm, both of which promote thoracic expansion.

27. 1. Ensuring a fluid intake of at least 3,000 mL is unnecessary. A fluid intake of approximately 2,000 mL is adequate.
2. Although providing for adequate pain relief is extremely important, it is not the priority.
3. **A tension pneumothorax may occur if the integrity of the chest drainage system becomes compromised (e.g., open to atmospheric pressure, clogged drainage tube, or mechanical dysfunction). Maintaining respiratory functioning is the priority.**

4. Although repositioning is done to promote drainage of secretions from lung segments and aeration of lung tissue, it is not the priority.

28. 1. **Postoperative clients often experience hypoventilation, immobility, and ineffective coughing that may lead to stasis of respiratory secretions and the multiplication of microorganisms, causing hypostatic pneumonia. Dyspnea results from decreased lung compliance, chest pain results from coughing and the increased work of breathing, and purulent sputum results from the presence of pathogens.**

2. Hypovolemic shock is characterized by tachycardia, tachypnea, and hypotension.

3. Thrombophlebitis is characterized by localized pain, swelling, warmth, and erythema. If a thrombus breaks loose and travels through the venous circulation to the lung (pulmonary embolus), it will cause dyspnea and chest pain, not purulent sputum.

4. Pneumothorax is characterized by a sudden onset of sharp pain on inspiration, dyspnea, tachycardia, and hypotension.

29. 1. Although muscle deterioration (atrophy) can occur with immobility, it is unrelated to hypercoagulability. Muscle atrophy is the decrease in the size of a muscle resulting from disuse.

2. **Immobility promotes venous vasodilation, venous stasis, and hypercoagulability of the blood, which can precipitate the formation of a clot in a vein of the leg (venous thrombus) and inflammation of the vein (phlebitis). This results in pain.**

3. Hypotension, an abnormally low systolic blood pressure (less than 100 mm Hg), is not related to hypercoagulability precipitated by immobility.

4. Bradypnea, abnormally slow breathing (less than 10 breaths per minute), is unrelated to hypercoagulability caused by immobility.

30. 1. A productive cough indicates that the person is managing respiratory secretions adequately and keeping the airway patent.

2. A sore throat indicates posterior oropharyngeal irritation or inflammation. This may or may not progress to respiratory distress.

3. **Orthopnea, the ability to breathe easily only in an upright (standing or sitting) position, is a classic sign of respiratory distress. The upright position permits maximum thoracic expansion because the abdominal organs do not press against the diaphragm and inspiration is aided by the principle of gravity.**

4. Eupnea is respirations that are quiet, rhythmic, and effortless within the expected rate per minute for age.

31. 1. The use of a toe for pulse oximetry can result in inaccurate results because of concurrent problems, such as vasoconstriction, hypothermia, impaired peripheral circulation, and movement of the foot.

2. **An earlobe is an excellent site to monitor pulse oximetry. It is least affected by decreased blood flow, has greater accuracy at lower saturations, and rarely is edematous. This site is used for intermittent, not continuous, monitoring.**

3. Soap and water will not resolve edema. In addition, attaching a pulse oximeter clip sensor to an edematous finger is contraindicated because interstitial fluid interferes with obtaining an accurate oxygen saturation level.

4. The cause of the edema must be identified first because range-of-motion exercises may be contraindicated.

32. 1. Tightening the strap around the head is unsafe because it can compress the capillaries under the strap, which may interfere with tissue perfusion and result in pressure ulcers.

2. Reapplying the mask every time the client pulls it off may increase the client's agitation and it is impractical.

3. Providing an explanation of why the oxygen is necessary will probably be ineffective because an agitated client often does not understand cause and effect.

4. **Agitated, confused clients generally tolerate a nasal cannula better than a face mask. A nasal cannula (nasal prongs) is less intrusive than a mask. Masks are oppressive and may cause a client to feel claustrophobic.**

33. 1. A hematocrit of 45% is within the expected range for hematocrit for men (42% to 52%). The expected hematocrit range for women is 36% to 48%.

2. **A hemoglobin of 10 g/dL is less than the expected range for hemoglobin for men (14.0 to 17.4 g/dL). The expected hemoglobin range for women is 12.0 to 16.0 g/dL.**

3. Adequate oxygen levels of more than 95% are necessary to meet the metabolic demands of activity that requires muscle contraction.

4. A white blood cell (WBC) count of 7,500 cells/mcL is within the expected range of 3,500 to 10,500 cells/mcL for WBCs. WBCs are not related to a client's oxygenation status; they are related to protecting the client from infection.

5. A red blood cell count of 4.8 million cells/mcL is within the expected range of 4.2 to 5.4 million cells/mcL for red blood cells for men.

34. 2. **Holding the incentive spirometer level prevents factors, such as friction and gravity, from altering the correct function of the device.**

5. **A firm seal around the mouthpiece is necessary during inhalation, but the mouthpiece should be removed during exhalation.**

1. **Inspiration should be accomplished through a slow, deep breath. A rapid, forceful inhalation can collapse the airway and is contraindicated.**

4. **When the visual indicator reaches the preset goal during inhalation, the inhalation should be maintained for 2 to 6 seconds to ensure ventilation of the alveoli.**

3. **Each exhalation should be an unforced, normal exhalation. A seal does not need to be maintained around the mouthpiece.**

35. **Answer: 408 mg.**
To solve this problem, first convert 150 pounds to its equivalent in kilograms by using the formula for ratio and proportion.

$$\frac{\text{Desired}}{\text{Have}} \quad \frac{150\ lb}{2.2\ lb} = \frac{x\ kg}{1\ kg}$$
$$2.2\ x = 150$$
$$x = 150 \div 2.2$$
$$x = 68.18\ kg$$

Round down to 68 because 0.18 is less than 0.5.
150 lb is equivalent to 68 kg.

Next, calculate the number of milligrams to be administered by multiplying the client's weight in kilograms by the prescribed dose per kilogram: 68 kg × 6 mg = 408 mg.

36. 1. In older adults, atrophy and thinning of both the epithelial and subcutaneous layers of tissue occur, collagenous attachments become less effective, sebaceous gland activity decreases, and interstitial fluid decreases. These changes lead to decreased skin elasticity and the potential to take longer for an incision to heal. However, these are not life-threatening complications associated with surgery and the aging process.

2. In older adults, bladder muscles weaken, bladder capacity decreases, the micturition reflex is delayed, emptying of the bladder becomes more difficult, and residual volume increases. However, these are not life-threatening complications associated with surgery and age-related changes.

3. In older adults, there is an increased threshold for sensations of pain, touch, and temperature because of age-related changes in the nerves and nerve conduction. This is not a life-threatening complication associated with surgery and the aging process.

4. **Age-related changes in older adults include calcification of costal cartilage (making the trachea and rib cage more rigid), an increase in the anteroposterior chest diameter, and weakening of thoracic muscles. These changes decrease respiratory excursion, which can result in multiple life-threatening postoperative complications such as atelectasis and hypostatic pneumonia.**

5. In older adults, there is a decrease in functioning capacity of the heart and vascular system. Atherosclerosis of the aorta, coronary arteries, and carotid arteries could decrease cardiac output, impair circulation to vital organs and distal extremities, and increase the workload of the heart at times of stress. These age-related changes are associated with life-threatening dysrhythmias, thrombophlebitis, and pulmonary emboli.

37. 1. These are the instructions for using an incentive spirometer. An incentive spirometer is designed to have a person deep breathe and expand the lungs to help prevent respiratory complications of immobility.

2. These are the instructions for using a nebulizer. A nebulizer is a medication delivery system that delivers aerosol spray, which is inhaled via a mouthpiece. Breathing deeply and slowly facilitates contact of the medication with the respiratory tract mucosa.

3. These are the instructions for assessing tidal volume. Tidal volume is the volume of air inhaled and exhaled with each normal breath; a tidal volume is approximately 500 mL.

4. **These are the instructions for using a peak expiratory flowmeter (PEFM), which is the device in the photograph. A PEFM measures the peak expiratory flow rate (PEFR). A PEFR is the volume of air that can be forcefully exhaled after taking a deep breath.**

38. 1. **Coughing and deep breathing should be encouraged because this helps to expand the lungs.**

2. Clamping the tube when providing for activities of daily living is contraindicated because clamping a chest tube may cause a tension pneumothorax.

3. **The chest drainage system should be kept below the level of the insertion site to promote the flow of drainage from the pleural space and prevent the flow of drainage back into the pleural space.**

4. **An airtight dressing seals the pleural space from the environment. If the pleural space is left open to the environment, atmospheric pressure causes air to enter the pleural space, which results in a tension pneumothorax.**

5. Emptying chest tube drainage every shift is unnecessary. Chest drainage systems are closed, self-contained systems that have a chamber for drainage. At routine intervals (as per hospital policy), the date, time, and nurse's initials mark the level of drainage on the drainage collection chamber.

6. **Avoiding using pins to secure tubing averts the risk of puncturing the tubing, which will cause an air leak.**

39. 1. Postural hypotension is unrelated to thrombophlebitis. Postural hypotension (orthostatic hypotension) is a decrease in blood pressure related to positional or postural changes from the lying down to sitting or standing positions.

2. **Dyspnea is a clinical manifestation of a pulmonary embolus, a life-threatening condition. A thrombus that breaks loose from a vein wall and travels through the circulation (embolus) eventually will obstruct a pulmonary artery or one of its branches (pulmonary embolus).**

3. Blanchable erythema is unrelated to thrombophlebitis. Blanchable erythema (reactive hyperemia) is a reddened area caused by localized vasodilation in response to lack of blood flow to the underlying tissue. The reddened area will turn pale with fingertip pressure.

4. Dependent edema is unrelated to thrombophlebitis. Although fluid will collect in the interstitial compartment (edema) around a thrombophlebitis, it is localized, not dependent, edema. Dependent edema is the collection of fluid in the interstitial tissues below the level of the heart; it occurs bilaterally and usually is caused by cardiopulmonary problems.

5. **Immobility promotes *venous stasis*, which, in conjunction with *hypercoagulability* and *injury to vessel walls*, predisposes clients to thrombophlebitis. These three factors are known as Virchow's triad. A thrombus can break loose from the vein wall and travel through the circulation (embolus), where eventually it obstructs a pulmonary artery or one of its branches and causes sudden, acute chest pain, dyspnea, coughing, and frothy sputum.**

40. 1. This is not the equipment used for the purpose of gastric lavage.

2. **The nurse is preparing to collect a sputum specimen via suctioning. The nurse is attaching a catheter to a sputum trap that attaches to the suction tubing.**

3. This is not the equipment used for gastric decompression.

4. This is not the equipment used to administer a nebulizer treatment.

41. 1. **A water-based lubricant will keep the nares supple. An oil-based lubricant should not be used because volatile, flammable substances can ignite in the presence of oxygen.**

2. Adjusting the flowmeter to the prescribed oxygen flow rate ensures that the client is receiving the accurate dose of oxygen.
3. Reassessing the client's skin for signs of pressure every 2 hours ensures that tissue irritation or capillary compression does not occur from the nasal prongs or tubing. The tubing should be snug enough to keep the nasal prongs from becoming displaced but loose enough not to compress or irritate tissue.
4. Placing the nasal prongs curving downward in the nares follows the natural curve of the nasal passages, preventing injury.
5. Looping the tubing over the client's ears and adjusting it gently under the chin is the correct placement of the tubing. A firm adjustment can cause pressure ulcers around the ears.

42. 1. A dysrhythmia, a heart rate with an irregular rhythm, can occur with hypoxia but it is a late response.
2. Hypoxia is insufficient oxygen anywhere in the body. An early sign of hypoxia is restlessness, which is caused by impaired cerebral perfusion of oxygen.
3. Irritability is an early sign of hypoxia caused by impaired cerebral perfusion of oxygen.
4. Cyanosis, a bluish discoloration of the skin and mucous membranes caused by reduced oxygen in the blood, is a late sign of hypoxia.
5. Apnea, a complete absence of respirations, is the cause of, not a response to, hypoxia.

43. 1. Simvastatin 20 mg once a day is within the expected dose range of 5 to 40 mg daily and is not a cause for concern. Simvastatin, a lipid-lowering agent, should be taken in the evening because the body produces the most cholesterol overnight.
2. A pulse rate of 100 beats per minute is within the expected range of 60 to 100 beats per minute and is not a cause for concern.
3. An oxygen saturation level of 85% is a cause for concern. An oxygen saturation level of 95% to 100% is considered

expected. An oxygen saturation level of less than 90% is considered low and is associated with hypoxemia.
4. A WBC count of 8,000 cells/mcL is within the expected range of 3,500 to 10,500 cells/mcL and is not a cause for concern.

44. 4. The first step is to attach the flowmeter to the wall oxygen source. The flowmeter controls the amount of oxygen delivered.
3. The second step is to attach the prefilled humidifier to the flowmeter. Humidification reduces drying of the respiratory system mucous membranes and is essential when oxygen delivery is 4 L or higher.
5. The third step is attaching the mask's tubing to the humidifier. This prepares the equipment for use.
6. The fourth step is turning on the oxygen flow rate to 6 L. This primes the tubing and mask with oxygen so that there is no delay once the mask is applied to the client's face.
1. The fifth step is placing the mask on the client's face. Applying it from the bridge of the client's nose to under the chin limits oxygen from leaking around the edges of the mask.
2. The sixth step is securing the elastic bands around the back of the client's head. This helps to hold the mask in position.

45. Answer: 2 tablets. First, determine the number of milligrams prescribed for each dose. Divide the daily dose (40 mg) by the number of times the medication should be administered (two times, once in the morning and once in the evening): 40 ÷ 2 = 20 mg per dose. The package insert for zafirlukast states that each tablet is 10 mg. Solve the problem by using the formula for ratio and proportion.

$$\frac{Desired}{Have} \frac{20\ mg}{10\ mg} = \frac{x\ tablet}{1\ tablet}$$
$$10\ x = 20\ mg$$
$$x = 20 \div 10$$
$$x = 2\ tablets$$

Urinary Elimination

KEYWORDS

The following words include English vocabulary, nursing/medical terminology, concepts, principles, and information relevant to content specifically addressed in the chapter or associated with topics presented in it. English dictionaries, nursing textbooks, and medical dictionaries, such as *Taber's Cyclopedic Medical Dictionary,* are resources that can be used to expand your knowledge and understanding of these words and related information.

Acidic urine

Anuria

Bacteriuria

Bladder cues

Bladder irritability

Bladder training

Catheter port

Commode chair

Credé maneuver

Cystoscopy

Detrusor muscles

Dysuria

Enuresis

Excretion

Foreskin

Fracture bedpan

Frequency

Glomerular filtration rate

Graduate

Hematuria

Hesitancy

Incontinence, types:
   Functional
   Overflow
   Reflex
   Stress
   Total
   Urge

Incontinent

Kegel exercises

Ketones

Micturition

Nocturia

Oliguria

Perineal care

Polyuria

Prostate

Pyuria

Reagent strips

Renal calculi

Renal perfusion

Residual urine

Retention

Specific gravity

Suprapubic distention

Trigone

Turbidity

Urea

Ureter

Urethra

Urgency

Urinary catheters:
   Condom (Texas)
   Indwelling (retention, Foley)
   Straight
   Suprapubic

Urinary diuresis

Urinary diversion

Urinary drainage system

Urinary meatus

Urinary obstruction

Urinary output

Urinary tract infection

Urine clarity

Urine specimens:
   24-hour urine collection
   Clean catch
   From a catheter port
   Urinalysis

Void

URINARY ELIMINATION: QUESTIONS

1. A nurse identifies that the client has overflow incontinence. Which factor contributes to this clinical manifestation?
   1. Coughing
   2. Mobility deficits
   3. Prostate enlargement
   4. Urinary tract infection

2. A nurse must measure the intake and output (I&O) of a client who has a urinary retention catheter. Which equipment is **most** appropriate to use to measure urine output from a urinary retention catheter accurately?
   1. Urinal
   2. Graduate
   3. Large syringe
   4. Urine collection bag

3. A client's urine is cloudy, is amber, and has an unpleasant odor. Which problem may this information indicate that requires the nurse to make a focused assessment?
   1. Urinary retention
   2. Urinary tract infection
   3. Ketone bodies in the urine
   4. High urinary calcium level

4. A nurse is caring for a debilitated female client with nocturia. Which nursing intervention is the **priority** when planning to meet this client's needs?
   1. Encouraging the use of bladder training exercises
   2. Providing assistance with toileting every 4 hours
   3. Positioning a bedside commode near the bed
   4. Teaching the avoidance of fluids after 5 p.m.

5. A primary health-care provider prescribes a urine specimen for culture and sensitivity via a straight catheter for a client. Which should the nurse do when collecting this urine specimen?
   1. Use a sterile specimen container.
   2. Collect urine from the catheter port.
   3. Inflate the balloon with sterile water.
   4. Have the client void before collecting the specimen.

6. A nurse reviews the results of a client's urinalysis. Which constituent found in urine indicates the presence of an abnormality that should be reported to the primary health-care provider?
   1. Electrolytes
   2. Protein
   3. Water
   4. Urea

7. A client reports burning on urination. Which question should the nurse ask to **best** obtain information about the client's dysuria?
   1. "Can you tell me about the problems you are having with urination?"
   2. "How would you describe your experience with incontinence?"
   3. "What are your usual bowel habits?"
   4. "What color is your urine?"

8. A nurse is caring for a group of clients with a variety of urinary problems. Which physical response identified by the nurse should cause the **most** concern?
   1. Anuria
   2. Dysuria
   3. Diuresis
   4. Enuresis

9. A nurse is performing a physical assessment on a newly admitted client who is experiencing urinary incontinence. Which problem identified by the nurse is often associated with this problem?
   1. Chronic pain
   2. Reduced fluid intake
   3. Disturbed self-esteem
   4. Insufficient knowledge

10. A nurse is caring for two clients. One client has reflex incontinence and the other has total incontinence. Which characteristic is common to both reflex incontinence and total incontinence?
    1. Small loss of urine after an increase in intra-abdominal pressure
    2. Loss of urine without awareness of bladder fullness
    3. Retention of urine with intermittent urine overflow
    4. Strong, sudden desire to pass urine

11. Which clinical manifestation can a nurse expect when a postoperative client experiences stress associated with surgery?
    1. Decreased urinary output
    2. Low specific gravity
    3. Reflex incontinence
    4. Urinary hesitancy

12. Which assessment is not related to monitoring both urine and stool?
    1. Constituents
    2. Urgency
    3. Shape
    4. Color

13. A nurse is assessing the urinary status of a client. Which sign indicates that additional nursing assessments are necessary?
    1. Aromatic odor
    2. Pale yellow urine
    3. Output of 50 mL hourly
    4. Specific gravity of 1.035

14. A client tells the nurse, "I have to urinate as soon as I get the urge to go." For which contributing factor to urinary urgency should the nurse implement a focused assessment?
    1. Anesthesia
    2. Dehydration
    3. Full bladder
    4. Urinary tract infection

15. Which is an effective nursing intervention to prevent urinary tract infections?
    1. Teach female clients to wipe from the back to the front after urinating.
    2. Advise clients to report burning on urination to health-care providers.
    3. Instruct clients to use bath powder to absorb perineal perspiration.
    4. Encourage clients to drink several quarts of fluid daily.

16. A client has urinary incontinence. Which is the **best** nursing intervention for this client?
    1. Providing skin care immediately after soiling
    2. Using a deodorant soap when providing skin care
    3. Drying the area well after providing perineal care
    4. Dusting the perineal area with a light film of cornstarch

17. A confused client is incontinent of urine and stool and smears the stool on the bed linens and bed rails. Which should be the **initial** client goal?
    1. The client will be clean and dry continuously.
    2. The client will become continent within a week.
    3. The client will stop soiling the environment immediately.
    4. The client will call for the bedpan whenever the urge to eliminate occurs.

18. A client has a urinary retention catheter. Which is **most** important when the nurse cares for this client?
    1. Applying an antimicrobial agent to the urinary meatus 2 times a day
    2. Ensuring that the catheter remains connected to the collection bag
    3. Wearing sterile gloves when accessing the specimen port
    4. Increasing fluid intake to 3,000 mL a day

19. Which information about a client is communicated when a nurse documents that the client has polyuria?
    1. Excreting excessive amounts of urine
    2. Experiencing pain on urination
    3. Retaining urine in the bladder
    4. Passing blood in the urine

20. A client is experiencing bladder irritability. Which fluid should the nurse teach the client to include in the diet?
    1. Beer
    2. Coffee
    3. Orange juice
    4. Cranberry juice

21. Which clinical manifestation identified by the nurse commonly is associated with excessive production of antidiuretic hormone (ADH)?
    1. Diuresis
    2. Oliguria
    3. Retention
    4. Incontinence

22. A nurse must obtain a urine specimen from a client. Which nursing intervention is the greatest help to **most** people who need to void for a urine test?
    1. Exerting manual pressure on the abdomen
    2. Encouraging a backward rocking motion
    3. Running water in the sink
    4. Providing for privacy

23. A client is admitted to the emergency department because of hypertension and oliguria. For which additional clinical manifestation associated with this cluster of information should the nurse assess the client?
    1. Thirst
    2. Retention
    3. Weight gain
    4. Urinary hesitancy

24. A nurse must obtain a clean-catch urine specimen from one client and a urine specimen via a straight catheterization from another. Which intervention is not performed for both when obtaining these specimens?
    1. Cleanse around the urinary meatus with antiseptic swabs.
    2. Send the specimen to the laboratory immediately.
    3. Use a sterile cup to collect the specimen.
    4. Wear sterile gloves during the procedure.

25. A primary health-care provider discusses the need for a cystoscopy with a client. Which is **most** important for the nurse to do when caring for this client before the cystoscopy?
    1. Monitor the client's I&O.
    2. Assess the client's urine routinely.
    3. Encourage the client to increase the intake of oral fluids.
    4. Have the client sign an informed consent form before the procedure.

26. An older adult with an indwelling urinary catheter is receiving 75 mL of 0.9% sodium chloride hourly. The client has had several hospital admissions in the last year for dehydration. The nurse is concerned about the client's renal function. What is the **best** intervention by the nurse to assess this client's renal functioning?
    1. Inspect the client's dependent areas for signs of edema.
    2. Calculate the client's intake and output every shift.
    3. Monitor the client's urine output hourly.
    4. Obtain the client's weight daily.

27. A nurse is inserting an indwelling urinary catheter into a male client. The nurse feels firm resistance while inserting the urinary catheter through the penis. What should the nurse do?
    1. Lower the penis until it is parallel to the length of the body.
    2. Inflate the balloon of the catheter with 10 mL of normal saline.
    3. Stop the procedure and notify the health-care provider about the resistance.
    4. Use a twisting motion and firmly advance the catheter 2 inches farther into the penis.

28. When a nurse assesses a client, which clinical manifestations **support** the presence of urinary retention? **Select all that apply.**
    1. _____ Nocturia
    2. _____ Hematuria
    3. _____ Bladder contractions
    4. _____ Suprapubic distention
    5. _____ Frequent small voidings

29. A nurse plans to clamp a client's urinary drainage system to obtain a urine specimen for a urine culture and sensitivity. Indicate with an X, on the figure below, where the nurse should clamp the catheter drainage system.

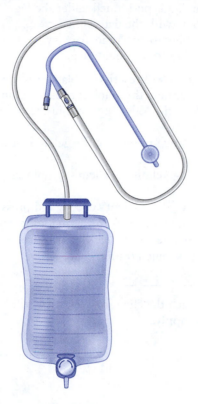

30. A nurse is caring for a client with a condom catheter. Which of the following is important to implement? **Select all that apply.**
1. _____ Avoiding kinks in the collection tubing
2. _____ Providing perineal care at least once a day
3. _____ Confirming that the adhesive band is not too tight
4. _____ Leaving 1 inch between the glans penis and drainage tubing
5. _____ Ensuring that the foreskin is over the glans penis before the catheter is applied

31. A primary health-care provider prescribes 250 mL 0.9% sodium chloride to be administered over 30 minutes to challenge a client's kidneys to produce urine. The nurse obtains an electronic infusion device to administer the solution. At what rate should the nurse program the infusion device? **Record your answer using a whole number.**

Answer: _____ mL/hr.

32. A nurse is caring for a female client on bedrest who has a urinary retention catheter. Which should the nurse do? **Select all that apply.**
1. _____ Position the tubing through the side rail of the bed.
2. _____ Ensure the tubing is positioned under the leg.
3. _____ Label the tubing with the date of insertion.
4. _____ Irrigate the tubing to ensure its patency.
5. _____ Secure the tubing to the client's leg.

33. A primary health-care provider prescribes a bladder ultrasound scan to be performed after a client voids to determine the amount of residual urine. The nurse explains the test to the client. Place the following steps in the order that they should be performed by the nurse.
1. Clean the client's abdomen to remove the gel and clean the scan head with isopropyl alcohol.
2. Put 5 mL of conducting gel on the client's symphysis pubis and place the scan head on the gel.
3. Aim the scan head toward the client's coccyx and press the scan head button.
4. Drape the client, exposing only the lower abdomen and suprapubic area.
5. Obtain the bladder volume and repeat the measurement several times.
6. Place the client in the supine position.

   Answer: _____

34. Which should a nurse teach the client to avoid that will help prevent urinary diuresis? **Select all that apply.**
1. _____ Narcotics
2. _____ Caffeine
3. _____ Activity
4. _____ Alcohol
5. _____ Protein

35. A primary health-care provider prescribes furosemide 40 mg to be added to 50 mL of D_5W to infuse at a rate of 3 mg/minute. Furosemide for IV infusion is 10 mg/mL. The nurse uses a secondary infusion set that has a drop factor of 10. How many drops per minute should the nurse administer?

   Answer: _____ drops/minute.

36. Which should the nurse implement to facilitate bladder continence for a male client who is cognitively impaired? **Select all that apply.**
1. _____ Offer toileting reminders every 2 hours.
2. _____ Apply a condom catheter in the morning.
3. _____ Provide clothing that is easy to manipulate.
4. _____ Encourage avoidance of fluids between meals.
5. _____ Explain the need to call for help with toileting every 4 hours.

37. When the nurse is planning nursing care, which factor in the client's history places the client at risk for stress incontinence? **Select all that apply.**
1. _____ Lumbar spinal cord injury
2. _____ Urinary obstruction
3. _____ Six vaginal births
4. _____ Menopause
5. _____ Obesity

38. A client returns from the surgical unit after a transurethral resection of the prostate gland. The nurse reviews the primary health-care provider's prescriptions, obtains the client's vital signs, and performs a focused client assessment. Which is the **best** intervention by the nurse?

1. Discontinue the continuous compression devices to the lower extremities.
2. Notify the surgeon of the status of the client's urinary drainage.
3. Obtain the client's temperature using a rectal thermometer.
4. Increase the flow rate of the continuous bladder irrigation.

CLIENT'S CLINICAL RECORD

Primary Health-Care Provider's Prescriptions

Regular diet
Vital signs every 4 hours
IV morphine via PCA pump: basal rate 1.5 mg/hour; PCA dose 1 mg; lockout interval
    12 minutes; maximum dose over 4 hours, 26 mg
IVF: 0.9% sodium chloride 125 mL/hour
Docusate sodium 100 mg PO once daily
Out of bed to chair in p.m., ambulate twice a day
Continuous compression devices to lower extremities when in bed
Continuous bladder irrigation 0.9% sodium chloride to run at rate to keep output pink

Client's Vital Signs

Temperature: 100.2°F, oral
Pulse: 88 beats per minute
Respirations: 20 breaths per minute
Blood pressure: 136/80 mm Hg

Focused Physical Assessment

IVF: 0.9% sodium chloride at 125 mL/hour, insertion site right forearm with no signs of infiltration or infection. Continuous compression devices in place. Pedal pulses palpable, toes pink and warm to touch. Client reporting abdominal pain of 2 on scale of 0 to 10 with occasional severe abdominal cramps. CBI in progress at 150 mL per hour. Urinary drainage is light red with numerous clots.

39. A client who had prostate surgery has a continuous bladder irrigation (CBI) in place. The nurse maintains the CBI at 200 mL/hour of GU irrigant as prescribed. The urine drainage bag was emptied several times during the course of the shift for a total of 3,200 mL. How many milliliters should the nurse calculate was urine at the end of the 12-hour shift? **Record your answer using a whole number.**

Answer: _____ mL.

40. A nurse must obtain a urine specimen for a culture and sensitivity test from a client who has an indwelling urinary catheter. Place the following steps in the order in which they should be performed.

1. Wash your hands and don clean gloves.
2. Remove the clamp from the drainage tubing.
3. Drain the urine in the tubing into the drainage bag.
4. Clamp the drainage tubing below the specimen port for 15 to 30 minutes.
5. Swab the specimen port with an antiseptic and aspirate urine via a sterile syringe.
6. Transfer the urine to a sterile specimen cup and discard the syringe into a sharps container.

Answer: _____

1. 1. Coughing, which raises the intra-abdominal pressure, is related to stress incontinence, not overflow incontinence.
  2. Mobility deficits, such as spinal cord injuries, are related to reflex incontinence, not overflow incontinence.
  3. **An enlarged prostate compresses the urethra and interferes with the outflow of urine, resulting in urinary retention. With urinary retention, the pressure within the bladder builds until the external urethral sphincter temporarily opens to allow a small volume (25 to 60 mL) of urine to escape (overflow incontinence).**
  4. Urinary tract infections are related to urge incontinence, not overflow incontinence.

2. 1. Although urinals have volume markings on the side, usually they occur in 100-mL increments that do not promote accurate measurements.
  2. **A graduate is a collection container with volume markings (usually at 25-mL increments) that promote accurate measurements of urine volume.**
  3. Using a large syringe is impractical. A large syringe is used to obtain a sterile specimen from a retention catheter (Foley catheter).
  4. A urine collection bag is flexible and balloons outward as urine collects. In addition, the volume markings are at 100-mL increments that do not promote accurate measurements.

3. 1. The clinical manifestations indicated in the question do not reflect urinary retention. Urinary retention is evidenced by suprapubic distention and lack of voiding or small, frequent voidings (overflow incontinence).
  2. **The urine appears concentrated (amber) and cloudy because of the presence of bacteria, white blood cells, and red blood cells. The unpleasant odor is caused by pus in the urine (pyuria).**
  3. The clinical manifestations indicated in the question do not reflect ketone bodies in the urine. A reagent strip dipped in urine will measure the presence of ketone bodies.
  4. The clinical manifestations indicated in the question do not reflect excessive calcium in the urine. Urine calcium levels are measured by assessing a 24-hour urine specimen.

4. 1. Although encouraging the use of bladder training exercises should be done, it is not the priority.

2. Toileting the client every 4 hours may be too often or not often enough for the client. Care should be individualized for the client.
3. **The use of a commode requires less energy than using a bedpan and is safer than walking to the bathroom. Sitting on a commode uses gravity to empty the bladder fully and thus prevents urinary stasis.**
4. Fluids may be decreased during the last 2 hours before bedtime, but they should not be avoided completely after 5 p.m. Some fluid intake is necessary for adequate renal perfusion.

5. 1. **A culture attempts to identify the microorganisms present in the urine, and a sensitivity study identifies the antibiotics that are effective against the isolated microorganisms. A sterile specimen container is used to prevent contamination of the specimen by microorganisms outside the body.**
  2. The urine from a straight catheter (single-lumen tube) flows directly into the specimen container. Collecting a urine specimen from a catheter port is necessary when the client has a urinary retention catheter.
  3. A straight catheter has a single lumen for draining urine from the bladder. A straight catheter does not remain in the bladder and therefore does not have a second lumen for water to be inserted into a balloon.
  4. Having the client void before collecting the specimen may result in no urine left in the bladder for the straight catheter to collect. A minimum of 3 mL of urine is necessary for a specimen for urine culture and sensitivity.

6. 1. Electrolytes are usual constituents of urine, and they fluctuate to help maintain fluid, electrolyte, and acid-base balance.
  2. **The presence of protein in the urine indicates that the glomeruli have become too permeable, which occurs with kidney disease. Most plasma proteins are too large to move out of the glomeruli, and the small proteins that enter the filtrate are reabsorbed by pinocytosis.**
  3. Urine usually is composed of 95% water.
  4. Urea is an expected constituent of urine. It is formed by liver cells when excess amino acids are broken down (deaminated) to be used for energy production.

7. **1.** **This open-ended question encourages the client to talk about the problem from a personal perspective. Follow-up questions can be more specific.**

    2. Dysuria is not necessarily related to incontinence.

    3. Dysuria is a problem associated with urine, not fecal, elimination.

    4. Although an abnormal color of urine may indicate a potential urinary tract infection, which is associated with dysuria, the question is too narrow because it focuses on only one issue.

8. **1.** **The inability to produce urine (anuria) is a life-threatening situation. If the cause is not corrected, the client will need dialysis to correct fluid and electrolyte imbalances and rid the body of the waste products of metabolism.**

    2. Although dysuria is a concern because it may indicate a urinary tract infection, it is not as serious as a response in another option.

    3. The secretion and excretion of large amounts of urine (diuresis) are a concern, but they are not as serious as a response in another option.

    4. Involuntary discharge of urine after an age when bladder control should be established (enuresis) is a concern, but it is not as serious as a response in another option.

9. **1.** Urinary incontinence usually is not related to chronic pain. Chronic pain is the state in which an individual experiences pain that is persistent or intermittent and lasts for longer than 6 months.

    2. Reduced fluid intake is unrelated to urinary incontinence. A reduced fluid intake places an individual at risk of experiencing vascular, interstitial, or intracellular dehydration.

    3. **Disturbed self-esteem is the state in which an individual experiences, or is at risk of experiencing, negative self-evaluation about self or capabilities. Incontinence may be viewed by a client as regressing to childlike behavior and has a negative impact on feelings about the self.**

    4. Urinary incontinence may be unpreventable and uncontrollable. Sufficient knowledge may not prevent or promote continence. Insufficient knowledge is the state in which an individual experiences a deficiency in cognitive information or psychomotor skills, concerning a condition or treatment plan.

10. **1.** Urination after an increase in intra-abdominal pressure is unrelated to both reflex and total incontinence. Urination after an increase in intra-abdominal pressure is related to stress incontinence, which is an immediate involuntary loss of a small volume of urine during an increase in intra-abdominal pressure.

    2. **Involuntary voiding and a lack of awareness of bladder distention are related directly to both reflex incontinence and total incontinence. Reflex incontinence is the predictable, involuntary loss of urine with no sensation of urgency, the need to void, or bladder fullness. Total incontinence is the continuous unpredictable loss of urine without distention or awareness of bladder fullness.**

    3. Retention of urine with overflow incontinence is related to urinary retention, which is the chronic inability to void followed by involuntary voiding (overflow incontinence).

    4. A strong, sudden desire to void is related to urge incontinence, which is an involuntary loss of urine associated with a strong, sudden desire to void.

11. **1.** **During surgery, because of the effects of the general adaptation syndrome, the posterior pituitary secretes antidiuretic hormone (ADH) that promotes water reabsorption in the kidney tubules. Also, the anterior pituitary secretes adrenocorticotropic hormone that stimulates the adrenal cortex to secrete aldosterone, which reabsorbs sodium and thus water.**

    2. A low specific gravity reflects dilute urine. With the stress response, urine will be concentrated and specific gravity will be elevated.

    3. The stress response is unrelated to reflex incontinence. Reflex incontinence is a predictable, involuntary loss of urine with no sensation of urgency, the need to void, or bladder fullness.

    4. The stress response is unrelated to urinary hesitancy. Hesitancy is the involuntary delay in initiating urination.

12. **1.** Both urine and stool have usual constituents. Urine has organic constituents (e.g., urea, uric acid, and creatinine) and inorganic constituents (e.g., ammonia, sodium, chloride, potassium, and calcium). Feces have waste residues of digestion (e.g., bile, intestinal secretions, and bacteria) and inorganic constituents (e.g., calcium and phosphorus).

2. A person can feel an overwhelming need to void as well as defecate.

3. **Only stool can be assessed regarding shape. Stool usually is tubular in shape. Urine is a liquid that assumes the shape of the container in which it is collected.**

4. Both urine and stool can be assessed for color. Stool usually is brown and urine usually is yellow, straw-colored, or amber, depending on its concentration.

13. 1. An aromatic odor is the usual odor of urine.

2. Urine usually is pale yellow, straw-colored, or amber, depending on its concentration.

3. Adequate renal perfusion and kidney function are reflected by an hourly urine output of 30 mL or more of urine.

4. **Specific gravity is the measure of the concentration of dissolved solids in the urine. The expected range is 1.001 to 1.029. A specific gravity of 1.035 indicates concentrated urine.**

14. 1. Anesthesia is a central nervous system depressant that tends to cause urinary retention, not urgency.

2. Dehydration causes a decrease in renal perfusion resulting in a diminished capacity to form urine (oliguria), not urgency.

3. The urinary bladder does not have to be full to precipitate the urge to void. The urge to void can be felt when 150 to 200 mL of urine collects and stimulates the trigone of the urinary bladder.

4. **Feeling the need to void immediately (urgency) occurs most often when the urinary bladder is irritated. In the adult, the usual bladder capacity is 400 to 600 mL of urine, although the desire to urinate can be sensed when it contains as little as 150 to 200 mL. As the volume increases, the bladder wall stretches, sending sensory messages to the sacral spinal cord, and parasympathetic impulses stimulate the detrusor muscle to contract rhythmically. Bladder contractions precipitate nerve impulses that travel up the spinal cord to the pons and cerebral cortex, where the person experiences a conscious need to void.**

15. 1. The opposite should be done to prevent microorganisms from the intestines (e.g., *Escherichia coli*) from being drawn from the anus toward the urinary meatus. Wiping from front to back follows the principle of clean to dirty.

2. Reporting burning on urination to a health-care provider will not prevent a urinary tract infection. Burning on urination (dysuria) is a response to acidic urine flowing over inflamed mucous membranes and is a sign of a urinary tract infection.

3. Bath powder should be avoided because it has been implicated as a precipitating cause of gynecological cancer and is a respiratory irritant.

4. **Drinking a minimum of 2,000 mL of fluid a day produces adequately dilute urine, washes out solutes, and flushes microorganisms from the distal urethra and urinary meatus.**

16. 1. **As soon as possible after an incontinence episode, the client should receive thorough perineal care with soap and water, and the area should be dried well. This action removes urea from the skin, which can contribute to skin breakdown.**

2. Plain soap, not deodorant soap, is all that is necessary when providing perineal care after urinary or bowel incontinence.

3. Although drying the area well after providing perineal care is done, it is not the best intervention of the options offered.

4. Dusting the perineal area with cornstarch should be avoided. Cornstarch can accumulate in folds of the skin and, when damp, can become like sandpaper, causing friction upon movement and then skin breakdown.

17. 1. **A client's basic physical needs should be given first priority. As soon as a client is incontinent of either urine or stool, the client should receive perineal care. Remaining "continuously" clean and dry meets the criterion of a time frame when writing a goal.**

2. The client may not have the physical, mental, or emotional ability to achieve the goal of becoming continent.

3. The client may not have the physical, mental, or emotional ability to achieve the goal of continence and stop soiling the environment.

4. The client may not have the physical or cognitive ability to achieve the goal of calling for a bedpan.

18. 1. Research demonstrates that cleansing the urinary meatus with soap and water daily is adequate to prevent an infection. An antimicrobial ointment provides no additional benefit. Also, it requires a prescription.
    2. **Maintaining the connection of the catheter to the collection bag prevents the introduction of microorganisms that can cause infection. A urinary retention catheter is a closed system that should remain closed.**
    3. Clean, not sterile, gloves should be worn. Surgical asepsis (use of a sterile syringe and alcohol swab) is necessary when accessing the specimen port on a urinary retention catheter.
    4. Although increasing fluid intake will increase urinary output, thereby flushing the bladder of microorganisms, it is not as important as another option.

19. 1. **Polyuria is an excessive output of urine. This is associated with problems such as diabetes mellitus, diabetes insipidus, the acute (diuresis) phase after a burn injury, and reduced levels of ADH.**
    2. Pain on urination is the description of dysuria, not polyuria.
    3. Retaining urine in the bladder is the description of urinary retention, not polyuria.
    4. Passing blood in the urine is the description of hematuria, not polyuria.

20. 1. Beer contains alcohol, which is irritating to the bladder.
    2. Coffee contains caffeine, which is irritating to the bladder.
    3. Orange juice, a citrus fruit, is irritating to the bladder. Citrus fruits are acidic.
    4. **Cranberries have no constituents that irritate the bladder. In addition, they produce a more acidic environment that is less conducive to the growth of microorganisms and prevents bacteria from adhering to the mucous membranes of the urinary tract, thus promoting bacterial excretion.**

21. 1. Diuresis occurs when there is inadequate ADH.
    2. **ADH increases the reabsorption of water by the kidney tubules, thus decreasing the amount of urine formed. Oliguria is diminished urinary output relative to intake (less than 400 mL in 24 hours).**
    3. With urinary retention, urine is formed, but it accumulates in the bladder and is not excreted.
    4. ADH is unrelated to incontinence.

22. 1. Manual bladder compression (Credé maneuver) is performed when a client has bladder flaccidity.
    2. This rocking motion is used to promote a bowel movement, not voiding.
    3. Although running water in the sink may be helpful, it is not as effective as an intervention in another option.
    4. **Tending to bodily functions is a personal, private activity in the North American culture. Providing privacy supports client dignity and generally promotes voiding.**

23. 1. Thirst is associated with dehydration, not hypertension and oliguria.
    2. Urinary retention is unrelated to hypertension and oliguria. Urinary retention is the inability to empty the bladder. It is caused by urethral obstruction, lesions involving the nerve pathways to and from the bladder or involving reflex centers in the brain or spinal cord, and medications. Urine is retained in the bladder when high urethral pressure inhibits complete emptying of the bladder or until increased abdominal pressure causes urine to be lost involuntarily.
    3. **Oliguria is the inability to produce more than 400 to 500 mL of urine daily. Expected daily urinary output is 1,000 to 3,000 mL, depending on the volume of fluid intake. If urine is not being produced in the presence of an average daily intake of 2,500 mL of fluid, then fluid will be retained and reflected in a gain in weight. One liter of fluid weighs 2.2 pounds. Excess fluid contributes to an increase in circulating blood volume, causing hypertension.**
    4. Urinary hesitancy is an involuntary delay in initiating urination and is unrelated to hypertension and oliguria. It often is related to an enlarged prostate gland.

24. 1. Both tests require the area around the urinary meatus to be swiped several times with an antiseptic solution. This limits the

presence of microorganisms that can contaminate the urine specimen, thus preventing inaccurate test results.

2. Both urine specimens should be sent to the laboratory immediately to prevent deterioration of the specimen that could result in inaccurate results. Casts in the urine will break down if urine is not tested for an extended time.

3. A sterile cup maintains the sterility of the specimen, a requirement of both tests.

4. **Sterile gloves must be worn when obtaining a urine specimen via a catheter. The nurse's hands touch the client and catheter tubing, which must remain sterile. Clean, rather than sterile, gloves are worn when obtaining a clean-catch urine specimen. Urine flowing out of the client is collected midstream into a sterile specimen cup.**

25. 1. Although monitoring the client's I&O may be done, it is not the priority when a cystoscopy is scheduled.

2. Although assessing the client's urine routinely should be done, it is not the priority before the procedure. The amount and color of urine are assessed after the procedure. Pink urine after a cystoscopy is common because of slight bleeding from irritation of the mucous membranes of the urinary tract.

3. Although encouraging the intake of oral fluid before and after the procedure should be done, it is not the most important thing a nurse should do when a cystoscopy is scheduled. Keeping the client well hydrated ensures that adequate intravascular fluid will pass through the kidneys, facilitating the production and passage of urine.

4. **During a cystoscopy, a fiberoptic instrument is inserted through the urethra and into the bladder. It is an invasive procedure that requires the client's written permission. The primary health-care provider's discussion with the client includes the purpose of the procedure, its risks and benefits, and alternatives.**

26. 1. Dependent edema is more of a reflection of cardiac output. Edema associated with renal disease usually is generalized rather than localized in dependent areas.

2. A shift generally is 8 to 12 hours long. A period of 8 to 12 hours is too long a time to wait to collect information.

3. **The kidneys should produce more than 30 mL/hour. The client has an indwelling urinary catheter that facilitates the assessment of urine output hourly. Clients without an indwelling urinary catheter should void a minimum of 240 mL of urine in 8 hours.**

4. Daily weights effectively monitor a client's fluid balance because 1 L of retained fluid weighs 2.2 pounds. However, a 24-hour period is too long a time to wait to collect information.

27. 1. Lowering the penis until it is parallel to the length of the body will increase the trauma to the mucous membranes of the urinary tract because placing the penis parallel to the length of the body will create a 90-degree angle in the urethra where the shaft of the penis meets the abdominal wall. The penis should be held perpendicular to the client's body during catheter insertion.

2. Inflating the balloon of the catheter in this situation will traumatize the urethra and inflict pain. The balloon is inflated once urine flows, and the catheter is advanced another 1 to 2 inches to ensure that it is completely inside the urinary bladder and not the urethra.

3. **Resistance indicates that there may be a blockage in the urethra (e.g., enlarged prostate, tumor). The procedure should be discontinued when firm resistance is felt, to prevent trauma to the urinary system. The event should be documented in the client's clinical record and the primary health-care provider notified.**

4. Using force or a twisting motion while advancing the catheter is contraindicated because it can traumatize the structures and mucous membranes of the urinary tract.

28. 1. Excessive urination at night is called nocturia. A person with urinary retention will have small, frequent voidings or dribbling (overflow incontinence) rather than a complete discharge of urine from the bladder.

2. Hematuria is the presence of red blood cells in the urine. It is associated with bladder inflammation, infection, or trauma, not urinary retention.

3. Urinary retention may produce an atonic bladder rather than bladder contractions.

4. The bladder lies in the pelvic cavity behind the symphysis pubis. When it fills with urine (600 mL), the bladder extends above the symphysis pubis, and when greatly distended (2,000 to 3,000 mL), it can reach to the umbilicus.

5. With urinary retention, the bladder fills with urine, causing distention. Eventually, the external urethral sphincter temporarily opens to allow a small volume of urine to pass out of the bladder (overflow incontinence, retention with overflow).

29.   The tubing from the collection bag that is attached to the catheter inserted into the bladder should be clamped 2 to 3 inches below the collection port. This location allows urine to collect above the port. The catheter inserted into the bladder should not be clamped to prevent trauma to the catheter lumen or the lumen leading to the inflated balloon.

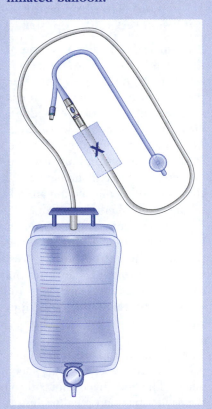

30. 1. Avoiding kinks in the tubing is essential so that urine flows unimpeded to the urine collection bag.
    2. Perineal hygiene should be performed at least once a day, after a bowel movement, and whenever the catheter is changed or replaced.

3. The anchoring device (e.g., adhesive band, elastic strip, or inflatable ring) must be snug enough to prevent the condom from falling off but not so tight that it interferes with blood circulation to the penis.

4. Placing the condom over and beyond the glans penis and leaving 1 inch between the glans penis and drainage tubing prevents pressure against the glans penis that could cause excoriation and skin trauma.

5. The foreskin should be over the glans penis. If the foreskin is left in the retracted position, it can constrict the penis, resulting in edema and tissue injury.

31.   Answer: 500 mL/hr. The electronic infusion device should be programmed for 500 mL/hr. An electronic infusion device uses milliliters (mL) per hour as the programmable infusion rate. The volume prescribed (250 mL) is to be infused over 30 minutes. Therefore, the nurse must double the infusion volume to 500 mL to maintain a rate that will infuse the 250 mL in 30 minutes.

32. 1. If retention catheter tubing is left on or through a side rail, the catheter may inadvertently be pulled out when the side rail is moved. In addition, the collection bag must be kept below the level of the bladder to promote the flow of urine from the bladder by gravity and prevent a flow of urine back into the bladder from the catheter.
    2. Positioning the tubing under the leg may put pressure on the drainage tubing that can interrupt the flow of urine from the bladder. The tubing should be maintained over, not under, the leg.
    3. Labeling the tubing with the date of insertion should be documented on the client's clinical record, not on the tubing.
    4. Irrigating the tubing is contraindicated because it may introduce microorganisms into the bladder that can cause an infection. Irrigation of a urinary retention catheter requires a prescription and is a dependent function of the nurse.
    5. Securing the tubing to the client's leg prevents tension on the urinary meatus.

33. 6. The supine position permits access to the client's lower abdomen and suprapubic area.

4. Draping the client and exposing just the lower abdomen and suprapubic area provide for client privacy.

2. The use of conducting gel or an ultrasound gel pad improves transmission of the ultrasound image.

3. The scan head should be placed approximately 1.5 inches (4 cm) above the pubic bone midline below the umbilicus (symphysis pubis) while aiming the scan head toward the coccyx. This permits visualization of the urinary bladder. In women, the bladder lies in front of and below the uterus. In men, the bladder can be partly obstructed by the pubic bone, and the scan head may require a slightly oblique angle to visualize the bladder.

5. Several measurements should be obtained to ensure accuracy of the results.

1. Removing the gel and washing the client's abdomen promote hygiene and comfort. Cleaning the scan head removes the gel on the end of the probe.

34. 1. Narcotics are central nervous system depressants that can cause urinary retention, not diuresis.

2. Drinks with caffeine (e.g., coffee, tea, and some carbonated beverages) promote the secretion and excretion of increased amounts of urine. This may be related to the inhibition of phosphodiesterases or antagonism of adenosine receptors (or both). Antagonism of adenosine receptors inhibits proximal tubular reabsorption, resulting in an increased urine output.

3. Although activity increases renal perfusion, which may increase urinary output, the increased fluid lost during activity usually is through insensible losses (e.g., perspiration, moisture in exhaled breaths).

4. Alcohol limits the production of vasopressin, a hormone that tells the kidneys to reabsorb water. Urine output increases because fluid is not reabsorbed in the kidneys.

5. Avoiding protein does not prevent diuresis. The presence of protein in the urine indicates that the glomeruli have become too permeable, which occurs in kidney disease. Most plasma proteins are too large to move out of the glomeruli, and the small proteins that enter the filtrate are reabsorbed by pinocytosis.

35. Answer: 40 drops per minute. Four mL of furosemide must be added to the diluent, yielding a total volume of 54 mL to be infused. First, determine how many milliliters contain 3 mg. Use ratio and proportion.

$$\frac{\text{Desired}}{\text{Have}} \quad \frac{3\text{ mg}}{40\text{ mg}} = \frac{x\text{ mL}}{54\text{ mL}}$$
$$40\,x = 162$$
$$x = 162 \div 40$$
$$x = 4.05\text{ mL}$$

Round 4.05 down to 4 because 0.05 is less than 0.5. Each 4 mL of solution contains 3 mg of furosemide.
Now determine how many drops 4 mL contains when the drop rate of the secondary infusion set is 10.
4 mL (mL to be administered in 1 minute) × 10 (drop factor of the infusion set) = 40 drops per minute.

36. 1. A cognitively impaired person may not be able to receive, interpret, or respond to cues for voiding. Reminding the person to void every 2 hours results in emptying of the bladder, which may limit episodes of incontinence.

2. Applying a condom catheter in the morning is unnecessary and intrusive. Also, it may create a safety issue because the client's mobility may be impaired by the tubing and urine drainage bag.

3. Cognitively impaired individuals may have problems handling clothing, particularly when attempting to respond to the urge to void. Clothing that is easy to manipulate, such as articles with elastic waistbands and zippers, will facilitate undressing and dressing to void.

4. Restriction of fluid intake is an inappropriate way to manage urinary incontinence. The body needs fluids throughout the day to maintain renal perfusion, kidney function, and fluid balance.

5. Toileting every 4 hours is too long a time to wait between opportunities to void and usually will result in an episode of incontinence. Also, a cognitively impaired individual may not understand cause and effect or be able to follow directions.

37. 1. A person with a spinal cord injury will experience reflex incontinence, not stress incontinence.
  2. A person with a urinary tract obstruction will experience urinary retention, not stress incontinence.
  3. Stress incontinence is an immediate, involuntary loss of urine during an increase in intra-abdominal pressure. It is associated with weak pelvic muscles and structural supports resulting from multiple pregnancies, age-related degenerative changes, and overdistention between voiding.
  4. Older women experience a weakening of the muscles surrounding the urinary and reproductive systems because of decreasing levels of estrogen associated with menopause.
  5. The relationship of obesity and stress incontinence is theorized to be that excess weight increases abdominal pressure. This, in turn, increases bladder pressure and mobility of the urethra. In addition, obesity may lead to chronic strain, stretching, and weakening of the nerves and muscles of the pelvic area.

38. 1. Discontinuing the continuous compression devices to the lower extremities is unsafe and may result in the client experiencing deep vein thrombosis and pulmonary embolus. Maintaining these devices is a dependent function of the nurse.
  2. Notifying the surgeon is unnecessary at this time. If the status of the client's urinary drainage intensifies, then the surgeon should be notified.
  3. Obtaining a rectal temperature from a client who has had a prostatectomy is contraindicated. The rectal probe could traumatize the surgical area.
  4. The surgeon's prescriptions indicate that the continuous bladder irrigation should be maintained at a flow rate that keeps the urinary drainage pink; this also implies the absence of clots.

39. Answer: 800 mL. To calculate the amount of urine output of a client receiving CBI, the total amount of the instilled irrigant must be subtracted from the total output. The client received 200 mL of GU irrigant per hour for 12 hours. To determine the total amount of GU irrigant received, multiply 200×12 (2,400). Subtract 2,400 mL from 3,200 mL (total amount of urinary drainage) to determine the amount of urine contained in the total output. 3,200 mL minus 2,400 mL equals 800 mL.

40. 3. Draining the urine ensures that previously produced urine is not collected for a current specimen.
  4. Clamping the drainage tubing allows urine to collect above the specimen port.
  1. Washing the hands limits the number of microorganisms on the hands. Clean gloves protect the nurse from the client's body fluids. Both practices are part of standard precautions.
  5. The use of an antiseptic swab removes microorganisms on the specimen port, and sterile equipment maintains the sterility of the closed urinary drainage system.
  6. The sterility of the specimen must be maintained to prevent contamination of the specimen, which can result in inaccurate results. Discarding the used syringe in a sharps container prevents accidental injury to self or others.
  2. Removing the clamp from the drainage tubing reestablishes the flow of urine from the client to the drainage bag. If it is left clamped, urine will not drain, causing bladder distention, and may precipitate a stasis-induced urinary tract infection.

Fluids and Electrolytes

KEYWORDS

The following words include nursing/medical terminology, concepts, principles, and information relevant to content specifically addressed in the chapter or associated with topics presented in it. English dictionaries, nursing textbooks, and medical dictionaries, such as *Taber's Cyclopedic Medical Dictionary*, are resources that can be used to expand your knowledge and understanding of these words and related information.

Acid
Active transport
Aldosterone
Anion
Antidiuretic hormone
Anuria
Base
Catheter
Cation
Colloid osmotic pressure, oncotic pressure
Dehydration
Diaphoresis
Diffusion
Diluent
Diuretic
Edema:
    Dependent
    Peripheral
    Pitting
    Sacral
Electrolytes:
    Calcium
    Magnesium
    Phosphorus
    Potassium
    Sodium
Fluid compartments:
    Extracellular
    Interstitial
    Intracellular
    Intravascular
    Third-compartment spacing
Fluid restriction

Fluid volume:
    Deficient
    Excess
Hydrostatic pressure
Hypercalcemia/hypocalcemia
Hyperkalemia/hypokalemia
Hypermagnesemia/hypomagnesemia
Hyperosmolar/hypo-osmolar
Hypertension/hypotension
Hypertonic/hypotonic
Hypervolemic/hypovolemic
Icteric
Infiltration
Infusion port
Insensible fluid loss
Ion
Irrigant
Isotonic
Macrodrip/microdrip
Milliequivalent
Osmolality
Osmolarity
Osmosis
Primary infusion line
Residual urine
Secondary infusion line
Sensible/insensible fluid loss
Skin turgor
Solute
Specific gravity
Tenting
Thirst
Vaporization

FLUIDS AND ELECTROLYTES: QUESTIONS

1. A nurse is caring for a critically ill client with a urinary retention catheter. Which hourly urine output should **first** alert the nurse that the primary health-care provider should be notified?
   1. 20 mL
   2. 30 mL
   3. 60 mL
   4. 120 mL

2. A nurse is caring for a client who has dependent edema. Which pressure has caused the excess fluid in the interstitial compartment?
   1. Oncotic pressure
   2. Diffusion pressure
   3. Hydrostatic pressure
   4. Intraventricular pressure

3. A nurse evaluates a client's fluid balance by monitoring the client's intake and output. Which must the nurse understand about the ratio of the client's fluid intake to output?
   1. Intake should be much higher than the fluid output.
   2. Intake should be slightly more than the output.
   3. Intake should be lower than the urine output.
   4. Intake should be equal to the urine output.

4. Hydrochlorothiazide, a diuretic, is prescribed for a client who is retaining fluid. The nurse should encourage the client to ingest nutrients that contain which electrolyte?
   1. Magnesium
   2. Potassium
   3. Calcium
   4. Sodium

5. Which should a nurse do to encourage a confused client to drink more fluid?
   1. Serve fluid at a tepid temperature.
   2. Explain the reason for the desired intake.
   3. Offer the client something to drink every hour.
   4. Leave a pitcher of water at the client's bedside.

6. A nurse suspects that an older adult may have a fluid and electrolyte imbalance. Which assessment **best** reflects fluid and electrolyte balance in an older adult?
   1. Serum laboratory values
   2. Intake and output results
   3. Condition of the skin
   4. Presence of tenting

7. A client has continuous bladder irrigation. Which should the nurse do with the irrigant on the I&O sheet when calculating the fluid balance for this client?
   1. Add it to the oral intake column.
   2. Deduct it from the total urine output.
   3. Subtract it from the intravenous flow sheet as output.
   4. Document the intake hourly in the urine output column.

8. A nurse is caring for two clients; one has oliguria and the other has polyuria. Which is the **priority** problem that is a concern for the nurse regarding both of these clients?
   1. Diarrhea
   2. Cachexia
   3. Deficient fluid volume
   4. Impaired skin integrity

9. A primary health-care provider prescribes a client's IV fluids to be discontinued. Which is an **essential** nursing intervention when discontinuing the client's intravenous infusion?
   1. Withdraw the intravenous catheter along the same angle of its insertion.
   2. Use an alcohol swab to scrub the insertion site.
   3. Flush the line with normal saline.
   4. Don sterile gloves.

10. A client is admitted to the hospital for a fever of unknown origin. The nursing assessment reveals profuse diaphoresis; dry, sticky mucous membranes; weakness; disorientation; and a decreasing level of consciousness. Which electrolyte imbalance do these data **support**?
    1. Hyperkalemia
    2. Hypercalcemia
    3. Hypernatremia
    4. Hypermagnesemia

11. A client exhibits an increasing blood pressure and 2-pound weight gain over 2 days. Which additional clinical manifestation can be clustered with these data?
    1. Decrease in heart rate
    2. Increase in skin turgor
    3. Increase in pulse volume
    4. Decrease in pulse pressure

12. An assessment of which of the following is **most** important when a nurse is caring for an adult client experiencing vomiting?
    1. Electrolyte values
    2. Bowel function
    3. Body weight
    4. Oral mucosa

13. A primary health-care provider prescribes an intravenous infusion containing potassium for a client. Which is the **most** important nursing intervention before administering this solution to the client?
    1. Assess the skin turgor.
    2. Obtain the blood pressure.
    3. Measure the depth of edema.
    4. Determine the presence of urinary output.

14. Which is the **best** choice for an appetizer when teaching a client about a 2-g sodium diet?
    1. Pigs in a blanket
    2. Stuffed mushrooms
    3. Cheese and crackers
    4. Fresh vegetable sticks

15. A nurse is documenting a client's I&O. Which should be recorded at approximately half its volume?
    1. Ice chips given by mouth
    2. A continuous bladder irrigation
    3. Solution used to maintain patency of a tube
    4. A tube feeding of half formula and half water

16. Several clients are taking supplemental calcium daily. The nurse teaches them to maintain their fluid intake at a minimum of 2,500 mL. The nurse explains that this intervention is designed to prevent which complication?
    1. Mobilization of calcium from bone
    2. Irritation of the bladder mucosa
    3. Occurrence of muscle cramps
    4. Formation of kidney stones

17. A client receiving an enteral feeding develops diarrhea. Which characteristic of the tube feeding formula does the nurse conclude precipitated the diarrhea?
1. Hypertonic
2. Hypotonic
3. Isotonic
4. Icteric

18. A nurse identifies that an older adult client may have a problem with excess fluid volume. Which characteristics of the client's skin **support** this conclusion?
1. Dry and scaly
2. Taut and shiny
3. Red and irritated
4. Thin and inelastic

19. When a client is under extreme stress, there is an increased production of antidiuretic hormone and aldosterone. The nurse plans to monitor the client routinely because an increase in these hormones will cause a **decrease** in which of the following?
1. Blood pressure
2. Urinary output
3. Body temperature
4. Sweat gland secretions

20. A nurse checks a meal tray for a client on a clear liquid diet. Which item is acceptable on this diet?
1. Ginger ale
2. Lemon sherbet
3. Vanilla ice cream
4. Cream of chicken soup

21. A nurse is caring for a client who has a reduced fluid intake. The nurse assesses the client for which response to this reduced fluid intake?
1. Urinary retention
2. Frequent urination
3. Incontinence of urine
4. Decreased urine output

22. A nurse is monitoring a client who is receiving IV fluid. Which clinical findings indicate that the client has a fluid overload?
1. Chills, fever, and generalized discomfort
2. Blood in the tubing close to the insertion site
3. Dyspnea, headache, and increased blood pressure
4. Pallor, swelling, and discomfort at the insertion site

23. The nurse is administering IV fluids to a client. Which complication should prompt the nurse to slow the rate of flow of the infusion rather than stop the infusion and remove the catheter?
1. Infiltration
2. Extravasation
3. Inflamed vein
4. Fluid overload

24. When a nurse evaluates the effectiveness of client teaching, which food selection by a client indicates understanding regarding an abundant source of calcium? **Select all that apply.**
1. _____ Bread
2. _____ Yogurt
3. _____ Spinach
4. _____ Green beans
5. _____ Peanut butter

25. A nurse is caring for a postoperative client over an 8-hour period. The client vomits 300 mL of greenish-yellow fluid. The client's IV fluid is infusing at 125 mL per hour. The client received two intermittent infusions of antibiotics each in 50 mL of solution, and they were infused at a different site than the IV fluid infusion. The client was given 8 ounces of ice chips, which were retained. The client urinated twice—250 mL and 400 mL. Which is the client's total fluid intake at the end of the 8-hour period? **Record your answer using a whole number.**

Answer: _____ mL.

26. A client's diet is progressed from clear liquid to full liquid. Which can the nurse include on the full-liquid diet that is not included on the clear-liquid diet? **Select all that apply.**
1. _____ Vanilla ice cream
2. _____ Cream of Wheat
3. _____ Cranberry juice
4. _____ Sport drinks
5. _____ Custard
6. _____ Milk

27. A nurse is caring for a client in the emergency department. The client's electrocardiogram (ECG) tracing is indicated below. Which additional response in the client that can be clustered with the results of this ECG tracing should be assessed by the nurse? **Select all that apply.**
1. _____ Bradycardia
2. _____ Flaccid paralysis
3. _____ Increased bowel sounds
4. _____ Ventricular dysrhythmias
5. _____ Decreased deep tendon reflexes

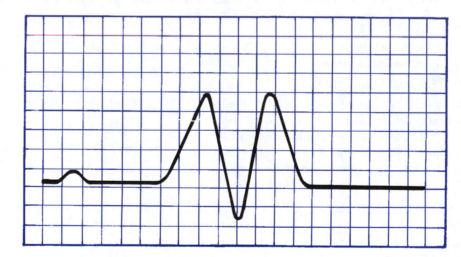

28. A nurse is assessing several clients for fluid and electrolyte imbalances. Which of the following is common to both excess fluid volume and deficient fluid volume? **Select all that apply.**
1. _____ Increased pulse amplitude
2. _____ Decreased blood pressure
3. _____ Difficulty breathing
4. _____ Mental confusion
5. _____ Muscle weakness

29. The illustration reflects a client's upper extremity while the nurse is obtaining the client's blood pressure. Which should the nurse do **next** after releasing the pressure in the sphygmomanometer cuff?
1. Notify the primary health-care provider of the client's response.
2. Assess the client's radial pulse in the affected arm.
3. Retake the client's blood pressure.
4. Tap over the client's facial nerve.

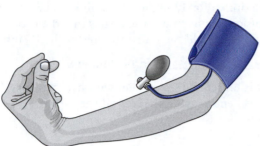

30. A nurse is monitoring a client who is receiving fluids intravenously. Which of the following at the insertion site indicates that the IV has infiltrated? **Select all that apply.**
1. _____ Redness
2. _____ Swelling
3. _____ Firmness
4. _____ Coolness
5. _____ Inflammation

31. An older adult is diagnosed with congestive heart failure and pulmonary edema, and the primary health-care provider prescribed furosemide 40 mg PO twice a day. The client has slight dysphagia as a result of a brain attack a year ago. The nurse obtains an oral solution of furosemide that states that there is 8 mg/mL. How many milliliters should the nurse administer? **Record your answer using a whole number.**

Answer: _____ mL.

32. A client receiving a diuretic is encouraged to increase the intake of potassium. Which food selected by the client indicates that the teaching is understood? **Select all that apply.**
1. _____ Pears
2. _____ Cabbage
3. _____ Cantaloupe
4. _____ Fresh salmon
5. _____ Chicken liver

33. A nurse must discontinue a client's intravenous infusion. The nurse shuts off the infusion, washes the hands, and dons clean gloves. Place the following steps in the order in which they should be performed.
1. Apply countertraction to the skin while loosening the tape at the venipuncture site.
2. Apply firm pressure to the site with sterile gauze for two to three minutes.
3. Apply a sterile dressing with tape over the venipuncture site.
4. Withdraw the needle/catheter along the line of insertion.
5. Examine the end of the needle/catheter.

Answer: _____

34. A nurse is assessing a client's fluid status. Which of the following assessments indicate that the client has a deficient fluid volume? **Select all that apply.**
    1. _____ Negative balance of intake and output
    2. _____ Increased body temperature
    3. _____ Decreased blood pressure
    4. _____ Flat neck veins
    5. _____ Weight loss

35. A client has a prescription for 1,000 mL of IV fluid to be administered over 12 hours. The infusion administration set states that the drop factor is 10. At how many drops per minute should the nurse administer the IV infusion?

    Answer: _____ drops/minute.

36. A 2-g sodium diet is prescribed for a client with hypertension. Which food should the nurse teach the client to avoid? **Select all that apply.**
    1. _____ American cheese
    2. _____ Canned tuna fish
    3. _____ Shredded wheat
    4. _____ Potatoes
    5. _____ Cashews

37. A nurse assesses a client for the clinical manifestations of electrolyte imbalances. Which of the following indicates that the client may have a potassium deficiency? **Select all that apply.**
    1. _____ Increased blood pressure
    2. _____ Irregular pulse rhythm
    3. _____ Muscle tension
    4. _____ Chest pain
    5. _____ Dry hair

38. A primary health-care provider prescribes 1,000 mL 0.9% sodium chloride to be infused over 6 hours. A gravity flow infusion set states that the drop factor is 15. At which rate should the nurse set the IV flow rate? **Record your answer using a whole number.**

    Answer: _____ drops/minute.

39. Which characteristic associated with touching an intravenous insertion site **supports** the conclusion that the insertion site may be inflamed? **Select all that apply.**
    1. _____ Warmth
    2. _____ Softness
    3. _____ Firmness
    4. _____ Coolness
    5. _____ Discomfort

40. A client in the hospital emergency department tells the nurse, "I feel lousy, and I've had diarrhea for several days. I have nausea, and I don't feel like eating or drinking." The nurse obtains the client's vital signs, performs a focused physical assessment, and reviews the results of laboratory studies. Which should the nurse conclude is the client's human response based on this information?

1. Hypokalemia
2. Hypervolemia
3. Metabolic acidosis
4. Respiratory alkalosis

CLIENT'S CLINICAL RECORD

Vital Signs
Temperature: 101.2°F, oral
Pulse: 92 beats per minute, regular, thready
Respirations: 26 breaths per minute, deep
Blood pressure: 100/60 mm Hg

Focused Physical Assessment
Weight loss of 4 pounds in 3 days
Tenting of the skin

Laboratory Values
Urine specific gravity: 1.036
Serum potassium: 5.3 mEq/L
Arterial blood gases:
  pH: 7.30
  $Paco_2$: 24 mEq/L
  HCO_3: 18 mEq/L

1. 1. The primary health-care provider should be notified long before the hourly urine output reaches 20 mL.
   2. **The circulating blood volume perfuses the kidneys, producing a glomerular filtrate of which varying amounts are either reabsorbed or excreted to maintain fluid balance. When a person's hourly urine output is only 30 mL, it indicates a deficient circulating fluid volume, inadequate renal perfusion, kidney disease, or all of these. The primary health-care provider should be notified.**
   3. An hourly urine output of 60 mL is close to the expected range of 1,400 mL to 1,500 mL/24 hours or 30 mL to 50 mL/hour.
   4. The primary health-care provider does not have to be notified about an hourly urine output of 120 mL. An hourly urine output of 120 mL indicates that there is adequate kidney perfusion.

2. 1. Oncotic (colloid osmotic) pressure is the force exerted by colloids (e.g., proteins) that pull or keep fluid within the intravascular compartment. Oncotic pressure is the major force opposing hydrostatic pressure in the capillaries.
   2. Diffusion is a continual intermingling of molecules with movement of molecules from a solution of higher concentration to a solution of lower concentration.
   3. **Hydrostatic pressure is the pressure exerted by a fluid within a compartment, such as blood within the vessels. Hydrostatic pressure moves fluid from an area of greater pressure to an area of lesser pressure. Hydrostatic pressure within vessels of the body moves fluid from the intravascular compartment into the interstitial compartment. Interstitial fluid is extracellular fluid that surrounds cells.**
   4. Intraventricular pressure is the pressure that exists in the left and right ventricles of the heart. These pressures do not move fluid from the intravascular compartment to the interstitial compartment.

3. 1. If the total intake is much higher than the total output, the client will develop an excess fluid volume.
   2. **The volume and composition of body fluids are kept in a delicate balance (total intake is slightly more than total output) by a harmonious interaction of the kidneys and the endocrine, respiratory, cardiovascular, integumentary, and gastrointestinal systems. In addition to urine output, the body has insensible fluid loss through the skin, in feces, and as water vapor in expired air.**
   3. If the total intake is lower than the urine output, the client will develop a deficient fluid volume.
   4. If intake and urine output are equal, the client will develop a deficient fluid volume because of fluid loss through routes other than the kidneys.

4. 1. Although loop and thiazide diuretics enhance magnesium excretion, which may produce mild hypomagnesemia, they do not require magnesium supplementation.
   2. **Most diuretics affect the renal mechanisms for tubular secretion and reabsorption of electrolytes, particularly potassium. Because of potassium's narrow therapeutic window of 3.5 to 5.0 mEq/L and its role in the sodium-potassium pump and muscle contraction, depleted potassium must be supplemented by increasing the dietary intake of foods high in potassium, the administration of potassium drug therapy, or both.**
   3. Serum calcium levels vary, depending on the diuretic. Thiazide diuretics, such as hydrochlorothiazide (HCTZ), decrease calcium excretion, which may produce hypercalcemia. Loop diuretics increase calcium excretion, which may produce hypocalcemia.
   4. Although sodium deficit (hyponatremia) may occur with diuretics, usually it is mild and does not require sodium supplementation.

5. 1. Fluids should be administered at the temperature usually associated with the fluid; for example, cool temperatures for juice, soda, and milk and warm temperatures for tea, coffee, and soup. Liquids should not be served hot for safety reasons.
   2. Explaining the reason for the desired intake probably will be ineffective because a confused person has difficulty understanding cause and effect.
   3. **Frequent, smaller volumes of fluid (50 to 100 mL per hour) are better tolerated**

physiologically and psychologically than infrequent larger volumes of fluid.

4. A confused client, having difficulty understanding cause and effect, may ignore a pitcher of water.

6. 1. **Laboratory studies provide objective measurements of indicators of fluid, electrolyte, and acid-base balance. Common diagnostic tests include serum blood studies of electrolytes (e.g., sodium, potassium, chloride, and calcium), osmolarity, hemoglobin, hematocrit, and arterial blood gases.**

2. Monitoring intake and output results assesses only fluid balance.

3. Assessment of the skin in the context of this question assesses only fluid balance. In addition, the changes in the integumentary system as a person ages complicate assessment of the skin for fluid balance disturbances in the older adult. Skin changes include loss of dermal and subcutaneous mass (thin and wrinkled), decreased secretion from sebaceous and sweat glands (dry skin), and less organized collagen and elastic fibers (wrinkles, decreased elasticity).

4. Presence of tenting assesses only fluid balance. Tenting occurs when the skin of a dehydrated person remains in a peak or tentlike position after the superficial layers of the skin are pinched together. Caution is advised when assessing an older person because some degree of tenting may occur even when hydrated because of the decrease in skin elasticity and tissue fluid associated with aging. The skin over the sternum is the area that should be tested for tenting in older adults.

7. 1. The irrigant of a continuous bladder irrigation is instilled into the urinary bladder, not the mouth.

2. **When continuous bladder irrigation is in use, drainage from the urinary bladder will consist of both urine and the instilled irrigant. To determine the client's urinary output, the amount of the irrigant instilled must be deducted from the total urinary output.**

3. The IV flow sheet should not contain any information regarding I&O other than the amount and type of fluid that is instilled into the circulatory system.

4. Intake anywhere in the body should be recorded in the appropriate intake column, not in the urinary output column.

8. 1. Frequent, loose, liquid stools, not oliguria or polyuria, are associated with diarrhea.

2. Oliguria and polyuria are related to fluid balance and kidney functioning, not nutrition. Cachexia is a profound state of malnutrition.

3. **The production of excessive amounts of urine by the kidneys (polyuria) without an increase in fluid intake can precipitate a deficient fluid volume. Oliguria, the production of excessively small amounts of urine by the kidney, is reflected as a negative balance in the intake and output. A negative balance of intake and output is a characteristic of deficient fluid volume.**

4. Oliguria and polyuria are related to fluid balance and kidney functioning, not skin integrity. However, because oliguria may be related to fluid retention and subsequent edema and polyuria may ultimately cause dehydration and dry skin, both clients may eventually be at risk for impaired skin integrity.

9. 1. **Removing an IV catheter by withdrawing it along the same path of its insertion minimizes injury to the vein and trauma to the surrounding tissue. This action limits seepage of blood and promotes healing of the puncture wound.**

2. Scrubbing the area with an alcohol wipe is unnecessary. The area should be compressed with a sterile gauze pad. Pressure helps stop the bleeding and prevents the formation of a hematoma. A sterile gauze pad provides for surgical asepsis, which prevents infection.

3. Flushing the line with normal saline is unnecessary.

4. Clean, not sterile, gloves should be worn by the nurse to prevent exposure to the client's body fluids.

10. 1. Although muscle weakness and lethargy are associated with hyperkalemia, the client's other responses are not.

2. Although weakness and lethargy are associated with hypercalcemia, the client's other responses are not.

3. **With profuse diaphoresis, the water loss exceeds the sodium loss, resulting in hypernatremia. Excess serum sodium precipitates changes in the musculoskeletal (weakness), neurological (disorientation and decreased level of consciousness), and integumentary**

(dry, sticky mucous membranes) systems.

4. Although muscle weakness, lethargy, and drowsiness are associated with hypermagnesemia, the client's other responses are not.

11. 1. With an excess fluid volume, the heart rate will increase, not decrease, in an attempt to maintain adequate cardiac output.
2. In the early stages of an excess fluid volume, a change in skin turgor may not be evident. One liter of fluid is equal to approximately 2.2 pounds.
3. **With an excess fluid volume, the amount of circulating blood volume increases, resulting in full, bounding peripheral pulses.**
4. The pulse pressure is the difference between the systolic and diastolic pressures of a blood pressure measurement, and the acceptable range is 30 to 50 mm Hg. With an excess fluid volume, the pulse pressure increases, not decreases.

12. 1. **Vomiting results in a loss of chloride (greatest amount), sodium (next greatest amount), and potassium (least amount, but of greatest importance because it can cause dysrhythmias and cardiac arrest).**
2. Although assessing bowel function will be done, it is not the priority.
3. Although obtaining a body weight will be done to assess deficient fluid volume (2.2 pounds equals approximately 1 L of fluid), it is not as critical as another assessment.
4. Although the mouth is assessed and oral care is provided, it is performed for comfort, not because there is a life-threatening problem.

13. 1. Assessing skin turgor is unnecessary for the administration of potassium. This is part of the assessment of a client's hydration status, particularly when the client is at risk for dehydration.
2. Although all the vital signs should be measured when a client is receiving any fluids or electrolytes, monitoring the heart rate and rhythm is a more significant assessment than the blood pressure in relation to the administration of potassium. Both a serum potassium decrease (hypokalemia) and an increase (hyperkalemia) cause cardiac dysrhythmias.

3. Measuring the depth of edema is unnecessary for the administration of potassium. This is part of the assessment when a client has an excess fluid volume in dependent tissues in which the hydrostatic capillary pressure is high.
4. **Serum potassium has a narrow therapeutic window (3.5 to 5.0 mEq/L). When kidney function is impaired, potassium can accumulate in the body and exceed the therapeutic level of 5.0 mEq/L, which can cause cardiac dysrhythmias and arrest.**

14. 1. One-tenth of a pound of frankfurters contains approximately 168 mg of sodium and should be avoided on a 2-g sodium diet.
2. Although mushrooms are low in sodium, when stuffed with seasoned bread crumbs (⅓ cup contains approximately 370 mg of sodium), they should be avoided on a 2-g sodium diet.
3. One ounce of cheese contains approximately 106 to 400 mg of sodium, depending on the cheese. Two crackers contain approximately 44 to 165 mg, depending on the product. These foods should be avoided on a 2-g sodium diet.
4. **As a food group, fresh vegetables have low sodium content. The sodium content of vegetables is as follows: 1 cup of broccoli, 17 mg; 1 cup of cauliflower, 20 mg; 1 carrot, 25 mg; 1 pepper, 2 mg; 1 radish, 1 mg; 1 cup of mushrooms, 3 mg; and 6 slices of cucumber, 1 mg.**

15. 1. **Ice chips are particles of frozen water that take up more volume when they are frozen than when they melt. When ice chips change from a solid to a liquid, the resulting fluid is approximately half the volume of the ice chips.**
2. The total amount of the irrigant instilled into the urinary bladder is accounted for as intake. The total volume that was instilled is then deducted from the total urinary output to determine the client's urinary output.
3. Whatever volume of solution is instilled into a catheter, the full volume used is recorded when the nurse documents the intervention.
4. When a tube feeding solution consists of half formula and half water, the final combined volume of the formula and water is recorded on the appropriate intake column of the I&O record.

16. 1. Calcium supplementation and weight bearing, not an increased fluid intake, prevent bone demineralization.
    2. Neither hypocalcemia nor hypercalcemia irritates the bladder mucosa.
    3. Excessive supplementation of calcium causes hypercalcemia. Muscle tremors and cramps are associated with hypocalcemia, not hypercalcemia.
    4. **A high fluid intake increases the volume of urine produced. The resulting frequent urination of dilute urine prevents the formation of renal calculi, which may occur because of the increased precipitation of calcium salts associated with calcium supplementation.**

17. 1. **Hypertonic solutions have a greater concentration of solutes than does the blood. The high osmolarity of a hypertonic enteral feeding exerts an osmotic force that pulls fluid into the gastrointestinal tract, resulting in intestinal cramping and diarrhea.**
    2. Hypotonic solutions have a lesser concentration of solutes than does the blood. A hypotonic enteral feeding will result in fluid being absorbed from the gastrointestinal tract into the intravascular and intracellular compartments.
    3. Isotonic solutions have the same concentration of solutes as the blood. With isotonic solutions, there is no net transfer of water across two compartments separated by a semipermeable membrane.
    4. Icteric is unrelated to enteral feedings and fluid shifts. Icteric is defined as pertaining to, or resembling, jaundice.

18. 1. Dry skin and scaly skin are signs of aging and dehydration, not excessive fluid volume.
    2. **With excessive fluid volume, the increased hydrostatic pressure moves fluid from the intravascular compartment into the interstitial compartment. As fluid collects in the interstitial compartment (edema), the skin appears taut and shiny.**
    3. Red skin and irritated skin are signs of the local inflammatory response, not of excessive fluid volume.
    4. Thin skin and inelastic skin are characteristics of skin in the older adult because of a loss of subcutaneous fat and a reduced thickness and vascularity of the dermis, not of excessive fluid volume.

19. 1. The blood pressure will increase, not decrease, when the circulating fluid volume increases in response to these hormones.
    2. **Both hormones are involved with water reabsorption, which conserves fluid and results in a decreased urinary output. With decreased kidney perfusion, the juxtaglomerular cells of the kidneys release angiotensin II, which stimulates the release of aldosterone from the adrenal cortex. Aldosterone promotes the excretion of potassium and reabsorption of sodium, which results in the passive reabsorption of water. As the concentration of the blood (osmolality) increases, the anterior pituitary releases antidiuretic hormone (ADH). ADH causes the collecting ducts in the kidneys to become more permeable to water, thus promoting its reabsorption into the blood.**
    3. ADH and aldosterone do not regulate body temperature.
    4. ADH and aldosterone influence the kidneys to maintain fluid balance. They do not affect insensible fluid loss through the skin, lungs, or intestinal tract.

20. 1. **Ginger ale is an easily ingested and digested liquid that is permitted on a clear liquid diet. It relieves thirst, prevents dehydration, and minimizes stimulation of the gastrointestinal tract.**
    2. Sherbet contains milk, which is not permitted on a clear liquid diet.
    3. When ice cream melts, it is not a clear liquid and therefore is not permitted on a clear liquid diet. Milk contains protein and lactose, which stimulate the digestive process; this is undesirable when a client is receiving a clear liquid diet.
    4. Cream of chicken soup contains milk and small particles of chicken, both of which are contraindicated on a clear liquid diet.

21. 1. The accumulation of urine in the bladder with an inability to empty the bladder (urinary retention) is unrelated to a decreased fluid intake.
    2. Frequent urination occurs with increased, not decreased, fluid intake.
    3. Involuntary urination (incontinence) is not associated with a reduced fluid intake.
    4. **When the serum osmolarity increases because of insufficient fluid intake,**

antidiuretic hormone increases the permeability of the collecting tubules in the kidneys, which increases the reabsorption of water and decreases urine output.

22. 1. These physiological responses indicate the presence of an infection, not excess fluid volume.
2. Blood in the tubing is unrelated to fluid overload; it occurs when the IV bag is held lower than the IV insertion site and is an undesirable occurrence.
3. **IV fluid flows directly into the circulatory system via a vein. Excess intravascular volume (hypervolemia) causes hypertension, pulmonary edema, and headache.**
4. These physiological responses indicate an IV infiltration, not excess fluid volume.

23. 1. The infusion should be stopped and the catheter removed when a client's IV infiltrates. When an IV catheter is displaced outside of a vein and IV fluid accidentally leaks into the interstitial compartment, it is called an infiltration. If the solution is just slowed, additional fluid will collect in the interstitial compartment and cause tissue damage.
2. The infusion should be stopped and the catheter removed when extravasation occurs. Extravasation occurs when an IV catheter is displaced outside of a vein and a vesicant solution accidentally leaks into the interstitial compartment. Vesicant solutions are extremely irritating solutions that cause tissues to blister, slough, and become necrotic.
3. The infusion should be stopped and the catheter removed when a client's vein becomes inflamed because of the presence of the catheter. Inflammation of a vein (phlebitis) can progress to an infection or promote the development of a thrombus at the site.
4. **When IV fluids are infused too rapidly or an excess amount of fluid is infused, the client can experience an overload of fluid in the intravascular compartment. The nurse should slow the rate of infusion to keep the venous access viable and notify the primary health-care provider for directions.**

24. 1. Grain products are not high in calcium. One slice of bread contains approximately 20 to 49 mg of calcium, depending on the type of grain.
2. **Yogurt is an excellent dietary source of calcium. Eight ounces of yogurt contains 415 mg of calcium.**
3. **Spinach is an excellent dietary source of calcium. One cup of cooked fresh spinach contains 245 mg of calcium.**
4. Green beans are not high in calcium. One cup of green beans contains approximately 60 mg of calcium.
5. Peanut butter is not high in calcium. One tablespoon of peanut butter contains approximately 5 mg of calcium.

25. **Answer: 1,220 mL. The client's IV fluid infused at 125 mL for 8 hours; therefore, $125 \times 8 = 1,000$ mL of IV fluids. The client received two intermittent infusions of 50 mL each; therefore, $50 \times 2 = 100$ mL of antibiotic solution. The client consumed 8 ounces of ice chips. When ice chips melt, they are half the volume of the original amount of ice chips; therefore, 8 ounces $\times$ 30 mL (amount of mL per ounce) = 240 (the total volume of ice chips before they melted). Then $240 \div 2 = 120$ mL to determine the amount of fluid in ice chips that the client consumed. Finally, to determine the total intake for 8 hours, add $1,000 + 100 + 120 = 1,220$ mL.**

26. 1. Vanilla ice cream is a liquid at room temperature and is permitted on a full-liquid diet, not a clear-liquid diet.
2. **Cooked, refined cereals, such as Cream of Wheat, cream of rice, oatmeal, grits, and farina, are permitted on a full-liquid diet, not a clear-liquid diet.**
3. Cranberry juice is a clear liquid.
4. Sport drinks are clear liquids.
5. **Custard contains milk, which has fat and proteins. Custard is permitted on a full-liquid diet, not a clear-liquid diet.**
6. Milk contains a high solute load, including fat and proteins. Milk is permitted on a full-liquid diet, not a clear-liquid diet.

27. 1. **The electrocardiogram (ECG) tracing indicates hyperkalemia (tall, thin T wave; prolonged PR interval, ST-segment depression; widened QRS; and loss of P wave). Bradycardia is associated with hyperkalemia.**

Potassium, an electrolyte, is part of the sodium-potassium pump that is involved in muscle contraction. The heart is a muscle.

2. The ECG tracing indicates hyperkalemia (tall, thin T wave; prolonged PR interval, ST-segment depression; widened QRS; and loss of P wave). Flaccid paralysis (muscles that lack tone and strength) is associated with hyperkalemia. Potassium, an electrolyte, is part of the sodium-potassium pump that is involved in muscle contraction.

3. The ECG tracing indicates hyperkalemia (tall, thin T wave; prolonged PR interval, ST-segment depression; widened QRS; and loss of P wave). Increased bowel sounds are associated with hyperkalemia because of hyperactivity of gastrointestinal smooth muscle.

4. Ventricular dysrhythmias are associated with hypokalemia, not hyperkalemia. The ECG tracing indicates hyperkalemia.

5. Decreased deep tendon reflexes are associated with hypokalemia, not hyperkalemia. The ECG tracing indicates hyperkalemia.

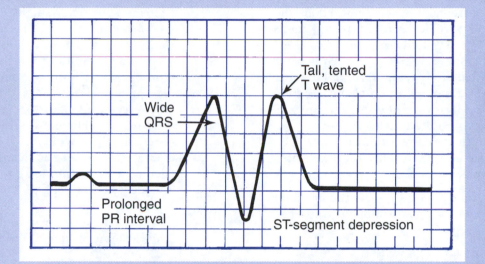

28. 1. The pulse amplitude is increased with excess fluid volume because of an increase in the circulating blood volume (hypervolemia). The pulse amplitude is decreased with deficient fluid volume because of a decrease in the circulating blood volume (hypovolemia).

2. A decrease in blood pressure is associated with deficient fluid volume, not excess, because of the decreased circulating blood volume.

3. Dyspnea is associated with excess fluid volume, not deficit, because fluid overload causes pulmonary congestion.

4. **Brain cells require a delicate balance of fluids and electrolytes. Too much fluid and too little fluid affect the appropriate balance of electrolytes, particularly sodium and potassium. Fluid and electrolyte imbalances cause cerebral changes such as headache, confusion, combative behavior, unconsciousness, and coma.**

5. **Muscle weakness is a musculoskeletal response to both increased fluid volume and decreased fluid volume because the fluid imbalances alter cellular and body metabolism.**

29. 1. Notifying the primary health-care provider is premature. The nurse should obtain additional information.

2. Obtaining the radial pulse is not necessary. Trousseau sign is a result of neuromuscular irritability, not a circulatory impairment.

3. It is not necessary to retake the client's blood pressure. Information already has been obtained from performing this procedure.

4. **When a carpopedal spasm results from compression of a client's arm by a sphygmomanometer cuff (Trousseau sign), it indicates that the client may have hypocalcemia. Tapping over the client's facial nerve will precipitate spasmodic spasms of the facial**

muscles (Chvostek sign) if the client has hypocalcemia. This intervention provides more data to support the conclusion that the client is hypocalcemic.

30. 1. When the insertion site of an IV is reddened, swollen, warm to the touch, and painful, the client has phlebitis, not an infiltration of an IV.
    2. **When an IV line moves out of a vein and into subcutaneous tissue, the IV fluid will begin to collect in the interstitial compartment, causing swelling.**
    3. When IV fluid flows into the tissue surrounding a vein (infiltration), the area will feel soft and spongy, not hard.
    4. **The IV fluid that is infusing is at room temperature, which is cooler than body temperature. Therefore, IV fluid collecting at the site of an infiltration will cause the site to feel cool to the touch.**
    5. When the area at the insertion site of an IV appears inflamed, the client has phlebitis, not an infiltration of an IV.

31. **Answer: 5 mL. Solve the problem by using the formula for ratio and proportion.**

$$\frac{\text{Desired}}{\text{Have}} \quad \frac{40 \text{ mg}}{8 \text{ mg}} = \frac{\text{x mL}}{1 \text{ mL}}$$
$$8 \text{ x} = 40$$
$$\text{x} = 40 \div 8$$
$$\text{x} = 5 \text{ mL}$$

32. 1. A half cup of pears contains only 100 mg or less of potassium.
    2. A half cup of cabbage contains only 100 mg or less of potassium.
    3. **Cantaloupe is an excellent source of potassium. One cup of cantaloupe contains 427 mg of potassium.**
    4. **Salmon is an excellent source of potassium. Three ounces of salmon contains 305 mg of potassium.**
    5. One cooked chicken liver contains only 28 mg of potassium.

33. 1. **Countertraction prevents pulling the skin and moving the needle/catheter, which can result in trauma and discomfort at the venipuncture site.**
    4. **Withdrawing the needle/catheter along the line of insertion prevents injury to the vein.**
    2. **Pressure prevents bleeding and the development of a hematoma at the** venipuncture site. Sterile gauze maintains sterility of the procedure and prevents the transfer of microorganisms to the client.
    5. **Examining the end of the needle/catheter ensures that it is intact and no portion remains in the client.**
    3. **A sterile dressing prevents exposure of the venipuncture site to the environment, limiting the risk of infection. The use of tape maintains pressure to prevent bleeding.**

34. 1. **A client has a negative balance of I&O when the output exceeds the intake. This is a characteristic of a deficient fluid volume.**
    2. **With deficient fluid volume, there is a reduced ability to sweat, thereby contributing to an elevated temperature.**
    3. **A decreased blood pressure is characteristic of a deficient fluid volume because of hypovolemia.**
    4. **Flat neck veins are associated with a deficient fluid volume as a result of the decreased circulating blood volume.**
    5. **Weight loss occurs with a deficient fluid volume; 1 liter of fluid weighs 2.2 pounds.**

35. **Answer: 14 drops/minute. Use the following formula to solve the problem.**

$$\text{Drops per minute} = \frac{\text{total mL to be infused} \times \text{drop factor}}{\text{total time in minutes}}$$

$$\frac{1{,}000 \text{ mL (total mL to be infused)} \times 10 \text{ (drop factor)}}{60 \text{ (minutes in an hour)} \times 12 \text{ hours (hours to be infused)}}$$

$$10{,}000 \div 720 = 13.8$$

Round 13.8 up to 14 because 0.8 of a drop cannot be administered and 0.8 is more than 0.5. The nurse should administer 14 drops/minute.

36. 1. **One ounce of American cheese contains 406 mg of sodium and should be avoided on a 2-g sodium diet.**
    2. **One and a half ounces of canned tuna fish contains approximately 400 mg of sodium and should be avoided on a 2-g sodium diet.**
    3. Two-thirds of a cup of shredded wheat cereal contains 3 mg of sodium and is permitted on a 2-g sodium diet.

4. One baked potato contains approximately 16 mg of sodium and is permitted on a 2-g sodium diet.
5. One ounce of roasted cashews, with no added salt, contains about 4 mg of sodium and is permitted on a 2-g sodium diet.

37. 1. Hypertension is associated with hypervolemia, not a potassium deficiency.
2. **Potassium is essential to the sodium-potassium pump that regulates muscle contraction. The heart is a major muscle. Hypokalemia can precipitate a weak, irregular pulse and ventricular dysrhythmias.**
3. Potassium is an essential component in the sodium-potassium pump, cellular metabolism, and muscle contraction. Responses associated with hypokalemia include muscle weakness, fatigue, lethargy, and depressed deep-tendon reflexes, not muscle tension.
4. Chest pain is associated with a myocardial infarction (heart attack) and pulmonary embolus, not a potassium deficiency.
5. Dry hair is associated with malnutrition and hypothyroidism, not hypokalemia.

38.   **Answer: 42 drops/minute. Solve the problem by using the following formula.**

$$\text{Drops per minute} = \frac{\text{total mL to be infused} \times \text{drop factor}}{\text{total time in minutes}}$$

$$\frac{1{,}000 \text{ mL (total mL to be infused)} \times 15 \text{ (drop factor)}}{60 \text{ (minutes in an hour)} \times 6 \text{ hours (hours to be infused)}}$$

$$15{,}000 \div 360 = 41.6$$

Round 41.6 up to 42 because 0.6 of a drop cannot be administered. The nurse should administer 42 drops/minute.

39. 1. **Vasodilation related to inflammation increases blood flow to the affected area, which causes the site to feel warm and look red (erythema).**
2. The site of an inflammation will feel firm, not soft.

3. **Edema related to inflammation causes the affected area to feel firm.**
4. Vasodilation related to inflammation increases blood flow to the affected area, which causes it to feel warm, not cool.
5. **Inflammation of a vein (phlebitis) causes a movement of fluid from the intravascular compartment into the interstitial compartment. Pressure of fluid on nerve endings causes local discomfort.**

40. 1. The client has hyperkalemia. The potassium is more than the acceptable range of 3.5 to 5.0 mEq/L.
2. The client has hypovolemia, not hypervolemia, because of dehydration. The pulse is rapid and thready, and the urine specific gravity is increased. An abrupt weight loss indicates fluid loss (2.2 pounds is equal to 1 L of fluid), and the client is exhibiting decreased intracellular and interstitial fluid, as evidenced by tenting of the skin. Also, the blood pressure is on the low extreme of the acceptable range of 90 to 119 mm Hg for systolic and 60 to 79 mm Hg for diastolic.
3. **Intestinal secretions distal to the pyloric sphincter contain large amounts of bicarbonate, which is lost through diarrhea. The arterial blood gases indicate uncompensated metabolic acidosis: the pH is less than the acceptable range of 7.35 to 7.45; the HCO_3 is less than the acceptable range of 21 to 28 mEq/L; and the $PaCO_2$ is within the acceptable range of 23 to 30 mEq/L.**
4. With respiratory alkalosis, the pH will be more than 7.45, the $PaCO_2$ will be less than 35 mm Hg, and the HCO_3 will be within the acceptable range of 21 to 28 mEq/L. Respiratory alkalosis usually is caused by hyperventilation precipitated by conditions such as anxiety, mechanical ventilation, early sepsis, and high fever.

Gastrointestinal System

KEYWORDS

The following words include English vocabulary, nursing/medical terminology, concepts, principles, and information relevant to content specifically addressed in the chapter or associated with topics presented in it. English dictionaries, nursing textbooks, and medical dictionaries, such as *Taber's Cyclopedic Medical Dictionary,* are resources that can be used to expand your knowledge and understanding of these words and related information.

Abdomen
Abdominal distention
Anus
Borborygmi
Bowel:
  Flora
  Habits
  Sounds
  Training
Cathartic
Colon
Colorectal
Constipation
Defecate
Diarrhea
Distention
Endoscopic
Enema:
  Cleansing
  Hypertonic
  Hypotonic
  Isotonic
  Large volume
  Oil retention
  Return flow (formerly Harris drip/
    Harris flush)
  Saline
  Soapsuds
  Tap water
Evacuate, evacuation
Fecal diversion:
  Colostomy
  Ileostomy

Fecal impaction
Feces
Flatus, flatulence
Fracture bedpan
Gastrocolic reflex
Hemoccult test, guaiac
Hemorrhoids
Hypermotility/hypomotility
Irrigation
Laxative
Mucosal
Nasogastric tube
Occult blood
Ova and parasites
Paralytic ileus
Perianal
Perineal
Peristalsis
Pinworms
Prolapse
Rectal tube
Rectum
Sigmoidoscopy
Sitz bath
Spastic colon
Sphincter
Steatorrhea
Stoma
Stool
Suppository
Tarry stool (melena)

GASTROINTESTINAL SYSTEM: QUESTIONS

1. Which statement by a client with an ileostomy alerts the nurse to the need for further education?
  1. "I don't expect to have much of a problem with fecal odor from the stoma."
  2. "I will have to take special precautions to protect my skin around the stoma."
  3. "I am going to have a bowel movement every morning when I irrigate the stoma."
  4. "I should avoid gas-forming foods like beans to limit funny noises from the stoma."

2. A primary health-care provider prescribes a return-flow enema (Harris flush/Harris drip) for an adult client with flatulence. When preparing to administer this enema, the nurse compares the steps of a return-flow enema with those for cleansing enemas. Which nursing intervention is unique to a return-flow enema?
   1. Lubricate the last 2 inches of the rectal tube.
   2. Insert the rectal tube about 4 inches into the anus.
   3. Raise the solution container about 12 inches above the anus.
   4. Lower the solution container after instilling about 150 mL of solution.

3. A nurse discourages a client from straining excessively when attempting to have a bowel movement. Which undesirable physiological response is the primary reason why straining on defecation should be avoided?
   1. Dysrhythmia
   2. Incontinence
   3. Fecal impaction
   4. Rectal hemorrhoid

4. A school nurse is planning a health class about bodily functions. Which information should be included regarding the purpose of mucus in the gastrointestinal tract?
   1. Activates digestive enzymes
   2. Protects the gastric mucosa
   3. Enhances gastric acidity
   4. Emulsifies fats

5. A nurse is caring for a client who is experiencing diarrhea. Which physiological response to diarrhea should the nurse be **most** concerned about?
   1. Dehydration
   2. Malnutrition
   3. Excoriated skin
   4. Urinary incontinence

6. A nurse identifies that a client's colostomy stoma is pale. Which should the nurse do?
   1. Notify the surgeon.
   2. Listen for bowel sounds.
   3. Wash the area with warm water.
   4. Gently massage around the stoma.

7. A nurse is caring for a group of clients. Which client factor should the nurse identify as placing a client at risk for bowel incontinence?
   1. Being ninety years old
   2. Taking a sedative for sleep
   3. Disoriented to time, place, and person
   4. Receiving multiple antibiotic medications

8. A client is admitted with lower gastrointestinal tract bleeding. Which characteristic of the client's stool should the nurse assess for that **supports** this medical diagnosis?
   1. Tarry stool
   2. Orange stool
   3. Green mucoid stool
   4. Bright red–tinged stool

9. A nurse determines that the teaching about a guaiac test of stool is understood when the client states that it identifies the presence of which of the following?
   1. Ova and parasites
   2. Hidden blood
   3. Bacteria
   4. Bile

10. A nurse must collect a specimen for the presence of pinworms. Which action is **essential** to ensure accuracy of the specimen?
1. Press the sticky side of nonfrosted cellophane tape across the anus before the client goes to bed at night.
2. Insert a swab beyond the internal anal sphincter and rotate it gently while removing it from the anus.
3. Perform the procedure the first thing in the morning before the first bowel movement.
4. Wash the rectal area gently with soap and water before performing the procedure.

11. Which client statement **supports** the nurse's conclusion that a client understands the need to reestablish bowel flora after a week of diarrhea?
1. "I must wean myself off of the antibiotics one day after my temperature is normal."
2. "I should eat a container of yogurt every day for a few days."
3. "I have to add rice to my diet in one meal each day."
4. "I ought to drink eight glasses of water a day."

12. A nurse is teaching a client with a history of constipation about the excessive use of laxatives. Which effect of laxatives should the nurse include as the **primary** reason why their use should be avoided?
1. Weakens the natural response to defecation
2. Results in distention of the intestines
3. Causes abdominal discomfort
4. Precipitates incontinence

13. A nurse identifies that a client has tarry stools. Which problem should the nurse conclude that the client is experiencing?
1. Upper gastrointestinal bleeding
2. Pancreatic dysfunction
3. Lactulose intolerance
4. Inadequate bile salts

14. A nurse is teaching a client with a cardiac condition to avoid the Valsalva maneuver. Which should the nurse teach the client to do?
1. Eat rice several times a week.
2. Take a cathartic on a regular basis.
3. Attempt to have a bowel movement every day.
4. Exhale while contracting the abdominal muscles.

15. A nurse is teaching a client how to irrigate a colostomy. The client asks, "Why is it necessary to use the cone attachment to the irrigation catheter?" What information should the nurse include in a response to this question?
1. Stops enema solution from flowing out of the bowel during the procedure
2. Prevents prolapse of the bowel during evacuation of the solution
3. Dilates the stoma so that the enema tube can be inserted
4. Facilitates the elimination of drainage from the colon

16. Which outcome of the options presented is **most** appropriate for a client with perceived constipation?
1. Have a bowel movement without the use of a laxative.
2. Explain the rationale for the use of laxatives.
3. Drink 8 glasses of water per day.
4. Defecate every day.

17. Which action is important for the nurse to teach clients about the intake of bran to facilitate defecation?
1. Ingest 3 tablespoons of bran each morning.
2. Drink at least 8 glasses of fluids daily when taking bran.
3. Attempt a bowel movement right after ingesting the bran.
4. Take a cathartic daily that will supplement the action of bran.

18. A primary health-care provider prescribes a tap-water enema for a client. The client asks about the purpose of the enema. Which specific information about the purpose of a tap-water enema should be included in the nurse's response?
1. "It reduces abdominal gas."
2. "It drains the urinary bladder."
3. "It empties the bowel of stool."
4. "It limits nausea and vomiting."

19. Which word is specific regarding how a soapsuds enema works on the mucosa of the bowel?
1. Dilating
2. Irritating
3. Softening
4. Lubricating

20. A nurse is caring for a client with an intestinal stoma. Which intervention is **most** important?
1. Cleansing the stoma with cool water
2. Spraying an air-freshening deodorant in the room
3. Selecting a bag with an appropriate-size stomal opening
4. Wearing sterile, nonlatex gloves when caring for the stoma

21. Which should the nurse do when administering a small-volume hypertonic enema to an adult?
1. Insert the rectal tube 1 to 1.5 inches into the anal canal.
2. Position the enema bottle 12 inches above the level of the client's anus.
3. Direct the rectal tube toward the vertebrae as it is inserted into the rectum.
4. Maintain the compression of the enema container until after withdrawing the tube.

22. Which should the nurse do before collecting a stool sample for occult blood?
1. Plan to collect the first specimen of the day.
2. Obtain a sterile specimen container.
3. Wash the client's perianal area.
4. Ask the client to void.

23. A nurse performs a physical assessment of a newly admitted client who is incontinent of stool. For which characteristic related to bowel incontinence should the nurse assess the client?
1. Frequent, soft stools
2. Involuntary passage of stool
3. Impaired anal sphincter control
4. Greenish-yellow color to the stool

24. A nurse is collecting a bowel elimination history from a newly admitted client with a medical diagnosis of possible bowel obstruction. Which question takes **priority**?
1. "Do you use anything to help you move your bowels?"
2. "When was the last time you moved your bowels?"
3. "What color are your usual bowel movements?"
4. "How often do you have a bowel movement?"

25. While providing a health history, the client tells the nurse, "I have gastroesophageal reflux disease." Which **most** serious consequence associated with this disorder should the nurse anticipate this client may develop?
1. Diarrhea
2. Heartburn
3. Gastric fullness
4. Esophageal erosion

26. A nurse is implementing a prescribed bowel preparation for a client who is scheduled for a colonoscopy. Which is the **most** serious consequence that is prevented by an effective bowel preparation?
    1. Psychological stress
    2. Wasted expense
    3. Misdiagnosis
    4. Discomfort

27. A nurse is assessing a client who has a distended abdomen resulting from flatulence. The client has a prescription for a regular diet and an activity prescription for "out of bed." Which can the nurse do to promote passage of the intestinal gas?
    1. Instruct the client to increase the amount of fluid intake.
    2. Suggest that the client avoid cruciferous foods.
    3. Obtain a prescription for a laxative.
    4. Encourage the client to ambulate.

28. A nurse should use a fracture bedpan for clients with which condition? **Select all that apply.**
    1. _____ Below the knee amputation
    2. _____ Peripheral vascular disease
    3. _____ Spinal cord injury
    4. _____ Dementia
    5. _____ Obesity

29. A nurse is performing a physical assessment of a client concerning the gastrointestinal system. Place the following interventions in the order in which they should be performed.
    1. Palpate the abdomen.
    2. Inspect the anus and perianal area visually.
    3. Percuss the abdomen for the quality of sounds.
    4. Auscultate the entire abdomen for bowel sounds.
    5. Observe the contour and symmetry of the abdomen.

    Answer: _____

30. A client is experiencing constipation. Which independent nursing action facilitates defecation of a hard stool? **Select all that apply.**
    1. _____ Applying a lubricant to the anus
    2. _____ Providing a sitz bath after defecation
    3. _____ Instilling warm mineral oil into the rectum
    4. _____ Placing a warm, wet washcloth against the perianal area
    5. _____ Encouraging the client to rock forward and back while defecating

31. A client is placed on a therapeutic regimen of an anticoagulant because of a history of deep vein thrombosis and an antihypertensive for an elevated blood pressure. Two weeks later, the client tells the nurse about eating a clove of garlic daily along with the prescribed medications. In addition to informing the primary health-care provider about the client's intake of garlic, what should the nurse teach the client about the client's medication regimen and the intake of garlic? **Select all that apply.**
    1. _____ Avoid taking garlic because it can cause excessive amounts of hemoglobin in your body.
    2. _____ Discontinue the intake of garlic two weeks before any surgery to prevent hemorrhage.
    3. _____ The risk of bruising and bleeding increases when garlic is taken concurrently with an anticoagulant.
    4. _____ Garlic increases the antihypertensive effects of medication taken to treat an elevated blood pressure.
    5. _____ Stop taking garlic and notify the doctor immediately if you experience a rash, itching, severe dizziness, trouble breathing, or swelling of the face, tongue, or throat.

32. A primary health-care provider prescribes docusate sodium in liquid form for a client who is constipated but has difficulty swallowing tablets. The prescription is for 200 mg daily to be divided into two doses, one in the a.m. and one at hour of sleep. The package insert states that there is 50 mg/5 mL. How much solution of docusate sodium should the nurse administer per dose? **Record your answer using a whole number.**

Answer: _____ mL.

33. A nurse is assisting a client with a regular bedpan. Which nursing action is **essential**? **Select all that apply.**
1. _____ Position the client slightly off the back edge of the bedpan.
2. _____ Fold the top linen out of the way when putting the client on the bedpan.
3. _____ Remain outside the curtains of the bed until the client is done using the bedpan.
4. _____ Elevate the head of the bed to the Fowler position after the client is on the bedpan.
5. _____ Raise the side rails on both sides of the bed after the client is positioned on the bedpan.

34. A nurse is providing dietary teaching to a client with acute diverticulitis who has a prescription for a low-fiber diet. Which food selected by the client indicates that the dietary teaching was understood? **Select all that apply.**
1. _____ White rice
2. _____ Split peas
3. _____ Soft tofu
4. _____ Turkey
5. _____ Pasta

35. A client is attending the health clinic for treatment of hemorrhoids. The nurse reviews the client's history, interviews the client, and performs a focused assessment. Which of the following in the client's history does the nurse conclude may have influenced the development of the hemorrhoids? **Select all that apply.**
1. _____ Stands for long periods of time at work
2. _____ Has had multiple pregnancies
3. _____ Tends to have constipation
4. _____ Has a disease of the liver
5. _____ Is obese

CLIENT'S CLINICAL RECORD

Client History
Married for 18 years
Has five children between the ages of 7 and 17: three single births and a set of twins
Works as a cashier 4 days a week
Has a history of liver disease

Client Interview
Client states that she drinks a glass of wine with dinner. When the hemorrhoids became increasingly painful and a continuous problem, she decided to do something about them. States she sometimes takes a stool softener when she is constipated.

Focused Assessment
Client is 60 pounds more than ideal body weight for height. Three external hemorrhoids are bright red, swollen, and oozing blood. Client states, "My rectal area is itchy and painful."

36. A nurse is caring for a group of clients with a variety of gastrointestinal problems. Which of the following can cause both diarrhea and constipation? **Select all that apply.**
1. _____ Inability to perceive bowel cues
2. _____ Cancer of the large intestines
3. _____ Side effects of medications
4. _____ High-solute tube feedings
5. _____ Increased metabolic rate

37. Which statement by a client with diverticulosis alerts the nurse that the client needs additional health teaching? **Select all that apply.**
1. _____ "I should avoid eating high-fiber cereal."
2. _____ "I sit on the toilet for 10 minutes after breakfast every day."
3. _____ "I am going to drink 8 glasses of water a day when I get home."
4. _____ "I should hold my breath and bear down when having a bowel movement."
5. _____ "I like to massage my lower abdomen when I'm trying to have a bowel movement."

38. A nurse is caring for a client with a colostomy, and the client's stool has a pasty consistency. Place an X over the area of the intestine where the nurse can expect a colostomy to produce stool with a pasty consistency.

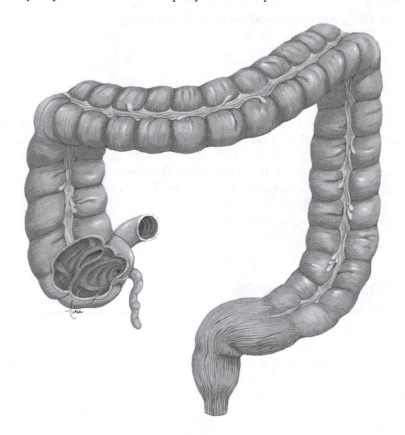

39. A client had a colonoscopy with several polyps excised for biopsies. The nurse teaches the client routine post-procedure expectations. Which of the following should the nurse instruct the client to report to the primary health-care provider? **Select all that apply.**

1. _____ Intermittent passage of gas from the anus
2. _____ Continuous abdominal cramping
3. _____ Some abdominal bloating
4. _____ Minimal rectal bleeding
5. _____ Mild fatigue

40. A nurse is to administer an oil-retention enema, a tap-water enema, and a return-flow enema to three different clients. Which of the following should be performed with all three enemas? **Select all that apply.**

1. _____ Use between 500 and 1,000 mL of solution.
2. _____ Place the client in the left side-lying position.
3. _____ Use water-soluble jelly to lubricate the tip of the rectal probe.
4. _____ Pull the curtain around the client's bed and drape the client.
5. _____ Hold the enema solution a minimum of 12 inches above the anus.

1. 1. The odor from drainage is minimal because fewer bacteria are present in the ileum compared with the large intestine. An ileostomy is an opening into the ileum (distal small intestine from the jejunum to the cecum).
   2. Cleansing the skin, skin barriers, and a well-fitted appliance are precautions to protect the skin around an ileostomy stoma. The drainage from an ileostomy contains enzymes that can damage the skin.
   3. **This statement is inaccurate in relation to an ileostomy and indicates that the client needs more teaching. An ileostomy produces liquid fecal drainage, not formed stool that requires irrigation.**
   4. An ileostomy stoma does not have a sphincter that can control the flow of flatus or drainage, resulting in noise.

2. 1. All rectal tubes should be lubricated to facilitate entry of the tube into the anus and rectum and prevent mucosal trauma.
   2. The anal canal is 1 to 2 inches (2.5 to 5 cm) long. Inserting the rectal tube 3 to 4 inches (7 to 10 cm) ensures that the tip of the tube is beyond the internal and external anal sphincters. This action is appropriate for all types of enemas.
   3. The solution container should be raised no higher than 12 inches for all enemas; this allows the solution to instill slowly, which limits discomfort and intestinal spasms.
   4. **Lowering the container of solution creates a siphon effect that pulls the instilled fluid back out through the rectal tube into the solution container. The return flow promotes the evacuation of gas from the intestines. This technique is used only with a return-flow enema. When performing a cleansing enema, the tubing is removed after all the solution is instilled.**

3. 1. **Straining on defecation requires the person to hold the breath while bearing down (Valsalva maneuver). This maneuver increases the intrathoracic and intracranial pressures, which can precipitate dysrhythmias, brain attack (stroke), and respiratory difficulties; all of these can be life-threatening.**
   2. The loss of the voluntary ability to control the passage of fecal or gaseous discharges through the anus (bowel incontinence) is caused by impaired functioning of the anal sphincters or their nerve supply, not straining on defecation.
   3. Fecal impaction is caused by the accumulation and prolonged retention of fecal material in the large intestine, not straining on defecation.
   4. Although straining on defecation can contribute to the formation of hemorrhoids, this is not the primary reason straining on defecation is discouraged. Hemorrhoids, although painful, are not life-threatening.

4. 1. The presence of fluid or food activates digestive enzymes, not mucus.
   2. **Mucus secreted by mucous membranes and glands is a viscous, slippery fluid containing mucin, white blood cells, water, inorganic salts, and exfoliated cells. Mucin, a mucopolysaccharide, is a lubricant that protects body surfaces from friction and erosion.**
   3. Mucus does not enhance gastric acidity. Gastric acidity enhances digestion.
   4. The low surface tension of bile salts contributes to the emulsification of fats in the intestine.

5. 1. **Usually digestive juices of 3.5 to 5.0 L are secreted and reabsorbed by the body daily. With diarrhea, the transit time through the intestine is decreased, interfering with the reabsorption of water, resulting in frequent, loose, watery stools and dehydration.**
   2. Although malnutrition may be related to diarrhea, particularly if it is prolonged, it is neither life-threatening nor the priority in comparison with another option.
   3. Although the skin may become excoriated in the presence of diarrhea because the enzymes in fecal material can erode the skin, it is neither life-threatening nor the priority in comparison with another option.
   4. Diarrhea is unrelated to urinary incontinence.

6. 1. **A pale stoma indicates that the circulation to the stoma is compromised, and viability of tissue is questionable without immediate intervention. The primary health-care provider should be notified immediately.**
   2. Although assessing bowel sounds might be done, it is not the priority. Active bowel sounds indicate peristalsis and the presence

of flatus in the small intestines, which can occur even if there is an impending problem in the large intestine.

3. Washing the area with warm water is inappropriate. This will not improve circulation to the stoma and will waste valuable time.

4. Massaging around the stoma is inappropriate. This will not improve circulation and may injure surrounding tissue.

7. 1. Constipation, not bowel incontinence, is more common in older adults than in other age groups. Constipation in older adults is caused by decreased bowel motility, inadequate hydration, lack of fiber, sedentary lifestyle, misuse of laxatives, and side effects of medications.

2. Sedatives depress the central nervous system, which may precipitate constipation, not bowel incontinence.

3. **When a person is disoriented to time, place, and person, the individual may not have the cognitive ability to perceive and interpret intestinal distention and rectal pressure cues to defecate, resulting in bowel incontinence.**

4. Antibiotic medications are known for causing diarrhea, not bowel incontinence.

8. 1. Tarry stools indicate upper gastrointestinal bleeding.

2. Orange stools indicate the presence of infection.

3. Green mucoid stools indicate the presence of infection.

4. **Bright red–tinged stools are the cardinal sign of lower gastrointestinal bleeding. When bleeding occurs close to the anus, enzymes have not digested the blood, so the blood has not turned black.**

9. 1. Ova and parasites are identified through microscopic examination of feces, not by the guaiac test.

2. **Testing the feces for occult blood is called the guaiac test. This test uses a chemical reagent to detect the presence of the enzyme peroxidase in the hemoglobin molecule. Occult blood is obscure (hidden) and may not be visible to the naked eye.**

3. Bacteria are identified in feces through a stool culture, not by the guaiac test.

4. Bile is an expected constituent of fecal material and is not detected with the guaiac test.

10. 1. Specimen collection is done immediately after awakening from sleep, not before sleep.

2. Inserting a swab beyond the internal anal sphincter and rotating it gently while removing it from the anus are unnecessary and can injure the anal and rectal mucosa.

3. **Performing the procedure the first thing in the morning before the first bowel movement ensures that there will be eggs available for collection at the perianal area. The adult pinworm (Enterobius vermicularis) exits the anus at night to lay eggs. The cellophane tape (Scotch tape) test is performed first thing in the morning before a bowel movement or bathing so that these eggs are not disrupted or removed before obtaining a specimen for testing.**

4. Washing the rectal area before collecting the specimen will remove any eggs that are present in the perianal area, which will interfere with accurate test results.

11. 1. Weaning off the antibiotic 1 day after the temperature is normal will not reestablish bowel flora. Discontinuing antibiotics before the full course of therapy is completed can result in a return of the original infection or precipitate the development of a superinfection.

2. **Yogurt is merely milk that is curdled by the addition of bacteria, specifically Lactobacillus bulgaricus and Streptococcus thermophilus. Eating yogurt helps to restore the bacterial balance of the resident flora of the intestine.**

3. Although rice helps to limit diarrhea, it will not reestablish bowel flora.

4. Although water is essential for all body processes, and to replace fluid lost in the diarrhea, it does not reestablish bowel flora.

12. 1. **Laxatives cause a rapid transit time of intestinal contents. When they are used excessively, the bowel's natural responses to intestinal distention and rectal pressure weaken, resulting in chronic constipation.**

2. Laxatives increase peristalsis, which helps evacuate the bowel, preventing, not promoting, abdominal distention from flatus or intestinal contents.

3. Although excessive laxative use can cause cramping, it is temporary and does not

have long-term implications, as does the problem in another option.

4. The loss of the voluntary ability to control the passage of fecal or gaseous discharges through the anus (bowel incontinence) is caused by impaired functioning of the anal sphincters or their nerve supply, not excessive laxative use.

13. 1. **When blood from bleeding in the upper gastrointestinal tract is exposed to the digestive process, the fecal material becomes black (tarry). In addition, ingestion of exogenous iron, red meat, and dark green vegetables can make the stool look black.**
2. Pancreatic dysfunction results in impaired digestion of fats (by lipase), protein (by trypsin and chymotrypsin), and carbohydrates (by amylase). Pancreatic dysfunction results in pale, foul-smelling, bulky stools, rather than tarry stools.
3. A reduction or lack of the secretion of lactase from the wall of the small intestine results in the inability of the body to break down lactose to glucose and galactose. Lactose intolerance causes diarrhea, gaseous distention, and intestinal cramping, not tarry stools.
4. Inadequate bile salts result in less bile entering the intestinal tract. The brown color of stool is caused by the presence of stercobilin and urobilin, which are derived from a pigment in bile (bilirubin). The stool will appear clay colored with inadequate bile salts.

14. 1. Rice thickens stool, which promotes the development of constipation. Constipation may result in straining on defecation, which employs the Valsalva maneuver.
2. Prescribing a cathartic is a dependent, not an independent, function of the nurse. Regular use of a cathartic is contraindicated because it leads to dependence.
3. Attempting to have a bowel movement every day may result in straining, which employs the use of the Valsalva maneuver. Also, the client may not need to have a daily bowel movement.
4. **Exhaling requires the glottis to be open, which prevents the Valsalva maneuver. The Valsalva maneuver is bearing down while holding the breath by closing the glottis, which increases intrathoracic pressure. The Valsalva maneuver briefly interferes with blood flow to the heart. When the glottis opens during exhalation, the pressure is released and a surge of blood flows to the heart, which may precipitate a dysrhythmia in a person with a cardiac condition.**

15. 1. **The cone advances into the stoma until it effectively fills the opening, which prevents a reflux of solution while the irrigating solution is being instilled. In addition, it helps prevent accidental perforation of the bowel with the rectal catheter.**
2. A cone will not prevent the prolapse of the bowel. If a prolapse should occur, the surgeon should be notified immediately.
3. Using a cone to dilate the stoma so that the enema tube can be inserted is not the purpose of the cone. The catheter is threaded through the center of the cone.
4. The cone is removed before the bowel evacuates its contents.

16. 1. **Having a bowel movement without the use of a laxative is the most appropriate outcome for a client with perceived constipation. People with perceived constipation believe that they should have a daily bowel movement and use laxatives, suppositories, enemas, or all of these to achieve this objective.**
2. Although knowledge is essential, behavioral outcomes determine if a desired outcome is achieved.
3. Drinking eight glasses of water per day is an intervention, not a desired outcome. Although desirable for everyone, it does not specifically relate to perceived constipation.
4. The need to have a bowel movement every day is unnecessary, unrealistic, and a myth. Patterns of bowel elimination vary considerably, depending on a multitude of factors.

17. 1. Eating 3 tablespoons of bran each morning is too stimulating for the intestines initially. Bran use should begin with 1 tablespoon and gradually increase as tolerated because it can cause flatus and distention.
2. **Bran is an insoluble fiber that increases bulk in the intestines. Eight glasses of water daily keep the body well hydrated and the stool soft. Intestinal elimination is dependent on the relationships among fiber, water, and activity.**

3. Attempting a bowel movement right after ingesting the bran is too soon to expect a physiological response to the bran.
4. Taking a cathartic daily is counterproductive. Cathartic use will weaken the bowel's natural responses to intestinal distention and rectal pressure, resulting in chronic constipation.

18. 1. A return-flow enema (Harris flush, Harris drip), not a tap-water enema, helps eliminate intestinal gas.
2. A urinary retention catheter (Foley), not a tap-water enema, drains the urinary bladder of urine.
3. **A tap-water enema instills fluid into the large intestine; the pressure of this volume stimulates peristalsis, causing the colon to evacuate stool.**
4. A tap-water enema will not affect nausea and vomiting; taking nothing by mouth or medication can be used to limit nausea and vomiting.

19. 1. High-volume (not soapsuds) enemas, such as tap-water or saline enemas, work by distending (dilating) the lumen of the intestine.
2. **Although a soapsuds enema works by increasing the volume in the colon, its unique attribute is that soap is irritating to the intestinal mucosa. Irritation of the mucosa precipitates peristalsis, which facilitates the evacuation of fecal material.**
3. An oil-retention enema, a small-volume enema, introduces oil into the rectum and sigmoid colon; this softens the feces and lubricates the rectum and anal canal, facilitating defecation.
4. An oil-retention enema, not a soapsuds enema, lubricates the rectum and anal canal, facilitating the passage of feces.

20. 1. Although a stoma can be cleaned with water as long as it is not at the extremes of hot or cold, it is not the priority.
2. Although spraying an air-freshening deodorant in the room might be done, it is not the priority.
3. **The opening of the appliance must be large enough to encircle the stoma to within ⅛ inch to protect the surrounding tissue from the enzymes present in the intestinal discharge without impinging on the stoma. Pressure against the stoma can damage delicate mucosal tissue or impede circulation to the**

stoma, both of which can impair the viability of the stoma.
4. Clean, not sterile, gloves should be worn when caring for a stoma. Medical, not surgical, asepsis should be practiced. Latex or nonlatex gloves can be worn as long as the client or nurse does not have a latex allergy.

21. 1. Inserting a rectal tube 1 to 1.5 inches into the anal canal will not permit safe administration of the enema solution. The rectal tube must be inserted 3 to 4 inches to ensure that the catheter is beyond both the external and internal anal sphincters.
2. A small-volume enema bottle is held directly outside the anus because the solution container is attached to the prelubricated nozzle. The container of a large-volume enema should not exceed a height of 12 inches above the anus.
3. Directing the rectal tube toward the vertebrae as it is inserted into the rectum will injure the intestinal mucosa. The catheter should be directed toward the umbilicus, not the vertebrae.
4. **Maintaining compression of the enema container until after withdrawing the tube prevents suctioning back of the fluid that has just been instilled. Releasing compression on the bottle causes a vacuum at the tip of the nozzle that can injure mucous membranes.**

22. 1. Collecting the first specimen of the day is unnecessary.
2. Using a sterile specimen container is unnecessary. Medical, not surgical, asepsis should be followed.
3. Washing the perineal area is unnecessary. However, the nurse may assist the client to perform perineal hygiene after the stool specimen is obtained.
4. **Emptying the urinary bladder before attempting to have a bowel movement prevents accidental contamination of the specimen by urine.**

23. 1. Frequent, soft stools are associated with diarrhea. Diarrhea is loose, liquid stools, increased frequency (three times a day or more) of stools, or both.
2. **An involuntary passage of stool is a major clinical finding associated with bowel incontinence, which is the state in which an individual experiences a**

change in usual bowel habits characterized by involuntary passage of stool.

3. Impaired anal sphincter control is not a characteristic a nurse can evaluate when performing a physical assessment.

4. A greenish-yellow color to the stool is unrelated to bowel incontinence. A green or orange color to the stool indicates intestinal infection.

24. 1. Although asking if anything is used to help move the bowels may be done, it is not the priority at this time.

2. A cardinal sign of a bowel obstruction is the lack of a bowel movement (obstipation).

3. Although asking about the color of bowel movements will be done, this information relates more to malabsorption, biliary problems, and gastrointestinal bleeding.

4. Although asking how often one has a bowel movement will be done to obtain baseline information about intestinal elimination, it is not specific to the presenting problem.

25. 1. Diarrhea is not associated with gastroesophageal reflux disease (GERD).

2. Pain occurring behind the sternum (heartburn) and sore throat are the predominant symptom of GERD. Although these responses are a concern, they can be treated.

3. Although feeling full, distended, or bloated can occur with GERD, it is not life-threatening, and the client can be taught interventions to limit its occurrence.

4. With GERD, a backflow of the contents of the stomach into the esophagus occurs. Gastric juices are acetic (pH less than 3.5), which can cause erosion of the mucous membranes of the esophagus. Cellular changes in the lining of the esophageal mucosa (Barrett's esophagus) are a risk factor for developing esophageal cancer.

26. 1. Although psychological stress is a serious consequence, it is not life-threatening.

2. Although a canceled or repeated colonoscopy may incur a wasted expense, this consequence is not life-threatening. A test may be canceled or performed a second time if the client has an ineffective bowel preparation.

3. Fecal material in the intestines can interfere with the visualization, collection, and analysis of data obtained through a colonoscopy, resulting in diagnostic errors.

4. Although discomfort may occur, it is not the most serious outcome of an inappropriate preparation for a colonoscopy.

27. 1. Increasing the amount of fluid intake will not facilitate the evacuation of intestinal gas.

2. Limiting the intake of cruciferous foods will prevent the development of intestinal gas, not promote its evacuation.

3. A laxative is an excessive intervention for a client with flatulence.

4. Ambulation increases metabolic activity, which increases intestinal peristalsis. Increased intestinal peristalsis moves intestinal gas toward the anus, where it can be expelled.

28. 1. A regular bedpan is appropriate for a client who has a below the knee amputation.

2. A regular bedpan is appropriate for a client with peripheral vascular disease.

3. A fracture bedpan has a low back that promotes functional alignment of the client's lower back while on the bedpan.

4. A regular bedpan is appropriate for a client with dementia.

5. A regular bedpan is appropriate for a client who is obese.

29. **5. Inspection should occur first because it is the least invasive assessment. The abdomen should be assessed before turning the client, which slightly rearranges the internal organs.**

2. The anus and the perianal area should be inspected after a less invasive assessment and before other assessment techniques that can alter the results of inspection.

4. Auscultation should occur after less invasive assessment techniques and before other more invasive assessment techniques that can alter the results of auscultation.

3. Percussion should occur after less invasive techniques but before a more invasive assessment technique that can alter the results of percussion.

1. Palpation should occur after less invasive assessment techniques are completed.

30. 1. A lubricant reduces friction, which facilitates the passage of a hard, dry stool through the anus. Nurses are legally permitted to diagnose and treat human responses. Constipation is a human response, and applying a water-soluble lubricant to the anus is an independent function of the nurse.
    2. A sitz bath requires a primary health-care provider's prescription and is a dependent, not independent, function of the nurse. A sitz bath will not promote the passage of a hard, dry stool, but it may promote hygiene and comfort after the bowel movement.
    3. An oil-retention enema softens the feces and lubricates the rectum and anus. However, it requires a primary health-care provider's prescription and is a dependent, not independent, function of the nurse.
    4. A warm, wet washcloth placed against the perianal area may facilitate defecation by relaxing the surrounding muscles and the external sphincter.
    5. Rocking forward and back when attempting to defecate increases both tension against the abdomen and intra-abdominal pressure; these facilitate the passage of stool from the rectum and anus.

31. 1. Garlic decreases, not increases, the production of hemoglobin. Also, it causes lysis of red blood cells.
    2. Because of garlic's antiplatelet properties, it should be discontinued 2 weeks before surgery to decrease the risk of bleeding.
    3. Garlic decreases platelet aggregation lengthening coagulation time. This antiplatelet action slows blood clotting, thereby increasing the risk of bruising and bleeding.
    4. Garlic decreases, not increases, the effectiveness of antihypertensive medication and should be avoided.
    5. These are serious allergic responses to the intake of garlic. The client may need immediate medical attention.

32. Answer: 10 mL. First, determine the amount of mg per dose of medication prescribed. 200 (total mg of medication daily) ÷ 2 (number of doses in the day) = 100 mg (amount of mg of medication per dose). Next, solve the problem by using the formula for ratio and proportion.

$$\frac{\text{Desired}}{\text{Have}} \quad \frac{100 \text{ mg}}{50 \text{ mg}} = \frac{x \text{ mL}}{5 \text{ mL}}$$
$$50 \text{ x} = 500$$
$$x = 500 \div 50$$
$$x = 10 \text{ mL}$$

33. 1. Positioning a client slightly off the back edge of a regular bedpan is unsafe and uncomfortable. The client should be positioned so that the buttocks rest on, not slightly off of, the smooth, rounded rim of a regular bedpan.
    2. Folding the top linen out of the way when putting the client on the bedpan is unnecessary. The top linen can be draped over the client in such a way as to promote placement of the bedpan while maintaining the privacy and dignity of the client.
    3. Remaining outside the curtains of the client's bed while the client is on the bedpan allows the nurse to be in close proximity to the client. The nurse is available to assist the client if needed, and it provides a sense of security for the client.
    4. Elevating the head of the bed so that the client is in the high-Fowler position assumes the familiar, usual position for having a bowel movement. A vertical position utilizes gravity, and hip flexion raises intra-abdominal pressure, both of which maximize evacuation of feces.
    5. Raising both side rails provides support on which the client can rest the upper extremities and maintains client safety. Raising the side rails before raising the head of the bed maintains safety.

34. 1. One cup of white rice contains just 0.6 g (grams) of fiber. Low-fiber foods limit the amount of material (residue) left in the intestines after the digestive process; this lessens the bulk of stool, which is less irritating to the intestinal mucosa.
    2. One cup of cooked split peas contains 16.3 g of fiber and should be avoided on a low-fiber diet.

3. One cup of soft tofu contains just 0.5 g of fiber.

4. Turkey contains no dietary fiber and is permitted on a low-fiber diet.

5. Refined white flour products (e.g., pasta) contain just 1.6 g or less of fiber per 1-cup serving.

35. 1. Prolonged standing or sitting increases pressure on the hemorrhoidal veins that can cause them to become dilated, enlarged, and inflamed.

2. Pregnancy increases intra-abdominal pressure, causing elevated systemic and portal venous pressure, which is transmitted to the anorectal veins. The added pressure of multiple births and having twins aggravates the problem. Eventually, the distended veins separate from the smooth muscle surrounding them, and prolapse of the hemorrhoidal vessels occurs.

3. Repeated straining on defecation because of constipation increases intra-abdominal pressure, eventually causing the anorectal veins to distend and become inflamed, resulting in hemorrhoids. Repeated straining causes them to enlarge.

4. Portal hypertension is associated with diseases of the liver. The veins of the intestine drain into the branches of the portal vein. Increased pressure in these veins results in distention and inflammation of the hemorrhoidal veins.

5. Increased intra-abdominal pressure associated with obesity causes elevated systemic and portal venous pressure, which is transmitted to the anorectal veins. Eventually, the veins distend and become inflamed, resulting in hemorrhoids.

36. 1. An inability to perceive bowel cues for defecation results in a lack of response that further weakens the defecation reflex, ultimately causing constipation, not diarrhea.

2. Cancer of the large intestine can cause constipation, diarrhea, alternating constipation and diarrhea, or all of these. The mass in the intestinal lumen may partially or totally obstruct the passage of stool, resulting in a condition that appears to be constipation. The leakage of stool around an intestinal tumor/lesion results in a condition that appears to be diarrhea.

3. Medications, depending on their physiological action, side effects, and toxic effects, can cause either constipation or diarrhea.

4. A high-solute tube feeding has a greater osmotic pressure than surrounding interstitial tissue; it draws fluid into the gastrointestinal tract, which may result in diarrhea, not constipation.

5. An increased metabolic rate will increase peristalsis and possibly result in an increased frequency of the passage of stools, not constipation.

37. 1. High-fiber foods are encouraged because they prevent constipation. Constipation increases intraluminal intestinal pressure, which promotes intestinal mucosal outpouching. Foods low in fiber are prescribed when a client has an acute inflammation of a diverticulum (diverticulitis) until the inflammation resolves.

2. Sitting on the toilet for 10 minutes after breakfast every day is an accepted practice. Bowel elimination should follow a familiar routine, and attempting to defecate after breakfast takes advantage of the gastrocolic reflex.

3. Drinking 8 glasses of water a day is desirable for effective bowel function. An adequate intake of fluid ensures that after water is reabsorbed through the large intestines for essential body processes, there is enough water left in the intestine to create a soft, formed stool.

4. The Valsalva maneuver increases intraluminal intestinal pressure, which promotes intestinal mucosal outpouching and should be avoided.

5. Massaging the lower abdomen when trying to have a bowel movement is an accepted practice. Light stroking of the skin (effleurage) reduces abdominal muscle tension, which may facilitate defecation.

38. An X anywhere along the highlighted area is the correct answer. Stool in the ascending colon is the most liquid, but as it travels through the transverse colon, fluid is reabsorbed and stool becomes pasty in consistency. In the descending colon, stool becomes more dry, solid, and formed.

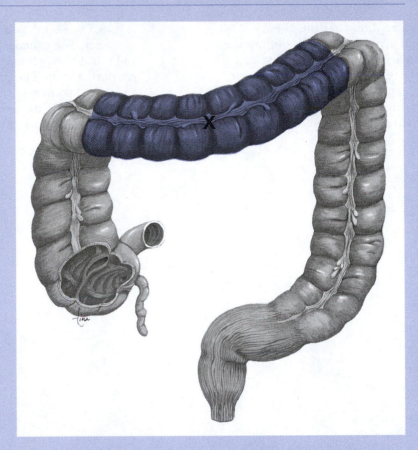

39. 1. This is an expected response after a colonoscopy. Carbon dioxide is inserted into the intestine (CO_2 insufflation) to distend the lumen, which permits visualization of internal intestinal structures. This gas will be passed through the anus for 24 to 48 hours after the procedure. Ambulation facilitates the passage of this gas.

2. Some abdominal cramping may occur from irritability of the intestine. However, it should not be severe or continuous. Severe abdominal cramping may indicate perforation of the intestinal wall.

3. Some abdominal bloating is expected after a colonoscopy. However, it should not be extensive. Abdominal bloating and distention that is excessive or continues beyond 24 hours after the test may indicate perforation of the intestinal wall.

4. Minimal rectal bleeding is expected after a colonoscopy when polyps are removed. When tissue is excised, the intestinal mucosa is traumatized, and the site will leak blood and body fluids. The client should be informed that an amount equal to several tablespoons of blood may exit the anus the day after the test.

5. Mild fatigue is expected after a colonoscopy. Fatigue results from the sedatives and conscious sedation used during the procedure.

40. 1. The amount of solution used depends on the type of enema prescribed. A tap-water enema uses 500 to 1,000 mL of tap water to distend the intestine and promote defecation. An oil-retention enema has 200 to 250 mL of an oil-based solution to soften feces and promote defecation. A return-flow enema begins with approximately 300 to 500 mL of tap water in the enema container. A small volume of the solution (e.g., 150 to 200 mL) is instilled, and the enema container is immediately lowered below the anus to withdraw fluid and gas into the collection container. The purpose of a return-flow enema is to reduce abdominal distention caused by intestinal gas.

2. The left side-lying position allows the fluid to flow via the principle of gravity as the fluid follows the normal curve of the anus, rectum, and sigmoid colon.

3. Lubrication of the tip of the catheter or probe limits trauma to the mucous membranes of the intestine.

4. **Enemas require that the client's perianal area be exposed. Pulling the curtain around the client's bed and draping the client provide for client privacy and dignity.**

5. Oil-retention enemas and hypertonic enemas are administered in small volumes (e.g., 4.5 to 7.8 mL) via a soft-sided container. The container is squeezed and rolled slowly from the distal to the proximal end until empty. With tap-water and soapsuds enemas, the solution is instilled holding the enema container 8 to 12 inches above the anus.

Pain, Comfort, Rest, and Sleep

The following words include nursing/medical terminology, concepts, principles, and information relevant to content specifically addressed in the chapter or associated with topics presented in it. English dictionaries, nursing textbooks, and medical dictionaries, such as *Taber's Cyclopedic Medical Dictionary,* are resources that can be used to expand your knowledge and understanding of these words and related information.

Addiction

Back rub

Bedtime routines

Biofeedback

Breakthrough pain

Circadian rhythm

Cold therapy

Continuous positive airway pressure (CPAP)

Contralateral stimulation

Distraction techniques

Enuresis

Epidural analgesia

Fatigue

Gate control theory

Grimacing

Guarding behaviors

Guided imagery

Heat therapy

Intensive care unit psychosis

Intrathecal analgesia

Massage

Meditation

Nocturia

Nonopioid

Opioid

Pain, characteristics:

  Aggravating factors

  Duration

  Intensity

  Onset

  Quality

  Relieving factors

Pain scale

Pain threshold

Pain tolerance

Pain, types:

  Acute

  Chronic

Episodic

Intermittent

Intractable

Malignant

Neuropathic

Phantom

Radiating

Remittent

Visceral

Patient-controlled analgesia (PCA)

Physical dependence

Placebo

Progressive muscle relaxation

Psychological dependence

Rest

Self-hypnosis

Self-splinting

Sleep:

  Non–rapid-eye-movement (NREM) sleep

  Rapid-eye-movement (REM) sleep

Sleep disorders:

  Bruxism

  Hypersomnia

  Insomnia

  Narcolepsy

  Night terrors

  Parasomnia

  Restless legs

  Sleep apnea

  Sleep deprivation

  Somnambulism

  Sleepiness

Sleep rituals

Snoring

Sundowning

Transcutaneous electrical nerve stimulation

PAIN, COMFORT, REST, AND SLEEP: QUESTIONS

1. A nurse is caring for a client who is experiencing pain. For which common psychological response to pain should the nurse assess the client?
   1. Concerned about loss of control and independence
   2. Withdrawing from social interactions with others
   3. Asking for medication to provide for relief
   4. Experiencing nausea and vomiting

2. Which is the appropriate client outcome for an adult who has disturbed sleep because of nocturia?
   1. Report fewer early morning awakenings because of a wet bed.
   2. Demonstrate a reduction in nighttime bathroom visits.
   3. Resume sleeping immediately after voiding.
   4. Use an incontinence device at night.

3. A client with a diagnosis of cancer of the ovary had her uterus and both ovaries and fallopian tubes removed (hysterectomy with bilateral salpingo-oophorectomy) and a surgical debulking via an abdominal incision 2 days ago. The client reports abdominal pain at level 5 on a 0-to-10 pain scale. After assessing the pain further, which should the nurse do **first**?
   1. Reposition the client.
   2. Offer a relaxing back rub.
   3. Use distraction techniques.
   4. Administer the prescribed analgesic.

4. A nurse is caring for a client who is diagnosed with narcolepsy. Which is the **most** serious consequence of this disorder?
   1. Inability to provide self-care
   2. Impaired thought processes
   3. Potential for injury
   4. Excessive fatigue

5. A client is experiencing discomfort associated with gastroesophageal reflux. In which position should the nurse teach the client to sleep?
   1. Right lateral
   2. Semi-Fowler
   3. Prone
   4. Sims

6. A client is experiencing anxiety. Which aspect of sleep should the nurse expect **primarily** will be affected as a result of the anxiety?
   1. Onset
   2. Depth
   3. Stage II
   4. Duration

7. A client requests pain medication for severe pain. Which should the nurse do **first** when responding to this client's request?
   1. Use distraction to minimize the client's perception of pain.
   2. Place the client in the most comfortable position possible.
   3. Administer pain medication to the client quickly.
   4. Assess the various aspects of the client's pain.

8. A nurse is planning a teaching program for a client with a diagnosis of obstructive sleep apnea. Which should the nurse plan to discuss with this client?
1. Using the prescribed device that supports airway patency
2. Placing two pillows under the head when sleeping
3. Requesting a sedative to promote sleep
4. Sleeping in the supine position

9. Which is the **most** important nursing intervention that **supports** a client's ability to sleep in the hospital setting?
1. Providing an extra blanket
2. Limiting unnecessary noise on the unit
3. Shutting off lights in the client's room
4. Pulling curtains around the client's bed at night

10. A client has a history of severe chronic pain. Which is the **most** important intervention associated with providing nursing care to this client?
1. Asking what is an acceptable level of pain
2. Providing interventions that do not precipitate pain
3. Focusing on pain management intervention before pain is excessive
4. Determining the level of function that can be performed without pain

11. Which concept should the nurse consider when assessing a client's pain?
1. The expression of pain is not always congruent with the pain experienced.
2. Pain medication can significantly increase a client's pain tolerance.
3. The majority of cultures value the concept of suffering in silence.
4. Most people experience approximately the same pain tolerance.

12. Which **most** common cause of sleep deprivation in the hospital should the nurse consider when planning care?
1. Fragmented sleep
2. Early awakening
3. Restless legs
4. Sleep apnea

13. A nurse is performing an admitting interview. Which client statement about pain should cause the **most** concern for the nurse?
1. "I try to pretend that it is not part of me, but it takes a lot of effort."
2. "My pain medication works, but I'm afraid of becoming addicted."
3. "At home, I take something for the pain before it gets too bad."
4. "They say my pain may get worse, and I can't stand it now."

14. A client has been in the intensive care unit (ICU) for 3 days. For which common adaptation indicating ICU psychosis associated with sleep deprivation should the nurse assess the client?
1. Hypoxia
2. Delirium
3. Lethargy
4. Dementia

15. Which concept associated with sleep should the nurse consider to plan nursing care for a hospitalized client?
1. People require eight hours of uninterrupted sleep to meet energy needs.
2. Frequency of awakenings during sleep decreases as people age.
3. Fear can interfere with the ability to relax and sleep.
4. Bedrest decreases the need for sleep.

16. A nurse is assessing a client in pain. Which word might the nurse use when documenting the pattern of a client's pain?
    1. Tenderness
    2. Moderate
    3. Episodic
    4. Phantom

17. A nurse is obtaining a health history from a newly admitted client. Which client statement about alcohol intake is based on a common physiological response?
    1. "After I go drinking, I have to urinate during the night."
    2. "When I drink, I get hungry in the middle of the night."
    3. "Falling asleep is hard, but once asleep I sleep great."
    4. "If I drink too much, I oversleep in the morning."

18. A nurse is assessing a client experiencing acute pain. Which characteristic is more common with acute pain than with chronic pain?
    1. Self-focusing
    2. Sleep disturbances
    3. Guarding behaviors
    4. Variations in vital signs

19. At which time does a nurse medicate a client for pain for it to be considered preemptive analgesia?
    1. Before a client goes to sleep
    2. At equally distant times around the clock
    3. As soon as a client reports the occurrence of pain
    4. Before doing a dressing change that has been painful in the past

20. A client is diagnosed with chronic fatigue syndrome. Which is **most** important for the nurse to explore in relation to the client's status?
    1. Ability to provide self-care
    2. Physical mobility
    3. Social isolation
    4. Gas exchange

21. Which is **most** important for nurses to understand when caring for clients in pain?
    1. Clients who are in pain will request pain medication.
    2. Clients usually are able to describe the characteristics of their pain.
    3. Clients need to know that the nurse believes what they say about their pain.
    4. Clients will demonstrate vital signs that are congruent with the intensity of their pain.

22. A client is experiencing lack of sleep because of pain. Which is the **most** appropriate goal for this client?
    1. The client will be provided with a back massage every evening before bedtime.
    2. The client will report feeling rested after awakening in the morning.
    3. The client will request less pain medication during the night.
    4. The client will experience four hours of uninterrupted sleep.

23. A nurse is helping a client who is experiencing mild pain to get ready for bed. Which nursing action is **most** effective to help limit pain?
    1. Assisting with relaxing imagery
    2. Obtaining a prescription for an opioid
    3. Encouraging the client to take a warm shower
    4. Recommending that the client be more active during the day

24. During which time frame do people tend to be the sleepiest?
    1. 12 noon and 2 p.m.
    2. 6 a.m. and 8 a.m.
    3. 2 a.m. and 4 a.m.
    4. 6 p.m. and 8 p.m.

25. Which client statement indicates that the client is experiencing bruxism?
   1. "I walk around in my sleep almost every night, but I don't remember it."
   2. "I annoy the whole family with the loud snoring noises I make at night."
   3. "I occasionally urinate in bed when I am sleeping, and it's embarrassing."
   4. "I am told by my wife that I make a lot of noise grinding my teeth when I sleep."

26. A nurse is caring for clients receiving a variety of interventions for pain management. Which pain relief method has the shortest duration of action?
   1. Client-controlled analgesia
   2. Intramuscular sedatives
   3. Intravenous narcotics
   4. Regional anesthesia

27. A nurse is teaching a community health education class about rest and sleep. Which concept related to sleep should the nurse include?
   1. Total time sleeping in bed decreases as one ages.
   2. Sleep needs remain consistent throughout the life span.
   3. Alcohol intake interferes with one's ability to fall asleep.
   4. Bedtime routines are associated with an expectation of sleep.

28. A nurse is teaching a client various techniques to promote sleep. Which internal stimulus that **most** commonly interferes with sleep should the nurse include in the teaching?
   1. Ringing in the ears
   2. Bladder fullness
   3. Hunger
   4. Thirst

29. A nurse is giving a back rub. Which stroke is **most** effective in inducing relaxation at the end of the procedure?
   1. Percussion
   2. Effleurage
   3. Kneading
   4. Circular

30. When the nurse is assessing a client, the client states, "The pain moves from my chest down my left arm." Which characteristic of pain is associated with this statement?
   1. Pattern
   2. Duration
   3. Location
   4. Constancy

31. A nurse is providing health teaching for a client with the diagnosis of obstructive sleep apnea. Which aspect of sleep should the nurse explain is **most** often affected?
   1. Amount
   2. Quality
   3. Depth
   4. Onset

32. A client is being admitted to the hospital, and the nurse is performing a complete assessment. Which is the **most** therapeutic question the nurse can ask about the quality of the client's sleep?
   1. "Does your bed partner complain about your sleep behaviors?"
   2. "Is the number of hours you sleep at night good for you?"
   3. "Do you consider your sleep to be restless or restful?"
   4. "How would you describe your sleep?"

33. A nurse strains a back muscle when moving a client up in bed. Which can the nurse do at home that utilizes the gate-control theory of pain relief to minimize the discomfort?
1. Use guided imagery.
2. Perform progressive muscle relaxation.
3. Apply a cold compress to the site for 20 minutes.
4. Take a nonsteroidal anti-inflammatory medication every 6 hours.

34. A client is having difficulty sleeping and may be experiencing shortened non–rapid-eye-movement (NREM) sleep. Which client assessment **supports** this conclusion? **Select all that apply.**
1. _____ Decreased pain tolerance
2. _____ Inability to concentrate
3. _____ Excessive sleepiness
4. _____ Irritability
5. _____ Confusion

35. A primary health-care provider prescribes oxycodone oral solution 15 mg every 6 hours. The drug is supplied in a 500-mL bottle that indicates 5 mg/5 mL. How much oral solution should the nurse administer? **Record your answer using a whole number.**

   Answer: _____ mL.

36. A 12-year-old boy is experiencing nocturnal enuresis. Which of the following should the nurse explore with the boy and his parents? **Select all that apply.**
1. _____ Limiting fluid intake after dinner
2. _____ Voiding immediately before going to bed
3. _____ Eliminating caffeinated beverages from the diet
4. _____ Thinking about waking up dry when going to bed
5. _____ Changing the wet bed linens using a nonchalant attitude

37. It is suspected that a client has acute appendicitis. The nurse assesses the client for rebound tenderness associated with this condition. Place an X on the body where the nurse should compress the abdomen to elicit this response.

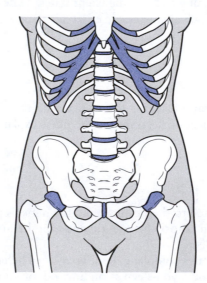

38. Which of the following statements associated with rest and sleep must the nurse consider when planning nursing care? **Select all that apply.**
1. _____ Energy demands increase with age.
2. _____ Metabolic rate increases during rest.
3. _____ Sleep requirements increase during stress.
4. _____ Catabolic hormones increase during sleep.
5. _____ Lack of awareness of the environment increases with sleep.

39. A nurse is caring for a client who is having difficulty sleeping. Which client response indicates that the client is not obtaining adequate rapid-eye-movement (REM) sleep? **Select all that apply.**
1. _____ Hyporesponsiveness
2. _____ Immunosuppression
3. _____ Irritability
4. _____ Confusion
5. _____ Vertigo

40. An older female adult explains to the nurse that she has insomnia. The nurse interviews the client and her husband and reviews the client's medication reconciliation form. Which of the following does the nurse conclude is associated with the client's insomnia? **Select all that apply.**
1. _____ Metformin
2. _____ Older adult
3. _____ Female gender
4. _____ Alcohol intake
5. _____ Diphenhydramine
6. _____ Several naps during the day

CLIENT'S CLINICAL RECORD

Interview with Client
Client reports having difficulty falling asleep, waking frequently during the night, and having difficulty falling back to sleep. Client states, "I never feel rested in the morning."

Interview with Client's Husband
"My wife's problem with sleeping has been going on for several months. She is so tired during the day that she takes several naps during the day. I encourage her to have a drink of whiskey to knock her out when she goes to bed."

Medication Reconciliation Form
Diphenhydramine 50 mg PO at hour of sleep
Metformin 100 mg PO twice a day

---

41. Which is important for a nurse to consider when a client reports the presence of pain? **Select all that apply.**
1. _____ The extent of pain is directly related to the amount of tissue damage.
2. _____ Fatigue decreases the intensity of pain experienced by the client.
3. _____ Behavioral adaptations are congruent with statements about pain.
4. _____ Giving opioids to a client in pain will lead to an addiction.
5. _____ The person feeling the pain is the authority on the pain.

42. Which statement by a client indicates a precipitating factor associated with pain? **Select all that apply.**
1. _____ "I usually feel a little dizzy and think I'm going to vomit when I have pain."
2. _____ "My pain usually comes and goes throughout the night."
3. _____ "I usually have pain after I get dressed in the morning."
4. _____ "My pain feels like a knife cutting right through me."
5. _____ "My abdominal incision hurts when I cough."

43. A nurse administers a back rub to a client after first providing for privacy and maintaining standard precautions. Place the following steps in the order in which they should be implemented.
1. Warm lotion in your hands.
2. Position the client in the side-lying position.
3. Assess the skin for color, turgor, and skin breakdown.
4. Arrange the gown and top linens so that the client's back is exposed.
5. Use a variety of strokes to massage the muscles of the back and sacral area.

Answer: _____

44. When assessing clients who have difficulty sleeping, the nurse assesses for which common physiological response to insomnia? **Select all that apply.**
1. _____ Vertigo
2. _____ Fatigue
3. _____ Irritability
4. _____ Headache
5. _____ Frustration

45. A nurse is assessing a client experiencing chronic pain. Which characteristic is more common with chronic pain than with acute pain? **Select all that apply.**
1. _____ Gradual onset
2. _____ Long duration
3. _____ Anticipated end
4. _____ Psychologically depleting
5. _____ Responds to conventional interventions

1. 1. **Psychological or affective responses to pain relate to feelings and emotional distress. Fear of being dependent on others and loss of self-control are psychological responses to pain.**
   2. Withdrawing from social interactions with others is a behavioral response to pain.
   3. Requesting pain medication is a behavioral response to pain.
   4. Nausea and vomiting are physiological responses to pain.

2. 1. Reporting fewer early morning awakenings because of a wet bed relates to enuresis, which is recurrent involuntary urination that occurs during sleep.
   2. **Demonstrating a reduction in night-time bathroom visits is an appropriate outcome for nocturia, which is voluntary urination during the night.**
   3. Resuming sleeping immediately after voiding relates to insomnia, which is difficulty initiating or maintaining sleep.
   4. Using an incontinence device at night is an intervention, not an outcome. In addition, the client is experiencing nocturia, not incontinence.

3. 1. Repositioning is effective for mild, not severe, pain.
   2. A back massage is ineffective for acute, severe pain; however, it may relax the client and increase the effectiveness of analgesic medication.
   3. Guided imagery is more effective for mild pain, not acute, severe pain.
   4. **Major abdominal surgery involves extensive manipulation of internal organs and a large abdominal incision that require adequate pharmacological intervention to provide relief from pain.**

4. 1. Although the overwhelming daytime sleepiness associated with narcolepsy may interfere with the ability to perform some self-care activities, this is not the major problem related to narcolepsy.
   2. Narcolepsy does not involve disturbed thought processes, which is the state in which an individual experiences a disruption in mental activities, such as conscious thought, reality orientation, problem solving, and judgment.
   3. **Narcolepsy is excessive sleepiness in the daytime that can cause a person to fall asleep uncontrollably at inappropriate**

times (sleep attack) and result in physical harm to self or others.
   4. Although a person with narcolepsy may report a lack of energy, this is not the primary concern associated with narcolepsy.

5. 1. The right-lateral position is a horizontal position that increases the pressure of the abdominal organs against the stomach and increases gastric reflux.
   2. **Gastric secretions increase during rapid-eye-movement (REM) sleep. The semi-Fowler position limits gastroesophageal reflux because gravity allows the abdominal organs to drop, which reduces pressure on the stomach and results in less stomach contents flowing upward into the esophagus.**
   3. The prone position is a horizontal position that increases the pressure of the abdominal organs against the stomach and increases gastric reflux. The abdomen rests on the mattress, and the body exerts direct pressure on the stomach.
   4. The Sims position is a horizontal position halfway between lateral and prone. Direct pressure exerted on the stomach, particularly in the left Sims position, promotes gastric reflux.

6. 1. **Anxiety increases norepinephrine blood levels through stimulation of the sympathetic nervous system, which results in prolonged sleep onset.**
   2. Clients with anxiety still reach the depth of stage IV non–rapid-eye-movement (NREM) sleep.
   3. Stage IV, not stage II, of NREM sleep is affected.
   4. The duration of sleep is affected indirectly, not directly, because of the prolonged onset of sleep.

7. 1. Distraction is not effective for severe pain.
   2. There is not enough information to indicate that this intervention may be effective. In addition, the position the client considers most comfortable may be contraindicated based on the provider's prescriptions or safety issues.
   3. Administering pain medication to the client quickly is a hasty, impulsive response that may or may not be necessary.
   4. **All the factors that affect the pain experience should be assessed, including location, intensity, quality, duration,**

pattern, aggravating and alleviating factors, and physical, behavioral, and attitudinal responses. Assessment must precede intervention.

8. 1. **A continuous positive airway pressure (CPAP) device worn when sleeping keeps the upper airway patent by maintaining an open pathway that facilitates gas exchange.**
   2. Positioning two pillows under the head flexes the neck, which narrows the upper airway and thus contributes to episodes of sleep apnea. Pillows under the upper shoulders and head or small blocks under the head of the bed may assist in keeping the upper airway open.
   3. Sedatives do not limit episodes of sleep apnea.
   4. Encouraging sleeping in the supine position increases the episodes of sleep apnea because the structures of the mouth and oropharynx (i.e., tonsils, adenoids, mucous membranes, uvula, soft palate, and tongue) drop by gravity and ultimately obstruct the airway.

9. 1. Although meeting the basic physiological need to feel warm is appropriate, a hospital's environment generally is warm, so a top sheet and spread are adequate.
   2. **Noise is a serious deterrent to sleep in a hospital. The nurse should limit environmental noise (e.g., distributing fluids, providing treatments, rolling drug and linen carts) and staff communication noise.**
   3. Shutting off lights in the client's room is unsafe. Dim the lights or put a night-light on to provide enough illumination for safe ambulation to the bathroom.
   4. Although pulling curtains around the bed at night provides privacy, it does not limit the factor that usually interferes with sleeping in a hospital.

10. 1. Although the nurse will ask this question to determine the client's level of pain tolerance, it is not the priority.
    2. Although the nurse will attempt to provide interventions that do not precipitate pain, there may be significant interventions that must be performed that may precipitate pain.
    3. **Administration of analgesics around the clock (ATC) administration at regularly scheduled intervals or by long-acting controlled-release transdermal**

patches maintains therapeutic blood levels of analgesics, which limit pain at levels of comfort acceptable to clients. This type of intervention helps to prevent pain from becoming excessive.
    4. Although the nurse and the client will determine the level of function that can be performed without pain, there may be unavoidable activities that may precipitate pain.

11. 1. **An obvious response to pain is not always apparent because psychosocio-cultural factors may dictate behavior. Fear of the treatment for pain, lack of validation, acceptance of pain as punishment for previous behavior, and the need to be strong, courageous, or uncomplaining are factors that influence behavioral responses to pain.**
    2. The opposite may be true. As a person experiences relief from pain, the person may be unwilling to endure previously acceptable levels of pain.
    3. This is not a true statement. Although a generalization, many members of Jewish, Italian, Greek, and Chinese ethnic groups, for example, are able to express pain.
    4. Pain tolerance varies widely among people and is influenced by experiential, psychological, and sociocultural factors.

12. 1. **Sleep deprivation occurs with frequent interruptions of sleep because the sleeper returns to stage I rather than to the stage that was interrupted. There is a greater loss of stage III and IV non-rapid-eye-movement (NREM) sleep, which is essential for restorative sleep.**
    2. Although early awakenings often do occur in hospital settings, they are not the most common cause of sleep deprivation in the hospital.
    3. Restless legs syndrome, an intrinsic sleep disorder, is not the most common cause of sleep deprivation in the hospital.
    4. Only 1% to 4% of the population has sleep apnea.

13. 1. This is not the statement of greatest concern. Nonpharmacological measures to relieve pain, such as imagery and self-hypnosis, use the mind-body (psyche-soma) connection to reduce pain. The nurse should encourage the use of these measures and validate the energy expended.

2. The concern of addiction is not the priority among these statements. The nurse can respond to this common concern through education and judicious medication administration.

3. This is desirable because it keeps pain under control before it becomes excessive.

4. **The level of pain tolerance is exceeded. The present pain must be relieved and the client assured that future pain also will be controlled.**

14. 1. Hypoxia is associated with obstructive sleep apnea because episodes of upper airway obstruction occur 50 to 600 times a night.

    2. **Melatonin regulates the circadian phases of sleep. Environmental triggers called synchronizers adjust the sleep-wake cycle to a 24-hour solar day. Intensive care units have bright lights and increased sensory input that cause disorientation to day and night and interrupt sleep. Interrupted sleep results in lability of mood, irritability, excitability, suspiciousness, confusion, and delirium.**

    3. Lethargy and fatigue are early signs of sleep deprivation, not ICU psychosis.

    4. Sleep deprivation may cause impaired memory, confusion, illusions, and visual or auditory hallucinations, not dementia.

15. 1. Although uninterrupted sleep is advantageous for restorative sleep, the number of hours required depends on the individual.

    2. In older adults, the length of stage IV sleep is markedly decreased; as a result, they awaken more frequently, and it takes them longer to go back to sleep.

    3. **Fear of loss of control, the unknown, and potential death results in the struggle to stay awake, which interferes with the ability to relax sufficiently to fall asleep.**

    4. Bedrest does not decrease the need for sleep. The body still needs stage IV restorative sleep. Often, the physiological problems requiring the bedrest increase the need for sleep.

16. 1. Tenderness is a sensory word that describes pain and is related to the quality of pain.

    2. The description of pain as being moderate is related to intensity of pain.

    3. **The word *episode* refers to an incident, occurrence, or time period; therefore,** the word episode refers to a pattern of pain and is concerned with time of onset, duration, recurrence, and remissions.

    4. Phantom pain is related to location of pain. Phantom pain is a painful sensation perceived in a body part that is missing.

17. 1. **Alcoholic beverages are fluids that have a mild diuretic effect. Frequent nighttime awakening to empty a full bladder is called nocturia.**

    2. Drinking may cause nausea and vomiting rather than hunger.

    3. Alcohol hastens, not delays, the onset of sleep.

    4. Alcohol disrupts sleep and causes early morning awakening.

18. 1. Self-focusing is associated with chronic, not acute, pain; because of chronic pain's unrelenting, prolonged nature, it interferes with pursuing a normal life. As a result, there may be changes in family dynamics, sexual functioning, financial status, and self-esteem that result in introspection and depression.

    2. Pain is an internal stimulus that can interrupt sleep. Because chronic pain is unrelenting and prolonged, over time, interrupted sleep results in sleep deprivation.

    3. Guarding behaviors occur in both acute and chronic pain. However, because of the unrelenting and prolonged nature of chronic pain, behavioral responses, such as guarding, stooped posture, and altered gait, may become permanent adaptations.

    4. **Acute pain stimulates the sympathetic nervous system, which responds by increasing pulse, respirations, and blood pressure. Chronic pain stimulates the parasympathetic nervous system, which results in lowered pulse and blood pressure.**

19. 1. Hour of sleep (h.s., *hora somni*) medications usually are sedatives that promote rest and sleep; they are not analgesics.

    2. Medications administered around the clock at regularly scheduled intervals usually maintain therapeutic drug levels regardless of other factors influencing the client.

    3. Medication administered when necessary at the client's request will have a primary health-care prescription that states prn (*pro re nata*).

4. The word *preemptive* means preventive, anticipatory, and defensive. Therefore, preemptive analgesia is administered before an activity or intervention that may precipitate pain in an attempt to limit the anticipated pain.

20. 1. **Chronic fatigue syndrome (also known as systemic exertion intolerance disease [SEID]) is a condition characterized by the onset of disabling fatigue. The fatigue is so overwhelming and consuming that it interferes with the activities of daily living.**
   2. Chronic fatigue syndrome does not impair mobility. Impaired physical mobility is the state in which an individual experiences limitation of physical movement but is not immobile.
   3. The fatigue of chronic fatigue syndrome may result in social isolation, which is a state in which an individual experiences or perceives a desire for increased involvement with others but is unable to make that contact. However, social isolation is not as significant a problem as an issue in another option.
   4. Chronic fatigue syndrome is not related to impaired gas exchange.

21. 1. Psychosociocultural factors may influence clients' lack of request for medication when experiencing pain. Clients may not request medication because they fear the possibility of addiction, consider the pain as punishment for previous behavior, or need to be strong, courageous, or uncomplaining.
   2. Clients, particularly children and those who are cognitively impaired, often have problems describing the characteristics of pain because of difficulty interpreting painful stimuli or having never experienced the sensation before.
   3. **Pain is a personal experience, and the nurse must validate its presence and severity as perceived by the client. This conveys acceptance and respect and promotes the development of trust.**
   4. Acute pain increases vital signs because of sympathetic nervous system stimulation, but chronic pain will not.

22. 1. This is a planned nursing intervention, not a goal.
   2. **Sleep is a sensory experience that restores cerebral and physical functioning. Evaluations related to sleep are** based on client reports because effectiveness of sleep is a subjective assessment.
   3. Just because the client requests less pain medication does not reflect whether the client is obtaining effective sleep.
   4. Four hours of sleep is not enough for most adults. Most adults require 6 to 8 hours of sleep.

23. 1. **Imagery, the internal experience of memories, dreams, fantasies, or visions, uses positive images to distract, which reduces stress, limits mild pain, and promotes relaxation and sleep.**
   2. The use of opioids should be a last resort. Nursing interventions or nonopioid medications usually are effective in limiting mild pain.
   3. Bathing preferences are highly individual, and the client may not prefer a shower. In addition, a shower is stimulating and may be counterproductive.
   4. Although daytime activity does promote sleep at night, clients with pain may be reluctant to be active.

24. 1. At this time of day, most people are engaged in stimulating activities and generally are not sleepy.
   2. By this time of the sleep cycle, most people have had sufficient sleep and are beginning to awaken.
   3. **Research demonstrates that most people experience sleep-vulnerable periods between 2 a.m. and 6 a.m. and between 2 p.m. and 5 p.m.**
   4. At this time of day, most people are engaged in stimulating activities, such as preparing and eating dinner.

25. 1. Somnambulism, sleepwalking, is a parasomnia that occurs during stages III and IV of non-rapid-eye-movement (NREM) sleep.
   2. Snoring relates to obstructive sleep apnea, which is a periodic cessation of airflow during inspiration that results in arousal from sleep.
   3. Nocturnal enuresis, bedwetting, is a parasomnia that occurs when moving from stages III to IV of non-rapid-eye-movement (NREM) sleep.
   4. **Bruxism, clenching and grinding of the teeth, is a parasomnia that occurs during stage II NREM sleep. Usually, it does not interfere with sleep for the affected individual but rather the sleeper's partner.**

26. 1. Patient-controlled analgesia routinely delivers a low dose of an opioid and additional doses on demand within safe limitations. Pain relief can be maintained for hours to days.
2. Intramuscular injections of analgesics usually are effective for 3 to 6 hours.
3. **Intravenous analgesics act within 1 to 2 minutes, but drug inactivation (biotransformation) also is fast, so there is a short duration of action.**
4. With regional anesthesia (e.g., nerve block, Bier block, spinal, epidural), an anesthetic agent is instilled around nerves to block the transmission of nerve impulses, thus reducing pain for many hours.

27. 1. The healthy older adult spends more time in bed, spends less time asleep, awakens more often, stays awake longer, and naps more often. Rapid-eye-movement (REM) sleep and stage IV non-rapid-eye-movement (NREM) sleep are reduced, resulting in less restorative sleep. Naps lead to desynchronization of the sleep-wake cycle.
2. The need for sleep varies and depends on factors such as age, activity level, and health.
3. Alcohol hastens the onset of sleep. Alcohol is associated with early awakening.
4. **An expectation of an outcome of behavior usually becomes a self-fulfilling prophecy. Bedtime rituals include activities that promote comfort and relaxation (e.g., music, reading, and praying) and hygienic practices that meet basic physiological needs (e.g., bathing, brushing the teeth, and toileting).**

28. 1. Although tinnitus can interfere with sleep, it is not the most common problem.
2. **Bladder fullness causes pressure in the pelvic area that interrupts sleep. Awakening to void during the night is a common occurrence, particularly in older adult men due to an enlarged prostate.**
3. Although hunger can interfere with sleep, it is not the most common problem. A light evening snack or glass of milk prevents hunger.
4. Although thirst can interfere with sleep, it is not the most common problem. Thirst is prevented by drinking water as part of the bedtime routine.

29. 1. Percussion involves gentle tapping of the skin. Percussion is stimulating and usually is performed during the middle of a back massage.
2. **Effleurage involves long, smooth strokes sliding over the skin. When performed slowly with light pressure at the end of a back rub, it has a relaxing, sedative effect.**
3. Kneading (pétrissage) involves squeezing the skin, subcutaneous tissue, and muscle with a lifting motion. Kneading is stimulating and usually is performed during the middle of a back rub.
4. Circular strokes usually are performed in the area around the buttocks, lower back, and scapulae. They are stimulating and are performed during the beginning of a back rub.

30. 1. The pattern of pain refers to time of onset, duration, recurrence, and remissions.
2. Duration refers to how long the pain lasts, which is an aspect of the pattern of pain.
3. **This is referred pain, which is pain felt in a part of the body that is at a distance from the tissues causing the pain. Referred pain is related to location of pain.**
4. Constancy refers to whether the pain is continuous or if there are periods of relief from pain, both of which relate to the pattern of pain.

31. 1. The amount of time spent sleeping usually is not affected.
2. **Sleep apnea is the periodic cessation of breathing during sleep. Episodes occur during rapid-eye-movement (REM) sleep (interfering with dreaming) and non-rapid-eye-movement (NREM) sleep (interfering with restorative sleep), both of which reduce the quality of sleep.**
3. Clients still reach the depth of stage IV NREM sleep.
4. Sleep apnea does not influence the onset of sleep.

32. 1. This direct question precipitates just a yes or no response about only one aspect of sleep.
2. This direct question precipitates just a yes or no response.
3. This direct question gathers information about only one aspect of sleep.
4. **This open-ended question requires clients to explore the topic of sleep as it relates specifically to their own experiences.**

33. 1. The gate-control theory of pain relief is not activated through guided imagery.

Guided imagery uses positive thoughts and emotions to promote relaxation and limit discomfort.

2. The gate-control theory of pain relief is not activated through progressive muscle relaxation. The performance of progressive muscle relaxation requires the mind to focus on an issue other than the pain. It interferes with the perception and interpretation of pain because the mind can process only a certain amount of information at a time.

3. **Thermal therapy (e.g., application of heat or cold) stimulates the large A-delta fibers that close the gate that allows the transmission of pain impulses to the central nervous system.**

4. Nonsteroidal anti-inflammatory medication, such as ibuprofen, inhibits prostaglandin synthesis. Nonsteroidal anti-inflammatory medications do not activate the gate-control theory of pain relief.

34. 1. **An increased sensitivity to pain is associated with disturbed NREM sleep. During NREM sleep, the body is engaged in restoring physiological properties of the body.**

2. An inability to concentrate is associated with disturbed rapid-eye-movement (REM) sleep. REM sleep is involved with cognitive and emotional restoration processes.

3. **During NREM sleep, the parasympathetic nervous system dominates and the vital signs and metabolic rate are low; also, growth hormone is consistently secreted, which provides for anabolism. Shortened NREM sleep decreases these restorative processes, resulting in fatigue, lethargy, and excessive sleepiness.**

4. Irritability and excitability are associated with disturbed REM, not NREM, sleep.

5. REM, not NREM, sleep is essential for maintaining mental and emotional equilibrium and, when interrupted, results in confusion, irritability, excitability, suspiciousness, delusions, and hallucinations.

35. **Answer: 15 mL. Solve the problem by using the formula for ratio and proportion.**

$$\frac{\text{Desired}}{\text{Have}} \quad \frac{15 \text{ mg}}{5 \text{ mg}} = \frac{\text{x mL}}{5 \text{ mL}}$$
$$5 \text{ x} = 75$$
$$\text{x} = 75 \div 5$$
$$\text{x} = 15 \text{ mL}$$

36. 1. **Limiting fluid intake after dinner reduces the amount of urine production while asleep.**

2. **Voiding empties the bladder and makes room for urine produced during the night.**

3. **Caffeine irritates the mucous membranes of the urinary system and stimulates the need to void.**

4. **Positive imagery supports self-esteem and may become a self-fulfilling prophesy.**

5. **Linens and clothing should be changed with a nonjudgmental, nonchalant demeanor to support the boy's self-esteem.**

37. **McBurney's point is located in the right lower quadrant one-third of the distance laterally drawn from the anterior superior iliac spine to the umbilicus (navel). Under normal conditions tenderness or pain should not occur when compression is released at this site. However, in some situations such as acute appendicitis rebound tenderness will occur.**

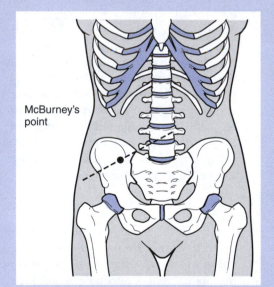

McBurney's point

38. 1. Energy requirements decrease with age as metabolic processes slow and older adults become more sedentary.

2. The metabolic rate decreases by 5% to 25% during rest.

3. **Stress precipitates the sympathetic nervous system, increasing cortisone, norepinephrine, and epinephrine, which increase the metabolic rate. Physical and psychic energy expended is restored through rest and sleep.**

4. Catabolic hormones (cortisol and epinephrine) increase with activity, not during sleep. Catabolism is the breaking down of muscle and lean body mass to produce glucose to meet energy needs (gluconeogenesis).

5. **Individuals experience varied levels of consciousness when asleep. There is a progressive lack of awareness of the environment as one passes from stages I through IV.**

39. 1. Hyporesponsiveness, withdrawal, apathy, flat facial expression, and excessive sleepiness are physiological responses associated with a lack of non-rapid-eye-movement (NREM) sleep.

2. A depressed immune system is a physiological response to a lack of NREM sleep.

3. **REM sleep is essential for maintaining mental and emotional equilibrium and, when interrupted, results in irritability and excitability.**

4. **REM sleep is essential for maintaining mental and emotional equilibrium and, when interrupted, results in confusion and suspiciousness.**

5. Shortened NREM sleep can result in vertigo, which is a physiological response to sleep deprivation.

40. 1. Metformin is an antidiabetic medication that decreases hepatic glucose production, decreases intestinal absorption of glucose, and increases sensitivity of cells to insulin. Side effects are abdominal bloating, diarrhea, nausea, and vomiting, not insomnia.

2. **Sleep patterns tend to change as one ages. Older people become sleepy earlier and wake up earlier (alteration in circadian rhythms), wake up more frequently (lower levels of growth hormone and melatonin), and experience less deep sleep (more rapid sleep cycles).**

3. **Hormonal shifts in women occur throughout life: monthly related to ovulation, during pregnancy, and during and after menopause. Hormonal changes can precipitate nausea, anxiety, weight gain, generalized discomfort, restless legs syndrome, acid reflux, and frequent urination. All of these physiological responses can precipitate insomnia.**

4. **Alcohol is a sedative that can help one fall asleep, but it prevents deeper stages of sleep and causes one to awaken frequently during the night and earlier in the morning.**

5. The medication diphenhydramine antagonizes the effects of histamine at H_1 receptor sites. It causes drowsiness and often is taken before retiring at night to treat insomnia.

6. **Naps that exceed 10 to 30 minutes can interfere with sleep at night, thus aggravating insomnia.**

41. 1. This statement may or may not be true.

2. Fatigue decreases a person's coping abilities, which increases the intensity of pain.

3. This statement may or may not be true. There may be behavioral signs of pain, such as guarding, grimaces, and clenching the teeth, at the same time that there are no verbal statements indicating the presence of pain. In some cultures, it is unacceptable to complain about pain, or tolerance of pain signifies strength and courage.

4. This is not a true statement. The judicious use of opioids does not necessarily result in addiction.

5. **Pain is a personal experience. Margo McCaffery, a pain researcher, has indicated that pain is whatever the person in pain says it is and exists whenever the person in pain says it exists.**

42. 1. These are physiological responses, not precipitating factors, associated with the pain experience.

2. This statement reflects the pattern (e.g., onset, duration, and intervals) of the pain experience.

3. **Anything that induces or aggravates pain is considered a precipitating factor of pain. For example, precipitating factors may be physical (e.g., exertion associated with activities of daily living, Valsalva maneuver), environmental (e.g., extremes in temperature, noise), or emotional (anxiety, fear).**

4. This statement reflects the quality of the pain. Descriptive adjectives, such as knifelike, burning, or cramping, explain how the pain feels.

5. **Anything that induces or aggravates pain is considered a precipitating factor of pain. Coughing raises intra-abdominal pressure, which can aggravate the pain of a surgical incision. Clients are taught to support the operative site with the hands or a**

pillow when coughing to limit the extent of pain.

43. **2.** The first step is to position the client in the side-lying position because this provides for a comfortable, supported position during the procedure.

   4. The second step is to arrange the gown and linens so that the client's back is exposed because this provides access to the client's back.

   3. The third step is to assess the skin to ensure that there are no indications of a problem that is a contraindication for having a back rub.

   1. The fourth step is to warm the lotion in your hands because warm lotion is more comfortable and supports muscle relaxation.

   5. A variety of strokes (e.g., effleurage, pétrissage, tamponage, small circular movements, and feathering) relieves muscle tension, promotes physical and emotional relaxation, and increases circulation to the area.

44. **1.** Shortened non-rapid-eye-movement (NREM) sleep can result in vertigo, which is a physiological response to sleep deprivation.

   2. Interrupted NREM sleep can result in fatigue, which is a physiological response to sleep deprivation.

   3. Irritability is a psychological response to sleep deprivation. As the difficulty of initiating or maintaining sleep continues, the person becomes progressively more upset about the lack of the amount and quality of sleep, further precipitating insomnia.

   4. Shortened NREM sleep can result in headache, which is a physiological response to sleep deprivation.

   5. Frustration is a psychological response to sleep deprivation.

45. **1.** Chronic pain has a gradual progressive onset because usually it is related to a long-term problem (e.g., diabetic neuropathy). Acute pain has a rapid onset because usually it is related to abrupt trauma to the body (e.g., surgical incision, damage from an automobile collision).

   2. Chronic pain is categorized as pain longer than 6 months' duration. Acute pain is categorized as pain shorter than 6 months' duration.

   3. An anticipated end is associated with acute pain. Chronic pain is associated with conditions that usually are lifelong with no anticipated end in sight.

   4. Chronic pain is psychologically depleting because it drains both physical and emotional resources; this is related to the unrelenting nature of the pain and that usually it continues for life.

   5. Chronic pain usually does not respond to conventional interventions such as back rub, imagery, distraction, and analgesics. Complementary and alternative modalities such as acupuncture, biofeedback, hypnosis, yoga, and therapeutic touch may provide some relief.

Perioperative Nursing

The following words include nursing/medical terminology, concepts, principles, and information relevant to content specifically addressed in the chapter or associated with topics presented in it. English dictionaries, nursing textbooks, and medical dictionaries, such as *Taber's Cyclopedic Medical Dictionary*, are resources that can be used to expand your knowledge and understanding of these words and related information.

Abdominal binder

Anesthesia, types:
  Epidural
  Conscious sedation
  General
  Local
  Nerve block
  Regional
  Spinal

Antiembolism stockings:
  Elastic
  Sequential compression devices

Bowel preparation

Collagen production

Deep breathing and coughing

Drains, types:
  Penrose
  Portable wound drainage systems:
    Hemovac
    Jackson-Pratt

Dressings, types:
  Alginates (exudate absorbers)
  Dry sterile dressing
  Hydrocolloids
  Impregnated
  Transparent
  Wet-to-damp/moist

Granulation

Hypostatic pneumonia

Informed consent

Laparoscopic

Latex allergy

Leg exercises

Medication reconciliation

Nasogastric decompression

Negative pressure

NPO status

Pain management

Patient-controlled analgesia (PCA)

Perioperative:
  Preoperative
  Intraoperative
  Postoperative

Postanesthesia care unit (PACU)

Postoperative complications:
  Aspiration
  Deep vein thrombosis
  Dehiscence
  Evisceration
  Malignant hyperthermia
  Pneumonia
  Postoperative ileus
  Pulmonary embolus, emboli
  Wound infection

Preoperative checklist

Residual limb

Skin preparation

Surgery, purposes of:
  Ablative
  Constructive
  Diagnostic
  Palliative
  Reconstructive
  Transplant

Surgery types:
  Ambulatory surgery
  Elective surgery
  Emergency surgery
  Major surgery
  Minor surgery
  Urgent surgery

Surgical asepsis

Verification processes:
  Client wrist band
  Preoperative check list
  Surgical time out, time out surgical
    check list

Wound drainage:
  Purulent
  Sanguineous
  Serosanguineous
  Serous

PERIOPERATIVE NURSING: QUESTIONS

1. There are discharge criteria for clients in the postanesthesia care unit (PACU) regardless of the type of anesthesia used and additional criteria for specific types of anesthesia. Which is the criterion specific for the client who has received spinal anesthesia?
   1. Oxygen saturation reaches the presurgical baseline.
   2. Motor and sensory function returns.
   3. Nausea and vomiting are minimal.
   4. Headache is reported as tolerable.

2. A client is admitted to the postanesthesia care unit. Which nursing action is **most** important during the client's stay in this unit?
   1. Monitoring urinary output
   2. Assessing level of consciousness
   3. Ensuring patency of drainage tubes
   4. Suctioning mucus from respiratory passages

3. A postoperative client is transferred back to the surgical unit with an abdominal dressing and a Penrose drain. Which is the **most** important nursing action associated with caring for a client with a Penrose drain?
   1. Removing the excess external portion until drainage stops
   2. Changing the soiled dressing carefully
   3. Maintaining the negative pressure
   4. Pinning the drain to the dressing

4. A client has abdominal surgery. Which should the nurse do to **best** assess for a sign of postoperative ileus in this client after surgery?
   1. Identify the time of the first bowel movement.
   2. Monitor the tolerance of a clear liquid diet.
   3. Palpate for abdominal distention.
   4. Auscultate for bowel sounds.

5. Four days after abdominal surgery, while being transferred from a bed to a chair, a client says to a nurse, "My incision feels funny all of a sudden." Which should the nurse do **first**?
   1. Take the vital signs.
   2. Apply an abdominal binder immediately.
   3. Place the client in the low-Fowler position.
   4. Encourage slow deep breathing by the client.

6. Which factor places a client at the **highest** risk for postoperative nausea and vomiting after receiving general anesthesia?
   1. Obesity
   2. Inactivity
   3. Hypervolemia
   4. Unconsciousness

7. On the second postoperative day after an above-the-knee amputation, the client's elastic dressing accidentally comes off. Which should the nurse do **first**?
   1. Wrap the residual limb with an elastic compression bandage.
   2. Apply a saline dressing to the residual limb.
   3. Notify the primary health-care provider.
   4. Place two pillows under the limb.

8. A nurse is caring for a postoperative client. Which action is effective in preventing postoperative urinary tract infections?
   1. Eating foods with roughage
   2. Taking sitz baths twice a day
   3. Drinking an adequate amount of fluid
   4. Increasing the intake of citrus fruit juices

9. A client received conscious sedation during a colonoscopy. Which should the nurse expect regarding the client's experience with this procedure?
   1. Client will be unresponsive and pain free.
   2. Client will be at risk for malignant hyperthermia.
   3. Client will be sleepy but able to follow verbal commands.
   4. Client will be positioned in the supine position to prevent headache.

10. Which client having emergency surgery should the nurse anticipate to be at the **highest** risk for postoperative mortality?
   1. Individual who has alcoholism
   2. Person who has epilepsy
   3. Middle-age adult
   4. Infant

11. A nurse is caring for a client who had an abdominal hysterectomy. Which intervention **best** prevents postoperative thrombophlebitis?
   1. Utilization of compression stockings at night
   2. Deep breathing and coughing exercises daily
   3. Leg exercises 10 times per hour when awake
   4. Elevation of the legs on 2 pillows

12. An obese client has abdominal surgery for removal of the gallbladder. Which should the nurse be **most** concerned about if exhibited by the client?
   1. Constipation
   2. Urinary retention
   3. Shallow breathing
   4. Inability to provide self-care

13. A client arrives in the postanesthesia care unit. Which is the **most** important information that the nurse needs to know?
   1. Anxiety level before surgery
   2. Type and extent of the surgery
   3. Type of intravenous fluids administered
   4. Special requests that were expressed by the client

14. Which client responses **best** support the decision to discharge the client from the postanesthesia care unit?
   1. Sao_2 of 95%, vital signs stable for 30 minutes, active gag reflex
   2. Tolerable pain, ability to move extremities, dry intact dressing
   3. Urinary output of 30 mL/hr, awake, turning from side to side
   4. Afebrile, adventitious breath sounds, ability to cough

15. How many days after surgery should the nurse anticipate that a postoperative client will begin to exhibit signs and symptoms of a wound infection if it should occur?
   1. Fifth day
   2. Third day
   3. Ninth day
   4. Seventh day

16. A nurse is assessing a client who had spinal anesthesia. For which common response should the nurse assess the client?
1. Headache
2. Neuropathy
3. Lower back discomfort
4. Increased blood pressure

17. A hospitalized client who has been receiving medications via a variety of routes for several days is scheduled for surgery at 10 a.m. Which should the nurse plan to do on the day of surgery?
1. Use an alternative route for the oral medications.
2. Withhold all the previously prescribed medications.
3. Withhold the oral medications and administer the other drugs.
4. Obtain directions from the primary health-care provider regarding the medications.

18. Which is the **most** common dietary prescription the nurse can anticipate after a client who had abdominal surgery exhibits a return of intestinal peristalsis?
1. Clear liquids
2. Full liquids
3. Low fiber
4. Regular

19. A nurse compares the advantages and disadvantages of a central venous catheter inserted into a peripheral vein and a central venous catheter inserted into a subclavian vein. Which of the following does the nurse conclude is the reason why a peripheral catheter is more desirable?
1. Because it will not be in the superior vena cava
2. Because it will not cause a tension pneumothorax
3. Because it will not prevent the development of an infection
4. Because it will not allow large volumes of fluid to be administered

20. A nurse is caring for a client who had abdominal surgery. Which type of incisional drainage should the nurse expect 4 hours after surgery?
1. Serous wound drainage
2. Purulent wound drainage
3. Sanguineous wound drainage
4. Serosanguineous wound drainage

21. A nurse is assessing a postoperative client. Which client response identified by the nurse indicates altered renal perfusion?
1. Oliguria
2. Cachexia
3. Yellow sclera
4. Suprapubic distention

22. A nurse is evaluating the effectiveness of nursing interventions for meeting the nutrient needs of clients during the first 2 days after abdominal surgery. Which outcome is **most** important?
1. Nausea and vomiting have not occurred.
2. Fluid and electrolytes are balanced.
3. Wound healing is progressing.
4. Oral intake is reestablished.

23. Which is the next **most** important assessment made by the nurse after ensuring a postoperative client has a patent airway?
    1. Condition of drains
    2. Level of consciousness
    3. Stability of the vital signs
    4. Location of the surgical dressing

24. A client's perineal area must be examined by the primary health-care provider prior to surgery. In which position should the nurse place the client for this physical assessment?
    1. Sims
    2. Supine
    3. Lithotomy
    4. Trendelenburg

25. A nurse is caring for two clients. One of the clients has a Jackson-Pratt drain and the other client has a Hemovac drain. Which does the nurse understand is the difference between these two drains?
    1. The size of the collection container
    2. How the pressure within the collection container is reestablished
    3. The type of pressure that promotes drainage to the collection container
    4. Where the collection container should be placed in relation to the insertion site

26. A nurse is caring for several clients who received general anesthesia. A client with which concurrent health problem poses the **highest** risk for the development of a postoperative complication?
    1. Gastroesophageal reflux disease
    2. Reduced reflexes
    3. Hypothyroidism
    4. Emphysema

27. A postoperative client experiences tachycardia, sudden chest pain, and low blood pressure. Which complication associated with the postoperative period should the nurse conclude that the client **most** likely experienced?
    1. Pulmonary embolus
    2. Hemorrhage
    3. Heart attack
    4. Pneumonia

28. A client spikes a fever during the first postoperative day after major abdominal surgery. The nurse suspects that the fever indicates an infection. Which site does the nurse conclude **most** likely is the source of the infection?
    1. Intestines
    2. Bladder
    3. Wound
    4. Lungs

29. A nurse is to apply a transparent wound barrier over a client's incision. Which nursing action is appropriate?
    1. Stretch the transparent dressing snugly over the entire wound.
    2. Clean the skin with normal saline before applying the dressing.
    3. Cover the transparent wound barrier with a gauze dressing and secure with paper tape.
    4. Ensure the reinforcing tape extends several inches beyond the edges of the transparent wound barrier.

30. A nurse is to position a client in the postanesthesia care unit. Which factor is **most** important for the nurse to consider?
    1. Allow for skeletal deformities.
    2. Prevent pressure on bony prominences.
    3. Provide for adequate thoracic expansion.
    4. Avoid stretching of neuromuscular tissue.

31. When should the nurse initiate planned interventions regarding a client's perioperative management?
    1. When the consent form is signed
    2. When the decision for surgery is made
    3. When the client is admitted for surgery
    4. When the client is transferred to the operating room

32. One hour after the reduction of a compound fracture of the ulna and radius and application of a cast, the nurse observes a centimeter circle of drainage on the client's cast. Which should the nurse do **first**?
    1. Inform the surgeon immediately.
    2. Reinforce the cast with a gauze dressing.
    3. Monitor the area frequently for expansion.
    4. Circle the spot with a pen and date, time, and initial the area.

33. A nurse is caring for a client with a nasogastric tube attached to suction. What is the **most** important nursing action in relation to the nasogastric tube?
    1. Using sterile technique when irrigating the tube
    2. Recording intake and output every 2 hours
    3. Providing oral hygiene every 4 hours
    4. Setting suction at the prescribed level

34. A nurse is considering the commonalities and differences of equipment used for gastric decompression. Which is the major advantage to using a double-lumen tube?
    1. Minimizes the risk of bowel obstruction
    2. Ensures drainage of the intestines
    3. Prevents gastric mucosal damage
    4. Promotes gastric rest

35. A nurse is performing preoperative teaching a week before surgery. The client is taking 650 mg of aspirin twice a day for arthritis. Which instruction should the nurse expect the surgeon to have the nurse include in the preoperative teaching?
    1. Continue to take the aspirin indefinitely.
    2. Stop taking the aspirin 5 days before surgery.
    3. Withhold the dose of aspirin on the morning of surgery.
    4. Reduce the dose of aspirin to 81 mg a day until after surgery.

36. A client has negative pressure wound therapy (vacuum-assisted closure [VAC]) after the amputation of a toe. The tubing is connected to intermittent negative pressure. What should the nurse do when the film over the wound collapses when negative pressure is exerted?
    1. Notify the primary health-care provider.
    2. Decrease the extent of negative pressure.
    3. Apply a new transparent film over the wound.
    4. Continue to observe the functioning of the device.

37. A primary health-care provider prescribes antiembolism stockings for a client. Place the following steps in the order in which they should be implemented when applying these stockings.
   1. Assess the client for contraindications to the use of antiembolism stockings.
   2. Apply the antiembolism stockings before getting the client out of bed in the morning.
   3. Ensure that the applied stockings are 1 to 2 inches below the popliteal fold (bend) in the back of the knee.
   4. Explain that antiembolism stockings are prescribed by the primary health-care provider and what is to be done and why.
   5. Measure the smallest circumference of the ankle, the largest circumference of the calf, and the length from the heel to 1 to 2 inches below the popliteal fold (bend) in the back of the knee.
   6. Turn the stocking inside out so that the foot portion is inside the stocking leg, stretch each side of the stocking and ease it over the toes, center the heel, and pull the stocking over the heel and up the leg.

   Answer: _____

38. A nurse is caring for a client recovering from abdominal surgery. Which nursing action is effective in facilitating ventilation? **Select all that apply.**
   1. _____ Encouraging fluid intake
   2. _____ Preventing abdominal distention
   3. _____ Positioning in the side-lying position
   4. _____ Implementing passive range-of-motion exercises
   5. _____ Ensuring that an incentive spirometer is used every hour when awake

39. A nurse is caring for a client in the ambulatory surgery unit who just had a laparoscopic cholecystectomy. The client reports the presence of pain that is commonly associated with the migration of CO_2 used to inflate the abdominal cavity to improve visualization during surgery. Shade in the location of this referred pain on the illustration.

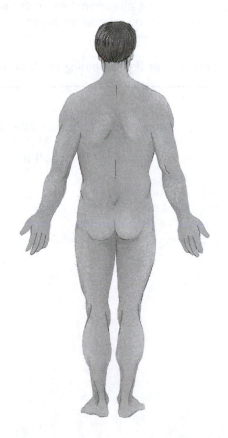

40. A client had a tonsillectomy and is on a soft diet. Which of the following should the nurse encourage this client to have during the first 24 hours after surgery? **Select all that apply.**

1. _____ Warm pudding
2. _____ Milk shakes
3. _____ Apple juice
4. _____ Ice pops
5. _____ Gelatin

41. A nurse in the postanesthesia care unit at 3 p.m. receives report from the nurse who is completing the day shift. The following information about a 65-year-old man who was admitted to the unit at 1:30 p.m. after repair of a double inguinal hernia is reported. Which information does not meet the standard criteria for discharge from the unit?

1. Stability of vital signs
2. Level of consciousness
3. Absence of bowel sounds
4. Presence of a urinary catheter

CLIENT'S CLINICAL RECORD

Vital Signs
Temperature: 99°F, temporal
Pulse: 98 beats per minute
Respirations: 30 breaths per minute
Blood pressure: 170/90 mm Hg

Physical Assessment
Abdominal dressing dry and intact; IV 0.9% sodium chloride at 125 mL per hour, site in left hand dry and intact, free of complications. Removed oral airway at 2 p.m.; gag reflex present; coughing, deep breathing and moving all extremities on command. Urinary catheter draining more than 50 mL per hour; bowel sounds absent.

Oxygen Status
Oxygen saturation 97% with nasal cannula at 2 L; breathing freely on own

42. A nurse is caring for a postoperative client. The client asks the nurse why vitamin C was prescribed by the primary health-care provider. Which information should the nurse include in a response to this question? **Select all that apply.**

1. _____ Facilitates healing
2. _____ Improves digestive processes
3. _____ Increases transport of oxygen to cells
4. _____ Encourages growth of red blood cells
5. _____ Minimizes formation of deep vein thrombosis

43. A nurse assesses the client on admission to the postanesthesia care unit and collects the following data: receiving 40% oxygen via a simple face mask; oxygen saturation 92%; opens eyes and responds to commands to move all four extremities; deep breathes and coughs; and vital signs are temperature—97.8°F, pulse—82 beats per minute, respirations—18 breaths per minute, and blood pressure—140/88 mm Hg, which is consistent with his previous blood pressures. Calculate the client's Aldrete score.
1. 10
2. 9
3. 8
4. 7

Aldrete Score			On Admission to PCAU	5 Min	15 Min	30 Min	45 Min	60 Min	At Discharge
Able to move 4 extremities voluntarily or on command	= 2	Activity							
Able to move 2 extremities voluntarily or on command	= 1								
Able to move 0 extremities voluntarily or on command	= 0								
Able to deep breathe and cough freely	= 2	Respiration							
Dyspnea or limited breathing	= 1								
Apneic	= 0								
BP ± 20% of pre-anesthetic level	= 2	Circulation							
BP ± 20%–50% of pre-anesthetic level	= 1								
BP ± 50% of pre-anesthetic level	= 0								
Fully awake	= 2	Consciousness							
Arousable on calling	= 1								
Not responding	= 0								
Able to maintain O_2 saturation >92% on room air	= 2	O_2 saturation							
Needs O_2 inhalation to maintain O_2 saturation >90%	= 1								
O_2 saturation <90% even with O_2 supplement	= 0								
		TOTAL							

44. A client has a right abdominal incision. Which should the nurse teach the client to do when getting out of bed? **Select all that apply.**
1. _____ Exit from the left side of the bed.
2. _____ Ask the nurse to apply an abdominal binder.
3. _____ Hold a pillow against the abdomen with both hands.
4. _____ Use the left arm to push up to a sitting position on the side of the bed.
5. _____ Sit on the side of the bed for a few minutes before moving to a standing position.

45. A nurse must initiate placement of a continuous passive motion machine after the client had a total knee replacement. Place the following steps in the order in which they should be implemented.
1. Position the extremity on the platform so the knee is centered over the break in the platform.
2. Set the degree of flexion, speed, and time on and off the machine as prescribed.
3. Ensure that the extremity is aligned with the client's hips and torso.
4. Assess the client's skin and provide skin care after the procedure.
5. Position sheepskin on the platform, especially at the gluteal fold.
6. Position the controller within easy reach of the client.

Answer: _____

46. A nurse is teaching a postoperative client the nutrients that are the **best** for supporting collagen production that promotes wound healing. Which food selected by the client indicates that the teaching was effective? **Select all that apply.**
1. _____ Yellow bell peppers
2. _____ Whole-grain bread
3. _____ Cantaloupe
4. _____ Oranges
5. _____ Kiwi

47. A nurse is caring for a client with the following type of portable wound drainage device. Which should the nurse do when caring for a client with this type of drainage system? **Select all that apply.**

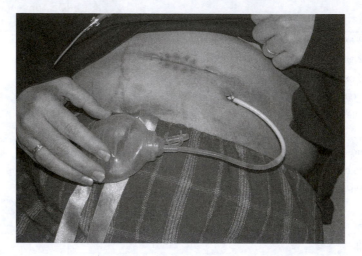

1. _____ Empty the container and then compress the collection container, close the port, and release hand compression.
2. _____ Wear sterile gloves when emptying the collection container.
3. _____ Keep the collection container below the insertion site.
4. _____ Shorten the length of the tubing by one inch daily.
5. _____ Empty the collection container when full.
6. _____ Attach tubing to clothing.

48. A nurse is caring for a postoperative client who had abdominal surgery. The client states, "The incision just felt like it gave way." The nurse identifies that the client had a dehiscence with slight evisceration. Which of the following should the nurse implement? **Select all that apply.**
1. _____ Instruct the client to avoid coughing or bearing down.
2. _____ Notify the primary health-care provider immediately.
3. _____ Position the client in the low-Fowler position.
4. _____ Cover the incision with a sterile dressing.
5. _____ Prepare the client for surgery.

49. Which of the following independent and dependent nursing interventions help prevent thrombophlebitis during the postoperative period? **Select all that apply.**
1. _____ Applying lower-extremity sequential compression devices when in bed
2. _____ Wearing antiembolism stockings when out of bed
3. _____ Walking in the hall several times a day
4. _____ Using an incentive spirometer
5. _____ Coughing and deep breathing
6. _____ Keeping the legs uncrossed

50. The primary health-care provider prescribes morphine sulfate 12 mg subcutaneously STAT for a postoperative client. The morphine sulfate vial states that there are 10 mg per mL. Indicate on the syringe the line to which it should be filled to administer the prescribed dose.

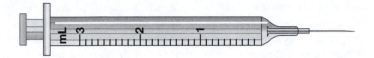

1. 1. The respiratory status of all postoperative clients should be stable and adequate regardless of the type of anesthesia used.
2. **The ability to move and feel sensations in all four extremities is especially important after receiving spinal anesthesia (subarachnoid block) because it indicates that nerve damage has not occurred because of the lumbar puncture necessary for the introduction of the anesthetic agent into the subarachnoid space.**
3. Nausea and vomiting are associated with general, not spinal, anesthesia.
4. Reporting that a headache is tolerable before discharge from the postanesthesia care unit is unrealistic. Although a headache may be associated with spinal anesthesia (subarachnoid block), it may manifest after discharge from the postanesthesia care unit and persist for several days until the cerebrospinal fluid pressure returns to an acceptable level.

2. 1. Although monitoring urinary output is done to ensure that urinary functioning is maintained, it is not the priority.
2. Although assessing level of consciousness is part of the routine assessment of a client recovering from anesthesia, particularly conscious sedation and general anesthesia, it is not the priority.
3. Although tubes and equipment are always monitored and maintained, the patency of drainage tubes is not the priority.
4. **Maintaining a patent airway always is the priority to prevent respiratory distress and hypoxia. This follows the ABCs (airway, breathing, circulation) of client care.**

3. 1. Although this is done, it is not the priority action associated with a Penrose drain. A Penrose drain, a small, pliable, flat tube, extends beyond the insertion site by approximately 2 inches. The end of the drain is placed between gauze 4 × 4s to absorb drainage. As a Penrose drain is shortened, it is withdrawn approximately 1 inch and cut to maintain the same 2-inch length outside the body.
2. **Changing a soiled dressing carefully is necessary to prevent inadvertent removal of the Penrose drain because it is placed between several layers of gauze 4 × 4s to absorb drainage.**
3. A Penrose drain functions by gravity, not negative pressure.
4. Pinning a Penrose drain to the dressing is contraindicated, to avoid removing the drain inadvertently during a dressing change. A safety pin is placed at the end of the drain to prevent the drain from being lost inside the insertion site.

4. 1. A bowel movement will occur long after the first signs of intestinal motility are evident.
2. Administration of fluids before intestinal motility has returned is unsafe and contraindicated. A clear liquid diet is not administered until there are definitive signs of intestinal motility.
3. Although palpating the abdomen for distention is done, it is not the best assessment for paralytic ileus. Abdominal distention can be caused by problems other than paralytic ileus, such as hemorrhage, peritonitis, and urinary retention.
4. **Expected bowel sounds are high-pitched gurgling sounds that vary in frequency, intensity, and pitch; they are caused by the propulsion of intestinal contents through the lower alimentary tract. These sounds are the first indication that intestinal motility is returning. Signs and symptoms of a postoperative ileus include a silent abdomen or minimal peristaltic sounds; abdominal distention; nausea; vomiting; anorexia; feeling of fullness; vague abdominal discomfort or cramping; and obstipation/constipation, passage of slight amounts of watery stool, or both.**

5. 1. Vital signs should be assessed eventually, but it is not the priority.
2. An abdominal binder may be used in high-risk clients to prevent, not treat, dehiscence and evisceration.
3. **The low-Fowler position, a back-lying position, permits inspection of the operative site and promotes retention of abdominal viscera by gravity if dehiscence has occurred. Also, slight flexion of the hips reduces tension on the abdominal musculature.**
4. Deep breathing is contraindicated because it increases intra-abdominal pressure, which could cause evisceration.

6. 1. **Obese people have excess adipose tissue that exerts pressure on the abdominal**

cavity, which raises intra-abdominal pressure. Increased intra-abdominal pressure exerts pressure on the gastrointestinal tract, increasing the risk of nausea and vomiting.

2. Although inactivity delays recovery of intestinal motility after surgery, a diligent activity and ambulation schedule should prevent postoperative ileus and its related nausea and vomiting.

3. Intestinal hypomotility, not hypervolemia, is related to postoperative nausea and vomiting. Hypervolemia is an increase in intravascular blood volume.

4. Unconsciousness is not related directly to postoperative nausea and vomiting.

7. 1. **Gentle compression is desirable because it prevents bleeding and promotes molding and shrinkage of the residual limb.**

2. A saline dressing is unsafe because soaking promotes the breakdown of connective tissue fibers (maceration), which impedes wound healing by primary intention.

3. Notifying the primary health-care provider should be done eventually, but caring for the client is the immediate priority.

4. Elevating the limb is unsafe because it promotes hip flexion contractures.

8. 1. Dietary roughage prevents constipation, not urinary tract infections.

2. A sitz bath can promote the development of a urinary tract infection if medical aseptic techniques are not followed.

3. **Adequate (2,000 to 3,000 mL/day) fluid intake daily promotes a dilute urine and more frequent emptying of the bladder, both of which limit the development of a urinary tract infection. The stasis of concentrated urine promotes microbial growth.**

4. The ingestion of citrus juice causes an alkaline urine, which provides a favorable environment for the multiplication of microorganisms and the development of a urinary tract infection.

9. 1. Unresponsiveness and being pain free occur with general anesthesia, not conscious sedation.

2. Life-threatening malignant hyperthermia is a rare, autosomal dominant–inherited syndrome that is precipitated by anesthetic inhalation agents and neuromuscular-blocking medications used to induce general anesthesia, not conscious sedation.

3. **Conscious sedation involves the use of IV opioids and sedatives to decrease the level of consciousness to a degree where the person can still maintain an airway, can respond to verbal commands, and cannot remember the procedure.**

4. Clients who have received spinal anesthesia (subarachnoid block), not conscious sedation, are placed in the supine position to limit leakage of cerebrospinal fluid from the needle insertion site. Bedrest in the supine position, hydration, and pressure against the infusion site limit headache associated with spinal anesthesia.

10. 1. **Chronic alcoholism disrupts the structure and function of the liver. A decrease in the synthesis of bile salts prevents the absorption of vitamin K, which is essential for the production of clotting factors II, VII, IX, and X. Therefore, clients with alcoholism are at risk for hemorrhage. In addition, malnutrition results in decreased protein synthesis, anemia, and vitamin deficiencies, all of which interfere with fluid and electrolyte balance and wound healing. Finally, the client will have to be medically managed to minimize the responses to alcohol withdrawal.**

2. Although clients with epilepsy have their own unique problems that must be considered, they are not at the greatest risk for postoperative mortality as a group in another option.

3. Middle-age adults are not at the greatest risk for postoperative mortality as a group in another option.

4. Although infants have a greater surgical risk than children and young to middle-age adults because they have a lower total blood volume, a larger percentage of body fluid, and difficulty maintaining body temperature as a result of an immature shivering reflex, they are not at the greatest risk for postoperative mortality as a group in another option.

11. 1. Although compression stockings at night are helpful, they will promote venous return for a limited amount of time (approximately 8 hours). The client will be at risk for the remaining time in the day (approximately 16 hours).

2. Deep breathing and coughing exercises help to prevent atelectasis and pneumonia, not thrombophlebitis; these exercises should be performed hourly when awake.

3. **Leg exercises are an active intervention by the client that contracts the muscles of the legs. This rhythmically compresses the veins, which promotes venous return and prevents venous stasis.**

4. Elevating the legs on two pillows is undesirable because pressure on the popliteal space constricts the vessels, which impedes venous return, promotes venous stasis, and injures tissues. Vessel injury, venous stasis, hypercoagulability, and dehydration all contribute to thrombophlebitis.

12. 1. Although constipation as a result of anesthesia is a concern, it is not life-threatening.

2. Although urinary retention as a result of anesthesia is a concern, it is not life-threatening.

3. **After abdominal surgery, clients frequently have shallow respirations because when the diaphragm contracts with a deep breath, it increases intra-abdominal pressure, which causes pain at the operative site. Shallow breathing may result in atelectasis, hypostatic pneumonia, or both.**

4. Although a person may experience an impaired ability to provide self-care during recovery from surgery, it is not life-threatening.

13. 1. The client's level of anxiety may be communicated; however, in the immediate postoperative period, the physiological needs of the client are the priority.

2. **The type and extent of the surgery are significant pieces of information because there are unique stressors and expected responses to various types of surgery that may direct the plan of care for the client.**

3. Although the type and amount of IV fluids prescribed are important and should be communicated, this is only one aspect of the client's care.

4. Although reasonable requests are honored, the status of the client or the environment may prohibit them.

14. 1. **These clinical findings are essential for discharge from the postanesthesia care unit because they reflect the body's vital functions, such as airway, breathing, and circulation.**

2. A dry dressing may be unrealistic. Some drainage from a surgical incision is expected in the immediate postoperative period. The other listed clinical findings are desirable.

3. A postoperative client may not be able to turn from side to side, but the client should be able to move all extremities. The other listed clinical findings are desirable for discharge.

4. The lack of a fever is not a criterion for discharge from the postanesthesia care unit because a low-grade fever is an expected response to the stress of surgery. Adventitious breath sounds are abnormal breath sounds (e.g., wheeze, crackles, and rhonchi) and indicate a respiratory problem. The ability to cough is desirable.

15. 1. A wound infection is less likely to occur 5 days after surgery because the proliferative or reconstructive phase of wound healing begins approximately 3 days after tissue damage. By the fifth postoperative day, the wound has filled with highly vascular fibroblastic connective tissue that protects the body from microorganisms.

2. **Microorganisms introduced into a surgical site take 72 hours to multiply and present local adaptations of pain, swelling, erythema, warmth, and purulent discharge and systemic adaptations of fever and tachycardia.**

3. A wound infection is less likely to occur at the ninth day because by the second postoperative week there is progressive collagen accumulation and the formation of the basic structure of the scar, which protect the body from microorganisms.

4. A wound infection is less likely to occur at the seventh day because by the seventh postoperative day the surface epithelium has an appropriate thickness and the subepithelial layers are bridged, which protect the body from microorganisms.

16. 1. **Leakage of cerebrospinal fluid from the needle insertion site reduces cerebrospinal fluid pressure, which causes a headache.**

2. Neuropathy, resulting from inflammation or degeneration of the peripheral nerves, is not a response to spinal anesthesia.

3. Although the needle insertion site may feel uncomfortable in some people, it is

not a common problem after spinal
anesthesia.

4. Anesthetic agents cause a decrease, not
increase, in blood pressure.

17. 1. Changing the route of a prescribed oral
medication is beyond the scope of the
legal practice of nursing.

2. Withholding medications without a significant reason is unsafe. These medications
may be essential to maintain the client's
physical or emotional status.

3. It is unsafe to withhold medications
without an important reason. The
withheld medications may be essential
to maintain the client's physical or
emotional equilibrium.

4. **This intervention meets the client's
needs and adheres to the laws that
govern the practice of nursing. A
change in the route of medication
delivery requires a prescription because medication administration is a
dependent function of the nurse.**

18. 1. **The molecules in clear liquids are less
complex and easier to ingest, tolerate,
and digest than those in a full-liquid
diet or food.**

2. A full-liquid diet is not the most common
diet prescribed postoperatively, although a
full-liquid diet frequently precedes solid
food.

3. A low-fiber diet is prescribed for specific
problems, such as intestinal inflammation
or infection. When able to be tolerated
postoperatively, dietary fiber promotes
intestinal motility and prevents
constipation.

4. A regular diet is not the most common
diet prescribed postoperatively, although
most initial postoperative diets eventually
progress to a regular diet.

19. 1. Both entry sites place the catheter in the
superior vena cava.

2. **A tension pneumothorax is not a
concern with a peripherally inserted
central venous catheter. Pneumothorax
is a complication of a central venous
catheter inserted into a subclavian
vein because of the close proximity
of its insertion site to the apex of the
lung.**

3. Both entry sites carry a risk of infection
because the first line of defense, the skin,
has been pierced.

4. Both entry sites allow for the administration of large volumes of fluid because the
distal ends of their catheters are both in
the superior vena cava.

20. 1. Serous exudate is a clear, watery fluid consisting mainly of serum. It is the exudate
expected before final wound healing.

2. Purulent exudate is a thick drainage
known as pus, which consists of leukocytes, liquefied dead tissue debris, and
bacteria. This is unexpected and indicates
the presence of a wound infection. Wound
infections generally become apparent 3 to
11 days postoperatively.

3. Sanguineous (hemorrhagic) exudate consists of large amounts of red blood cells
and is associated with open wounds or
hemorrhage.

4. **Serosanguineous exudate, a combination of serous and sanguineous
drainage, consists of plasma and red
blood cells and is pale red and watery.
This is the initial drainage expected
after surgery.**

21. 1. **Oliguria is diminished urine secretion
in relation to fluid intake, which is
indicated by a negative balance in the
intake and output record or an hourly
urine output of less than 30 mL.
Oliguria is caused by decreased renal
perfusion or kidney disease.**

2. Cachexia is not an adaptation related to
altered renal perfusion. Cachexia is
malnutrition and emaciation associated
with serious diseases, such as cancer.

3. Yellow sclera indicates jaundice. Jaundice
is the accumulation of bile pigments in
tissue, which is associated with liver or
biliary problems, not altered renal
perfusion.

4. Suprapubic distention indicates urinary
retention, which is an inability of the
bladder to empty, not a problem with
renal perfusion. If it occurs, usually it
becomes evident 6 to 8 hours after
surgery.

22. 1. Avoiding nausea and vomiting is an
unrealistic expectation after abdominal
surgery, considering all the stressors that
can contribute to these problems. Essential nutrient needs can be met despite the
presence of nausea and vomiting.

2. **Fluid is the most basic nutrient of the
body, and it contains compounds such**

as electrolytes. Electrolytes help maintain fluid balance, contribute to acid-base balance, and facilitate enzyme and neuromuscular reactions. The narrow safe limits of the volumes and composition of fluid compartments are essential for the life-sustaining processes of nutrition, metabolism, and excretion.

3. Wound healing takes time, and it is difficult to evaluate during the inflammatory phase, which lasts 1 to 4 days.

4. Oral intake should not be reestablished until intestinal motility returns, which may take several days.

23. 1. Although the condition of drains ultimately will be assessed, the physiological status of the client is the priority.

2. Although the client's level of consciousness eventually will be assessed, it is not the priority at this time.

3. Assessment in acute situations always follows the ABCs: airway, breathing, and circulation. Respirations and pulse reflect the cardiopulmonary status of the client.

4. Both the location and status of the dressing should be assessed, but not until more critical assessments are completed.

24. 1. The Sims position will not adequately expose the perineal area for examination.

2. The supine position will not expose the perineal area for examination

3. The lithotomy position, back-lying with the hips and knees flexed and the legs supported in stirrups, provides optimal visualization of and access to the perineal area for a physical examination.

4. A client's legs are adducted when in the Trendelenburg position, which does not permit visualization of the perineal area.

25. **1. A Hemovac is designed to accommodate 100, 400, or 800 mL of drainage, depending on the system used, whereas a Jackson-Pratt system accommodates volumes of less than 100 mL of drainage.**

2. Both create a vacuum by closing the drainage port while compressing the device.

3. Both work by gentle negative pressure that draws fluid from the tissues to the collection chamber.

4. Both collection chambers should be placed below the site of insertion to allow gravity to work in conjunction with the negative pressure within the self-contained systems.

26. 1. Gastroesophageal reflex disease is not a problem with general anesthesia because of interventions such as NPO status before surgery, use of a cuffed endotracheal tube, and positioning.

2. Although reduced reflexes are significant to know when monitoring a client throughout the surgical experience, they do not place a client at the greatest risk.

3. Although a decreased metabolism is taken into consideration when monitoring reflexes during the induction, maintenance, and reversal phases of anesthesia, hypothyroidism does not place a client at the greatest risk.

4. Respiratory problems complicate the administration of inhalation anesthesia. Emphysema is characterized by destruction of alveoli, loss of elastic recoil, and narrowing of bronchioles, which result in alveolar hyperinflation and increased airflow resistance.

27. **1. These are the classic clinical manifestations of a pulmonary embolus. Chest pain results from local tissue hypoxia, tachycardia from systemic hypoxia, and hypotension from decreased cardiac output. A pulmonary embolus is caused by an embolus lodging in a vessel in the pulmonary circulation, occluding blood supply to the capillary side of the alveolar-capillary membrane.**

2. Although tachycardia and hypotension occur with hemorrhage, chest pain does not.

3. Although tachycardia and chest pain occur with a myocardial infarction (heart attack), the blood pressure probably will increase, not decrease. If cardiogenic shock occurs, the blood pressure decreases eventually.

4. Pneumonia, inflammation of the lung with consolidation and exudation, is associated with tachycardia and chest discomfort. However, it does not have a sudden onset and the blood pressure will increase, not decrease.

28. 1. The absence of intestinal motility (paralytic ileus), not infection, is the intestinal response that can occur during the first 24 to 36 hours after surgery. Abdominal distention and absent bowel sounds, not a fever, indicate this problem.

2. A urinary catheter usually is inserted before major abdominal surgery. A bladder infection will not be apparent during the first 24 hours after catheterization because microorganisms take at least 72 hours to multiply sufficiently to manifest symptoms.

3. Microorganisms introduced into the incision at the time of surgery take at least 72 hours to multiply sufficiently to manifest symptoms.

4. **When postoperative pneumonia (an inflammation of the lung with consolidation and exudation) occurs, client symptoms are evident usually any time within 36 hours after surgery.**

29. 1. Stretching a transparent dressing snugly over an entire incision restricts mobility and may exert undue pressure on the surface of the wound. The dressing should be laid gently over the wound and the edges pressed against the skin to ensure adherence.

2. **Cleansing the skin with normal saline before applying the dressing removes exudate and ensures adhesion of the dressing. Transparent adhesive films are semipermeable (allows oxygen exchange) and nonabsorbent (impermeable to water and bacteria).**

3. Covering a transparent wound barrier with a gauze dressing and securing it with paper tape defeats one of the purposes of a transparent dressing, which is the ability to visualize the wound.

4. A transparent dressing has an adhesive backing and therefore does not require reinforcing tape.

30. 1. Although allowing for skeletal deformities is always taken into consideration when positioning a client, another option is the priority.

2. It is impossible to prevent all pressure on bony prominences in the postanesthesia care unit. Turning as well as positioning devices and padding are used to minimize pressure.

3. **Maintaining an airway and facilitating respirations and oxygenation always are the priorities in the postanesthesia care unit.**

4. Although stretching of neuromuscular tissue should be avoided, another option is the priority.

31. 1. Significant nursing care must be provided before this point in time. The operative consent form is signed during the preoperative phase of the perioperative experience.

2. **The surgical experience begins as soon as the decision for surgery is made. Perioperative nursing responsibilities begin immediately and continue throughout the preoperative, intraoperative, and postoperative phases.**

3. A nurse is negligent if nursing care begins at this point in the surgical experience.

4. The nurse is negligent if nursing care begins only at this point in the surgical experience. This is the intraoperative phase of the perioperative experience.

32. 1. Informing the surgeon is premature because some drainage is expected with a compound fracture.

2. Reinforcing the cast with a gauze dressing is undesirable because it impedes the ability to assess the site in the future.

3. The determination of expansion is a subjective assessment without objective parameters and is undesirable as a form of measurement.

4. **Circling the spot with a pen and indicating the date, time, and initials is appropriate. This determines objectively the time and extent of the bleeding and the person who performed the assessment. The extent of progression of the bleeding can be established objectively using the original circle as a standard.**

33. 1. The implementation of medical, not surgical, asepsis is the standard because a nasogastric tube enters the stomach, which is not a sterile cavity.

2. It is unnecessary to monitor the intake and output (I&O) this frequently. The I&O must be recorded at routine intervals as per hospital policy, usually every 8 and 24 hours.

3. Oral hygiene should be provided more frequently than every 4 hours. Because there is no food or fluid to stimulate salivary gland secretion and the tube in the nose may interfere with breathing, precipitating mouth breathing, the mouth becomes dry.

4. **The level of suctioning is part of the primary health-care provider's**

prescription for nasogastric decompression. Low suction pressure is between 80 and 100 mm Hg, and high suction pressure is between 100 and 120 mm Hg. Suctioning must be maintained continuously with a double-lumen tube (e.g., Salem sump) to prevent reflux of gastric secretions into the vent lumen, which will obstruct its functioning and result in mucosal damage. A single-lumen tube requires low intermittent suction to prevent the tube from adhering to the stomach mucosa.

34. 1. A double-lumen tube will not minimize the risk of a bowel obstruction.
2. All nasogastric tubes attached to suction remove drainage from the stomach, not the intestine. Nasointestinal tubes attached to suction remove fluid from the intestine.
3. **A double-lumen tube has two lumens: one allows stomach secretions to be removed by suction (first lumen) and the other allows air to be drawn into the stomach (second lumen). The second lumen (blue pigtail) is open to environmental (atmospheric) air, which is drawn into the stomach to equalize the outside pressure with the pressure inside the stomach. This prevents the catheter tip from attaching to the gastric mucosa when the drainage lumen is attached to suction, limiting mucosal damage.**
4. All nasogastric tubes attached to suction empty the stomach contents in an effort to promote gastric and intestinal rest. Gastric glands produce up to 4 to 5 liters of fluid a day that stimulate the intestine unless removed.

35. 1. Continuing the aspirin is unsafe. Acetylsalicylic acid (aspirin) is a salicylate that inhibits thromboxane, which binds platelet molecules together. Continuing the aspirin can interfere with platelet aggregation and may result in hemorrhage.
2. **Acetylsalicylic acid (aspirin) is a salicylate that inhibits thromboxane, which binds platelet molecules together. It has a half-life of 15 to 30 hours. It should be discontinued at least 5 days before surgery. Some providers advocate discontinuing aspirin 7 days before surgery.**

3. It is unsafe to continue to take aspirin until the evening of surgery. On the day of surgery, there will still be chemical properties of aspirin in the client's body that inhibit platelet aggregation, which may result in hemorrhage.
4. The dose of 81 mg of aspirin will still interfere with platelet aggregation, which may result in hemorrhage on the day of surgery. Also, changing the dose of a medication is not within the legal practice of nursing.

36. 1. It is not necessary to notify the primary health-care provider because this is an expected response when negative pressure is applied to the device.
2. It is not necessary to change the setting of the negative pressure. Changing the setting of the negative pressure requires a prescription; it is a dependent function of the nurse. The pressure can be continuous or intermittent and set between 5 and 123 mm Hg.
3. Changing the transparent film is not necessary because the device is intact. The film is expected to collapse when negative pressure is exerted.
4. **The device is functioning appropriately. The transparent film will collapse or wrinkle as negative pressure is applied to the wound. This indicates that there are no leaks in the dressing and the negative pressure is functioning.**

37. 4. **Clients have a right to know what is going to be done and why.**
1. **Antiembolism stockings should not be applied to a client with such conditions as excessive peripheral edema or lower extremity arterial disease because doing so may make these conditions worse.**
5. **Antiembolism stockings must fit the size of the client for compression to be effective. If the stockings are too loose, they will not provide adequate compression to facilitate venous return, and if they are too tight, they will have a tourniquet effect.**
2. **The supine position facilitates venous return via gravity, thereby limiting trapping of blood pooled in the lower extremities. When the legs are dependent, they can develop dependent edema. Antiembolism stockings should be applied before the client gets out of**

bed in the morning before dependent edema has a chance to occur. Antiembolism stockings are elastic garments worn around the leg; they exert pressure against the legs, thus reducing the diameter of the veins. When the diameter of veins is reduced, the volume and velocity of blood flow increase, preventing venous stasis. Venous stasis promotes the formation of a thrombus.

6. **Turning the stocking inside out and stretching each side make it easier to get the elastic over the toes and heel. Centering the heel keeps the stocking straight, providing for even compression.**

3. **Avoiding placement of antiembolism stockings over the popliteal fold prevents damage to nerves and blood vessels in the popliteal area.**

38. 1. **Increasing fluid intake will make respiratory secretions less viscous and easier to expectorate, thereby facilitating ventilation.**

2. **Abdominal distention raises the pressure within the abdominal cavity, which exerts pressure against the diaphragm, impeding its contraction and limiting thoracic excursion.**

3. When the client is in a side-lying position, aeration of the dependent side of the lung is limited because of pooling of secretions and the weight of the body compressing the dependent part of the body.

4. Passive range-of-motion exercises do not facilitate respirations; they help prevent contractures.

5. **An incentive spirometer will help increase depth of inspirations, preventing stasis of secretions in the respiratory tract, which in turn will facilitate ventilation.**

39. The carbon dioxide used to insufflate the abdominal cavity during a laparoscopic cholecystectomy that is not released or absorbed by the body can be trapped in the subdiaphragmatic recesses. It can irritate the diaphragm, causing referred pain to the right shoulder and scapular area. In addition, the retained carbon dioxide can irritate the phrenic nerve, causing dyspnea. Positioning the client in the left Sims position may help move the gas away from the diaphragm. The nurse should

encourage the client to walk and periodically breathe deeply once fully recovered from anesthesia.

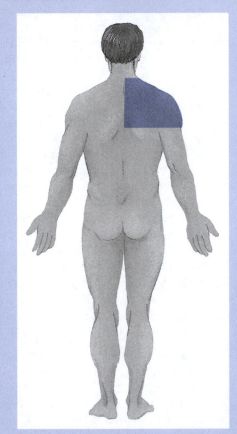

40. 1. Warm liquids and food are contraindicated during the first several days after a tonsillectomy because they cause vasodilation, which may increase bleeding from the vascular mucous membranes of the oropharynx.

2. Milk and milk products are avoided during recovery from oral surgery because some health-care professionals believe milk increases the consistency of phlegm.

3. **Apple juice is a clear liquid that, when cool, will promote vasoconstriction and limit bleeding from the operative site.**

4. **An ice pop is a frozen clear liquid that promotes vasoconstriction and limits bleeding from the operative site. However, flavors that have a red color are contraindicated because they complicate assessing for bleeding.**

5. **Cool gelatin desserts promote vasoconstriction, limiting bleeding from the operative site. Flavors that have a red color are contraindicated because they complicate assessing for bleeding.**

41. 1. The client's vital signs are not stable. Respirations at a rate of 30 are too rapid. A pulse rate of 98 is within the expected range of 70 to 100; however, it is in the high range of normal, and the blood pressure of 170/90 mm Hg is higher than the expected range of 150/90 mm Hg for an older adult. The client should be monitored further.
    2. The client's level of consciousness meets the criteria for discharge from the postanesthesia care unit. The client is easily aroused, as indicated by "coughing and deep breathing on command and able to move all extremities on command."
    3. The absence of bowel sounds is an expected response to surgery and the use of anesthesia. The presence of bowel sounds is not a criterion for discharge from the postanesthesia care unit.
    4. Urinary retention catheters frequently are in place postoperatively. The ability to void is not a criterion for discharge from a postanesthesia care unit.

42. 1. Vitamin C (ascorbic acid) promotes collagen production, an essential component of the proliferative phase of wound healing. In addition, vitamin C enhances capillary formation, decreases capillary fragility, increases the tensile strength of the wound, and provides a defense against infection because of its role in the immune response.
    2. Vitamin C does not improve digestion.
    3. Vitamin C does not increase transport of oxygen to cells. The hemoglobin in red blood cells transports oxygen to body cells.
    4. Vitamin B_{12} (cobalamin), folic acid, and iron promote red blood cell production, not vitamin C.
    5. Vitamin C promotes the strength of capillaries, not large veins. Ambulation, leg exercises, and hydration prevent deep vein thrombosis.

43. 1. Ten is not the client's Aldrete score.
    2. Nine is not the client's Aldrete score.
    3. Eight is the client's Aldrete score. The client received 2 points for moving all four extremities on command, 2 points for breathing deeply and coughing freely, 2 points for a blood pressure consistent with preanesthetic levels, 1 point for being aroused on command, and 1 point for oxygen saturation of 92% while on oxygen inhalation.
    4. Seven is not the client's Aldrete score.

44. 1. When exiting from the left side of the bed, the left-lateral side of the abdomen will be compressed against the bed by body weight. The left, not right, side of the abdomen will absorb the majority of the muscular strain exerted by the transfer.
    2. Although an abdominal binder might be applied for clients at high risk for dehiscence, abdominal binders are not used routinely because they increase intra-abdominal pressure; this exerts a force against the diaphragm that impedes maximum respiratory excursion.
    3. Holding a pillow against the abdomen with both hands is unsafe. At least one upper extremity should be used to help raise the body to a sitting position and promote balance during the transfer out of bed.
    4. Using the left arm to assist in lifting the body to a sitting position on the side of the bed places less strain on abdominal muscles in the area of the incision.
    5. Sitting on the side of the bed for a few minutes before moving to a standing position allows the blood pressure to adjust to the change in position, thus avoiding orthostatic hypotension.

45. 5. Positioning sheepskin on the platform, especially at the gluteal fold, provides a soft base on which to position the extremity. The site of the gluteal fold is the site that is most at risk for excess pressure.
    1. Positioning the extremity on the platform so that the knee is centered over the break in the platform ensures that flexion occurs at the site of the knee joint when the device is in motion.
    3. Ensuring that the extremity is aligned with the hips and torso prevents stress and strain on the muscles, bones, joints, ligaments, and tendons of the body.
    2. Setting the degree of flexion, speed, and time on and off the machine as prescribed ensures that the plan of care is implemented as prescribed.
    6. Positioning the controller within easy reach of the client allows the client to turn off the device if unable to tolerate the procedure.

4. Assessing the skin once the extremity is removed from the device ensures that a skin problem is immediately identified. Providing skin care keeps skin clean, dry, and moisturized, which helps to keep skin supple and intact.

46. 1. **Selecting yellow bell peppers indicates learning. A half a cup of yellow bell peppers contains approximately 170 mg of vitamin C. Vitamin C promotes collagen production, which is essential in the proliferative and maturation phases of wound healing.**
   2. Selecting whole-grain bread does not indicate learning. Whole grains contain trace amounts or no vitamin C necessary for collagen production. Whole grains are noted primarily for containing vitamin E and potassium.
   3. **Selecting cantaloupe indicates learning. A cup of cantaloupe contains approximately 68 mg of vitamin C. Vitamin C promotes collagen production, which is essential in the proliferative and maturation phases of wound healing.**
   4. **Selecting an orange indicates learning. One medium orange contains approximately 69 mg of vitamin C. Vitamin C promotes collagen production, which is essential in the proliferative and maturation phases of wound healing.**
   5. **Selecting kiwi indicates learning. One kiwi contains approximately 72 mg of vitamin C. Vitamin C promotes collagen production, which is essential in the proliferative and maturation phases of wound healing.**

47. 1. **Compressing the collection container, closing the port, and releasing hand compression after emptying the container establish negative pressure within the collection container.**
   2. Clean, not sterile, gloves should be worn when emptying a Jackson-Pratt drain. Although the nurse should maintain sterile technique when emptying a Jackson-Pratt drain, it can be accomplished without wearing sterile gloves. Clean gloves are worn by the nurse to protect the nurse from the client's blood or body fluids.
   3. **Keeping the collection container below the insertion site augments the negative pressure of the system.**
   4. A primary health-care provider may prescribe that a Penrose drain be shortened

daily, not the tubing of a Jackson-Pratt drain.
   5. The collection container should be emptied when half full, not when full. This action prevents the weight of the bulb pulling on the tubing and helps maintain negative pressure. The amount of negative pressure decreases as drainage in the collection container increases.
   6. **Attaching tubing to clothing prevents tension on the tubing.**

48. 1. **Coughing or bearing down will increase tension on the suture line, potentially extending the dehiscence and evisceration, and should be avoided.**
   2. **The client needs emergency surgical care, and the primary health-care provider should be notified immediately.**
   3. **The client should be placed in the low-Fowler position with the knees slightly flexed to reduce stress on the suture line.**
   4. **Covering the wound with a sterile dressing protects the open wound from contamination.**
   5. **The client should be prepared for surgery because the surgeon will most likely return the client to the operating room for surgical repair of the incision.**

49. 1. **Sequential compression devices apply pressure progressively from the ankles to the thighs, promoting venous return. Volume and velocity of blood flow in the superficial and deep veins in the legs increase, preventing venous stasis. Venous stasis promotes the development of a thrombus.**
   2. **Antiembolism stockings are elastic garments worn around the leg; they exert pressure against the legs, reducing the diameter of the veins. When the diameter of veins is reduced, the volume and velocity of blood flow increases, preventing venous stasis. Venous stasis promotes the formation of a thrombus.**
   3. **Walking contracts the muscles of the lower extremities and increases cardiac output. Both increase the volume and velocity of blood flow through the veins of the lower extremities, preventing venous stasis and thrombus formation.**
   4. Using an incentive spirometer prevents atelectasis, not thrombophlebitis.

5. Coughing and deep breathing prevent atelectasis, not thrombophlebitis.

6. Keeping the legs uncrossed eliminates pressure against the calves or behind the knee (popliteal space), depending on where the legs are crossed. Pressure to these areas impairs venous return, which promotes venous stasis and thrombus formation.

50. Solve the problem using the formula for ratio and proportion.

$$\frac{\text{Desired}}{\text{Have}} \quad \frac{12 \text{ mg}}{10 \text{ mg}} = \frac{x \text{ mL}}{1 \text{ mL}}$$

$$10\, x = 12$$
$$x = 12 \div 10$$
$$x = 1.2 \text{ mL}$$

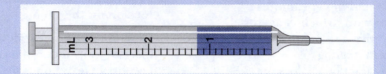

Alternate Item Formats

6

National Council Licensure Examinations (NCLEX®) include multiple-choice questions and alternate item format questions. A typical multiple-choice question (one answer) presents a statement or situation and requires the test taker to identify the correct answer from among four presented options. Alternate item formats use the benefits of computer technology to assess knowledge via various methods. Alternate item formats include questions that require test takers to do the following: identify multiple answers (multiple-response items); identify a location on a presented image (hot-spot items); perform a mathematical calculation (fill-in-the-blank calculation items); respond to a question in relation to an image such as a picture, table, photograph, or illustration (graphic items); identify priorities (drag and drop/ordered response items); and answer a question in relation to a client situation that presents data, such as information from a client's clinical record (exhibit items). All item types may include multimedia, such as illustrations, charts, tables, audio, or video technology, to present information in the question. Alternate item formats are able to measure entry-level nursing competence in ways that are different from those used in the typical multiple-choice format. It is believed that some nursing content is more readily and authentically evaluated using alternate item formats.

This chapter includes 60 questions that use formats other than multiple-choice questions. For specific test-taking techniques for answering alternate item questions, see *Test Success: Test-Taking Techniques for Beginning Nursing Students*. This is an F.A. Davis textbook written by Nugent and Vitale.

ALTERNATE ITEM FORMATS: QUESTIONS

Multiple-Response Items

A multiple-response item presents a statement or situation that asks a question that has more than one answer among presented options. The test taker is required to select all options that correctly answer the question.

1. A client comes to the emergency department with a lacerated thumb. For which of the following associated with the local adaptation syndrome (LAS) should the nurse assess the client? **Select all that apply.**
   1. _____ Pain
   2. _____ Heat
   3. _____ Erythema
   4. _____ Increased heart rate
   5. _____ Decreased blood pressure
   6. _____ Elevated blood glucose level

2. A nurse is assisting a postoperative client to ambulate. Which postoperative complication will ambulation help prevent? **Select all that apply.**
   1. _____ Hypovolemia
   2. _____ Constipation
   3. _____ Atelectasis
   4. _____ Dehiscence
   5. _____ Infection

3. A client is learning self-care in relation to a 2-g sodium diet. Which food high in sodium selected by the client indicates to the nurse that further teaching is necessary? **Select all that apply.**
   1. _____ Apple juice
   2. _____ Feta cheese
   3. _____ Corned beef
   4. _____ Canned soup
   5. _____ Broccoli spears

4. A nurse is monitoring a client's IV infusion. Which information is necessary to determine that the IV is "on time"? **Select all that apply.**
   1. _____ Drip rate per minute
   2. _____ Time the bag was hung
   3. _____ Solution indicated on the IV bag
   4. _____ Volume of solution in the IV bag
   5. _____ Milliliters per hour that was prescribed

5. A client who was in an automobile collision is brought to the emergency department by ambulance. The client is exhibiting signs and symptoms of multiple trauma. For which common response to hemorrhage should the nurse assess the client? **Select all that apply.**
   1. _____ Tachypnea
   2. _____ Tachycardia
   3. _____ Pale skin color
   4. _____ Thready pulse
   5. _____ Delayed capillary refill

6. A nurse is caring for several postoperative clients who require common therapeutic interventions that involve the principle of gravity. Which of the following is associated with the principle of gravity? **Select all that apply.**
   1. _____ Foley catheter
   2. _____ Penrose drain
   3. _____ Tap-water enema
   4. _____ Gastric decompression
   5. _____ Portable wound drainage system

7. A nurse is supervising a nursing team consisting of two nurses and two nursing assistants. Which task can the nurse delegate to the nursing assistants? **Select all that apply.**
   1. _____ Helping a client who is constipated walk to the bathroom
   2. _____ Pushing a client in a wheelchair to the x-ray department
   3. _____ Applying antifungal cream to unbroken skin
   4. _____ Weighing a client using a bed scale
   5. _____ Emptying a urine collection bag

8. Which action is based on the principles of surgical asepsis? **Select all that apply.**
   1. _____ Washing hands
   2. _____ Keeping a sterile field dry
   3. _____ Holding sterile objects below the waist
   4. _____ Wearing personal protective equipment when providing care
   5. _____ Considering the outer half inch of the sterile field as contaminated

9. A newly admitted client's respiratory status is assessed by a nurse, who identifies the presence of gurgles and a productive cough. For which of the following associated with this data cluster should the nurse assess the client? **Select all that apply.**
1. _____ Dyspnea
2. _____ Purulent sputum
3. _____ Decreased blood pressure
4. _____ Decreased pulse oximetry level
5. _____ Bronchovesicular breath sounds

10. A nurse is caring for a client who is receiving continuous formula feedings through a nasogastric tube. Which nursing intervention **supports** comfort? **Select all that apply.**
1. _____ Check tube patency frequently.
2. _____ Administer oral hygiene every 2 hours.
3. _____ Apply lubricant after cleaning the nares.
4. _____ Ensure that the tube is secured to the nose.
5. _____ Instill 30 mL of water into the tube every 4 to 6 hours.

11. A client is receiving a diuretic that contributes to the loss of potassium, and the nurse provides dietary teaching. Which food that contains more than 800 mg of potassium per serving selected by the client indicates an understanding of excellent sources of potassium? **Select all that apply.**
1. _____ Hard-cooked egg
2. _____ Baked potato
3. _____ Green beans
4. _____ Bran flakes
5. _____ Lean meat

12. A nurse is caring for a client who has the following medication prescribed by the primary health-care provider: albuterol sulfate inhalation aerosol 90 mcg, 2 puffs via a metered-dose inhaler with a spacer, every 12 hours. Which should the nurse teach the client to implement when using this inhaler? **Select all that apply.**
1. _____ Seal the lips around the mouthpiece of the spacer.
2. _____ Exhale fully through the nose before taking a dose.
3. _____ Breathe in deeply and quickly after activating the canister.
4. _____ Rinse the mouth with water and spit it out after the procedure.
5. _____ Remove the cap, shake it well, and spray it into the air three times when using a metered-dose inhaler for the first time.

13. A nurse is providing dietary teaching for a client with the diagnosis of osteoporosis. Which food selected by the client indicates that the teaching about foods high in calcium was understood? **Select all that apply.**
1. _____ Cheese
2. _____ Lettuce
3. _____ Peppers
4. _____ Oranges
5. _____ Sardines

14. Which nursing action is important when applying antiembolism stockings? **Select all that apply.**
1. _____ Eliminating the wrinkles in the stockings
2. _____ Ensuring the toe window is properly positioned
3. _____ Applying the stockings after the client is out of bed
4. _____ Flexing the knee as the stocking is pulled over the knee
5. _____ Removing the stocking once a day for at least thirty minutes

Hot-Spot Items

A hot-spot item asks a question in relation to an illustration. The test taker must identify a location on the illustration that answers the question.

1. A client with a primary health-care provider's prescription for bedrest consistently lies in the right-lateral position. Place an X over the bony prominence the nurse should assess because it has the **highest** risk for the development of a pressure ulcer.

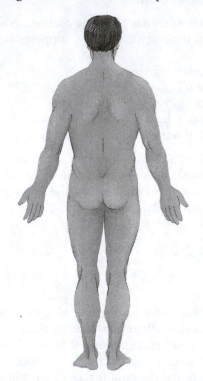

2. A nurse is caring for a client who had the creation of a colostomy. Place an X over the large intestine that produces the **most** liquid stool, thereby placing the client at risk for skin breakdown.

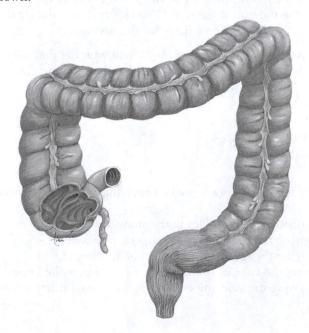

3. A nurse is to administer an intermittent tube feeding via a nasogastric tube. A nurse obtains gastric contents via the nasogastric tube and then assesses the client's abdomen with a stethoscope when returning the gastric contents. Mark an X where the nurse should place the stethoscope when double-checking placement of the nasogastric tube.

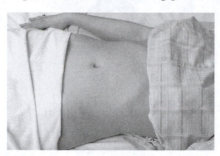

4. A primary health-care provider prescribes heparin 5,000 units subcutaneously twice a day. Place an X over the site that is **most** commonly used by the nurse to administer this medication.

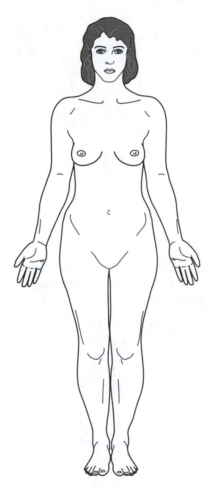

5. Two nurses are performing CPR on a postoperative client. One nurse performs sternal compressions, and the other delivers breaths and monitors the client. Place an X over the preferred site to obtain this client's pulse.

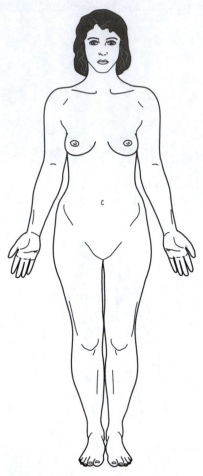

6. After assessing a client and taking the temperature, the nurse determines that the client is experiencing pyrexia. Put an X within the range of temperatures on the thermometer scale that reflects pyrexia.

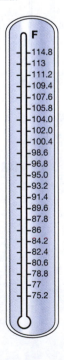

7. A primary health-care provider prescribes diphenhydramine 25 mg PO four times a day to minimize allergy symptoms. Diphenhydramine is supplied as a syrup 12.5 mg/5 mL. Put an X at the point on a graduated medicine cup that indicates the dose of diphenhydramine the nurse must dispense.

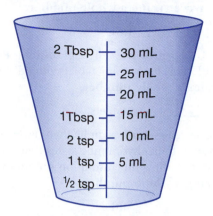

8. A nurse is caring for a client who is receiving airborne precautions because of tuberculosis. Place an X within the chain of infection when the nurse wears a particulate filter mask (N95 respirator).

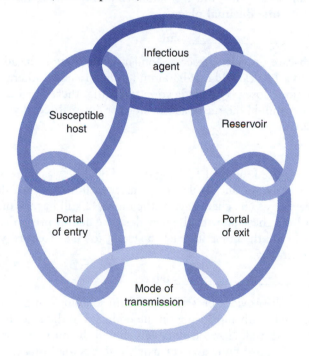

Fill-in-the-Blank Calculation Items

A fill-in-the-blank item asks a question that requires the test taker to perform a calculation. Fill-in-the-blank items are associated with pharmacological and parenteral therapies and other situations requiring a calculation.

1. A primary health-care provider prescribes an antidysrhythmic medication of 2 g in 1,000 mL D_5W at 4 mg/min. At what rate should the nurse set the infusion pump? **Record your answer using a whole number.**

Answer: _____ mL/hr.

2. A primary health-care provider prescribes an antibiotic of 400,000 units IV piggyback (IVPB) every 6 hours. The medication vial contains 1 million units with the following directions: add 4.6 mL of diluent to yield a concentrated solution of 200,000 units/mL. How much solution of the antibiotic should the nurse prepare to be added to IVPB solution? **Record your answer using a whole number.**

Answer: _____ mL.

3. A primary health-care provider prescribes digoxin 0.25 mg PO once daily. Tablets are available that contain 0.125 mg. How many tablets should the nurse administer? **Record your answer using a whole number.**

Answer: _____ tablets.

4. A primary health-care provider prescribes diphenhydramine elixir 25 mg PO twice a day for 3 days. The bottle of diphenhydramine states that there are 12.5 mg/mL. When preparing the first dose, how much solution should the nurse administer? **Record your answer using a whole number.**

Answer: _____ mL.

5. A primary health-care provider prescribes epoetin 100 units/kg/dose subcutaneously three times a week for a client who weighs 110 pounds. The medication states that there are 2,000 units/mL. How much solution should the nurse administer? **Record your answer using one decimal place.**

Answer: _____ mL.

6. A primary health-care provider prescribes ondansetron 6 mg to be administered via oral suspension to a 12-year-old child 30 minutes before chemotherapy and then every 8 hours for two more doses. The medication states that there are 4 mg/5 mL. How much oral solution should the nurse administer per dose? **Record your answer using one decimal place.**

Answer: _____ mL.

7. A client initially received ramipril 1.25 mg daily. The dose was increased to 2.5 mg once a day for several days, and finally the primary health-care provider increases the dose to 5 mg every day. The client says to the nurse, "I still have a lot of 1.25-mg tablets left. Can I use these up with the new dose the doctor prescribed?" How many 1.25-mg tablets should the nurse instruct the client to take? **Record your answer using a whole number.**

Answer: _____ tablets.

8. A primary health-care provider prescribes warfarin sodium 10 mg PO once a day on the even days of the month and 15 mg on the odd days of the month. The 10-mg tablets supplied are scored. How many tablets should the nurse administer on the fifth day of the month? **Record your answer using one decimal place.**

Answer: _____ tablets.

9. A primary health-care provider prescribes an IV infusion of 1,000 mL of D_5W with 20 mEq of potassium chloride to be administered at 125 mL/hr. The infusion set has a drop factor of 15. At how many drops per minute should the nurse set the IV infusion? **Record your answer using a whole number.**

Answer: _____ drops/min.

10. A client has a prescription for regular insulin. The prescription states: administer regular insulin before meals and at bedtime based on the client's glucose monitoring results.

Blood glucose 71 to 150: no insulin
151 to 200: 3 units
201 to 250: 5 units
251 to 300: 7 units
301 to 350: 9 units
351 to 400: 11 units and call the primary health-care provider

The client's blood glucose at 11:30 a.m. is 230. How many units of regular insulin should the nurse administer? **Record your answer using a whole number.**

Answer: _____ units.

11. A nurse is calculating a client's intake and output for an 8-hour period of time. The client has 1,000 mL of 0.9% sodium chloride infusing intravenously at 75 mL/hr. The client received two intermittent doses of an intravenous antibiotic in 50 mL of solution each. The intravenous antibiotic solutions were administered over 20 minutes each via a secondary intravenous line that was hung higher than the primary infusion of sodium chloride. For breakfast, the client had 4 ounces of coffee and 6 ounces of orange juice. For lunch, the client ingested 240 mL of beef broth. Later, the client experienced nausea and vomited 300 mL of greenish fluid. The client consumed 8 ounces of ice chips. What was the client's total fluid intake? **Record your answer using a whole number.**

Answer: _____ mL.

12. A client who is taking a prescribed liquid oral medication at home calls the clinic for instructions. The dose prescribed is 30 mL, but a measuring device is not supplied with the medication. How many tablespoons of the liquid medication should the nurse instruct the client to take? **Record your answer using a whole number.**

Answer: _____ tablespoons.

13. A client with the diagnosis of anorexia nervosa is admitted to the hospital. A nurse is calculating the total calories that the client ingested for lunch. The client ate 10 g of carbohydrates, 4 g of protein, and 3 g of fat. How many calories did the client consume with lunch? **Record your answer using a whole number.**

Answer: _____ calories.

14. A primary health-care provider prescribes a medication for a client that should be administered based on body weight. The prescription states to administer 0.5 mg per kilogram of body weight once a day. The client weighs 160 pounds. How many milligrams of medication should be administered per dose? **Record your answer using one decimal place.**

Answer: _____ mg.

Graphic Items (Items Using a Graphic, Chart, Table, or Illustration)

An item using a chart, table, or graphic image requires the test taker to refer to the illustration presented to arrive at the correct answer. It tests the ability to identify, calculate, analyze, or interpret data from a chart, table, or graphic image to arrive at the correct answer.

1. A nurse is reviewing a client's temperatures over the course of hospitalization. What was the client's temperature on June 7th at 4 p.m.?
   1. 97.8°F
   2. 99.2°F
   3. 101.2°F
   4. 102.6°F

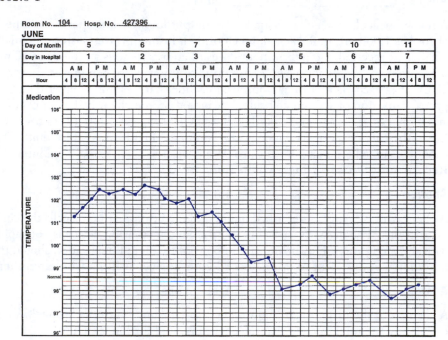

2. A nurse is caring for a client who has a prescription for intake and output. Referring to the intake and output flow sheet, what was the client's total output for the hours between 7 a.m. and 3 p.m.?
   1. 355
   2. 720
   3. 1,300
   4. 1,405

DAILY INTAKE AND OUTPUT RECORD

DATE JUNE 5

Time	Bottle	Amount	Solution	Medication and Dosage	* ABS.	⊤ LIB	ORAL	URINE	EMESIS	N.G. TUBE	HÆMOVAC
8	1	1000	NS	20 mEq KCl				650			
8:30							360				
10:00							120				
11:30							240	150			
12:00									160		
1:40									90		60
2:15								250			
3:00						525	475				45
7-3 TOTAL		8-HR TOTAL									
3-11 TOTAL		8-HR TOTAL									
11-7 TOTAL		8-HR TOTAL									
24 HOUR TOTAL											

INTAKE GRAND TOTAL [   ]   OUTPUT GRAND TOTAL [   ]

* ABS. = amount absorbed   ⊤ LIB = Left in bag

3. A nurse is making rounds at the beginning of a shift and enters the room of the client depicted in the photograph. What should the nurse do? **Select all that apply.**

1. _____ Move the straps of the mask to above the client's ears.
2. _____ Put a second pillow under the client's head.
3. _____ Obtain the client's oxygen saturation level.
4. _____ Elevate the head of the client's bed.
5. _____ Place a hospital gown on the client.

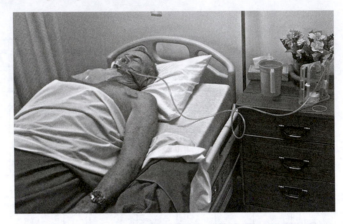

4. A client is admitted to the emergency department for treatment after stepping on a rusty nail at a job site. The primary health-care provider prescribes tetanus immune globulin 250 units IM STAT. Which illustration indicates the angle at which this injection should be administered by the nurse?

1. A
2. B
3. C
4. D

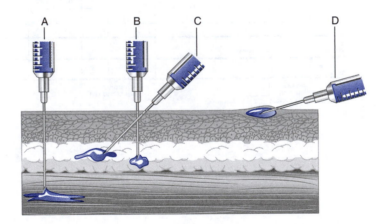

5. A client is admitted to an extended care facility after initially recovering from a brain attack resulting in right-sided hemiplegia. The nurse begins passive range-of-motion exercises on the client's right upper and lower extremities. Which movement is indicated in the illustration?
1. Inversion
2. Adduction
3. Supination
4. Opposition

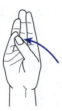

6. Which illustration indicates the type of thermometer that the nurse should use to obtain a temperature of an alert and active 2-year-old child?
1. A
2. B
3. C
4. D

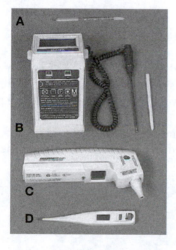

7. Review the illustration, and identify which site the nurse is landmarking for the administration of an intramuscular injection.
1. Dorsogluteal
2. Ventrogluteal
3. Rectus femoris
4. Vastus lateralis

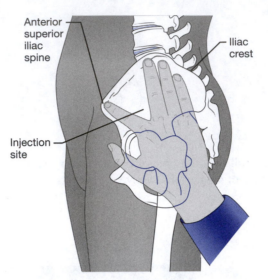

8. What instructions should the nurse give a client who is using the device in the illustration?
1. Breathe out slowly and completely, seal your mouth around the mouthpiece, press down on the canister, slowly inhale, and hold your breath for ten seconds.
2. Hold the device, seal your mouth around the mouthpiece, and breathe in and out slowly and deeply.
3. Seal your mouth around the mouthpiece and breathe in and out normally.
4. Take a deep breath and forcefully exhale through the mouthpiece.

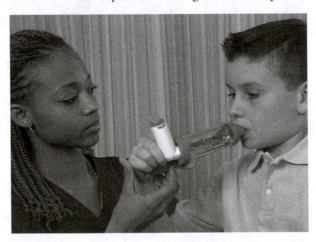

Drag and Drop/Ordered Response Items

A drag and drop/ordered response item presents a situation followed by a list of statements. The test taker is asked to place the statements in order of priority.

1. At the beginning of a 7 a.m. to 7 p.m. shift, a nurse receives a report, which is completed by 7:20 a.m. Place in order of priority the tasks that should be performed by the nurse.
   1. Give a prn pain medication to a client in pain.
   2. Change a client's dressing that must be done two times a day.
   3. Obtain the vital signs of a client reporting shortness of breath.
   4. Administer the prescribed 8 a.m. medications to the clients on the unit.

   Answer: _____

2. When assessing a client's abdomen, nurses should follow a logical sequence. Place these assessments in the order in which they should be performed.
   1. Percuss the suprapubic area to determine bladder distention.
   2. Auscultate the four quadrants of the abdomen for bowel sounds.
   3. Observe the abdomen for contour and visible signs of peristalsis.
   4. Palpate the abdomen to determine the presence of tenderness and fluid.

   Answer: _____

3. A nurse always must be prepared for, and ready to respond to, a fire that may occur on a hospital unit. Place the following activities in the order in which they should be implemented.
   1. Know the location and use of alarms and extinguishers.
   2. Rescue clients in danger when a fire is identified.
   3. Pull the fire alarm to notify others about the fire.
   4. Close doors and windows on the unit.
   5. Be alert for the signs of a fire.

   Answer: _____

4. A nurse plans to reposition an unconscious client from the supine position to the right side-lying position. Initially, the nurse explains the care to the client, closes the door for privacy, and performs hand hygiene before touching the client. Place the following nursing actions in the order in which they should be performed.
   1. Move the right shoulder and arm forward and downward.
   2. Place the client's arms across the chest and the left foot over the right foot.
   3. Place pillows behind the client's back and under the head, left arm, and left leg.
   4. Roll the client toward the right side, using one hand behind the client's shoulder and the other behind the client's hip.

   Answer: _____

5. A primary health-care provider prescribes a soapsuds enema for an adult client. The nurse explains the procedure to the client and arranges for the bathroom to be available. The nurse then performs hand washing, collects the equipment, and begins to prepare the enema equipment. Arrange the following interventions in the order in which they should be performed.
   1. Add soap to the container, and gently rock the enema bag to disperse the soap.
   2. Lubricate the catheter tip with water-soluble jelly.
   3. Fill the container with 1,000 mL of 110°F water.
   4. Flush the tubing with water.
   5. Clamp the tubing.

   Answer: _____

6. A client who had a total abdominal hysterectomy 2 days ago is ambulating and reports shortness of breath and stabbing chest pain on inspiration. A nursing assessment reveals a pulse of 110 beats per minute and respirations of 35 breaths per minute. Place the nursing interventions in priority order.
   1. Administer oxygen.
   2. Assess breath sounds.
   3. Notify the rapid response team.
   4. Return the client to bed by wheelchair.
   5. Place the client in the high-Fowler position.

   Answer: _____

7. A nurse receives the following information about clients at the change-of-shift report. The nurse plans to assess the following clients in priority order depending on the importance of their needs. List the clients in order based on which client should be assessed first, progressing to the client who should be assessed last.
   1. A client who reported feeling nauseated
   2. A client who just was informed of having cancer
   3. A client who is receiving a titrated medication via an infusion pump
   4. A client whose vital signs include an irregular pulse and labored respirations
   5. A client who received an analgesic by mouth for pain immediately before report

   Answer: _____

8. An older adult experienced a number of events during the last year while living in an assisted-living residence. Place the following events in order progressing from the first-level need to the last-level need according to Maslow's Hierarchy of Needs theory.
   1. Learning how to use a computer
   2. Falling while walking in a hallway
   3. Having an episode of shortness of breath
   4. Being the honoree at a family birthday party
   5. Winning an art contest at the assisted-living residence

   Answer: _____

Exhibit Items

An exhibit item asks a question that requires the test taker to analyze and interpret data, which are organized into sections such as a client's clinical record, physical assessment results, and results of client/family member interviews. The test taker must review all of this information to arrive at a conclusion to answer the question.

1. An older adult with multiple health problems is admitted to the hospital after a fainting episode. An electrocardiogram reveals a dysrhythmia, and the client is scheduled for a cardiac catheterization. Twelve hours after admission, a nurse reads the collected information about the client and performs a physical assessment. Which response does the nurse conclude that the client is exhibiting?
   1. Systemic infection
   2. Anaphylactic shock
   3. Excess fluid volume
   4. Orthostatic hypotension

CLIENT'S CLINICAL RECORD

Health History
Health problems: atherosclerosis, heart failure
Daily medications: digoxin, furosemide

Vital Signs on Admission
Temperature: 100.2°F, oral
Pulse: 94 beats per minute, irregular
Respirations: 24 breaths per minute
Blood pressure: 150/92 mm Hg

Physical Assessment
Subjective
   Headache
   Extreme fatigue
   Short of breath
Objective
   1+ pitting edema of ankles
   Crackles in base of lungs
   Vital signs
      Pulse: 100 beats per minute
      Respirations: 26 breaths per minute
      Blood pressure: 170/96 mm Hg

2. A 75-year-old man who had been having transient ischemic attacks (TIAs) is admitted to the hospital after experiencing a brain attack (stroke, cerebrovascular accident). The client is semicomatose and has right hemiplegia. The nurse reviews the client's clinical record. Which complication is this client at the **highest** risk of developing?
   1. Diarrhea
   2. Hemorrhage
   3. Pressure ulcers
   4. Excessive serum glucose

CLIENT'S CLINICAL RECORD

Physical Assessment
Right hemiplegia
Muscle flaccidity
Urinary and fecal incontinence
Responsive only to painful stimuli

Health History
Atherosclerosis
Iron-deficiency anemia

Laboratory Tests
RBC: 3.5 million cells/mcL
WBC: 9,000 cells/mcL
Hb: 10.0 g/dL
Ferritin: 14 ng/mL
Fasting blood glucose: 85 mg/dL

3. A nurse is monitoring a client who had major abdominal surgery. At 11 a.m., the client reports difficulty breathing. The nurse reviews the client's previous vital signs, performs a focused physical assessment, and obtains current vital signs. Which complication should the nurse conclude that the client may be experiencing?
   1. Pulmonary embolus
   2. Respiratory infection
   3. Subcutaneous emphysema
   4. Postoperative hemorrhage

CLIENT'S CLINICAL RECORD

Vital Signs Record
10:30 a.m.: P—72 beats per minute, R—16 breaths per minute, BP—120/72 mm Hg
10:45 a.m.: P—70 beats per minute, R—20 breaths per minute, BP—118/74 mm Hg

Physical Assessment
Diaphoresis
Blood-tinged sputum
Right-sided chest pain
Dyspnea, decreased breath sounds on right side
Abdomen flat and nontender, abdominal dressing dry and intact

Current Vital Signs—11 a.m.
Temperature: 100.2°F, temporal
Pulse: 92 beats per minute, regular
Respirations: 28 breaths per minute, shallow, labored
Blood pressure: 160/92 mm Hg

4. A nurse is caring for a client who had abdominal surgery at 8 a.m., 12 hours ago. An abdominal dressing, two Jackson-Pratt drains, an IV of 1,000 mL of 0.95% NaCl with 20 mEq of KCl at 125 mL/hr, a PCA pump with an analgesic, and a urinary catheter are present. The nurse reviews the client's clinical record and performs a physical assessment. Which response does the nurse conclude that the client is experiencing?
   1. Pain
   2. Hemorrhage
   3. Urinary retention
   4. Excess fluid volume

CLIENT'S CLINICAL RECORD

Vital Signs
4 p.m.: P—76 beats per minute, R—18 breaths per minute, BP—116/72 mm Hg
6 p.m.: P—80 beats minute, R—20 breaths per minute, BP—120/76 mm Hg

I&O: 8 a.m. to 8 p.m.
Intake: IVF—1,500 mL
Output: urine—1,050 mL; wound drainage systems—210 mL

Physical Assessment at 8 p.m.:
Dressing dry and intact
Pain of 8 on a scale of 0 to 10
IVF intact and infusing at 125 mL/hr
Retention catheter draining clear amber urine, no suprapubic distention
Vital signs: P - 86 beats per minute, R - 24 breaths per minute, BP - 136/80 mm Hg

5. An older adult who is dehydrated is to receive rehydration therapy. The nurse collects a health history, obtains the vital signs, and performs a physical assessment. Which complication is this client at the **highest** risk for developing?
   1. Infection
   2. Aspiration
   3. Malnutrition
   4. Constipation

CLIENT'S CLINICAL RECORD

Health History
Brain attack 6 months ago
Flu and pneumonia vaccines in past 4 months

Vital Signs
Temperature: 99.6°F, oral
Pulse: 88 beats per minute, regular rhythm
Respirations: 22 breaths per minute, shallow
Blood pressure: 109/68 mm Hg

Physical Assessment
Lethargic
Dysphagia
Dysarthria
Diminished gag reflex
Skin dry, exhibiting "tenting"
Borborygmi auscultated in all four quadrants

6. An older adult is admitted to the hospital after several days of nausea, vomiting, and diarrhea. The nurse performs an assessment and reviews the client's clinical record. Which does the nurse conclude that the client is experiencing based on the data collected?
   1. Hypokalemia
   2. Hypocalcemia
   3. Hypernatremia
   4. Hypermagnesemia

CLIENT'S CLINICAL RECORD

Physical Assessment
Client reports muscle weakness and leg cramps
Decreased bowel sounds
Weak irregular pulses
Weight loss of 5 pounds over the past few days

Laboratory Tests
Serum potassium: 3.1 mEq/L
Serum sodium: 138 mEq/L
Serum magnesium: 2.2 mEq/L
Serum calcium: 9 mg/dL

Medications
Furosemide 40 mg, PO, once daily
Simvastatin 20 mg, PO, at hour of sleep

7. A client returns to the surgical unit from the postanesthesia care unit after surgical resection of the colon and removal of numerous regional lymph nodes. Two hours later, after a change-of-shift report, the oncoming nurse reviews the client's vital signs record, performs a physical assessment, and interviews the client. Which client complication does the nurse identify after considering all the information?

1. Pain
2. Atelectasis
3. Hemorrhage
4. Constipation

CLIENT'S CLINICAL RECORD

Vital Signs
3 p.m.: P—86 beats per minute, R—20 breaths per minute, BP—116/70 mm Hg
4 p.m.: P—102 beats per minute, R—26 breaths per minute, BP—100/60 mm Hg

Physical Assessment—5 p.m.
Vital signs: P—126 beats per minute, R—28 breaths per minute, BP—86/60 mm Hg
Urinary retention catheter draining clear amber urine, 50 mL in collection bag
Intravenous solution infusing at 125 mL/hr
Absence of bowel sounds, no bowel movement
Two portable wound drainage devices in abdomen: #1 = 250 mL of sanguineous
    drainage; #2 = 300 mL of sanguineous drainage
Abdominal dressing dry and intact
Vesicular, bronchovesicular, and bronchial breath sounds heard on auscultation of lungs
Appears restless (e.g., moving around in bed, clenching and unclenching fists)

Client Interview
Reports pain as 4 on a 0 to 10 numerical pain scale
Reports feeling anxious

8. A client who sustained trauma to the right lower extremity in an automobile collision is placed in traction and scheduled for surgery in the morning. The nurse on the orthopedic unit obtains the client's vital signs, interviews the client, and reviews the client's laboratory results. Which data should cause the nurse the **most** concern?

1. Sadness over death of his wife
2. Avoidance of prostate surgery
3. Pulse and respiratory rates
4. Smoking history

CLIENT'S CLINICAL RECORD

Vital Signs
Temperature: 97.8°F, temporal
Pulse: 96 beats per minute, regular rhythm
Respirations: 24 breaths per minute
Blood pressure: 150/88 mm Hg

Client Interview
The client is a 70-year-old retired man whose wife of 42 years died 4 months ago. He stated, "I miss her terribly, and I'm so sad." He has three married sons and eight grandchildren. He looks forward to playing with his grandchildren every day. He stated, "I am relatively healthy, but I smoke two packs of cigarettes a day, am 40 pounds overweight, and drink a glass of wine every night." He has urinary hesitancy and a slow stream from an enlarged prostate but refused surgery. When asked about his current situation, he stated, "I am not happy about having surgery for my leg, but I really don't have a choice."

Laboratory Results
Hb: 16 g/dL
Hct: 45%
WBC: 8,000 cells/mcL

ALTERNATE ITEM FORMATS: ANSWERS AND RATIONALES

Multiple-Response Items

1. 1. Pain is caused by irritation of nerve tissue by chemical substances and the pressure of fluid congestion in the area of local trauma.
   2. Heat is caused by an increased blood flow in response to release of histamine at the site of local trauma.
   3. Erythema is caused by an increased blood flow in response to release of histamine and an increased capillary permeability in response to kinins at the site of local trauma or infection.
   4. An increased heart rate is unrelated to the local adaptation syndrome (LAS). An increased heart rate is associated with activation of the sympathetic nervous system related to the general adaptation syndrome (GAS).
   5. A decreased blood pressure is unrelated to the LAS. An increased, not a decreased, blood pressure is associated with activation of the sympathetic nervous system related to the GAS.
   6. An elevated blood glucose level is unrelated to the LAS. An elevated blood glucose level occurs in response to secretion of glucocorticoids in the GAS.

2. 1. Ambulation will not prevent blood loss that results in hypovolemia. Providing adequate hydration and assessing for early signs of hemorrhage help prevent hypovolemia.
   2. **Ambulation promotes intestinal peristalsis that may result in a bowel movement.**
   3. **Ambulation promotes deep breathing that helps alveoli to expand, preventing the collapse of alveoli (atelectasis).**
   4. Ambulation will not help prevent dehiscence. Supporting the incisional site during coughing, deep breathing, and activity helps prevent dehiscence.
   5. Ambulation will not help prevent infection. The use of sterile technique and hand washing help prevent infection.

3. 1. Apple juice contains approximately 7 mg of sodium per cup and is permitted on a 2-g sodium diet.
   2. **A quarter cup of crumbled feta cheese contains approximately 418 mg of sodium and should be avoided on a 2-g sodium diet.**
   3. **Corned beef contains approximately 800 mg of sodium per 3 ounces and**

should not be included on a 2-g sodium diet.
   4. **Most canned soups contain between 800 and 1,000 mg of sodium per cup and are contraindicated on a 2-g sodium diet. Even soups stipulated as low sodium or heart healthy may contain significant amounts of sodium.**
   5. One broccoli spear contains approximately 20 mg of sodium and is permitted on a 2-g sodium diet.

4. 1. It is not necessary to know the drip rate per minute when determining whether an IV is "on time."
   2. **The time that the IV bag was hung is essential for the nurse to know when determining whether an IV is "on time." The nurse must identify how many minutes/hours the IV has been running and then multiply this number by the milliliters of solution prescribed by the primary health-care provider per minute/hour. This volume is then deducted from the original volume in the IV bag. The actual volume in the bag should be compared with the volume that should be in the bag. If the volumes match, the IV is "on time"; if there is more fluid than should be in the bag, then the IV is "behind schedule"; and if there is less fluid than should be in the bag, then the IV is "ahead of schedule."**
   3. The solution indicated on the IV bag is necessary to know to ensure that it is identical to the solution prescribed by the primary health-care provider, not to determine whether an IV is "on time."
   4. **The volume of solution in the IV bag is essential for the nurse to know to determine whether an IV is "on time." The nurse must identify how many minutes/ hours the IV has been running and then multiply this number by the milliliters of solution prescribed by the primary health-care provider per minute/hour. This volume is then deducted from the original volume in the IV bag. The actual volume that is in the bag should be compared with the volume that should be in the bag. If the volumes match, the IV is "on time"; if there is more fluid than should be in the bag, then the IV is "behind schedule"; and if there is less fluid than should be in the bag, then the IV is "ahead of schedule."**

5. The number of milliliters per hour prescribed by the primary health-care provider is essential for the nurse to know to determine whether an IV is "on time." The nurse must identify how many minutes/hours the IV has been running and then multiply this number by the milliliters of solution prescribed by the primary health-care provider per minute/hour. This volume is then deducted from the original volume in the IV bag. The actual volume that is in the bag should be compared with the volume that should be in the bag. If the volumes match, the IV is "on time"; if there is more fluid than should be in the bag, then the IV is "behind schedule"; and if there is less fluid than should be in the bag, then the IV is "ahead of schedule."

5. 1. Tachypnea occurs in response to sympathetic nervous system stimulation as the body attempts to deliver more oxygen to body tissues. Tachypnea is more than 20 breaths per minute.
   2. Tachycardia occurs in response to sympathetic nervous system stimulation as the body attempts to deliver more oxygen to body tissues. Tachycardia is a heart rate of more than 100 beats per minute.
   3. The skin becomes pale and cold in response to hemorrhage as peripheral vasoconstriction occurs in an attempt to shunt blood to vital organs of the body.
   4. A weak, thready pulse is related to hypovolemia. The circulating blood volume decreases with hemorrhage.
   5. Delayed capillary refill occurs in response to peripheral vasoconstriction in an attempt to shunt blood to vital organs.

6. 1. Gravity is the force that pulls mass toward the center of the earth. Urine flows by gravity out of the bladder through a tube (indwelling catheter, Foley catheter) into a collection bag placed below the level of the bladder.
   2. A Penrose drain is a flexible, collapsible tube with a potential diameter of approximately 1 inch that drains fluid from inside a surgical site to a dressing via gravity.
   3. Enema fluid flows from a container through a rectal tube into the large intestine via gravity. The force of the flow is regulated by raising or lowering the height of the enema bag in relation to the anus. Raising the bag increases the force; lowering the bag decreases the force.
   4. A nasogastric tube removes fluid from the stomach via negative pressure, not gravity.
   5. A portable wound drainage system is a closed system that uses negative pressure, not gravity, to drain secretions from an incisional site.

7. 1. Helping a client who is constipated walk to the bathroom is within the scope of practice of a nursing assistant. Clients who have a stable respiratory and circulatory status can be ambulated by a nursing assistant.
   2. Pushing a client in a wheelchair is within the scope of practice of a nursing assistant. Nursing assistants are taught how to perform this skill safely.
   3. Applying an antifungal cream includes assessment of the area and correct application requiring the knowledge and skill of a nurse. Antifungal cream is a topical medication that requires a primary health-care provider's prescription, and applying it is a dependent function of the nurse.
   4. Weighing a client using a bed scale is within the scope of practice of nursing assistants. Nursing assistants can collect vital statistics such as a client's weight, temperature, pulse, respiration, and intake and output. However, it is the responsibility of the nurse to interpret the results.
   5. Emptying a urine collection bag is within the scope of practice of nursing assistants. Nursing assistants have been taught to implement medical aseptic principles and standard precautions. Once the nursing assistant documents the output on the intake and output (I&O) flow sheet, it is the responsibility of the nurse to interpret the results.

8. 1. Hand washing is based on principles of medical, not surgical, asepsis.
   2. Keeping a sterile field dry requires actions based on the principles of surgical asepsis. Moisture contaminates a sterile field by facilitating the movement of microorganisms from the unsterile surface below the field to the sterile field by capillary action.
   3. Holding sterile objects below the waist is considered contaminated because they may

be out of the visual field of the nurse. Holding sterile objects above the waist is based on the principle of surgical asepsis that states that all sterile objects must be within the visual field of the caregiver.

4. Wearing personal protective equipment protects the caregiver and is a principle of medical, not surgical, asepsis.

5. A 1-inch, not a ½-inch, border of a sterile field is considered contaminated. This is based on a principle of surgical, not medical, asepsis.

9. 1. **The presence of gurgles and a cough indicates respiratory impairment. Difficult or uncomfortable breathing (dyspnea) is a clinical manifestation associated with impaired respiratory function.**

2. **The presence of gurgles and a cough indicates respiratory tract impairment. These clinical manifestations, along with purulent sputum, may indicate the presence of a respiratory tract infection. A respiratory tract infection can be confirmed with a chest radiograph and a sputum culture.**

3. The presence of gurgles and a cough indicates impaired respiratory function. The blood pressure does not decrease with impaired respiratory function. However, it may increase with respiratory distress because of the influence of the sympathetic nervous system. A decreased blood pressure is associated with a decreased circulating blood volume, which is often caused by dehydration or hemorrhage.

4. **A pulse oximeter is a device that measures a client's arterial blood oxygen saturation (SaO_2) via a sensor attached to the client (e.g., via finger or earlobe). A value that is less than 95% indicates respiratory impairment.**

5. Bronchovesicular breath sounds are expected sounds associated with an uncompromised respiratory function.

10. 1. Checking tube patency does not contribute to comfort. Checking tube patency ensures that the client is receiving the prescribed volume of formula.

2. **Administering oral hygiene every 2 hours helps prevent drying of the oral mucosa, may relieve thirst, and supports oral comfort.**

3. **Applying lubricant after cleaning the nares helps prevent drying of the**

respiratory mucosa of the nares, which supports comfort.

4. **Ensuring that the tube is secured to the nose helps reduce friction and trauma to the nares by the tube, which supports comfort.**

5. Flushing the tubing helps maintain tube patency; it does not contribute to comfort. In addition, flushing the tubing is based on the primary health-care provider's prescription or a hospital policy.

11. 1. A hard-cooked egg contains approximately 63 mg of potassium.

2. **A baked potato is an excellent source of potassium. A baked potato, depending on its size, contains approximately 844 to 955 mg of potassium.**

3. A half cup of green beans provides less than 100 mg of potassium.

4. Bran flakes do not contain potassium.

5. Depending on the type of meat, 3 ounces of meat contains only 57 to 323 mg of potassium, and this is not the best choice of the options offered.

12. 1. **Sealing the lips around the mouthpiece prevents medication from escaping from around the mouth and mouthpiece and allows delivery of an accurate dose.**

2. The client should exhale through the mouth. Back pressure occurs when exhaling through the nose because the nostrils are smaller than the mouth. When a client is using an inhaler, it is important to empty the lungs of as much air as possible to make a larger surface area available to come into contact with the subsequent inhaled medication.

3. Breathing in deeply is a correct action because it delivers medication deep into the lungs. However, inhalation should be slow, not quick. Inhaling slowly allows for even contact of the medication with the lining of the respiratory tract.

4. **Medication in a metered-dose inhaler may cause irritation of the oral mucosa or a fungal infection of the oral cavity. A swish and spit procedure with water reduces the exposure of the oral mucosa to the medication and reduces the risk of irritation to or a fungal infection of the oral cavity.**

5. **Removing the cap, shaking it well, and spraying it into the air, repeating this three times before using it for the first time, primes the inhaler and ensures**

that the user is getting the correct dose. Also, this should be done when the inhaler has not been used for 14 or more days or when it has been dropped.

13. 1. Cheese, a dairy product, is an excellent dietary source of calcium. One ounce of cheese contains 150 to 406 mg of calcium, depending on the type of cheese. Calcium is essential to maintain bone structure in addition to several neuromuscular, cardiac, and coagulation functions.

   2. Lettuce is not high in calcium. One cup of shredded leaf lettuce contains approximately 38 mg of calcium.

   3. Peppers are not high in calcium. One pepper contains approximately 4 mg of calcium.

   4. Oranges are not high in calcium. One orange contains approximately 52 mg of calcium.

   5. Sardines are high in calcium because they contain soft, edible bones. Three ounces of sardines (about seven fish) contains approximately 320 mg of calcium.

14. 1. Wrinkles create ridges, causing unnecessary pressure that can lead to tissue injury.

   2. The toe window should be positioned over the toes or sole of the feet, depending on the manufacturer. This ensures that the stocking is aligned correctly and the distal portion of the foot can be accessed to perform the blanch test to assess peripheral circulation.

   3. The stockings should be applied before, not after, the client gets out of bed. Standing permits the development of dependent edema because of the force of gravity. Putting antiembolism stockings on while still in bed helps prevent dependent edema. If stockings are applied after getting out of bed, they will compress edematous tissues and cause tissue injury.

   4. Flexion of the knee impedes, while extension of the knee promotes, application of an antiembolism stocking. Most

antiembolism stockings are knee high rather than thigh high.

   5. Removing the stocking once a day for at least 30 minutes is inadequate. Antiembolism stockings should be removed every 8 hours for 30 minutes. This permits inspection and physical hygiene.

Hot-Spot Items

1.   This site is at risk because it is dependent when the client is lying in a right-lateral position; the majority of body mass overlies the greater trochanter. The area over the greater trochanter has limited subcutaneous tissue, and when exposed to pressure more than 32 mm Hg, the capillaries are compressed, and blood does not bring oxygen and nutrients to the tissues.

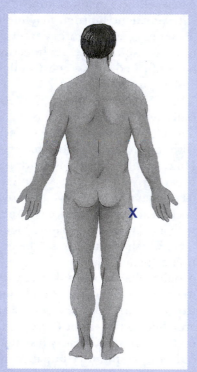

2.   An X anywhere along the highlighted area is the correct answer. This site is the ascending colon, which contains the most liquid stool because it is at the beginning of the large intestine. As stool moves through the large intestine,

fluid is reabsorbed, and stool becomes more dry and formed as it approaches the anus.

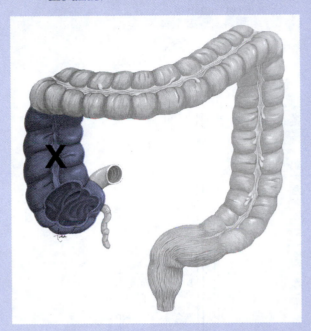

3. Auscultating over the left upper quadrant slightly to the left of the midsternal line will detect whooshing, gurgling, or bubbling sounds in the stomach as gastric content or air is instilled through the nasogastric tube.

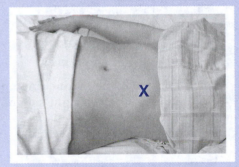

4. An X anywhere within the shaded area of the illustration is a correct answer. The abdomen, level with or below the level of the umbilicus, is the preferred site for a subcutaneous injection of 5,000 units of heparin. The nurse must avoid the area 2 inches around the umbilicus. The abdomen generally provides a layer of fat located below the dermis and above the muscle for heparin to be administered deep into the subcutaneous tissue. Also, it allows for faster absorption than subcutaneous sites on thighs and buttocks. A large area of subcutaneous tissue, which generally is found over the abdomen, is preferred because heparin may cause a hematoma and pain if accidentally administered intramuscularly.

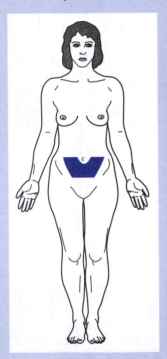

5. An X over either the right or left carotid artery is a correct answer. The nurse performing sternal contractions is next to the client's chest and abdomen. The nurse delivering breaths and monitoring the client is next to the client's head. The preferred site to assess the pulse is the carotid artery on the side in which the nurse delivering breaths is positioned because the nurse is next to the client's head.

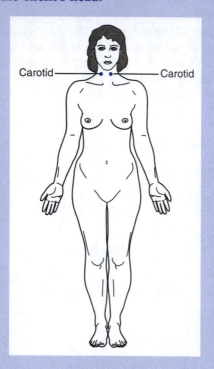

6. A temperature in the range of 100.4°F to 105.8°F is called pyrexia, or fever. An X placed anywhere within this range is a correct answer.

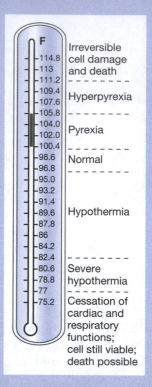

7. Solve for x using ratio and proportion.

$$\frac{\text{Desired}}{\text{Have}} \quad \frac{25 \text{ mg}}{12.5 \text{ mg}} = \frac{x \text{ mL}}{5 \text{ mL}}$$

$$12.5 \, x = 125$$
$$x = 125 \div 12.5$$
$$x = 10 \text{ mg}$$

The 10 mL line is the second line up from the bottom on the right side of the medicine cup.

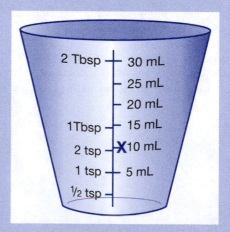

8. When a nurse wears a particulate filter mask (N95 respirator), the nurse is protected from exposure to the client's respiratory pathogen, *Mycobacterium tuberculosis*. The nurse's nose and mouth are portals of entry.

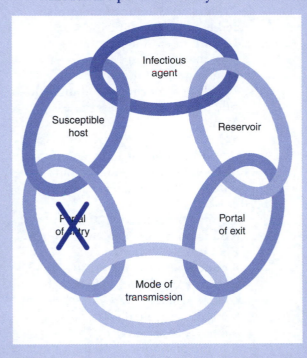

Fill-in-the-Blank Calculation Items

1. Answer: 120 mL/hr.
The nurse has to calculate how many milliliters to administer per minute to deliver 4 mg/min. Solve for x by using ratio and proportion after converting 2 g to its equivalent of 2,000 milligrams.

$$\frac{\text{Desired}}{\text{Have}} \quad \frac{4\ mg}{2,000\ mg} = \frac{x\ mL}{1,000\ mL}$$
$$2,000\ x = 4,000$$
$$x = 4,000 \div 2,000$$
$$x = 2\ mL\ (2\ mL$$
$$\text{contains 4 mg)}$$

The hourly volume to be infused is calculated by multiplying the milliliters per minute (2) by the number of minutes (60). Therefore, the infusion pump should be set at 120 mL per hour.

2. Answer: 2 mL.
Solve for x by using ratio and proportion.

$$\frac{\text{Desired}}{\text{Have}} \quad \frac{400,000\ units}{200,000\ units} = \frac{x\ mL}{1\ mL}$$
$$200,000\ x = 400,000$$
$$x = 400,000 \div 200,000$$
$$x = 2\ mL\ \text{of the}$$
$$\text{antibiotic solution}$$

3. Answer: 2 tablets.
Solve for x by using ratio and proportion.

$$\frac{\text{Desired}}{\text{Have}} \quad \frac{0.25\ mg}{0.125\ mg} = \frac{x\ tablets}{1\ tablet}$$
$$0.125\ x = 0.25$$
$$x = 0.25 \div 0.125$$
$$x = 2\ tablets$$

4. Answer: 10 mL.
Solve for x by using ratio and proportion.

$$\frac{\text{Desired}}{\text{Have}} \quad \frac{25\ mg}{12.5\ mg} = \frac{x\ mL}{1\ mL}$$
$$12.5\ x = 125$$
$$x = 125 \div 12.5$$
$$x = 10\ mL$$

5. Answer: 2.5 mL.
Use ratio and proportion to convert 110 pounds to kilograms.

$$\frac{\text{Desired}}{\text{Have}} \quad \frac{110\ pounds}{2.2\ pounds} = \frac{x\ kg}{1\ kg}$$
$$2.2\ x = 110$$
$$x = 110 \div 2.2$$
$$x = 50\ (50\ kg\ \text{is equal}$$
$$\text{to 110 pounds)}$$

Now calculate the number of units of medication required by using ratio and proportion.

$$\frac{\text{Desired}}{\text{Have}} \quad \frac{50\ kg}{1\ kg} = \frac{x\ units}{100\ units}$$
$$1\ x = 50 \times 100$$
$$x = 5,000\ units$$

Now calculate the amount of solution needed to administer the prescribed dose of 5,000 units by using ratio and proportion.

$$\frac{\text{Desired}}{\text{Have}} \quad \frac{5,000\ units}{2,000\ units} = \frac{x\ mL}{1\ mL}$$
$$2,000\ x = 5,000$$
$$x = 5,000 \div 2,000$$
$$x = 2.5\ mL$$

6.   **Answer: 7.5 mL.**
Solve the problem by using ratio and proportion.

$$\frac{\text{Desired}}{\text{Have}} \quad \frac{6 \text{ mg}}{4 \text{ mg}} = \frac{x \text{ mL}}{5 \text{ mL}}$$

$$4x = 30 \text{ mL}$$
$$x = 30 \div 4$$
$$x = 7.5 \text{ mL}$$

7.   **Answer: 4 tablets.**
Solve the problem by using ratio and proportion.

$$\frac{\text{Desired}}{\text{Have}} \quad \frac{5 \text{ mg}}{1.25 \text{ mg}} = \frac{x \text{ tablets}}{1 \text{ tablet}}$$

$$1.25x = 5$$
$$x = 5 \div 1.25$$
$$x = 4 \text{ tablets}$$

8.   **Answer: 1.5 tablets.**
Solve the problem by using ratio and proportion. Five is an odd-numbered day.

$$\frac{\text{Desired}}{\text{Have}} \quad \frac{15 \text{ mg}}{10 \text{ mg}} = \frac{x \text{ tablets}}{1 \text{ tablet}}$$

$$10x = 15$$
$$x = 15 \div 10$$
$$x = 1.5 \text{ tablets}$$

9.   **Answer: 31 drops/min.**
Solve the problem by using the following formula.

$$\frac{\text{Total volume to be infused} \times \text{Drop factor}}{\text{Total time in minutes}}$$

$$\frac{125 \text{ (volume to be infused)} \times 15 \text{ (drop factor)}}{1 \text{ hour} \times 60 \text{ minutes}}$$

$$\frac{1,875}{60} = 31.25 \text{ drops/min}$$

Because 0.25 is less than half a drop, round the answer down to 31 drops/min.

10.   **Answer: 5 units of regular insulin.**
According to the prescription, the nurse should give 5 units of regular insulin when the blood glucose level is between 201 and 250 mg/dL.

11.   **Answer: 1,310 mL.**
Compute the amount of IV solution received.
The client's IV fluid was prescribed at 75 mL/hr. Over an 8-hour period, the client should have received 600 mL of sodium chloride. Every 20 minutes, 25 mL of the solution of the primary infusion should have infused. However, the primary infusion was interrupted for 40 minutes while the intermittent antibiotic infusions were administered.

Therefore, for 40 minutes the client received 100 mL of antibiotic solution rather than 50 mL of the primary solution of sodium chloride.
Add the amount of IV solution the client received.
    7 hours at 75/hour of the primary sodium chloride infusion = 525 mL.
    100 mL of antibiotic solution (two doses of 50 mL each) over 40 minutes = 100 mL.
    25 mL of the primary sodium chloride infusion over 20 minutes = 25 mL.
    525 + 100 + 25 = 650 mL of IV solution (total amount of IV solution).
Now compute the client's amount of oral intake. One ounce is equal to 30 mL.
    4 ounces of coffee = 120 mL.
    6 ounces of orange juice = 180 mL.
    Beef broth = 240 mL.
    8 ounces of ice chips = 120 mL. Ice chips are calculated as half their volume when melted. Therefore, 8 ounces of ice chips is equal to 4 ounces of water.
Add the amount of oral fluid the client received.
    120 + 180 + 240 + 120 = 660 mL.
To determine the total fluid intake for the client over 8 hours, add the total IV intake (650 mL) and the total oral fluid intake (660 mL):
    650 mL + 660 mL = 1,310 mL.

12.   **Answer: 2 tablespoons.**
There are 15 mL of solution in 1 tablespoon; this is a memorized equivalent. Therefore, 2 tablespoons contain 30 mL of solution. Also, you can solve this problem by using ratio and proportion.

$$\frac{\text{Desired}}{\text{Have}} \quad \frac{30 \text{ mL}}{15 \text{ mL}} = \frac{x \text{ tablespoons}}{1 \text{ tablespoon}}$$

$$15x = 30$$
$$x = 30 \div 15$$
$$x = 2 \text{ tablespoons}$$

13.   **Answer: 83 calories.**
There are 4 calories per gram of carbohydrate; therefore, $10 \times 4 = 40$ calories of carbohydrate.
There are 4 calories per gram of protein; therefore, $4 \times 4 = 16$ calories of protein. There are 9 calories per gram of fat; therefore, $3 \times 9 = 27$ calories.
Total the number of calories:
$40 + 16 + 27 = 83$ calories.

14.   Answer: 36.4 mg.
       First, determine how many kilograms
       are equal to 160 pounds by using a
       formula for ratio and proportion.

$$\frac{\text{Desired}}{\text{Have}} \quad \frac{160 \text{ pounds}}{2.2 \text{ pounds}} = \frac{\text{x kilograms}}{1 \text{ kilogram}}$$

$$2.2 \text{ x} = 160$$
$$\text{x} = 160 \div 2.2$$
$$\text{x} = 72.72 \text{ kilograms is}$$
$$\text{equal to 160 pounds.}$$

Next, multiply 72.72 kilograms by
the prescribed dose of 0.5 mg to
determine the total dose to be administered. 72.72 × 0.5 = 36.36 mg. Round
the dose up to 36.4 because the
6 following the 3 is more than 5.
Therefore, the dose is 36.4 mg.

Graphic Items (Items Using a Graphic, Chart, Table, or Illustration)

1. 1. A temperature of 97.8°F occurred on the
      sixth day of hospitalization (June 10) at
      4 a.m.
   2. A temperature of 99.2°F occurred on the
      fourth day of hospitalization (June 8) at
      4 p.m.

3. Find the box in the top left that indicates "Day of Month." Read toward the
   right across the row until you see the
   box with the 7 (indicating the seventh
   day of the month, also called the third
   day in hospital, as indicated in the box
   below it). Look two rows down below
   the box with the 7 until you see the box
   with p.m. Now look below the p.m. box
   for the box with the 4. Guide your eye
   down the column until you find a dot on
   a line. From the dot on the line, guide
   your eye left across the row until you
   reach the numbers running along the
   left end of the graph. The nearest dark
   line below the row with the dot that indicates a full degree of temperature
   is 101. The dot in the 4 p.m. column
   is one light-colored line above the
   101 line, indicating two-tenths of a
   degree of temperature. Therefore,
   the dot in the 4 p.m. column indicates a
   temperature of 101.2°F.
4. A temperature of 102.6°F occurred on the
   second day of hospitalization (June 6) at
   4 p.m.

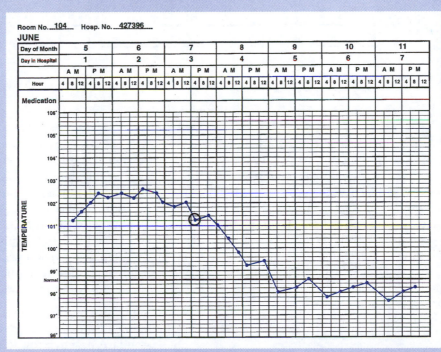

2. 1. 355 mL is an incorrect calculation.
2. 720 mL is an incorrect calculation.
3. 1,300 mL is an incorrect calculation.
4. **The total output between the hours of 7 a.m. and 3 p.m. is 1,405 mL. The nurse must first calculate the urine, emesis, and Hemovac totals and insert** the amounts in the "7 to 3 Total" row under the appropriate column. Then the nurse must add the totals of the three columns (1,050 + 250 + 105 = 1,405) to arrive at the overall total output for the hours between 7 a.m. and 3 p.m.

DAILY INTAKE AND OUTPUT RECORD

DATE   JUNE 5

Time	Bottle	Amount	Solution	Medication and Dosage	* ABS.	∓ LIB	ORAL	URINE	EMESIS	N.G. TUBE	HEMOVAC
8	1	1000	NS	20 mEq KCl				650			
8:30							360				
10:00							120				
11:30							240	150			
12:00									160		
1:40									90		60
2:15					↓			250			
3:00							525	475			45
7-3 TOTAL		8-HR TOTAL					525	475	720	1050	250	105
3-11 TOTAL		8-HR TOTAL									
11-7 TOTAL		8-HR TOTAL									
24 HOUR TOTAL											

INTAKE GRAND TOTAL [ ]   OUTPUT GRAND TOTAL [ ]

* ABS. = amount absorbed   ∓ LIB = Left in bag

3. 1. **Moving the straps of the mask to above the ears should be done to ensure that the mask is correctly positioned over the client's nose and mouth.**
2. Two pillows under the head will flex the neck, causing stress and strain on the anatomical structures of the neck, which should be avoided. One pillow is sufficient to ensure functional alignment of the head and neck in relation to the torso.
3. **Monitoring a client's oxygen saturation level is an objective assessment of a client's respiratory status. This is an important assessment to make at the beginning of a shift and routinely throughout the shift of a client with an oxygenation problem.**
4. **A client who has a medical condition impairing respiratory function and requiring oxygen therapy should be positioned in the mid-Fowler or high-Fowler position. These Fowler positions cause abdominal structures to move down and away from the diaphragm via gravity, facilitating respiratory exertion.**
5. **A gown should be applied to provide for client comfort and privacy.**

4. 1. **This illustration indicates a medication being administered into a muscle. The standard practice for an intramuscular injection is to use a 1.5-inch needle that is administered at 90 degrees into muscle tissue.**
2. This illustration indicates a medication being administered with a ⅝-inch needle

inserted at 90 degrees into subcutaneous tissue. A ½-inch needle inserted at 90 degrees into subcutaneous tissue is also an acceptable technique. Both are considered standard practice.

3. This illustration indicates a medication being administered with a ⅝-inch needle inserted at 45 degrees into the subcutaneous tissue and is considered standard practice.

4. This illustration indicates an intradermal injection whereby solution is injected just beneath the skin surface.

5. 1. Inversion is when the foot is turned inward medially.

2. Adduction is when a body part (e.g., leg, arm) is moved toward the midline.

3. Supination is when the forearm and hand are turned facing upward.

4. **Opposition is when the thumb is moved so that it touches the tip of each finger.**

6. 1. A plastic thermometer that requires insertion into the mouth or rectum is inappropriate for a 2-year-old child. A 2-year-old child does not have the cognitive ability to follow instructions or the behavioral ability to remain still during the 3 minutes required to obtain an accurate temperature.

2. An electronic thermometer that requires the insertion of a probe into the mouth for the temperature to register is inappropriate for a 2-year-old child. A 2-year-old child does not have the cognitive ability to follow instructions or the behavioral ability to remain still during the 15 to 30 seconds required to obtain an accurate temperature.

3. **An electronic infrared tympanic membrane thermometer is most appropriate from among the options presented for a 2-year-old child because it takes only 2 to 5 seconds to register a temperature. Its ease of use and rapid measurement make it an effective choice for taking the temperature of an alert and active 2-year-old child.**

4. A plastic digital thermometer requires the insertion of a probe into the mouth or rectum for 10 or more seconds for an accurate result and is inappropriate for a 2-year-old child. A 2-year-old child does not have the cognitive ability to follow instructions or the behavioral ability to remain still during the 10 or more seconds required to obtain an accurate temperature.

7. 1. This is not an illustration landmarking the dorsogluteal site. To landmark the

dorsogluteal site, the nurse palpates the posterior superior iliac spine and then draws a line to the greater trochanter. The dorsogluteal site is superior to halfway along this line.

2. **This is an illustration landmarking the ventrogluteal site. Place the heel of the hand on the greater trochanter with the fingers toward the client's head. Use the right hand for the client's left hip and the left hand for client's right hip. Place the index finger on the client's anterior superior iliac spine, and stretch the middle finger dorsally (toward the buttocks), palpating the iliac crest and then pressing below it. The triangle formed by the third finger, the index finger, and the edge of the crest of the ilium is the ventrogluteal site.**

3. This is not an illustration of the rectus femoris site. The rectus femoris is on the anterior aspect of the thigh.

4. This is not an illustration landmarking the vastus lateralis site. To landmark the vastus lateralis, the nurse identifies the middle third of the vastus lateralis muscle that is on the anterior lateral aspect of the thigh. It is within a rectangular area between a handbreadth above the knee and a handbreadth below the greater trochanter of the femur.

8. 1. **These are the instructions for using a metered-dose inhaler, which is the device in the photograph. A prefilled, pressurized canister delivers a measured dose of medication, which is inhaled by the client. Breathing out completely expels air from the lungs that, if retained, will interfere with the volume that can be inspired during the procedure. Sealing the mouth around the mouthpiece ensures that the dose is completely inhaled rather than lost to the atmosphere around the mouthpiece. The client must coordinate pushing the canister while inhaling the medication. The breath should be held for 10 seconds to maximize contact of the medication with the respiratory mucosa. This photograph exhibits a metered-dose inhaler with an extender (spacer). Instead of delivering a dose via a mouthpiece directly into the client's mouth, a dose is pumped into the extender's chamber, where it is then inhaled by the client. An extender can increase the volume of medication that moves deep into the lungs.**

2. These are the instructions for using a nebulizer. A nebulizer is a medication delivery system that produces an aerosol spray that is inhaled via a mouthpiece. Breathing deeply and slowly facilitates contact of the medication with the respiratory tract mucosa.

3. These are instructions for assessing tidal volume. Tidal volume is the volume of air inhaled and exhaled with each normal breath, which is approximately 500 mL.

4. These are the instructions for using a peak expiratory flowmeter (PEFM), which measures the peak expiratory flow rate (PEFR). A PEFR is the volume of air that can be forcefully exhaled after a deep inspiration.

Drag and Drop/Ordered Response Items

1. 3. The basics of assessment should follow the ABCs (airway, breathing, and circulation). Shortness of breath reflects a potential respiratory or cardiac problem, and a further assessment is the priority.

1. Relieving pain is a basic physiological and safety/security need. Relief from pain is not as high a priority as maintaining a client's respiratory status but is more important than routine tasks.

4. Administering medications is a dependent function of the nurse. It is accepted practice that medications prescribed for 8 a.m. can be dispensed up to 1 hour before or 1 hour after the prescribed time.

2. A task prescribed twice a day gives the nurse a range in the time frame in which it must be performed. Among the tasks presented, this task can be performed last because the others have greater priority.

2. 3. Inspection uses purposeful observation in a systematic manner. It does not require touching the client; therefore, it will not precipitate a response that will influence future assessments.

2. Auscultation involves listening to sounds produced within the body. It requires the gentle placement of a warmed stethoscope progressively over all four quadrants of the abdomen; it will minimally influence future assessments.

4. Palpation is the use of touch to assess temperature, turgor, texture, dampness, vibration, shape, and presence of fluid.

Areas of tenderness are palpated last in the palpation process. Light palpation may cause responses that influence future assessments, but it is less invasive than another assessment listed.

1. Percussion is striking a part of the body with short, sharp blows of the fingers. The sound obtained helps to determine the size, position, and density of the underlying body parts. It should be performed last in the assessment process because it is the most disruptive.

3. 1. Knowing where fire alarms/extinguishers are located saves time in the event of a fire.

5. By identifying a fire early, it may be extinguished quickly before it becomes a danger to clients.

2. Once the presence of a fire is identified, clients in danger must be removed from the immediate area to prevent injury.

3. The fire alarm should be activated once clients in the immediate vicinity of the fire are removed from danger.

4. After clients in danger are moved to safety and the fire alarm is activated, the nurse should close all doors and windows on the unit to contain the fire.

4. 2. Crossing the arms facilitates turning and protects the client's arms. Crossing the left leg over the right leg uses the client's weight to facilitate movement.

4. Turning the client with the hands spread apart and at strategic points of the client's anatomy permits the body to turn along its vertical axis, minimizing strain on the client's vertebral column.

1. Moving the right shoulder and arm forward and downward minimizes pressure on the ball-and-socket joint and rotator cuff of the shoulder.

3. Pillows under the head and extremities keep them in functional alignment. A pillow behind the back maintains the client on the side and keeps the vertebral column in functional alignment.

5. 5. Clamping the tubing allows the water to collect in the container once it is added.

3. A soapsuds enema for an adult should be 500 to 1,000 mL of water at 105°F to 110°F. The volume is sufficient to distend the intestinal lumen, and the temperature is slightly more than body temperature to provide for comfort.

4. This action expels air from the tubing and prevents air from entering the intestine.
1. Soap is added after the container is filled to prevent the formation of bubbles and after the tubing is flushed to ensure that the soap is diluted in the total volume of solution (3 to 5 mL of soap per 1,000 mL of water). Gently rocking the enema bag prevents bubble formation while dispersing the soap evenly throughout the fluid. Usually a mild and gentle soap such as Castile soap is used for a soapsuds enema.
2. The catheter is lubricated to limit trauma as the catheter is inserted into the client's anus and rectum.

6. 4. The client most likely experienced a pulmonary embolus. Using a wheelchair limits muscle activity. Activity can contribute to more emboli and increase the demand on the heart and lungs.
5. The high-Fowler position facilitates thoracic expansion and respirations, which are necessary to promote pulmonary functioning.
1. Administering oxygen is essential to provide more oxygen for gas exchange, which will increase oxygen to body cells.
2. After initial interventions, the nurse can take the time to auscultate breath sounds to collect information that may be helpful to the primary health-care provider when making a medical diagnosis.
3. After emergency nursing interventions are performed to assess and facilitate respirations, the rapid response team should be activated and the primary health-care provider notified.

7. 4. A client with an irregular pulse and labored respirations should be assessed first. These vital signs are outside the expected range; these adaptations may indicate a life-threatening situation.
2. A client who was just informed of having cancer should be assessed second. The diagnosis of cancer may have precipitated a crisis for this client. Psychosocial needs of clients are as important as physiological needs.
1. A client who reports feeling nauseated should be assessed third. Although nausea should be assessed, it is not life-threatening. Other clients are a greater priority.

3. A client who is receiving a titrated medication via an infusion pump should be assessed fourth. Infusion pumps deliver fluid volumes safely. Other client situations are a greater priority.
5. A client who received an analgesic by mouth for pain immediately before report should be assessed last. An analgesic by mouth takes approximately 30 minutes to be effective. This client's response to the medication can be evaluated after other clients' needs are met.

8. 3. Having an episode of shortness of breath is related to physiological needs, the first step of Maslow's Hierarchy of Needs theory.
2. Experiencing a fall is related to safety and security needs, the second step of Maslow's Hierarchy of Needs theory.
4. Being the honoree at a family birthday party is related to loving and belonging needs, the third step of Maslow's Hierarchy of Needs theory.
5. Winning an art contest at the assisted-living residence is related to self-esteem needs, the fourth step of Maslow's Hierarchy of Needs theory.
1. Learning how to use a computer is related to self-actualization needs, the fifth step of Maslow's Hierarchy of Needs theory.

Exhibit Items

1. Answer: 3. Excess fluid volume
1. Although the client is manifesting increases in temperature, pulse, respirations, and blood pressure, which are associated with a systemic infection, the client is not experiencing the other classic responses to a systemic infection, which include chills, diaphoresis, malaise, and change in mental status.
2. Anaphylactic shock, caused by exposure to an allergen, is manifested by anxiety, tachypnea, throat tightness, stridor, diaphoresis, flushing, and urticaria. Except for tachypnea, none of the other responses are exhibited by the client.
3. Excess fluid volume in this situation is caused by the inefficient pumping action of the heart. A decreased cardiac output results in decreased renal perfusion that stimulates a renin/angiotensin response; this precipitates vasoconstriction and the

increased release of aldosterone, which causes sodium and fluid retention, resulting in an excess fluid volume. The client has a history of heart failure and has been receiving digoxin, which slows and strengthens the heart rate and acts as a mild diuretic, and furosemide, which is a loop diuretic. Objective data: the vital signs have increased, particularly the blood pressure, which indicates an increase of fluid in the intravascular compartment, and the pulse and respirations, which indicate an attempt to increase the amount of oxygen being delivered to body cells. Pitting edema results because of the movement of excess fluid from the intravascular to the interstitial compartment. Crackles in the lungs indicate pulmonary edema associated with fluid moving from the capillaries in the lung into the alveoli. Subjective data: these clinical manifestations all support an excess fluid volume as the body responds to the excess accumulated fluid.**

4. Orthostatic hypotension, caused by inefficient vasomotor responses in the circulatory system, is manifested by light-headedness, vertigo, weakness, and diaphoresis when transferring from lying to sitting or from sitting to standing positions. The client is not experiencing these physiological responses.

2. **Answer: 3. Pressure ulcers**
   1. The client is unable to control the passage of stool (fecal incontinence) and does not have diarrhea. Diarrhea is the passage of three or more liquid or unformed stools a day.
   2. No data indicate the presence of hemorrhage. The brain attack (stroke, cerebrovascular accident) may be related to the development of a thrombus or embolus associated with the history of atherosclerosis and TIAs.
   3. **The client is anemic. Older men should have a red blood cell count of 3.7 to 6.0 million cells/mcL, a Hb level of 11.0 to 17.0 g/dL, and a serum ferritin value of 18 to 270 ng/mL. The client is underweight and has less subcutaneous fat because of aging. Urine and feces are irritating to the skin because of their acidity and enzyme content, respectively. The presence of inadequate nutrition, the inability to move the right side of**

the body, the potential presence of urine and feces on the skin, and the characteristics of skin in older adults all create an increased risk for pressure ulcers.
   4. The client's serum glucose is within the acceptable range for an older adult (70 to 120 mg/dL).

3. **Answer: 1. Pulmonary embolus**
   1. **When an embolus obstructs an artery in the lung, it interrupts gas exchange at the cellular level. This precipitates unilateral chest pain, blood-tinged sputum (hemoptysis), and respirations that become rapid, shallow, and labored (dyspnea). Decreased breath sounds occur over the affected alveoli as a result of the lack of gas exchange. Diaphoresis and an increase in vital signs occur as a result of the release of epinephrine.**
   2. Although the client is in respiratory distress, the client responses do not support the presence of a respiratory infection. With a respiratory infection, the sputum would be yellow or green rather than blood tinged unless the infection was severe and prolonged, which is unlikely because of preoperative testing. Also, the temperature would be elevated. A temperature of 100.2°F is common after the stress of surgery.
   3. The client is not exhibiting manifestations of subcutaneous emphysema. Tenderness and crackling occur when suspect tissue is palpated. Subcutaneous emphysema is the presence of air in the subcutaneous tissue; this may occur with an open pneumothorax or around the site of a thoracotomy tube.
   4. The client is not experiencing postoperative hemorrhage. The dressing is dry and intact, and the abdomen is flat and nontender. Also, the blood pressure increased rather than decreased. If the client were hemorrhaging, the blood pressure would decrease as a result of hypovolemia.

4. **Answer: 1. Pain**
   1. **The client is in pain, as evidenced by a rating of 8 on a pain scale of 0 to 10. The increase in the pulse, respirations, and blood pressure reflects the response to stress-related catecholamines.**
   2. The client is not hemorrhaging. If the client were hemorrhaging, the blood pressure should have decreased, not increased, the portable wound drainage systems would contain more than 210 mL, and the dressing may have evidence of blood.

3. The client is not experiencing urinary retention. The urinary retention catheter is draining clear amber urine, the suprapubic area is not distended, and the I&O are approximately equal, taking into consideration the fluid lost during surgery.
4. If the client were experiencing excess fluid volume, the blood pressure would be much higher, and the fluid intake would exceed the output on the I&O record.

5. **Answer: 2. Aspiration**
   1. Although older adults have a diminished immune system, the client is not at high risk for an infection compared with the risk for the other options presented.
   2. **The client is exhibiting imperfect articulation of speech (dysarthria), difficulty swallowing (dysphagia), a diminished gag reflex, and lethargy, all which are associated with brain attack (stroke, cerebrovascular accident). These clinical manifestations place the client at high risk for aspiration. Airway is the priority as per the ABCs (airway, breathing, and circulation) of client assessment.**
   3. With a mechanical soft diet and supervision during meals, the client should ingest adequate nutrients to prevent malnutrition.
   4. Although constipation may occur in the client because of lethargy and decreased peristalsis associated with aging, the complication of constipation is not as likely as a complication in another option. The client has borborygmi in all four quadrants of the abdomen, indicating the presence of intestinal peristalsis. Also, if constipation occurs, it can be diminished with stool softeners.

6. **Answer: 1. Hypokalemia**
   1. **Muscle weakness, leg cramps, decreased bowel sounds, and a weak, irregular pulse are all clinical manifestations of hypokalemia. The serum potassium level of 3.1 mEq/L is below the expected range of 3.5 to 5.0 mEq/L. Furosemide is a diuretic that prevents the reabsorption of water and electrolytes from the tubules of the kidney into the bloodstream. When fluid is lost in response to furosemide, potassium is also eliminated, increasing the risk for hypokalemia. In addition, potassium is lost via vomiting and diarrhea. Weight loss occurs with dehydration.**
   2. The client is not experiencing hypocalcemia. The serum calcium level of 9 mg/dL is within the expected range of 8.5 to

10.5 mg/dL. The client is not exhibiting the following clinical manifestations of hypocalcemia: depressed deep tendon reflexes, bone pain, polyuria, lethargy, and a positive Chvostek or Trousseau sign.
   3. The client is not experiencing hypernatremia. The serum sodium level of 138 mEq/dL is within the expected range of 135 to 145 mEq/L. Although the client has nausea, vomiting, and muscle weakness, which are associated with hypernatremia, the client is not exhibiting the following clinical manifestations of hypernatremia: thirst; dry, sticky mucous membranes; red, dry, swollen tongue; confusion; and agitation.
   4. The client is not experiencing hypermagnesemia. The serum magnesium level of 2.2 mEq/L is within the normal range of 1.5 to 2.5 mEq/L. The client is not exhibiting the following clinical manifestations of hypermagnesemia: peripheral vasodilation, flushing, paralysis, hypotension, bradycardia, lethargy, and respiratory depression.

7. **Answer: 3. Hemorrhage**
   1. A 4 on a pain scale of 0 to 10 usually indicates that the client can tolerate the pain and perform essential activities.
   2. Atelectasis is an incomplete expansion of the lung. Although restlessness and anxiety may accompany atelectasis, other clinical findings should include dyspnea, diminished breath sounds over the affected area, crackles, and cyanosis. Vesicular, bronchovesicular, and bronchial breath sounds heard on auscultation of the lungs are expected breath sounds and indicate effective pulmonary functioning.
   3. **Hemorrhage is an excessive loss of blood. It is evidenced by sympathetic nervous system–precipitated responses such as tachycardia (heart rate more than 100 beats per minute), tachypnea (respiratory rate more than 20 breaths per minute), presence of behavioral signs of restlessness, and reports of feeling anxious. The decrease in the systolic and diastolic blood pressures reflects the decrease in the circulating blood volume. The inadequate urinary output in relation to the fluid intake reflects a decrease in kidney perfusion and the kidney's attempt to conserve fluid because of the decreased circulating blood volume. The collection of 550 mL of blood in the portable wound drainage**

systems is excessive. The client is experiencing internal hemorrhage.

4. Constipation is infrequent bowel movements (fewer than two per week) or hard, dry feces. After abdominal surgery, particularly surgery involving the intestine, peristalsis will be interrupted temporarily because of the effects of anesthesia and the manipulation of the intestines. The absence of bowel sounds and a bowel movement is not significant at this time.

8. **Answer: 4. Smoking history**
   1. The client's sadness over the death of his wife is within the realm of expected grieving because the death occurred only 4 months ago. His statement that he looks forward to playing with his grandchildren every day indicates that he is looking toward the future.
   2. Although the client's avoidance of prostate surgery may be a concern in the future, it is not the priority at this time.

3. A pulse of 96 beats per minute and respirations of 24 breaths per minute most likely are in response to anxiety associated with the scheduled surgery. Although the client is unhappy with the need for surgery and the nurse should explore the client's feelings, they are not as much a concern as another option.

4. **On the basis of Maslow's hierarchy of needs, the client's smoking history poses a serious physiological concern about his respiratory status. The reduced respiratory compensatory reserve associated with aging, the two-pack a day smoking history, and need for general anesthesia during surgery to repair his right leg place him at risk for impaired oxygenation.**

Comprehensive Final Book Exam

This 100-item examination provides an opportunity to take a test that integrates content from among the topics included in Chapters 2 through 5. It includes alternate item formats that reflect the questions presented in Chapter 6. The answer(s) and rationales are provided to enhance your knowledge concerning the information being tested in each question. A Critical-Thinking Strategy (the RACE model), which is described in Chapter 1, is applied to every question to illustrate a methodical approach to analyze questions, eliminate options, and arrive at the correct answer.

COMPREHENSIVE FINAL BOOK EXAM

1. Which early response indicates to the nurse that the client is experiencing hypoxia? **Select all that apply.**
   1. _____ Increased heart rate
   2. _____ Difficulty breathing
   3. _____ Restlessness
   4. _____ Bradypnea
   5. _____ Irritability

2. A nurse determines that a client's IV infusion has infiltrated. Which should the nurse do **next**?
   1. Clamp the tubing and initiate an incident report.
   2. Remove the infusion and start it in another site.
   3. Slow the infusion to a rate just to keep the vein open.
   4. Notify the primary health-care provider of the situation.

3. A nurse is assessing several clients who had surgery the previous day. Which sudden client response should the nurse identify as a potential life-threatening event?
   1. Slightly elevated temperature
   2. Separation of wound edges
   3. Edema of the legs
   4. Chest pain

4. A client states, "I like to have a bowel movement every morning." Which additional information collected by the nurse **supports** a concern regarding perceived constipation?
   1. Hard, dry stools defecated daily
   2. Laxatives used excessively
   3. Abdominal distention
   4. Straining at stool

5. A nurse must administer a sedative to a client before surgery. Which should the nurse do **first**?
   1. Verify that the preoperative checklist is completed.
   2. Check that the surgical consent is signed.
   3. Ensure an intravenous line is in place.
   4. Assess vital signs.

6. A primary health-care provider prescribes 500 mg of an antibiotic to be administered IV piggyback (IVPB) every 6 hours for a client with an infection. The vial dispensed by the hospital pharmacist contains 1 g of the prescribed antibiotic in powder form. The instructions on the vial state, "Instill 9.6 mL to yield 10 mL." How many milliliters of the antibiotic should the nurse add to the IVPB bag? **Record your answer using a whole number.**

   Answer: _____ mL.

7. A nurse in charge of a surgical unit is reviewing the progress of a variety of clients from the date of surgery to predict the potential date of discharge from the unit. Which of the following should the nurse use to assess the clients' progress as a cost-containment strategy in managed care?
   1. Primary nursing
   2. Critical pathways
   3. Functional method
   4. Quality improvement

8. A nurse is assisting with a bed bath for a client who has moderate cognitive deficits. Which is important for the nurse to do?
   1. Explain in detail everything that will be done during the bath before beginning.
   2. Arrange the basin within the center of the client's visual field.
   3. Encourage attention to each task of bathing.
   4. Check the client every few minutes.

9. When the nurse is interviewing the wife of a client, which statement about the client's husband **supports** the presence of obstructive sleep apnea? **Select all that apply.**
   1. _____ "He snores and gasps all night long and wakes me up."
   2. _____ "He falls asleep sometimes when he drives, so now I do all the driving."
   3. _____ "He kicks and thrashes so much that the bed linen is upside down by morning."
   4. _____ "He has nightmares that are so scary that he wakes me up because he is afraid."
   5. _____ "He has these episodes and never wakes up, but I do, and then I can't get back to sleep."

10. A nurse identifies that a client's breath has a sweet, fruity odor. Which of the following should the nurse do **next**?
    1. Take the client's blood pressure.
    2. Review the client's intake and output record.
    3. Obtain a blood sample for a serum glucose level.
    4. Assess for clinical manifestations of hyperglycemia.

11. A nurse is caring for a client who has had diarrhea for several weeks. For which common problem associated with prolonged diarrhea should the nurse assess the client?
    1. Skin breakdown
    2. Self-care deficit
    3. Sexual dysfunction
    4. Disturbed body image

12. A nurse causes harm to a hospitalized client because of improper use of a mechanical lift. Based on which specific tort can this client pursue legal action?
   1. Battery
   2. Assault
   3. Negligence
   4. Malpractice

13. A client with type 2 diabetes is experiencing blurred vision, generalized weakness, and fatigue. A nurse receives a report from the nurse on the previous shift and obtains additional information from the client's clinical record. Which should the nurse conclude that the client is experiencing?
   1. Fluid retention
   2. Kidney impairment
   3. Hyperglycemic event
   4. Hypertensive episode

CLIENT'S CLINICAL RECORD

Laboratory Results
BUN: 18 mg/dL
Creatinine: 1.2 mg/dL
Hemoglobin A_{1c}: 8%
Serum glucose: 350 mg/dL

I&O Record (past 24 hours)
Intake: 2,400 mL
Output: 4,200 mL

Progress Note
10 a.m.—Client reports being thirsty and urinating a lot; has lost 20 pounds over the past 2 months; has "tenting" of skin; and has dry mucous membranes.

14. Nurses on a unit are personally and professionally mature and motivated. Which one of the following classic leadership styles should the nurse manager employ when working with this group?
   1. Directive
   2. Autocratic
   3. Democratic
   4. Laissez-faire

15. A nurse transfers a client from a bed to a wheelchair. Which should the nurse do after placing the client in the wheelchair?
   1. Ensure the client's popliteal areas are not touching the seat edge.
   2. Attach the client's transfer belt to clips on the wheelchair.
   3. Support the client's back with a pillow.
   4. Put the client's feet flat on the floor.

16. A nurse identifies a client's perception of health. Which should the nurse do as a result of obtaining this information?
   1. Help the client prevent the occurrence of physiological responses to disease.
   2. Identify the client's needs based on Maslow's Hierarchy of Human Needs.
   3. Choose a place for the client along the health-illness continuum.
   4. Cluster this data with related data when assessing the client.

17. An older adult asks the nurse, "I want to make sure I get enough vitamin A to keep my eyes healthy. Which fruits can I eat because I am not fond of vegetables?" Which of the following should the nurse explain is an excellent source of vitamin A? **Select all that apply.**
1. _____ Cantaloupe
2. _____ Apricots
3. _____ Peaches
4. _____ Raisins
5. _____ Prunes

18. A nurse is caring for several clients who have different cultural backgrounds and are under stress. Which is an important concept that the nurse must consider when making assessments about these clients' nonverbal behavior?
1. It is controlled by the conscious mind.
2. It carries less weight than what the client says.
3. It does not have the same meaning for everyone.
4. It is a poor reflection of what the client is feeling.

19. A nurse is administering an intramuscular injection at the client's ventrogluteal site. Which action should the nurse implement to help landmark this site?
1. Locate the lower edge of the acromion and the midpoint of the lateral aspect of the arm.
2. Identify the line from the posterior superior iliac spine to the greater trochanter.
3. Place the heel of the hand on the greater trochanter.
4. Palpate the anterior lateral aspect of the thigh.

20. A nurse is caring for a group of four clients. The client with which clinical manifestation requires immediate attention from the nurse?
1. Temperature of 101.6°F with a diagnosis of pneumonia
2. Pulse of 90 beats per minute 2 hours after abdominal surgery
3. Decrease of 10 mm Hg in the systolic blood pressure upon standing
4. Respiratory rate of 25 breaths per minute after resting for 3 minutes following activity

21. A client has a diagnosis of osteoporosis. Which of the following should the nurse encourage this client to eat? **Select all that apply.**
1. _____ Rice
2. _____ Milk
3. _____ Yogurt
4. _____ Sardines
5. _____ Almonds
6. _____ Tomatoes

22. A nurse must obtain a urine specimen from a client with a urinary retention catheter (Foley) and explains the procedure to the client. Which should the nurse do **next**?
1. Cleanse the exit tube at the bottom of the drainage bag with an alcohol swab.
2. Use a clamp to constrict the tubing slightly below the collection port.
3. Position the client in the high-Fowler position.
4. Don a pair of sterile gloves.

23. A nurse is caring for a client who is incontinent of stool. Which action should the nurse implement?
1. Wear a pair of sterile gloves when collecting the client's stool for culture and sensitivity.
2. Apply a moisture barrier to the client's perianal area.
3. Encourage the client to drink cranberry juice daily.
4. Toilet the client before each meal.

24. Which should the nurse teach a client when the primary health-care provider prescribes ibuprofen, an NSAID, for pain? **Select all that apply.**
    1. _____ "Remain in an upright position for 15 to 30 minutes after taking the drug."
    2. _____ "Use this medication carefully because it is addictive."
    3. _____ "Eat food when you take this medication."
    4. _____ "Drink 8 ounces of water with each dose."
    5. _____ "Monitor your blood pressure every day."

25. A primary health-care provider prescribes a 2-g sodium diet for a client. Which fluid should the nurse teach is high in sodium? **Select all that apply.**
    1. _____ Cocoa
    2. _____ Seltzer
    3. _____ Lemonade
    4. _____ Low-fat milk
    5. _____ Tomato juice

26. A nurse is caring for a client in the postanesthesia care unit. For which **most** serious complication of intubation associated with the administration of general anesthesia should the nurse assess this client?
    1. Stomatitis
    2. Atelectasis
    3. Sore throat
    4. Laryngeal spasm

27. A nurse is assessing a client who is experiencing pain. Which statement by the client does the nurse determine reflects the quality of the client's pain?
    1. "This pain is excruciating."
    2. "The pain is just below my ribs."
    3. "The pain feels like something is on fire."
    4. "The pain gets worse as the day progresses."

28. A nurse places a client who had abdominal surgery in the semi-Fowler position. The client states, "I prefer to lie flat when in bed. I feel like I am almost sitting up." Which is an appropriate response by the nurse?
    1. "Raising the head of your bed supports your breathing."
    2. "Increasing the height of the top of the bed promotes your passing gas."
    3. "Keeping your upper body elevated encourages your urinary elimination."
    4. "Lifting your chest above your abdomen facilitates drainage in your wound drains."

29. A nurse is coordinating discharge planning for an older adult who is recovering from a neurological event that left the client with significant right-sided weakness. The client and the spouse express concerns about the limitations of their health insurance, the rehabilitation process, and the prescribed low-cholesterol, 2-g sodium diet. Which individual should the nurse include in a health-care team conference when planning for this client's discharge needs? **Select all that apply.**
    1. _____ Client
    2. _____ Social worker
    3. _____ Registered dietitian
    4. _____ Respiratory therapist
    5. _____ Home health-care nurse
    6. _____ Home health nurse's aide

30. A primary health-care provider writes the prescription *Client may shower* for a client receiving home care. When the nurse is preparing the client for the shower, the client reports feeling weak and very dizzy. The nurse determines that the client will not tolerate standing for a shower safely. Which should the nurse do?
    1. Have the client sit on a commode chair in the shower.
    2. Assist the client with a bath while the client is in bed.
    3. Place the client in a chair in front of a sink.
    4. Transfer the client into a bathtub.

31. A nurse arrives on the unit during the last 5 minutes of a 20-minute change-of-shift report for the second time within a week. How should the nurse in charge handle this situation?
    1. Document the lateness in an incident report.
    2. Ignore the lateness, but intervene if it should happen again.
    3. Include the lateness in the nurse's yearly performance evaluation.
    4. Discuss the lateness with the nurse in private immediately after the report.

32. A nurse hangs an IV piggyback (IVPB) of an antibiotic. Within a few minutes, the client reports a thickening of the back of the tongue and swelling under the chin. Place the following interventions in the order in which they should be implemented.
    1. Turn off the IV piggyback.
    2. Maintain an airway and administer oxygen.
    3. Instruct a colleague to initiate the rapid response team.
    4. Pull the bedside call light out of the wall to initiate an emergency alarm.
    5. Assign a colleague to hang a new intravenous tubing and an isotonic solution.
    6. Prepare emergency medications according to protocol and await arrival of the members of the rapid response team.

    Answer: _____

33. A newly admitted client arrives on the unit. Which is **most** important for the nurse to do to help minimize the development of this client's anxiety?
    1. Validate anxious feelings.
    2. Teach relaxation techniques.
    3. Minimize environmental stimuli.
    4. Explain procedures to the client.

34. A home health-care nurse is providing care for a client who was discharged from the hospital after receiving acute care for a brain attack (i.e., stroke, cerebrovascular accident). The client has left-sided hemiparesis, difficulty swallowing, and anxiety. Which nursing intervention reflects the nurse's role of being a resource person?
    1. Helping the client to negotiate the health-care system within the community
    2. Encouraging the client to chew food thoroughly before swallowing
    3. Teaching the client to use deep breathing exercises when anxious
    4. Instructing the client on how to use a walker when ambulating

35. Which client statement indicates to the nurse that an older adult understands the teaching about how to care for dry skin effectively?
    1. "I will increase the amount of water that I drink."
    2. "I can use baby powder on my skin rather than lotion."
    3. "I should have a bath every day using a moisturizing soap."
    4. "I ought to wear clothing made of wool rather than cotton."

36. A client has a prescription for a vaginal suppository. Which of the following should the nurse perform when administering this medication? **Select all that apply.**
    1. _____ Lubricate the suppository and the index finger of a gloved hand before insertion of the suppository.
    2. _____ Instruct the client to remain flat in bed for 20 minutes after insertion of the suppository.
    3. _____ Irrigate the vagina with normal saline before inserting the suppository.
    4. _____ Place the client in the dorsal recumbent position for the procedure.
    5. _____ Advance the suppository along the posterior vaginal wall.
    6. _____ Insert the suppository while wearing clean gloves.

37. A nurse is taking a client's temperature using the instrument in the illustration. Place the following steps in the order in which they should be implemented.
1. While holding the button down and keeping the probe flat against the forehead, slide the instrument across the forehead, stopping when the hairline on the side of the face is reached.
2. Position the probe flat on the middle of the forehead halfway between the hairline and the eyebrow and hold the button down.
3. While continuing to hold the button, touch the probe to the soft area behind the earlobe and below the mastoid.
4. Clean the probe, following the manufacturer's directions.
5. Release the button.

Answer: _____

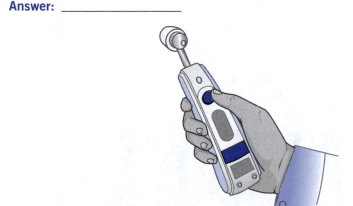

38. A first aid nurse at a beach is caring for a client who sustained a soft tissue injury of the right shoulder after being hit by a surfboard. Which should the nurse do to limit the stress of both edema and bleeding into tissue?
1. Apply a cold compress.
2. Exert direct pressure.
3. Provide massage.
4. Elevate the arm.

39. A nurse is caring for a group of clients in the postanesthesia care unit. Which response by a client in the postanesthesia care unit is the **priority** concern for the nurse?
1. Pain
2. Nausea
3. Reduced level of consciousness
4. Excessive loss of fluid through indwelling drains

40. A client's double-lumen nasogastric tube for decompression becomes obstructed. Which should the nurse do?
1. Instill 10 mL of air into the vent lumen.
2. Place the client in the high-Fowler position.
3. Position the vent below the level of the stomach.
4. Withdraw 30 mL of gastric contents from the drainage lumen.

41. Which scenario requires a nurse to complete an incident report? **Select all that apply.**
1. _____ A client refused to go to physical therapy that was prescribed by a primary health-care provider.
2. _____ A client climbed over raised side rails and fell but was not injured.
3. _____ A visitor ambulated a client who should have been on bedrest.
4. _____ A nurse left work early without reporting to the supervisor.
5. _____ A client did not receive a prescribed medication.
6. _____ A nurse fell in the hall and broke an arm.

42. A client who has a transdermal analgesic patch for cancer experiences breakthrough pain with activity. Which is **most** important for the nurse to do?
1. Encourage the avoidance of moving around.
2. Seek a dose increase in the long-acting opioid.
3. Administer the prescribed shorter-acting opioid.
4. Obtain a prescription for an antianxiety medication.

43. A nurse must perform a procedure and is unsure of the exact steps of the procedure. Which should the nurse do **first**?
1. Refer to a fundamentals of nursing skills textbook.
2. Call the staff education department for assistance.
3. Check the nursing policy and procedure manual.
4. Refuse to do the nursing procedure.

44. A nurse sees the stable client walking down the hall, as depicted in the photograph. What should the nurse instruct the client to do **first**?
1. Switch hands holding the IV pole and urine collection bag.
2. Hold the urine collection bag below the waist.
3. Raise the height of the IV pole.
4. Put on shoes and a bathrobe.

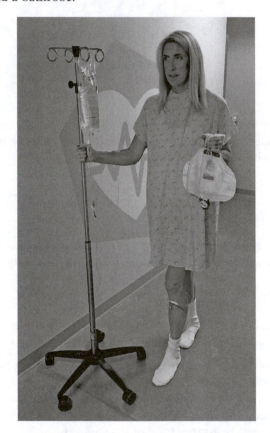

45. At which date and time did the client have a respiratory rate of 15 breaths per minute?
1. 9-9 at 04
2. 9-9 at 08
3. 9-10 at 08
4. 9-10 at 16

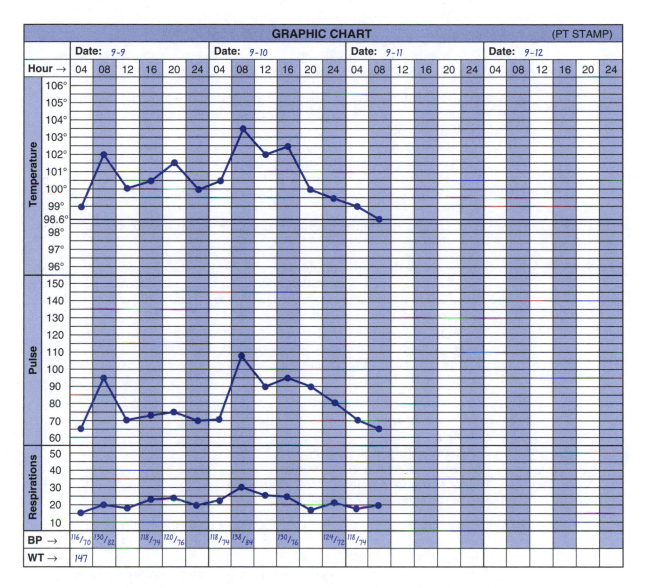

46. A client appears agitated and states, "I'm not sure that I want to go through with this surgery." Which response by the nurse uses the technique of paraphrasing?
1. "Are you saying that you want to postpone the surgery?"
2. "Are you undecided about having this surgery?"
3. "You seem upset about this surgery."
4. "Tell me more about your concerns."

47. A nurse is planning to apply a transdermal patch to a client. Which of the following should the nurse implement? **Select all that apply.**
   1. _____ Use a different site each time to limit skin irritation and excoriation.
   2. _____ Rub the area to promote comfort and vasodilation before applying the patch.
   3. _____ Shave the area to facilitate adherence of the patch and medication absorption.
   4. _____ Wear clean gloves to protect one's self from absorbing the medication through the hands.
   5. _____ Remove the old patch an hour after applying the new patch to ensure a therapeutic blood level of the drug.

48. A nurse is evaluating a nursing assistant changing the linen on an unoccupied bed. Which action by the nursing assistant reflects acceptable medical aseptic technique? **Select all that apply.**
   1. _____ Containing soiled linen in a pillowcase resting on a bedside chair
   2. _____ Positioning a soiled-linen hamper inside the doorway to a client's room
   3. _____ Holding soiled linen away from touching the nursing assistant's uniform
   4. _____ Washing the hands after disposing of a client's linen in a soiled-linen hamper
   5. _____ Using sterile gloves when changing linen soiled by a client's sanguineous drainage

49. A client is told by the primary health-care provider that the client has metastatic lung cancer and is seriously ill. After the provider leaves the room, the client has a severe episode of coughing and shortness of breath and says, "This is just a cold. I'll be fine once I get over it." How should the nurse respond?
   1. "What did you just find out about having a serious illness?"
   2. "Didn't you receive some bad news today?"
   3. "This is not a cold; it's lung cancer."
   4. "Tell me more about your illness."

50. A client develops diarrhea after receiving several intermittent enteral tube feedings. Which should the nurse consider is the cause of the diarrhea before responding to this situation?
   1. A high osmolarity of the feeding
   2. An inadequate volume of the feeding
   3. Failure to test for a residual before the feeding
   4. Use of the high-Fowler position during the feeding

51. While in a restaurant, a pregnant woman exhibits a total airway obstruction because of a bolus of food. How should the nurse modify the thrusts of the abdominal thrust (Heimlich) maneuver for this woman?
   1. Perform them when the woman is in the supine, rather than the standing, position.
   2. Use the pinkie finger side of the fist, rather than the thumb side, against the woman's body.
   3. Compress against the middle of the woman's sternum rather than between the umbilicus and xiphoid process.
   4. Initiate the procedure after the woman becomes unconscious, and discontinue it after six tries if unsuccessful.

52. A nurse in charge is making assignments for a nursing team. Which intervention should the nurse in charge assign to the registered nurse? **Select all that apply.**
   1. _____ Assessing the skin of a newly admitted client
   2. _____ Offering apple juice to a client on a clear liquid diet
   3. _____ Assisting a client out of bed for the first time after surgery
   4. _____ Explaining how a client should self-administer a hypertonic enema
   5. _____ Measuring the urinary output of a client with an indwelling urinary catheter

53. A nurse is providing dietary teaching for a client who follows a plant-based (pure) vegan diet. Which food combination that is a substitute for a complete protein should the nurse include in the dietary teaching? **Select all that apply.**
    1. _____ Pasta and peas
    2. _____ Yogurt and fruit
    3. _____ Bread and cheese
    4. _____ Legumes and rice
    5. _____ Peanut butter and jelly

54. A construction worker comes to the emergency department with an injury that occurred 3 days ago. The client has an open wound of the right calf that has purulent drainage. The medical professional decides to admit the client to the hospital for IV antibiotic therapy and prescribes contact precautions. Which should the nurse in the emergency department do before transporting the client to a room?
    1. Arrange for an airborne infection isolation room.
    2. Cover the wound with a sterile dressing.
    3. Administer the prescribed antibiotic.
    4. Don a gown, gloves, and goggles.

55. A nurse is going to instill medicated drops into the ear of an adult. Which should the nurse do to ensure that the medication flows toward the eardrum?
    1. Pull the pinna of the ear backward and downward.
    2. Insert the drops into the center of the auditory canal.
    3. Press the tragus of the ear several times after insertion.
    4. Roll the client from the side-lying to the supine position.

56. A nurse is caring for a client on bedrest. Which client statement should alert the nurse to assess for indications of immobility-induced thrombophlebitis?
    1. "The skin on my legs is very dry."
    2. "One of my calves looks swollen."
    3. "I have tingling sensations in my feet."
    4. "The toes on my left foot feel cool when I touch them."

57. A nurse is obtaining a client's blood pressure. Which of the following will result in an accurate blood pressure measurement? **Select all that apply.**
    1. _____ Positioning the arm at the level of the heart
    2. _____ Wrapping the lower edge of the cuff over the antecubital space
    3. _____ Pumping the cuff about 30 mm Hg above the point where the brachial pulse is lost on palpation
    4. _____ Releasing the valve on the cuff so that the pressure decreases at the rate of 2 to 3 mm Hg per second
    5. _____ Deflating the cuff completely and waiting 2 minutes before reinflating the blood pressure cuff to take the pressure again

58. A nurse is caring for a client who is unconscious. Which should the nurse use to **best** clean this client's oral cavity?
    1. Gauze-wrapped tongue blades with a saline solution
    2. Half-strength mouthwash and saline
    3. Packaged glycerin swabs
    4. Nonfoaming toothpaste

59. A client is admitted to the hospital with the diagnosis of diverticulitis. Which is the **best** question the nurse should ask when obtaining an admission history from this client?
    1. "What did you eat yesterday?"
    2. "How long have you had diverticulitis?"
    3. "What led up to your coming to the hospital today?"
    4. "Have you ever had any previous episodes of diverticulitis?"

60. A primary health-care provider prescribes peak and trough levels for a client receiving an IV antibiotic. What time should the nurse obtain a blood sample to determine a trough level when the antibiotic was administered at 12 noon?
    1. 11:00 a.m.
    2. 11:30 a.m.
    3. 12:30 p.m.
    4. 1:00 p.m.

61. A nurse is monitoring a client who is receiving an IV infusion because of dehydration. Which client response **most** specifically indicates that the IV fluid replacement is adequate?
    1. Moist lips
    2. Bounding pulse
    3. Urinary output of 50 mL/hr
    4. Blood pressure of 96/60 mm Hg

62. A nurse is teaching a group of clients about correct body mechanics. Which action reflects teaching about the principle, *the greater the base of support, the more stable the body*? **Select all that apply.**
    1. _____ "Use a cane when you walk."
    2. _____ "Lock the wheels of your wheelchair."
    3. _____ "Seek assistance when you get out of bed."
    4. _____ "Hold objects close to your body when you walk."
    5. _____ "Keep your back straight when you lift an object."

63. A nurse is caring for a client who has been having difficulty sleeping. Which should the nurse do because it is the **most** effective nursing intervention to promote sleep that is appropriate for a client in any situation?
    1. Provide a back rub.
    2. Play relaxing music.
    3. Offer a glass of warm milk.
    4. Follow a routine at bedtime.

64. A nurse is performing an assessment of a client. Place an X on the figure of the body where the nurse should place the stethoscope to assess for the presence of borborygmi.

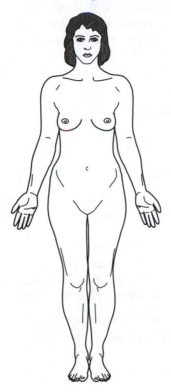

65. A nurse is caring for clients who are on a medical/surgical unit in a hospital. Which should the nurse do to **best** prevent clients from falling due to physical hazards?
1. Position the telephone within easy reach.
2. Store belongings in a safe place.
3. Ensure adequate lighting.
4. Use an over-bed table.

66. A client prefers and excessively maintains the supine position. For which potential problem associated with this position should the nurse assess the client?
1. Pressure against the heels
2. Internal rotation of the hips
3. Flexion contracture of the knees
4. Compression of tissue over the trochanters

67. A client is using the call bell numerous times an hour and requesting assistance with activities that the client is capable of achieving independently. Which should the nurse do to help this client?
1. Set limits verbally.
2. Alternate care with another nurse.
3. Point out the behavior to the client.
4. Attempt to see the situation from the client's perspective.

68. A nurse going off duty is making rounds with the nurse coming on duty and provides a report about each client in the district. Which information reported by the nurse is the **most** complete?
1. The client was given an antiemetic an hour ago and reports resolution of the nausea.
2. The client's family members just visited and the client appears happy.
3. The client seems less anxious than earlier in the day.
4. The client's blood pressure is now stable.

69. A nurse is bathing a client. Which action is associated with medical asepsis? **Select all that apply.**
1. _____ Washing from the inner canthus to the outer canthus of the eye
2. _____ Replacing the top covers with a clean flannel bath blanket
3. _____ Changing the bathwater after washing the perineal area
4. _____ Having the client void before beginning the bed bath
5. _____ Wearing clean gloves when washing the perineum

70. A nurse is assessing the oxygen status of a dark-skinned client. Where should the nurse assess for cyanosis in this client?
1. Lower legs
2. Sclera of eyes
3. Nailbeds of toes
4. Oral mucous membranes

71. A client who self-administers an aerosol medication by a metered-dose inhaler reports a "nasty taste to the medication." Which should the nurse encourage the client to do?
1. Suck on a hard candy after the procedure.
2. Shake the cartridge longer before using it.
3. Perform oral hygiene before inhalation of medication.
4. Attach an aerosol chamber to the metered-dose cartridge.

72. A nurse is meeting a client for the first time. Which should the nurse do during the orientation phase of this therapeutic relationship?
1. Collect data.
2. Build rapport.
3. Identify problems.
4. Establish priorities.

73. A client has a temperature of 102°F and reports feeling cold. For which additional response should the nurse assess the client during this onset phase (cold or chill phase) of a fever? **Select all that apply.**
1. _____ Lethargy
2. _____ Pale skin
3. _____ Shivering
4. _____ Diaphoresis
5. _____ Dehydration

74. A nurse is delegating an assignment to a nursing assistant. Which client who will benefit the **most** from soaking the feet for several minutes as part of a bath should the nurse assign to the nursing assistant?
1. A client who has a personal preference for taking showers
2. A client who has lower-extremity arterial disease
3. A client who was living in an abandoned car
4. A client who has a prescription for bedrest

75. A nurse is assessing the skin of an older adult. Which condition is of **most** concern to the nurse?
1. Flat, brown spots on the skin
2. Thin, translucent skin
3. Tenting of the skin
4. Dry, flaky skin

76. A nurse is caring for a client who is using an incentive spirometer. Which client behavior observed by the nurse indicates that the teaching was effective? **Select all that apply.**
    1. _____ Inhales slowly and deeply using the spirometer
    2. _____ Tilts the incentive spirometer while breathing in
    3. _____ Raises the inspiratory goal on the spirometer once a day
    4. _____ Takes several regular breaths before using the spirometer again
    5. _____ Exhales while keeping the mouth sealed firmly around the mouthpiece

77. A nurse on a postpartum unit is teaching a class for new mothers about umbilical cord care. The nurse identifies that one mother does not become involved with the discussion and is withdrawn. Which is the **best** action by the nurse to help this new mother learn about umbilical cord care?
    1. Give the mother written material about cord care.
    2. Invite the mother to the next class about cord care.
    3. Bring an audiovisual cassette about cord care into the mother's room.
    4. Provide informal, individual instruction for the mother about cord care.

78. A nurse is teaching a client with dysphagia how to eat safely. Which should the nurse encourage the client to do? **Select all that apply.**
    1. _____ Tilt the head backward when swallowing.
    2. _____ Drink fluids when eating bites of solid food.
    3. _____ Reduce environmental stimuli to a minimum.
    4. _____ Make sure that the mouth is empty after eating.
    5. _____ Keep food in the front of the mouth when chewing.

79. A nurse is assessing a client for clinical manifestations of an altered serum potassium level. Which clinical manifestation is common to both hypokalemia and hyperkalemia? **Select all that apply.**
    1. _____ Increased bowel sounds
    2. _____ Muscle weakness
    3. _____ Dysrhythmias
    4. _____ Confusion
    5. _____ Nausea

80. A nurse in charge is delegating assignments to a registered nurse and a nursing assistant on the nursing team. Which assignment should be delegated to only the registered nurse? **Select all that apply.**
    1. _____ Evaluating a client's response to activity
    2. _____ Taking the pulse of a client with a dysrhythmia
    3. _____ Teaching a client how to change a colostomy bag
    4. _____ Applying a condom catheter on a client who is incontinent
    5. _____ Changing the linen on an occupied bed for a comatose client

81. A nurse is caring for a client who recently received a diagnosis of diabetes. The nurse institutes all of the following interventions. Which nursing action reflects teaching self-management in the affective domain?
    1. Providing the client with a list of signs and symptoms of a high blood glucose level
    2. Encouraging the client to express feelings about this new medical challenge
    3. Instructing the client about which foods are high in glucose
    4. Coaching the client on how to self-administer insulin

506 FUNDAMENTALS SUCCESS

82. A nurse is caring for a client with an infected leg ulcer. Which common systemic response to an infection should the nurse assess for when monitoring this client? **Select all that apply.**
    1. _____ Pain
    2. _____ Edema
    3. _____ Hyperthermia
    4. _____ Increased heart rate
    5. _____ Increased white blood cell count

83. A client with terminal cancer says to the nurse, "I've been fairly religious, but sometimes I wonder if the things I did were acceptable to God." How should the nurse respond?
    1. "Not knowing what the future brings can be an unsettling thought."
    2. "God will appreciate that you went to religious services."
    3. "If you were good, you have nothing to fear."
    4. "In life, all we have to do is try to be good."

84. A nurse is administering a lozenge to a client's buccal area of the mouth. Which should the nurse do? **Select all that apply.**
    1. _____ Ensure the client stays awake while the lozenge dissolves.
    2. _____ Instruct the client to take occasional sips of water.
    3. _____ Place the medication under the client's tongue.
    4. _____ Use the same cheek when placing the lozenge.
    5. _____ Administer the lozenge just before meals.

85. The nurse is assessing a client who is in pain. Which question should the nurse ask to assess the client's pain tolerance?
    1. "At what point on a scale of 0 to 10 do you feel that you must have pain medication?"
    2. "What activities help distract you so that you don't feel the need for medication?"
    3. "How intense on a scale of 0 to 10 is the pain that you feel right now?"
    4. "Do you take pain medication frequently?"

86. An obese client asks the nurse, "What should I do to help myself lose weight?" How should the nurse respond while considering the **best** behavior modification strategy for controlling food intake?
    1. "Ask family members not to bring tempting food into the house."
    2. "Post pictures of thin people on the refrigerator."
    3. "Avoid snacks between meals."
    4. "Maintain a daily food diary."

87. A primary health-care provider prescribes diltiazem (Cardizem) 75 mg by mouth three times a day. The scored diltiazem tablets are labeled 30 mg/tablet. How many tablets should the nurse administer? **Record your answer using one decimal place.**

    Answer: _____ tablets.

88. A primary health-care provider prescribes the insertion of an indwelling urinary catheter (retention, Foley) as part of the client's preoperative prescriptions. Place the following steps of the procedure in the order in which they should be performed by the nurse.
    1. Don sterile gloves.
    2. Open the catheterization package.
    3. Place a fenestrated drape over the client's perineal area.
    4. Maintain spread of labia while swiping directly over the urinary meatus.
    5. Maintain spread of labia while swiping each labium with a separate cotton ball.

    Answer: _____

89. A client's vital signs are: apical heart rate—100 beats per minute, radial heart rate—84 beats per minute, respirations—20 breaths per minute, blood pressure—140/84 mm Hg. What is the client's pulse deficit? **Record your answer using a whole number.**

Answer: _____

90. A client is admitted to the emergency department after sustaining a crushing injury at work. For which characteristic of blood pressure should the nurse assess the client to identify impending shock?
1. Rising diastolic
2. Decreasing systolic
3. Widening pulse pressure
4. Robust Korotkoff's sounds

91. A client's primary health-care provider prescribes antiembolism stockings to be worn when out of bed. Which is an important action about antiembolism stockings that the nurse should teach the client?
1. Massage the feet and legs with body lotion before putting them on.
2. Put them on before the legs are in a dependent position.
3. Ensure that the top band is rolled slightly for comfort.
4. Remove and reapply them every four hours.

92. A nurse must perform a straight catheterization of a client to obtain a urine specimen. The nurse opens the prepackaged straight catheter kit. Place an X on the item in the kit that the nurse should touch **first.**

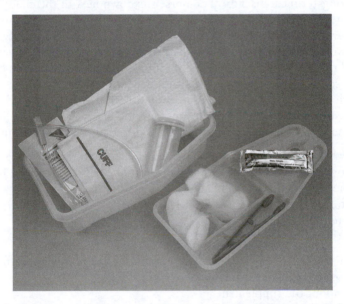

93. A primary health-care provider prescribes 1 g of an antibiotic to be administered via the intramuscular route twice a day. The nurse implements all of the following actions. Which nursing action reflects the planning step of the nursing process?
1. Verifying the client's allergies in the chart and on the client's allergy band
2. Ensuring that the prescription was received by the pharmacy
3. Identifying body landmarks before giving the injection
4. Deciding times when the medication should be given

94. A nurse working in a nursing home routinely administers digoxin 0.125 mg by mouth to a client every morning. Which of the following should alert the nurse to withhold the medication? **Select all that apply.**
1. _____ Diplopia
2. _____ Vomiting
3. _____ Tachypnea
4. _____ Bradycardia
5. _____ Dysrhythmias

95. A nurse is giving a client a bed bath. Which should the nurse do to **increase** circulation?
1. Wash the extremities with firm strokes toward the heart.
2. Soak the feet in warm water for at least 20 minutes.
3. Expose just the areas that are being washed.
4. Ensure that the water is 120°F to 125°F.

96. A nurse is planning a teaching program for a client regarding the learning of a new skill. The nurse assesses each of the following. Which factor does the nurse conclude is **most** relevant when predicting success of the teaching program?
1. Level of education
2. Interest of the client
3. Extent of family support
4. Cognitive ability of the client

97. A client who immigrated with her family to the United States 15 years ago is residing in a long-term care facility. The nurse sits down next to the client, who is crying. Eventually, the client states, "Our son is 30 years old and still is not married. My husband and I want to arrange a marriage for him, but he refuses. My husband and I have a wonderful marriage, and we had an arranged marriage 35 years ago. Arranged marriages are accepted in our culture." What is the nurse's **best** response?
1. "Your son is disregarding your cultural beliefs."
2. "The length of your marriage is a tribute to arranged marriages."
3. "It must be troublesome when a son does not agree with your beliefs."
4. "You may have to accept that your son is developing his own point of view."

98. A client who is secretly smoking in bed falls asleep, and the cigarette ignites the client's gown. Which should the nurse do **first** after discovering the fire?
1. Smother the flames with a blanket.
2. Roll the client from side to side.
3. Activate the fire alarm.
4. Close the door.

99. A nurse discovers that a client is taking natural herbal remedies. Which intervention is **most** important for the nurse to do?
1. Learn about the supplements.
2. Think of the supplements as drugs.
3. Communicate the supplement use to the primary health-care provider.
4. Include the details about supplement use in the client's health history.

100. A client sustained a traumatic brain injury resulting in neurological deficits after falling off a ladder at work. Which setting is **most** appropriate for the nurse to explore with the client and the family to assist this client to learn how to live with neurological limitations?
1. Assisted-living residence
2. Extended care facility
3. Acute care setting
4. Hospice program

COMPREHENSIVE FINAL BOOK EXAM: ANSWERS AND RATIONALES

1.

CRITICAL-THINKING STRATEGY

Recognize keywords.	Which **early response** indicates to the nurse that the client is experiencing **hypoxia**?
Ask what the question is asking.	Which is an early sign of hypoxia?
Critically analyze each option in relation to the question and the other options.	Examine each option from the perspective of whether or not the response is associated with reduced oxygen in the body. This requires an understanding of physiological responses to reduced oxygen and why each occurs. **Rationales:** 1. **A heart rate of more than 100 beats per minute (tachycardia) is an early response to hypoxia. Hypoxia is insufficient oxygen anywhere in the body. To compensate for this lack of oxygen, the heart increases its rate to improve cardiac output, thereby increasing oxygen to all body cells.** 2. Difficulty breathing (dyspnea) is a late, not early, sign of hypoxia. 3. **Restlessness is an early sign of hypoxia. Restlessness occurs with hypoxia because of a decrease in oxygen to the brain.** 4. An increase in respirations to more than 20 breaths per minute (tachypnea), not a decrease in respirations less than 12 breaths per minute (bradypnea), occurs as the body attempts to deliver more oxygen to body cells. 5. **Irritability is an early sign of hypoxia. Irritability occurs with hypoxia because of a decrease in oxygen to the brain.**
Eliminate incorrect options.	Options 2 and 4 are late signs of hypoxia and can be eliminated.

2.

CRITICAL-THINKING STRATEGY

Recognize keywords.	A nurse determines that a client's **IV** infusion has **infiltrated. Which should the nurse do next**?
Ask what the question is asking.	What should the nurse do when an IV infiltrates?
Critically analyze each option in relation to the question and the other options.	Explore what will happen when the action in each option is implemented. Identify options that are unnecessary or unsafe. **Rationales:** 1. Not only should the infusion be clamped, but it also should be removed. An incident report is unnecessary. 2. **The IV catheter moves out of the vein and into interstitial tissue (extravasation) when an IV infiltrates. The infusion must be discontinued and restarted at another site, preferably another extremity.** 3. Slowing the infusion rate to just keep the vein open is unsafe because fluid will continue to collect in the interstitial compartment. 4. The primary health-care provider does not have to be notified. However, the situation must be documented in the client's clinical record.
Eliminate incorrect options.	The actions in options 1 and 4 are unnecessary. The action in option 3 is unsafe. Eliminate options 1, 3, and 4.

3.

CRITICAL-THINKING STRATEGY

Recognize keywords.	A nurse is assessing several clients who had **surgery the previous day**. Which **sudden client response** should the nurse identify as a potential **life-threatening** event?
Ask what the question is asking.	Which clinical finding indicates a possible life-threatening event?
Critically analyze each option in relation to the question and the other options.	Critically review several expected or potential problems related to the stress of surgery. Then identify the one complication that is life-threatening. **Rationales:** 1. A slight elevation of body temperature is expected after surgery because of the body's response to the stress of surgery. 2. Dehiscence, separation of the wound edges, is more likely to occur between the fifth and eighth postoperative days, and it is not life-threatening. 3. Dependent edema indicates problems, such as a fluid and electrolyte imbalance, impaired kidney function, or decreased cardiac output. All are serious but generally manageable. **4. An acute onset of chest pain within 24 hours of surgery may indicate myocardial infarction in response to the stress of surgery. Also, it can be caused by a pulmonary embolus, although this is more likely to occur between the 7th and 10th postoperative days. Both of these complications are life-threatening.**
Eliminate incorrect options.	Option 1 is an expected outcome; options 2 and 3 are complications that are not as life-threatening as chest pain. Chest pain may indicate a myocardial infarction, which is a life-threatening condition. Options 1, 2, and 3 can be eliminated.

4.

CRITICAL-THINKING STRATEGY

Recognize keywords.	A client states, **"I like to have a bowel movement every morning."** Which **additional information** collected by the nurse **supports** a concern regarding **perceived constipation**?
Ask what the question is asking.	Which is a clinical finding associated with perceived constipation?
Critically analyze each option in relation to the question and the other options.	Analyze the differences between constipation and perceived constipation. **Rationales:** 1. The passage of hard, dry stools supports the presence of constipation, not perceived constipation. **2. The expectation of a daily bowel movement at the same time every day with the resulting overuse of laxatives, enemas, or suppositories (or all of these) supports a concern regarding perceived constipation.** 3. Abdominal distention supports the presence of constipation, not perceived constipation. 4. Straining at stool supports the presence of constipation, not perceived constipation.

Continued

Eliminate incorrect options.	Perceived constipation has no relationship with the characteristics of stool, but it is related to the use of an enema or laxative to ensure a daily bowel movement. The clinical findings in options 1, 3, and 4 are associated with characteristics related to actual, not perceived, constipation. Options 1, 3, and 4 can be eliminated.

5.

CRITICAL-THINKING STRATEGY

Recognize keywords.	A nurse must administer a **sedative** to a client **before surgery. Which should the nurse do first**?
Ask what the question is asking.	Which intervention is necessary before giving a preoperative sedative?
Critically analyze each option in relation to the question and the other options.	Review the components of a preoperative checklist and the legal implications of a preoperative consent form in relation to the administration of a sedative. **Rationales:** 1. Although checking the preoperative checklist is done, it is not the priority. Usually, it is done last before the intraoperative period. **2. The consent for surgery must be signed before preoperative medications are administered because they depress the central nervous system, impairing problem-solving and decision-making.** 3. Ensuring placement of an IV line is unnecessary. This can be done at any time during the preoperative phase or at the beginning of the intraoperative phase of surgery. 4. Although assessing vital signs is done, it is not the priority.
Eliminate incorrect options.	Options 1, 3, and 4 are unrelated to when a presurgical sedative is administered; all these interventions can be done immediately before surgery and before or after the sedative is administered. Options 1, 3, and 4 can be eliminated.

6.

CRITICAL-THINKING STRATEGY

Recognize keywords.	A primary health-care provider prescribes **500 mg** of an antibiotic to be administered IV piggyback (IVPB) every 6 hours for a client with an infection. The **vial dispensed** by the hospital pharmacist **contains 1 g** of the prescribed antibiotic in powder form. The instructions on the vial state, "**Instill 9.6 mL to yield 10 mL.**" How many milliliters of the antibiotic should the nurse **add to the IVPB bag**? Record your answer **using a whole number.**
Ask what the question is asking.	Compute the dose of the prescribed medication.

Continued

Continued

| Critically analyze each option in relation to the question and the other options. | Use a mathematical formula to convert milligrams to grams. Then use a mathematical formula to compute the correct dose of medication prescribed. The information you need to insert into the formula is the Desired (prescribed: 500 mg [0.5 g]) dose and what you Have (how the medication is supplied: 1 g/10 mL).

Rationale:
Answer: 5 mL.
Use ratio and proportion to first convert 500 mg to its equivalent in grams. In the formula, the "have" is the memorized equivalent of 1,000 milligrams and is equal to 1 gram.

$$\frac{\text{Desired}}{\text{Have}}\ \frac{500\ mg}{1{,}000\ mg} = \frac{x\ gram\ (g)}{1\ g}$$
$$1{,}000x = 500$$
$$x = 500 \div 1{,}000$$
$$x = 0.5\ g\ (\text{is equal to } 500\ mg)$$

Now proceed to solve the problem by using ratio and proportion. In the formula, the "have" is the dose (1 g) in the resulting solution in the vial (10 mL).

$$\frac{\text{Desired}}{\text{Have}}\ \frac{0.5\ g}{1\ g} = \frac{x\ mL}{10\ mL}$$
$$1x = 0.5 \times 10$$
$$x = 5\ mL$$ |
| Eliminate incorrect options. | There is no need to eliminate options because this is a fill-in-the-blank question. |

7.

CRITICAL-THINKING STRATEGY

Recognize keywords.	A nurse in charge of a surgical unit is reviewing the progress of a variety of clients from the date of surgery to predict the potential date of discharge from the unit. Which of the following should the nurse use to **assess the clients' progress** as a **cost-containment strategy** in managed care?
Ask what the question is asking.	Which is a cost-containment measure that manages and documents a client's progress through the health-care system?
Critically analyze each option in relation to the question and the other options.	Recall the definition and components of each of the presented options. Determine which is a strategy that facilitates tracking a client's progress as a cost-containment measure. **Rationales:** 1. Primary nursing is not a cost-containment strategy in managed care but rather a nursing-care delivery system that ensures a comprehensive and consistent approach to identifying and meeting clients' needs. Primary nursing occurs when one nurse is assigned the 24-hour responsibility for the planning and delivery of nursing care to a specific client for the duration of the client's hospitalization.

Continued

	2. **Critical pathways are a case management system that identifies specific protocols and timetables for care and treatment by various disciplines that are designed to achieve expected client outcomes within a specific time frame. The purpose is to discharge clients sooner, thereby reducing the cost of health care.**
	3. Functional method refers to a model of nursing-care delivery that assigns a specific task for a group of clients to one person. Although it is efficient, it is impersonal and contributes to fragmentation of care because it is task oriented rather than client centered.
	4. Quality improvement refers to a program designed to increase the quality of care delivered to clients. Also, it includes an educational component to support growth and provide for corrective action.
Eliminate incorrect options.	Options 1 and 3 are two different types of nursing-care delivery and are not strategies that track a client's progress through the health-care system. Option 4 addresses ongoing activities designed to improve the quality of health care. Options 1, 3, and 4 can be eliminated.

8.

CRITICAL-THINKING STRATEGY

Recognize keywords.	A nurse is **assisting with a bed bath** for a client who has **moderate cognitive deficits**. Which is **important** for the nurse **to do**?
Ask what the question is asking.	Which must the nurse do to safely ensure that a client with moderate cognitive deficits receives an adequate bath?
Critically analyze each option in relation to the question and the other options.	Integrate what a client with moderate cognitive deficits can and cannot do, that daily-living activities must be accomplished adequately and safely, and that nursing care must address a client's physical, emotional, and mental needs. **Rationales:** 1. Explaining about the bath in detail may precipitate anxiety. A client with moderate cognitive deficits does not have the cognitive ability or attention span to comprehend a detailed explanation before a procedure. 2. The client has a problem with cognition, not vision. 3. **Give simple, direct statements when progressing through each aspect of the bath to limit the number of incoming stimuli at one time. This will promote comprehension and self-care.** 4. Clients with moderate cognitive deficits do not have the cognitive ability to perform a procedure independently. The client should be supervised.
Eliminate incorrect options.	Options 1 and 4 are unrealistic for a client with moderate cognitive deficits. Although option 2 should be done, it will not ensure an adequate bath. Options 1, 2, and 4 can be eliminated.

9.

CRITICAL-THINKING STRATEGY

Recognize keywords.	When the nurse is interviewing the wife of a client, **which statement** about the client's husband **supports** the presence of **obstructive sleep apnea**?
Ask what the question is asking.	Which statement describes a clinical finding related to obstructive sleep apnea?
Critically analyze each option in relation to the question and the other options.	Distinguish among behaviors associated with obstructive sleep apnea versus other sleep disorders. **Rationales:** 1. **Episodes of sleep apnea begin with loud snoring followed by silence, during which the person struggles to breathe against a blocked airway. Decreasing oxygen levels cause the person to awaken abruptly with a loud snort.** 2. Falling asleep abruptly describes narcolepsy, which is a sudden overwhelming sleepiness (hypersomnia) in the daytime. 3. Kicking and thrashing describe restless legs syndrome, a feeling of creeping or itching sensation occurring in the lower extremities that causes an irresistible urge to move and kick the legs. 4. Dreams that cause fear describe nightmares. Nightmares are vivid, frightening dreams that occur during rapid eye movement sleep and awaken the sleeper. 5. **Clients with obstructive sleep apnea usually are not aware of awakening during an episode.**
Eliminate incorrect options.	Options 2, 3, and 4 are descriptions of narcolepsy, restless legs syndrome, and nightmares, respectively. Options 2, 3, and 4 can be eliminated.

10.

CRITICAL-THINKING STRATEGY

Recognize keywords.	A nurse identifies that a client's **breath has a sweet, fruity odor**. **Which** of the following **should the nurse do next**?
Ask what the question is asking.	What should the nurse do first after identifying that the client has a sweet, fruity odor to the breath?
Critically analyze each option in relation to the question and the other options.	Recall that a sweet, fruity odor to the breath is a clinical manifestation of hyperglycemia by using inductive reasoning (i.e., making a broad generalization from a specific observation). Once you identify that the client may be experiencing hyperglycemia, examine all the options in light of this conclusion. **Rationales:** 1. Hyperglycemia does not affect the blood pressure. However, the heart rate may be increased. 2. Although this eventually may be done, it is not the first nursing intervention because it will take time to review the intake and output record. With hyperglycemia, the client will have a negative fluid balance; the output will exceed the intake.

Continued

	3. Although this eventually may be done, it is not the first nursing intervention. It will take time to collect the equipment for this procedure and perform the procedure. Of course, a serum glucose level will confirm the presence of hyperglycemia. **4. Sweet, fruity-smelling breath is an indicator of ketoacidosis, which can result from hyperglycemia. The nurse is at the bedside and should assess the client for additional clinical manifestations of hyperglycemia, such as fatigue, weakness, headache, thirst, blurred vision, nausea, and confusion.**
Eliminate incorrect options.	After examining all the options, focus on option 4 because it is global in nature. Options 2 and 3 may be done to identify clinical manifestations of hyperglycemia, and therefore these interventions fall under the action identified in option 4. Eliminate option 1 because a change in blood pressure is not directly related to hyperglycemia.

11.

CRITICAL-THINKING STRATEGY

Recognize keywords.	A nurse is caring for a client who has had diarrhea for several weeks. For which **common problem associated with prolonged diarrhea** should the nurse assess the client?
Ask what the question is asking.	Which common problem is caused by prolonged diarrhea?
Critically analyze each option in relation to the question and the other options.	Explore the consequences of diarrhea and identify the most common human response to diarrhea. Consider Maslow's Hierarchy of Needs when analyzing these options. **Rationales:** **1. Diarrhea is related directly to a risk for damage to epidermal and dermal tissue. The gastric and intestinal enzymes present in feces are acids capable of eroding the skin.** 2. Diarrhea is unrelated to the ability to provide self-care. The inability to care for self is the state in which the individual experiences an impaired motor or cognitive function, causing a decreased ability to perform the activities of daily living (e.g., bathing, grooming, dressing, and eating). 3. Diarrhea is not related directly to sexual dysfunction, which is the state in which an individual experiences, or is at risk of experiencing, a change in sexual function that is viewed as unrewarding or inadequate. 4. Diarrhea is not related directly to body image disturbance, which is the state in which an individual experiences, or is at risk of experiencing, a disruption in the way one perceives one's body image.
Eliminate incorrect options.	Preventing skin breakdown in option 1 is addressing a physiological need, which is a first-level need when compared with later-level needs, such as sexuality and body image. Just because a client has diarrhea does not mean that the person cannot provide self-care, and there are no data that indicate the client is dependent. Eliminate option 2. Although sexual dysfunction and disturbed body image can occur with prolonged diarrhea, they are not as common as skin breakdown. Options 3 and 4 can be eliminated.

12.

CRITICAL-THINKING STRATEGY

Recognize keywords.	A nurse causes harm to a **hospitalized client** because of **improper use of a mechanical lift**. Based on **which specific tort** can this client **pursue legal action**?
Ask what the question is asking.	Which tort is associated with unsafe care administered to a hospitalized client that results in harm to the client?
Critically analyze each option in relation to the question and the other options.	Review the definitions and examples of situations that relate to the torts in each option. Identify which tort relates to the client situation presented in the question. **Rationales:** 1. This situation is not an example of battery. Battery is the purposeful, angry, or negligent touching of a client without consent. 2. This situation is not an example of assault. Assault is an attempt, or threat, to touch another person unjustly. 3. Although negligence occurs when a nurse's actions do not meet appropriate standards of care and result in injury to another, this term is not as specific as another term. **4. Malpractice is misconduct via an act of commission or omission performed in professional practice that results in harm to another. Under a malpractice charge, the nurse and the client have a professional nurse-client relationship.**
Eliminate incorrect options.	Options 1 and 2 include intentional behaviors that are a threat to touch another unjustifiably (assault) or actual touching another unjustifiably (battery). Option 3 is a tort that does not address behaviors within a professional relationship. Options 1, 2, and 3 can be eliminated.

13.

CRITICAL-THINKING STRATEGY

Recognize keywords.	A client with **type 2 diabetes** is experiencing **blurred vision, generalized weakness, and fatigue**. A nurse receives a report from the nurse on the previous shift and obtains **additional information from the client's clinical record. Which should the nurse conclude that the client is experiencing**?
Ask what the question is asking.	Which physiological response in the client is based on the information presented in the clinical record?
Critically analyze each option in relation to the question and the other options.	Analyze the information presented in the laboratory results, I&O record, and nursing progress record and determine if any of them are outside the norm. Then consider the information outside the norm in relation to each option to arrive at the correct answer. **Rationales:** 1. The client is not experiencing fluid retention. The urine output is almost twice the volume of the intake. With fluid retention, the skin is taut and shiny, the mucous membranes are moist, and the client will gain weight.

Continued

	2. Kidney impairment can be ruled out because the 4,200 mL of urinary output indicates that the kidneys are functioning. Also, with kidney impairment, generally there is weight gain, not loss. The blood uria nitrogen and creatinine levels are within the expected range and indicate that the kidneys are not impaired.
	3. The serum glucose value of 350 mg/dL is excessive and indicates a hyperglycemic event; the acceptable range is less than 110 mg/dL. A hemoglobin A$_{1c}$ level of 8% indicates inadequate glucose control over the past 90 to 120 days. The acceptable value for hemoglobin A$_{1c}$ for a person with diabetes mellitus is less than 7% (American Diabetes Association) or less than 6.5% (American Association of Clinical Endocrinologists). The acceptable range for hemoglobin A$_{1c}$ in a person without diabetes mellitus is 4.0% to 5.5%.
	4. There are no data to support the conclusion that this event is a hypertensive episode. With the degree of polyuria, "tenting of skin," and dry mucous membranes, hypotension resulting from dehydration, not hypertension, is expected.
Eliminate incorrect options.	The data presented do not support the problems in options 1, 2, and 4. See rationales for explanations. Eliminate options 1, 2, and 4.

14.

CRITICAL-THINKING STRATEGY

Recognize keywords.	**Nurses** on a unit are personally and **professionally mature and motivated. Which one** of the following **classic leadership styles should the nurse manager employ** when working with this group?
Ask what the question is asking.	Which classic leadership style works best when nurses are mature and motivated?
Critically analyze each option in relation to the question and the other options.	Review the descriptions of leadership styles and explore the situations in which each works best. Then select the style that works best in the situation presented. **Rationales:** 1. Directive is not one of the four classic leadership styles. 2. The autocratic leadership style probably is the least effective style to use with a professionally mature and motivated staff. Autocratic leaders give orders and make decisions for the group. There is little freedom and a large degree of control by the leader, which frustrates motivated, professionally mature staff members. 3. The democratic leadership style is the second-best style from among the presented options to use when staff is motivated and professionally mature. The democratic style offers fewer opportunities for autonomy for staff members who are mature and motivated than a leadership style in another option. **4. The laissez-faire leadership style is appropriate for a group of individuals who have an internal locus of control and desire autonomy and independence. Individuals who are professionally mature and motivated more often have an internal locus of control.**

Continued

Continued

| Eliminate incorrect options. | Option 1 is not a leadership style. Option 2 is too dictatorial for individuals with an internal locus of control. Although option 3 is more independent than an autocratic style, it is more restricted than a laissez-faire style. Eliminate options 1, 2, and 3. |

15.

CRITICAL-THINKING STRATEGY

Recognize keywords.	A nurse transfers a client from a bed to a wheelchair. **Which should the nurse do after** placing the **client in the wheelchair**?
Ask what the question is asking.	Which action is essential when a client is in a wheelchair?
Critically analyze each option in relation to the question and the other options.	List the steps of the procedure—transferring a client from a bed to a wheelchair. Then compare the steps in the procedure to the behavior in each option. Finally, you must identify the option that reflects a safe, correct action by the nurse. **Rationales:** 1. **Pressure on the popliteal areas can cause damage to nerves and interfere with circulation; it must be avoided.** 2. The transfer belt should be removed after the transfer is completed. 3. A pillow will move the client too close to the front of the seat and is unsafe. 4. The client's feet should be positioned flat on the footrests of the wheelchair, not the floor, to protect the feet if the wheelchair is moved.
Eliminate incorrect options.	Options 3 and 4 are both unsafe interventions and may jeopardize the client. Option 2 is unnecessary and may be uncomfortable for the client. Eliminate options 2, 3, and 4.

16.

CRITICAL-THINKING STRATEGY

Recognize keywords.	A nurse identifies a **client's perception of health.** **Which should the nurse do as a result of obtaining this information**?
Ask what the question is asking.	Which should a nurse do after learning about the client's beliefs about health?
Critically analyze each option in relation to the question and the other options.	Appreciate that health beliefs are specific to the individual. This concept must be analyzed in relation to the theories of Maslow's Hierarchy of Human Needs and the health-illness continuum. **Rationales:** 1. A healthy lifestyle can promote health and prevent some illness or even minimize complications; however, understanding a person's perceptions of health may not prevent responses to disease.

Continued

	2. A client's perceptions are only one part of the data that must be collected before the nurse can establish the priority of the client's needs. Maslow's Hierarchy of Human Needs helps the nurse to determine the client's needs in order of priority based on the collected data. 3. Only a client, not a nurse, can choose a client's place along the health-illness continuum. How people perceive themselves is subjective and is influenced by their own attitudes, values, and beliefs. **4. Health perception reflects a person's knowledge, behavior, and attitudes regarding illness, disease prevention, health promotion, and what constitutes a healthy lifestyle. This information, in addition to related information, captures the uniqueness of each individual and provides essential data that must be considered before needs are identified and a plan formulated.**
Eliminate incorrect options.	Options 1, 2, and 3 are incorrect statements, as indicated in their rationales, and can be eliminated.

17.

CRITICAL-THINKING STRATEGY

Recognize keywords.	An older adult asks the nurse, "I want to make sure I get enough vitamin A to keep my eyes healthy. Which fruits can I eat because I am not fond of vegetables?" **Which of the following** should the nurse explain **is an excellent source of vitamin A?**
Ask what the question is asking.	Which fruit is high in vitamin A content?
Critically analyze each option in relation to the question and the other options.	Recall how much vitamin A is contained in each nutrient and then compare and contrast the nutrients among the options. The options with high vitamin A content are the correct answers. **Rationales:** **1. Cantaloupe is an excellent source of vitamin A. A half cup of melon balls contains approximately 2,993 International Units of vitamin A.** **2. Apricots are an excellent source of vitamin A. A 3½-ounce serving of apricots contains approximately 7,240 International Units of vitamin A.** **3. Peaches are an excellent source of vitamin A. A 3½-ounce serving of peaches contains approximately 2,160 International Units of vitamin A.** 4. Raisins are not high in vitamin A. A 3½-ounce serving of raisins contains approximately 10 International Units of vitamin A. **5. Prunes are an excellent source of vitamin A. A 3½-ounce serving of prunes contains approximately 1,990 International Units of vitamin A.**
Eliminate incorrect options.	Option 4 can be eliminated because raisins contain only small amounts of vitamin A. Larger amounts of vitamin A are contained in the fruits in options 1, 2, 3, and 5.

18.

CRITICAL-THINKING STRATEGY

Recognize keywords.	A nurse is caring for several clients who have different cultural backgrounds and are under stress. Which is an **important concept** that the nurse must consider **when making assessments about these clients' nonverbal behavior**?
Ask what the question is asking.	Which statement about nonverbal behavior that influences nursing assessments is important?
Critically analyze each option in relation to the question and the other options.	Review these statements about nonverbal behavior, and determine their accuracy. Then select the option that is a true statement. **Rationales:** 1. Nonverbal behavior is controlled more by the unconscious than by the conscious mind. 2. Nonverbal behavior carries more, not less, weight than verbal interactions because nonverbal behavior is influenced more by factors not under the client's control. **3. Transculturally, nonverbal communication varies widely. For example, gestures, facial expressions, eye contact, and touch may reflect opposite messages among cultures and among individuals within a culture.** 4. The opposite is true. Nonverbal behaviors often directly reflect feelings.
Eliminate incorrect options.	Options 1, 2, and 4 can be eliminated because the statements in the options are incorrect, as indicated in the rationales.

19.

CRITICAL-THINKING STRATEGY

Recognize keywords.	A nurse is administering an intramuscular injection at the client's **ventrogluteal site**. Which action should the nurse implement to help **landmark this site**?
Ask what the question is asking.	Which action helps to identify where a ventrogluteal intramuscular injection should be inserted?
Critically analyze each option in relation to the question and the other options.	List the steps in the procedure that landmark the ventrogluteal injection site. Then identify the specific action included in one of the options that relates to the ventrogluteal site. **Rationales:** 1. The lower edge of the acromion and the midpoint of the lateral aspect of the arm are anatomical landmarks that help to identify the deltoid muscle. 2. The line from the posterior superior iliac spine to the greater trochanter is an anatomical landmark that helps to identify the dorsogluteal site. **3. Placing the heel of the hand on the greater trochanter is the initial placement of the hand when identifying landmarks for the ventrogluteal site.** 4. Palpating the anterior lateral aspect of the thigh is associated with identifying the vastus lateralis site. It is between one handbreadth above the knee and one handbreadth below the greater trochanter on the anterior lateral aspect of the thigh.
Eliminate incorrect options.	Options 1, 2, and 4 are options that present steps that are related to sites other than the ventrogluteal site and can be eliminated.

20.

CRITICAL-THINKING STRATEGY

Recognize keywords.	A nurse is caring for a group of four clients. The client with **which clinical manifestation requires immediate attention** from the nurse?
Ask what the question is asking.	Identify the vital sign that indicates a problem based on the information in the related option scenario.
Critically analyze each option in relation to the question and the other options.	Identify the expected range of each vital sign. Identify the vital signs that are outside the expected range. Examine the situations associated with each vital sign that is outside the expected range and determine if the response is consistent with the situation and not a cause for concern. Identify the unexpected vital sign that indicates a problem in light of the information in the option scenario. Refer to the concepts associated with the ABCs (Airway, Breathing, and Circulation) to help you focus on the correct answer. No option is associated with Airway, but option 4 is associated with breathing. **Rationales:** 1. An elevated temperature is expected with an infection because the hypothalamus is responding to the pathogens that are present. 2. In the immediate postoperative period, the pulse may be elevated because of blood loss. This pulse should be assessed in conjunction with the blood pressure. 3. This is an expected response when one moves from the sitting to the standing position, because venous return slows as blood pools in the lower extremities until the vasomotor response of the body compensates. **4. The expected respiratory rate is 12 to 20 breaths per minute. The respiratory rate should return to baseline within 3 minutes after activity. A respiratory rate greater than 24 breaths per minute after 3 minutes of rest following activity indicates activity intolerance.**
Eliminate incorrect options.	The clinical manifestations in options 1, 2, and 3 are not unexpected based on the information presented in each option scenario. Option 4 is the correct answer because an elevated respiratory rate after 3 minutes of rest is unexpected and indicates an activity intolerance.

21.

CRITICAL-THINKING STRATEGY

Recognize keywords.	A client has a diagnosis of **osteoporosis**. **Which of the following** should the nurse encourage this client to **eat**?
Ask what the question is asking.	Which nutrient facilitates bone maintenance?
Critically analyze each option in relation to the question and the other options.	Recall that osteoporosis is the reduction of bone mass and that an increase in calcium will support bone maintenance. Recall how much calcium is contained in each nutrient, and then compare and contrast the nutrients among the options. The options with the higher calcium content are the correct answers.

Continued

Continued

	Rationales:
	1. Rice, regardless of the type, is not high in calcium. One cup of rice contains approximately 5 to 33 mg of calcium.
	2. Milk and products made with milk, such as various forms of cheese, are an excellent source of calcium. Eight ounces of 1% low-fat milk contain approximately 290 mg of calcium. Eight ounces of 2% reduced-fat milk contain approximately 285 mg of calcium.
	3. Yogurt is an excellent source of calcium. Eight ounces of yogurt contain approximately 400 mg to 450 mg of calcium.
	4. Sardines, which contain soft, edible bones, are an excellent source of dietary calcium. Three ounces of sardines contain approximately 371 mg of calcium.
	5. Almonds are an excellent source of calcium. One ounce of almonds (about 24) contains approximately 75 mg of calcium.
	6. Tomatoes are not high in calcium. One tomato (2¾ inches in diameter) contains approximately 9 mg of calcium.
Eliminate incorrect options.	Options 1 and 6 can be eliminated because these foods contain small amounts of calcium compared with the amounts of calcium in foods from options 2, 3, 4, and 5.

22.

CRITICAL-THINKING STRATEGY

Recognize keywords.	A nurse must obtain a **urine specimen** from a client with a **urinary retention catheter** (Foley) and **explains the procedure** to the client. **Which should the nurse do next?**
Ask what the question is asking.	What should the nurse do first when collecting a urine specimen from a urinary retention catheter?
Critically analyze each option in relation to the question and the other options.	List the step-by-step procedure for collecting a specimen from a urinary retention catheter. Then analyze the four options and select the option that reflects the next step of the procedure after explaining the procedure to the client.
	Rationales:
	1. Urine specimens from a retention catheter should not come from the urine collection bag because this urine has been collected over time and is not reflective of the client's present status.
	2. The drainage tubing should be clamped 1 to 2 inches below the aspiration port for 15 to 20 minutes to allow urine to accumulate. This urine is the most recently excreted urine and will reflect the client's present status.
	3. Positioning the client in the high-Fowler position is unnecessary. Positioning the client in the semi-Fowler position is done later in the procedure if necessary. The semi-Fowler position moves urine toward the triangular area at the base of the bladder where the urethra enters the bladder (trigone). The urinary retention catheter passes through the urinary meatus and the urethra and remains in place in the area of the trigone after inflation of the catheter balloon.

Continued

	4. Sterile gloves are not necessary to perform this procedure. However, the nurse should wear clean gloves. Wearing personal protective equipment, such as clean gloves, is a medical asepsis practice. Gloves protect the nurse from the client's body fluids because the catheter is close to the perineal area and there is a potential for exposure to urine during the procedure.
Eliminate incorrect options.	Options 1 and 4 are not steps in this procedure. Option 3 is a step that is performed later in the procedure. Options 1, 3, and 4 can be eliminated.

23.

CRITICAL-THINKING STRATEGY

Recognize keywords.	A nurse is caring for a client who is **incontinent of stool**. Which **action** should **the nurse implement**?
Ask what the question is asking.	Which nursing intervention is needed because microorganisms and enzymes are irritating to the skin?
Critically analyze each option in relation to the question and the other options.	This statement requires the integration of several concepts: microorganisms are irritating to the skin; enzymes are irritating to the skin; and moisture barriers can protect the skin from irritating substances. To eliminate the other options, identify that they are either an inaccurate statement or are unrelated to the consequence of fecal incontinence. **Rationales:** 1. Clean gloves are adequate. **2. A skin barrier protects the skin from the digestive enzymes in feces.** 3. Cranberry juice makes urine more alkaline; it does not influence bacteria and enzymes in stool. 4. Clients should attempt to have a bowel movement after a meal to take advantage of the gastrocolic reflex.
Eliminate incorrect options.	The focus is on the connection between factors that irritate the skin and what can be done to prevent it. Option 1 is an inaccurate statement because sterile gloves are not necessary to obtain a stool specimen for culture and sensitivity. Option 3 may help minimize the risk of a urinary tract infection but is unrelated to preventing irritation of the skin due to fecal incontinence. Option 4 is unrelated to preventing irritation of the skin. Toileting before meals is more appropriate for promoting urinary elimination so that the need to void does not interrupt the meal. Toileting after meals often is done to promote fecal elimination by taking advantage of the gastrocolic reflex. Options 1, 3, and 4 can be eliminated.

24.

CRITICAL-THINKING STRATEGY

Recognize keywords.	Which should the nurse **teach a client** when the primary health-care provider prescribes **ibuprofen, an NSAID,** for pain?
Ask what the question is asking.	What should the nurse teach the client about ibuprofen?
Critically analyze each option in relation to the question and the other options.	Recall concerns associated with the intake of NSAIDs. Identify the statements in options that are applicable to the intake of ibuprofen (an NSAID). **Rationales:** 1. **Remaining in an upright position keeps the medication in the stomach, which prevents regurgitation. If ibuprofen dissolves in the esophagus, it will irritate the lining of the esophagus.** 2. Ibuprofen is not addictive. 3. Food interferes with the absorption of ibuprofen. Ibuprofen should be taken 30 minutes before a meal or 2 hours after a meal. If gastrointestinal disturbances occur, then it can be taken with food to minimize gastric irritation. Not all clients develop gastrointestinal disturbances. 4. **Water ensures that the medication reaches the stomach and dilutes the medication in the stomach.** 5. It is not necessary to monitor the blood pressure daily because ibuprofen does not affect the blood pressure.
Eliminate incorrect options.	Eliminate options 2, 3, and 5 because these statements are incorrect in relation to ibuprofen. Eliminate options 2, 3, and 5.

25.

CRITICAL-THINKING STRATEGY

Recognize keywords.	A primary health-care provider prescribes a **2-g sodium diet** for a client. Which **fluid** should the nurse teach is **high in sodium**?
Ask what the question is asking.	Which fluid is high in sodium content?
Critically analyze each option in relation to the question and the other options.	Identify the sodium content of a variety of fluids. Compare and contrast the fluids in the options presented, and identify the options with the high sodium content. **Rationales:** 1. **Cocoa powder, containing nonfat dry milk, contains approximately 173 mg of sodium when mixed with 6 ounces of water and should be avoided when on a 2-g sodium diet.** 2. Seltzer contains no sodium and is permitted on a 2-g sodium diet. 3. Twelve fluid ounces of lemonade contains approximately 12 mg of sodium and is permitted on a 2-g sodium diet. 4. **One cup of low-fat milk contains approximately 103 mg of sodium and should not be included in large amounts on a 2-g sodium diet.** 5. **One cup of tomato juice contains approximately 877 mg of sodium and should be avoided on a 2-g sodium diet.**
Eliminate incorrect options.	Options 2 and 3 can be eliminated because these fluids contain no sodium or small amounts of sodium compared with the large amounts of sodium in the fluids presented in options 1, 4, and 5.

26.

CRITICAL-THINKING STRATEGY

Recognize keywords.	A nurse is caring for a client in the postanesthesia care unit. For which **most serious complication of intubation** associated with the administration of general anesthesia should the nurse assess this client?
Ask what the question is asking.	What is the most serious potential consequence of intubation?
Critically analyze each option in relation to the question and the other options.	First, define each problem and recall the cause of each. Then explore each problem in relation to the stress of intubation. Finally, compare and contrast the problems and determine which is the most serious. The concept of airway, breathing, and circulation can be applied when the question requires you to prioritize information. **Rationales:** 1. Although inflammation of the mouth (stomatitis) can occur from irritation caused by the tube used for delivering general anesthesia, it is uncommon and not life-threatening. 2. Although atelectasis is serious, it is not as serious as a response in another option. Anesthesia delivered by intubation can interfere with the action of surfactant, resulting in the collapse of alveoli (atelectasis). 3. Although the tube used for intubation commonly does irritate the posterior oropharynx, resulting in a sore throat, a sore throat is not as serious as a response in another option. **4. Laryngeal spasm is a potentially life-threatening complication because it prevents the exchange of gases between the lungs and the atmosphere. Laryngeal spasm can result from irritation caused by the presence of the intubation tube in the space between the vocal cords (glottis) during surgery.**
Eliminate incorrect options.	All of the options can occur, but their consequences vary in severity. Options 1 and 3 can be eliminated first because they are similar and not life-threatening. Although atelectasis (in option 2) will compromise respiratory function, it is not an obstruction of the airway and therefore can be eliminated.

27.

CRITICAL-THINKING STRATEGY

Recognize keywords.	A nurse is assessing a client who is experiencing pain. **Which statement** by the client does the nurse determine **reflects the quality of** the client's **pain**?
Ask what the question is asking.	Which client statement is related to the quality of pain?
Critically analyze each option in relation to the question and the other options.	First, review the characteristics of pain; for example, intensity, location, quality, pattern (i.e., onset, duration, exacerbation, and remission). Then identify the characteristic of pain that is reflected in each client statement. Compare and contrast the statements to identify the one that reflects the quality of pain.

Continued

Continued

	Rationales:
	1. This statement reflects the intensity of pain. The intensity of pain refers to the strength or amount of pain experienced, which often is rated from mild to excruciating. Pain scales (e.g., numerical scale, Wong-Baker FACES Rating Scale) can facilitate the assessment of the intensity of pain.
	2. This statement reflects the location of pain. Location refers to the actual site where the pain is felt.
	3. This statement reflects the quality of pain. Quality refers to the description of the pain sensation.
	4. This statement refers to the pattern of pain. The pattern of pain is concerned with the time of onset, duration, recurrence, and remissions associated with the pain experience.
Eliminate incorrect options.	Option 1 relates to the intensity or severity of the pain. Option 2 is related to the location of pain. Option 4 relates to onset and duration of pain. Options 1, 2, and 4 can be eliminated because none of them refers to the quality of pain.

28.

CRITICAL-THINKING STRATEGY

Recognize keywords.	A nurse places a client who had **abdominal surgery** in the **semi-Fowler position**. The client states, "I **prefer to lie flat** when in bed. I feel like I am almost sitting up." Which is an **appropriate response by the nurse**?
Ask what the question is asking.	Why is it beneficial for a client who had abdominal surgery to be placed in the semi-Fowler position?
Critically analyze each option in relation to the question and the other options.	First, establish the relationship between abdominal surgery and the semi-Fowler position. Then explore nursing interventions that achieve the outcome identified in each option. Then connect the information among abdominal surgery, the semi-Fowler position, and each option. **Rationales** **1. In the semi-Fowler position, the abdominal organs drop by gravity, which permits maximum thoracic excursion. In addition, slight flexion of the hips reduces abdominal muscle tension, which limits pressure on the suture line and facilitates diaphragmatic (abdominal) breathing.** 2. Resting in bed in any position promotes flatus retention. Ambulation promotes intestinal motility, which promotes the passage of flatus. 3. Resting in bed in any position results in decreased detrusor muscle tone, incomplete bladder emptying, and urinary stasis. Ambulation uses gravity and activity to promote urinary elimination. Activity increases circulation to the kidneys, which increases the glomerular filtration rate, resulting in an increase in urine excretion. 4. The semi-Fowler position does not facilitate drainage via a portable wound drainage system. Although negative pressure creates the vacuum that draws fluid into a portable wound drainage system, the collection container should be lower than the insertion site because its negative pressure does not have to work against gravity.

Continued

Eliminate incorrect options.	For each option, compare your list of nursing interventions that should accomplish the objective stated in the option. If the semi-Fowler position was not on your list, that option can be eliminated. Eliminate options 2, 3, and 4.

29.

CRITICAL-THINKING STRATEGY

Recognize keywords.	A nurse is coordinating discharge planning for an older adult who is recovering from a neurological event that left the client with **significant right-sided weakness**. The client and the spouse express **concerns about** the limitations of their **health insurance, the rehabilitation process, and the prescribed low-cholesterol, 2-g sodium diet. Which individual should the nurse include in a** health-care **team conference when planning for this client's discharge needs**?
Ask what the question is asking.	According to the client's needs identified in the scenario, which professional health team member is educationally prepared to participate in developing a plan of care?
Critically analyze each option in relation to the question and the other options.	Recall the role and scope of practice of each individual identified in the options. Recall whether each is professionally educated to be involved in planning to meet the needs of a client after discharge. Identify only the health-care professionals required to address the discharge concerns presented in the scenario. **Rationales:** 1. **The client is the center of the health-care team and is the most essential participant in discharge planning. The spouse also may be invited to participate because the spouse will be instrumental in caring for the client.** 2. **A social worker is an important member of the client's health-care team. This professional can assist the couple to identify resources to help with their needs and finances.** 3. **A registered dietitian is an important member of the client's health-care team because the client and the spouse express concerns about the prescribed diet. The couple will need assistance in learning to identify foods to avoid those that are high in cholesterol and sodium.** 4. A respiratory therapist is a nonessential professional needed at this time. No data indicate that the client or the spouse is concerned about the client's respiratory status. 5. **The home health-care nurse should be included in discharge planning because this nurse will be responsible for coordinating the members of the home health-care team as well as fulfilling many roles, such as counselor, teacher, caregiver, and, most importantly, advocate.** 6. Although a home health nurse's aide is a member of the health-care team, this person does not have the education necessary to be involved in the planning phase of this client's discharge planning. The home health-care nurse is responsible for assigning a home health nurse's aide to implement nonprofessional activities such as bathing, toileting, ambulating, and feeding the client.

Continued

Continued

Eliminate incorrect options.	Eliminate option 4 (respiratory therapist) because no data in the scenario support the claim that the client has a respiratory problem. Eliminate option 6 (home health nurse's aide) because developing a client's discharge plan is outside the scope of practice of a home health nurse's aide. Only health-care professionals are educationally prepared to engage in planning activities.

30.

CRITICAL-THINKING STRATEGY

Recognize keywords.	A primary health-care provider writes the **prescription** *Client may shower* for a client receiving home care. When the nurse is preparing the client for the shower, the **client reports feeling weak and very dizzy**. The nurse determines that the client will not tolerate standing for a shower safely. **Which should the nurse do**?
Ask what the question is asking.	Which change in the client's hygiene plan of care ensures safety when the client reports feeling weak and very dizzy?
Critically analyze each option in relation to the question and the other options.	Explore the ramifications of each type of bath for a client who reports feeling weak and very dizzy. Determine which bath is most appropriate to ensure safety while still supporting independence. **Rationales:** 1. Transferring a client who is weak and dizzy to a commode chair for a shower is unsafe because the client may fall. Also, warm water flowing over the entire body will dilate blood vessels, increasing blood flow to the periphery rather than to central organs and the brain. This effect can increase the physical demands on the body and intensify the dizziness, and it may even result in unconsciousness. **2. The client should remain in bed because feeling weak and dizzy are contraindications for getting out of bed. Assisting the client with the bath allows the client to remain as independent as possible while ensuring that the client's hygiene needs are met. The nurse changed the plan of care based on the current status of the client.** 3. Transferring a client who is weak and dizzy to a chair in front of a sink is unsafe because the client may fall. 4. Assisting this client into a bathtub is unsafe because the client is weak and dizzy and may fall. A bath in a bathtub requires a prescription.
Eliminate incorrect options.	Eliminate option 1 because this action fosters dependence rather than independence. Eliminate options 3 and 4 because these options are unsafe when considering the reported weakness and feelings of dizziness.

31.

CRITICAL-THINKING STRATEGY

Recognize keywords.	A **nurse arrives** on the unit **during the last 5 minutes of a 20-minute change-of-shift report** for the **second time** within a week. **How should the nurse in charge handle this situation**?
Ask what the question is asking.	How should the nurse in charge respond to an employee who arrives late for work several times?
Critically analyze each option in relation to the question and the other options.	Examine each option, recognizing that the nurse manager must address the nurse's lateness immediately. A delayed response may be perceived by the offender as acceptance of the negative behavior. Recall the purpose of an incident report. **Rationales:** 1. An incident report is not the appropriate format to document this event. Incident reports are used to document unusual events associated with the performance of health-care activities. They include events such as falls, medication or treatment errors, omissions of care, and any situations that cause an injury to a client, visitor, or staff member. 2. The nurse's lateness should not be ignored because it is the second time it has happened. 3. Waiting for a nurse's yearly performance evaluation is too long a time to wait to address the nurse's lateness. **4. The nurse's behavior should be addressed by the nurse manager and the expected behavior reinforced. Counseling sessions with employees should be confidential and conducted in private as soon as possible after the offending event.**
Eliminate incorrect options.	Option 1 can be eliminated because personnel matters are not documented in an incident report. Options 2 and 3 delay addressing the nurse's lateness. Eliminate options 1, 2, and 3.

32.

CRITICAL-THINKING STRATEGY

Recognize keywords.	A nurse hangs an IV piggyback (IVPB) of an **antibiotic**. Within a few minutes, the **client reports a thickening of the back of the tongue and swelling under the chin**. **Place** the following **interventions in** the **order** in which they should be implemented.
Ask what the question is asking.	What should a nurse do in order of priority when a client has an allergic reaction to an IV antibiotic?
Critically analyze each option in relation to the question and the other options.	Recall the steps that should be implemented in the event that the client has an allergic response to an IV antibiotic. Examine the options presented and compare them with your list of recalled steps. Place the options in order after this comparison. **Rationales:** **1. Discontinuing the IVPB should be implemented first because this is the agent that is causing the client's allergic response.**

Continued

Continued

	4. Pulling the bedside call light out of the wall generally initiates an emergency alarm and should be done second. Staff members are educated to immediately respond to such an alarm because it indicates a need for urgent assistance. The nurse requires help in implementing additional interventions.
	2. Once the first two interventions are implemented, the nurse must ensure that the client's airway is maintained and oxygen is administered.
	3. Instructing another staff member to call the rapid response team is the fourth intervention. Because a nurse should never leave the bedside of a client during an emergency, the nurse should instruct another staff member to initiate the rapid response team and bring the crash cart to the bedside. The rapid response team consists of a team of professionals representing various disciplines, such as a licensed medical professional, an anesthesiologist, a respiratory therapist, and a clinical nurse specialist. This team of professionals assembles quickly and delivers critical care in instances when a client's status deteriorates outside of a critical care area.
	5. Instructing another nurse to hang new IV tubing and an isotonic solution is the fifth intervention. This ensures that the IV line is free of the offending medication and available for the administration of emergency medication; in addition, the isotonic solution is nonoffensive.
	6. Preparing emergency medication according to protocol should be done last. This provides for a quick administration of emergency medication when prescribed by the appropriate licensed professional on the rapid response team.
Eliminate incorrect options.	No options are eliminated in an ordered-response item.

33.

CRITICAL-THINKING STRATEGY

Recognize keywords.	A newly admitted client arrives on the unit. Which is **most important** for the nurse to do to **help minimize the development of** this client's **anxiety**?
Ask what the question is asking.	Which action will limit anxiety in a newly hospitalized client?
Critically analyze each option in relation to the question and the other options.	The interventions in all the options may help reduce anxiety. The words *newly admitted* set a focus that must be addressed when analyzing the options. You are being asked to identify a priority action in relation to a parameter.
	Rationales:
	1. Although validating a client's feelings will help the client feel accepted, understood, and credible, there is no information indicating that the client is experiencing anxiety.
	2. Relaxation techniques are effective ways to reduce the autonomic nervous system response to a threat. However, they are not as effective as an intervention in another option.

Continued

	3. Minimizing environmental stimuli may support rest and sleep, which is an essential aspect of stress management in any setting. However, it is not as helpful as another option.
	4. Anxiety is a response to an unknown threat to the self or self-esteem. Therefore, explaining what, how, why, when, and where of procedures to the client will prevent and reduce anxiety by minimizing the unknown.
Eliminate incorrect options.	Option 1 may minimize anxiety after it occurs, not before. Options 2 and 3 are general interventions that address anxiety in any situation. Options 1, 2, and 3 can be eliminated.

34.

CRITICAL-THINKING STRATEGY

Recognize keywords.	A home health-care nurse is providing care for a client who was discharged from the hospital after receiving acute care for a brain attack (i.e., stroke, cerebrovascular accident). The client has left-sided hemiparesis, difficulty swallowing, and anxiety. **Which nursing intervention** reflects the **nurse's role of being a resource person**?
Ask what the question is asking.	Which nursing intervention is an example of the nurse working as a resource person?
Critically analyze each option in relation to the question and the other options.	Explore the behaviors of a nurse who is functioning as a resource person. Your list of behaviors should parallel the behavior in the correct option. **Rationales:**
	1. The health-care delivery system in the United States is complex and can be confusing at a time when a client has the least energy to explore and negotiate intervention options. When functioning as a resource person, the nurse identifies resources, provides information, and makes referrals.
	2. Encouraging the client to chew food thoroughly reflects the nurse's role of teacher.
	3. Teaching the client to use deep breathing exercises reflects the nurse's role of teacher.
	4. Instructing the client on how to use a walker reflects the nurse's role of teacher.
Eliminate incorrect options.	Review each option in relation to the list of behaviors you identified as related to being a resource person for a client. A resource person provides information and facilitates movement through the multidisciplinary health-care system. Options 2, 3, and 4 can be eliminated because these behaviors all are related to the nurse's role of a teacher.

35.

CRITICAL-THINKING STRATEGY

Recognize keywords.	Which client statement indicates to the nurse that an older adult understands the teaching about **how to care for dry skin effectively**?
Ask what the question is asking.	How should an older adult care for dry skin?
Critically analyze each option in relation to the question and the other options.	Only one option is correct because you are not asked to identify a priority action. Explore interventions that can prevent or care for dry skin, particularly in the older adult. Compare your list to the options presented. **Rationales:** 1. **The percentage of body water dramatically decreases with age, and older adults have altered thirst mechanisms that place them at risk for inadequate fluid intake and dehydration. In addition, the skin of older adults is drier because of a decreased ability to sweat and a decreased production of sebum.** 2. Lotion is preferable to baby powder because lotion lubricates the skin. Also, baby powder should be avoided because, when aerosolized, it is a respiratory irritant. 3. Having a bath daily, even when using a moisturizing soap, is drying to the skin of older adults. Bathing two to three times a week is adequate for an older adult who is continent of urine and feces. 4. Wool fabrics are coarse and irritate the skin; therefore, they should be avoided.
Eliminate incorrect options.	Option 2 can be eliminated because lotion is preferable to baby powder, which is a respiratory irritant. Having a daily bath is too drying for the skin of older adults. Eliminate option 3. Eliminate option 4 because it is an incorrect statement.

36.

CRITICAL-THINKING STRATEGY

Recognize keywords.	A client has a prescription for a **vaginal suppository. Which of the following should the nurse perform when administering** this medication?
Ask what the question is asking.	Which is a step in the procedure for administering a vaginal suppository?
Critically analyze each option in relation to the question and the other options.	List the steps in the procedure for administering a vaginal suppository. Compare the statements in the options with your list. **Rationales:** 1. **Lubricating the suppository and the index finger of a gloved hand facilitates insertion and limits trauma to vaginal mucous membranes.** 2. **Having the client remain flat in bed for 20 minutes will maintain the medication in place, which facilitates absorption.** 3. Perineal care, not a vaginal irrigation, should be performed before inserting a vaginal suppository. 4. **The client should be placed in the supine position with the knees flexed (dorsal recumbent) to facilitate insertion of a vaginal suppository.**

Continued

	5. Advancing the suppository along the posterior vaginal wall facilitates the placement of the vaginal suppository just outside the cervical os so that when it melts it will eventually disperse through the entire vaginal canal. 6. The vagina is not a sterile cavity. Only medical asepsis is required for the insertion of a vaginal suppository.
Eliminate incorrect options.	Delete from consideration those options that do not correlate to your list of steps for administering a vaginal suppository. Eliminate option 3.

37.

CRITICAL-THINKING STRATEGY

Recognize keywords.	A nurse is taking a client's **temperature** using the **instrument in the illustration**. Place the following **steps in** the **order** in which they should be **implemented**.
Ask what the question is asking.	List the steps of using a temporal thermometer.
Critically analyze each option in relation to the question and the other options.	Identify the sequential steps when using a temporal thermometer. Refer to your list as you examine the options presented. Order the steps presented according to the sequence you identified. **Rationales:** 4. Cleaning the probe minimizes cross-contamination from one client to another. This should be done before and after the procedure. 2. Placing the temporal artery scanner in the middle of the forehead positions the instrument so that it is over the temporal artery as it is moved across the forehead and down toward the hairline on the side of the face. 1. The temporal artery is close to the skin and provides easy access to measure true body temperature accurately. Holding the probe flat against the forehead keeps the instrument in contact with the skin and provides for a more accurate reading. 3. Touching the probe to the soft area just behind the earlobe helps to ensure an accurate reading if a person is sweating. Sweating causes cooling of the skin, and a reading given by a temporal scanner may be low. Research demonstrates that gently positioning the probe on the neck directly behind the earlobe below the mastoid provides accurate results. 5. Releasing the button instructs the instrument to display the temperature reading on the liquid-crystal display (LCD) display screen on the instrument.
Eliminate incorrect options.	There are no incorrect options.

38.

CRITICAL-THINKING STRATEGY

Recognize keywords.	A first aid nurse at a beach is caring for a client who sustained a soft tissue injury of the right shoulder after being hit by a surfboard. **Which** should the nurse do to **limit** the stress of **both edema and bleeding** into tissue?
Ask what the question is asking.	Which intervention limits both edema and bleeding?
Critically analyze each option in relation to the question and the other options.	Explore the purpose and outcomes of a cold compress, direct pressure, massage, and elevation of a body part. Then consider this information in relation to just edema, just bleeding into tissue, and both edema and bleeding into tissue. **Rationales:** 1. **Cold lowers the temperature of the skin and underlying tissue, which causes vasoconstriction, reducing blood flow to the area. This controls bleeding and slows the passage of fluid from the intravascular to the interstitial compartment, which limits edema.** 2. Direct pressure may limit bleeding by compressing injured blood vessels, but it will not affect edema. 3. Cutaneous stimulation (massage) will not limit edema or bleeding into tissues. However, massage uses the gate-control theory of pain to limit pain. 4. Although elevating an extremity will reduce edema, it is contraindicated in this situation because it may cause additional injury to the right shoulder joint and surrounding tissue. The nurse should place the right arm in a sling, secure it close to the client's body, and then refer the client for medical attention.
Eliminate incorrect options.	Pressure only limits bleeding. Eliminate option 2. Massage does not influence bleeding or edema. Eliminate option 3. Elevation of the right arm may cause additional damage and is contraindicated. Eliminate option 4.

39.

CRITICAL-THINKING STRATEGY

Recognize keywords.	A nurse is caring for a group of clients in the postanesthesia care unit. **Which response** by a client in the **postanesthesia care unit** is the **priority concern** for the nurse?
Ask what the question is asking.	Which client response places a client at the highest risk for a postoperative complication?
Critically analyze each option in relation to the question and the other options.	Explore the consequences of the client responses in each option. Analyze the severity of each response in relation to the other responses. Identify the response that may be life-threatening. Analyze these options in relation to the ABCs (airway, breathing, and circulation) of client assessment and needs. **Rationales:** 1. Although the physical trauma of surgery causes pain, which must be relieved, pain is not the priority. 2. Although general anesthesia can cause nausea, nausea is not the priority problem in the postanesthesia care unit.

Continued

	3. With an altered level of consciousness, the pharyngeal, laryngeal, and gag reflexes may be impaired. The inability to cough or swallow can result in aspiration of oral secretions. When a nurse is considering the ABCs of nursing intervention (airway, breathing, and circulation), the airway has priority. 4. Excessive fluid loss through indwelling drains may indicate hemorrhage and cause a deficient fluid volume. Although this issue is very serious, the nurse has time to meet this need safely.
Eliminate incorrect options.	Pain and nausea are not life-threatening issues in a postanesthesia care unit. Although deficient volume has the potential to be a life-threatening problem if it is related to hemorrhage, it is a lower priority than another option because surgical clients are supported with IV fluids during and after surgery. Options 1, 2, and 4 can be eliminated.

40.

CRITICAL-THINKING STRATEGY

Recognize keywords.	A client's **double-lumen nasogastric tube** for decompression **becomes obstructed. Which should the nurse do**?
Ask what the question is asking.	How do you correct an obstruction in a double-lumen nasogastric tube?
Critically analyze each option in relation to the question and the other options.	Distinguish between what the nurse should do regarding routine care of a double-lumen nasogastric tube versus what specifically should be done when the tube is clogged. **Rationales:** 1. **The only way to reestablish patency of the air vent lumen of a double-lumen nasogastric tube is to instill air into the lumen. The injected air will push the secretions blocking the lumen back into the stomach, where the fluid can be removed by the drainage lumen. Keeping the end of the air vent lumen higher than the stomach prevents reflux of gastric contents into the air vent lumen.** 2. Repositioning the client will not reestablish patency of the air vent lumen. The client is placed in this position as the tube is being inserted to facilitate its passage into the stomach. 3. Placing the vent below the level of the stomach will draw fluid from the stomach into the air vent lumen by the principle of gravity. 4. Withdrawing 30 mL of gastric contents from the drainage lumen will not reestablish patency of the air vent lumen. Withdrawing 30 mL of gastric contents via the drainage lumen is done to ensure that the catheter is in the correct anatomical location.
Eliminate incorrect options.	Options 2, 3, and 4 are nursing interventions that will not clear the air vent of gastric fluid. Eliminate these options.

41.

CRITICAL-THINKING STRATEGY

Recognize keywords.	**Which scenario requires** a nurse to complete **an incident report**?
Ask what the question is asking.	Identify a situation that requires an incident report.
Critically analyze each option in relation to the question and the other options.	Recall and make a list of the variety of situations that require an incident report. Compare the situations presented in the options to your identified list of situations. Identify parallel situations.
	Rationales:
	1. An incident report is unnecessary when a client refuses treatment. Clients have the right to refuse care; however, the client's refusal of care and the reasons for the refusal should be documented in the client's clinical record.
	2. Any incident such as a fall that either results in harm to a client, employee, or visitor or does not result in an injury must be documented in an incident report.
	3. An incident report does not have to be completed when a visitor ambulates a client who should have been on bedrest. The incident should be documented in the client's clinical record.
	4. A nurse leaving work early without reporting to the supervisor does not require an incident report. The nurse manager should discuss this behavior with the nurse and may document it in the nurse's personnel file.
	5. Not receiving a prescribed medication may have the potential to cause harm. Therefore, an incident or adverse occurrence report should be completed to document the incident. This adds to the data so that similar situations can be prevented in the future.
	6. Any incident such as a fall that either results in harm to a client, employee, or visitor or does not result in an injury must be documented in an incident report.
Eliminate incorrect options.	Clients have a right to refuse care. Visitors violating a primary health-care provider's prescription should have their actions documented in progress notes rather than in an incident report. A nurse leaving work early without reporting to the supervisor describes an ethical situation that does not require an incident report. Options 1, 3, and 4 can be eliminated.

42.

CRITICAL-THINKING STRATEGY

Recognize keywords.	A client who has a transdermal **analgesic patch** for cancer experiences **breakthrough pain** with activity. Which is **most important** for the nurse **to do**?
Ask what the question is asking.	Which action will relieve intractable breakthrough pain?
Critically analyze each option in relation to the question and the other options.	Explore the outcome of the interventions in each option. Compare and contrast the benefits among the proposed interventions. Identify the priority nursing intervention that will relieve the client's pain immediately.

Continued

	Rationales: 1. Limiting movement is ineffective in relieving intractable pain. Encouraging the avoidance of moving can result in destructive effects of immobility and may interfere with the quality of life. 2. Seeking a dose increase in the long-acting opioid is not the priority. Although this may eventually be necessary, the client's pain must be relieved immediately. **3. Intermittent episodes of pain that occur despite continued use of an analgesic (breakthrough pain) can be managed by administering an immediate-release analgesic to reduce pain (rescue dosing). This reduces pain during an unanticipated pain episode without unnecessarily raising the dosage of the long-acting analgesic.** 4. Antianxiety medication will be ineffective in this situation. The client has intractable (resistant to treatment) pain that requires an opioid at this time.
Eliminate incorrect options.	Transdermal patches are administered for the intractable pain associated with cancer; therefore, limiting movement will be ineffective to prevent severe pain. Eliminate option 1. Options 2 and 4 involve requesting additional medication. One is not better than the other, and it will take time to obtain a prescription. Options 2 and 4 can be eliminated.

43.

CRITICAL-THINKING STRATEGY

Recognize keywords.	A nurse must perform a procedure and is **unsure of** the exact **steps of the procedure. Which should the nurse do first**?
Ask what the question is asking.	Which should be done first when the nurse is unsure of the steps of a procedure?
Critically analyze each option in relation to the question and the other options.	All of the interventions in the options may eventually be done. Analyze each option in relation to the others to identify what should be done first. You are being asked to set a priority. If you cannot identify what should be done first, eliminate the option that would be done last. Repeat this process with the remaining three options. Make a final selection when you are down to two options. **Rationales:** 1. Fundamental nursing textbooks are not the best source for a step-by-step review of a nursing skill. Generally, fundamental nursing textbooks do not address every nursing skill in a step-by-step approach, nor do they include intermediate or advanced skills. 2. Calling the staff education department for assistance should not be the first thing to do when one is unsure of the steps in a nursing procedure. Another action should be implemented first. **3. Checking the nursing policy and procedure manual is the first resource the nurse should use when unsure of the steps in a nursing procedure. A review of the procedure in the manual may refresh the memory or support the confidence of the nurse so that it is safe to proceed.** 4. Refusing to do the procedure is premature. Another action should be implemented first.

Continued

Continued

Eliminate incorrect options.	A fundamentals of nursing textbook does not provide comprehensive coverage of nursing procedures. Staff education personnel may not be available immediately. Refusing to perform a procedure is a behavior of last resort. Options 1, 2, and 4 can be eliminated.

44.

CRITICAL-THINKING STRATEGY

Recognize keywords.	A nurse sees the **stable client walking** down the hall, as depicted in the photograph. **What should the nurse instruct the client to do first**?
Ask what the question is asking.	When seeing this client, which should the nurse instruct the client to do first?
Critically analyze each option in relation to the question and the other options.	Examine the options in light of the consequences associated with each instruction by the nurse if the instruction is not implemented. Then compare and contrast the seriousness of the potential complications you identified. Then identify the instruction that will reduce the risk of the most serious complication. **Rationales:** 1. It is unnecessary to change hands to push the IV pole with the left hand and hold the urine collection bag with the right hand. A stable client with an IV in the right forearm can safely push an IV pole with the right hand. An unstable client should not be holding onto an IV pole when ambulating; nor should an unstable client be walking independently. **2. Instructing the client to hold the urine collection bag below the level of the waist is the first thing that the nurse should do in this scenario. Holding the urine collection bag below the level of the waist allows urine to flow from the bladder to the collection bag by gravity. This prevents urine from flowing back into the bladder, thus decreasing the risk of a urinary tract infection.** 3. Although the height of the IV pole should be increased to prevent a backflow of blood from the intravascular compartment into the IV tubing, it is not the first thing the nurse should do in this scenario. 4. Although the client should be assisted to put on shoes and a bathrobe, they are not the first things that the nurse should instruct the client to do in this scenario.
Eliminate incorrect options.	Option 1 is unnecessary. Options 3 and 4 are less of a serious concern than option 2, which is the correct answer.

45.

CRITICAL-THINKING STRATEGY

Recognize keywords.	At **which date and time** did the client have a **respiratory rate of 15 breaths per minute**?
Ask what the question is asking.	Interpret a graphic record to identify the date and time at which a client had a respiratory rate of 15 breaths per minute.
Critically analyze each option in relation to the question and the other options.	Identify the location of the date and time for each option at the top of the graphic chart, and carefully proceed down the column to identify the rate of respirations indicated by the position of the dot. Repeat this action for each date and time indicated in each option. Identify the option that has a dot on the line that indicates 15 respirations. **Rationales:** 1. **On 9-9 at 04, the client's respiratory rate was 15 breaths per minute.** 2. On 9-9 at 08, the client's respiratory rate was 20 breaths per minute. 3. On 9-10 at 08, the client's respiratory rate was 30 breaths per minute. 4. On 9-10 at 16, the client's respiratory rate was 25 breaths per minute.

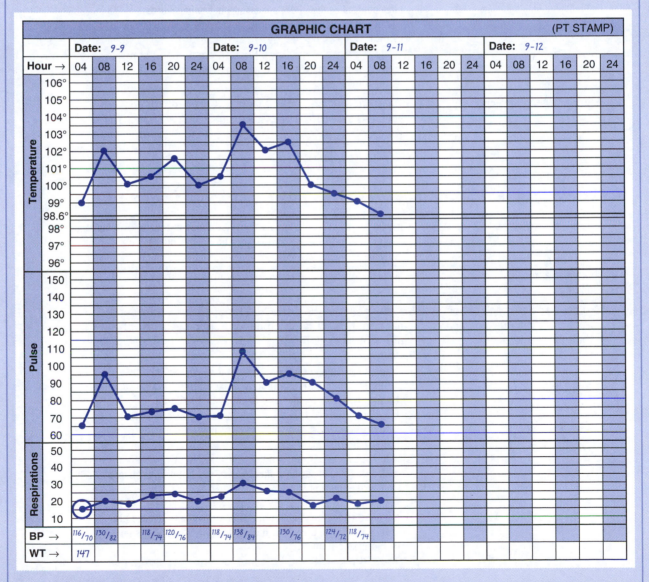

Eliminate incorrect options.	Eliminate the three options where the dot is located on a line that indicates more than 15 respirations.

46.

CRITICAL-THINKING STRATEGY

Recognize keywords.	A client appears agitated and states, **"I'm not sure that I want to go through with this surgery." Which response** by the nurse uses the technique of **paraphrasing**?
Ask what the question is asking.	Which nursing response uses the technique of paraphrasing?
Critically analyze each option in relation to the question and the other options.	Define *paraphrasing*. Identify the communication technique being used in each nursing response. Make a correlation between the definition of paraphrasing and the nursing response that restates the content of what the client said. **Rationales:** 1. This response is clarifying, not paraphrasing. In addition, to respond more accurately when using clarification, the nurse should have said, "Are you saying that you do not want to have this surgery?" Not wanting surgery and postponing surgery are two different concepts. **2. This response is an example of paraphrasing, which restates the content of the client's message in similar words.** 3. This response is an example of reflective technique, which focuses on feelings. 4. This response is an example of an open-ended statement, which invites the client to elaborate on the stated concern.
Eliminate incorrect options.	Option 1 uses clarification. Option 3 uses reflection. Option 4 is an open-ended statement. Eliminate options 1, 3, and 4.

47.

CRITICAL-THINKING STRATEGY

Recognize keywords.	A nurse is planning to apply a **transdermal patch** to a client. **Which** of the following **should the nurse implement**?
Ask what the question is asking.	Which step is associated with applying a transdermal patch?
Critically analyze each option in relation to the question and the other options.	List the steps of the procedure for applying a transdermal patch. Identify which options are on your list of interventions. **Rationales:** **1. Sites for a transdermal patch should be rotated because doing so limits skin irritation and excoriation. Also, rotation allows time for the site to recover if irritated.** 2. Both irritation of the skin and vasodilation can result from rubbing the skin, which can alter absorption of the medication. **3. A hairless site will ensure that there is effective contact with the skin, ensuring adherence of the patch and absorption of medication.** **4. When preparing and applying the patch, the nurse may be exposed to the medication on the patch. Clean gloves provide a barrier and protect the nurse from absorbing some of the medication.** 5. The old patch should be removed before the new patch is applied.
Eliminate incorrect options.	Option 2 may harm the client and is contraindicated. Permitting two patches to remain on the skin concurrently may result in absorption of excessive medication, which may harm the client. Eliminate options 2 and 5.

48.

CRITICAL-THINKING STRATEGY

Recognize keywords.	A nurse is evaluating a nursing assistant **changing the linen on an unoccupied bed**. Which **action** by the nursing assistant **reflects acceptable medical aseptic technique**?
Ask what the question is asking.	Which action related to changing bed linens is based on a principle of medical asepsis?
Critically analyze each option in relation to the question and the other options.	Examine each option and determine whether or not the action is based on a principle of medical aseptic technique. **Rationales:** 1. Containing soiled linen in a pillowcase resting on a client's bedside chair violates medical asepsis because it contaminates the chair. Soiled linen should be placed immediately into the soiled-linen hamper. 2. Positioning a soiled-linen hamper inside the doorway to a client's room violates medical asepsis. A soiled-linen hamper should be kept outside the door to a client's room. **3. Holding soiled linen away from one's uniform protects the uniform from becoming contaminated.** **4. The hands should be washed whether or not gloves were worn during the procedure. This prevents the transmission of microorganisms to the nurse and to others. Clean gloves should be worn if there is potential to be exposed to excretions or secretions.** 5. Medical, not surgical, asepsis should be followed when changing soiled linen. Clean gloves are adequate. Sterile gloves are unnecessary.
Eliminate incorrect options.	The actions in options 1 and 2 violate principles of medical aseptic technique. In option 5, clean, not sterile, gloves may be worn if the linen being replaced is soiled with blood or body fluids. Eliminate options 1, 2, and 5.

49.

CRITICAL-THINKING STRATEGY

Recognize keywords.	A **client is told** by the primary health-care provider that the client **has metastatic lung cance**r and is seriously ill. After the provider leaves the room, the client has a severe episode of coughing and shortness of breath and says, **"This is just a cold. I'll be fine once I get over it." How should the nurse respond**?
Ask what the question is asking.	Which response will encourage a client in denial to talk further about the topic being discussed?
Critically analyze each option in relation to the question and the other options.	Examine each option and identify if the statement is therapeutic or not therapeutic. **Rationales:** 1. This response is a challenging statement and is inappropriate. It may take away the client's coping mechanism and cut off communication; the client is using denial to cope with the diagnosis. Also, it does not address what the client thinks or feels about the diagnosis.

Continued

Continued

	2. This response may take away the client's coping mechanism, is demeaning, and may cut off communication. The use of the word "bad" may precipitate anxiety. The client is using denial to cope with the diagnosis.
	3. This response is too direct and demeaning and may cut off communication. The client is using denial to cope with the diagnosis.
	4. This provides an opportunity to discuss the illness; eventually, a developing awareness will occur, and the client will move on to other coping mechanisms.
Eliminate incorrect options.	Options 1, 2, and 3 are challenging and not therapeutic. Responses should not take away a client's coping mechanism. Eliminate options 1, 2, and 3.

50.

CRITICAL-THINKING STRATEGY

Recognize keywords.	A client develops diarrhea after receiving several **intermittent enteral tube feedings.** Which should the nurse consider is the **cause of** the **diarrhea** before responding to this situation?
Ask what the question is asking.	Why can intermittent enteral tube feedings cause diarrhea?
Critically analyze each option in relation to the question and the other options.	Review the physiological response of the body to a hypertonic solution and an inadequate volume of enteral feedings. Explore why testing for a residual is performed before and a high-Fowler position is used during an intermittent enteral tube feeding. Compare and contrast the information you gathered in your review with the reasons for diarrhea presented in each option.
	Rationales:
	1. An enteral tube feeding formula usually is hypertonic, which exerts an osmotic force that pulls fluid into the stomach and intestine, resulting in intestinal cramping and diarrhea.
	2. An inadequate volume of the enteral feeding may result in a deficient fluid volume and malnutrition, not diarrhea.
	3. Failure to test for a residual before the enteral feeding may result in vomiting, not diarrhea. If there is still fluid remaining from the previous enteral feeding, failure to test for a residual before administering an enteral tube feeding can result in adding more fluid than the client's stomach can tolerate.
	4. Placing a client in the high-Fowler position during the administration of an enteral tube feeding is done to prevent aspiration of the formula and will not cause diarrhea.
Eliminate incorrect options.	Options 1 and 2 address the formula (osmolarity and volume, respectively). Options 3 and 4 address nursing interventions during the procedure. Option 2 is related to fluid and nutritional deficiencies, not diarrhea. Failure to test for a residual in option 3 may result in vomiting, not diarrhea. A high-Fowler position in option 4 prevents aspiration, not diarrhea. Eliminate options 2, 3, and 4.

51.

CRITICAL-THINKING STRATEGY

Recognize keywords.	While in a restaurant, a **pregnant woman** exhibits a **total airway obstruction** because of a bolus of food. How should the nurse **modify** the thrusts of the **abdominal thrust** (Heimlich) maneuver for this woman?
Ask what the question is asking.	How should the abdominal thrust maneuver be adapted for a pregnant woman?
Critically analyze each option in relation to the question and the other options.	List the steps of the abdominal thrust maneuver. Recall the physiological changes in a woman's body when pregnant. Compare these physiological changes with the steps of the procedure, and determine what step may harm the woman or the fetus. Identify the modification of the procedure that will help dislodge the obstruction while protecting the woman and the fetus. **Rationales:** 1. Placing the client in the supine position is unnecessary. This is done when the person is unconscious. 2. The thumb side of the hand should always be against the person's body when performing the abdominal thrust maneuver. **3. This is the appropriate modification of the abdominal thrust (Heimlich) maneuver for a pregnant woman. This provides thoracic compression while preventing pressure against the uterus that can result in trauma to the woman or the fetus.** 4. Waiting until the person becomes unconscious wastes valuable time and is unsafe. Delaying or discontinuing the maneuver before the obstruction is cleared will result in death.
Eliminate incorrect options.	Options 1 and 4 delay the initiation of the procedure. Eliminate options 1 and 4. Option 2 will be physically difficult to perform and will still compress the woman's abdominal area, which may harm the woman or the fetus. Eliminate option 2.

52.

CRITICAL-THINKING STRATEGY

Recognize keywords.	A nurse in charge is making assignments for a nursing team. **Which intervention** should the nurse in charge **assign to the registered nurse**?
Ask what the question is asking.	Which nursing action is within the scope of practice of a registered nurse?
Critically analyze each option in relation to the question and the other options.	Recall that interventions associated with assessment, planning, and evaluation require the knowledge and judgment of a registered nurse. In addition, professional interventions that require a complex level of interaction with the client or that have the potential for harm as well as a need for problem-solving abilities are within the scope of practice of a registered nurse. Examine each option in relation to the recalled information.

Continued

Continued

	Rationales:
	1. **A task of this complexity requires the knowledge and judgment of a registered nurse. This task has great potential for harm if the caregiver does not perform an accurate assessment of the client's condition. It requires an assessment of numerous systems and risk factors, a complex level of interaction with the client, and problem-solving abilities. In addition, it requires innovation in the form of an individually designed plan of care that addresses protecting the client's skin.**
	2. Offering apple juice to a client on a clear liquid diet is not a complex task, has little potential for harm, requires only simple problem-solving skills, involves a predictable outcome, employs a simple level of interaction with the client, and is within the scope of practice of a nursing assistant.
	3. **Registered nurses have the knowledge required to ambulate clients who may not be stable. Clients after surgery are at risk for falls because of weakness, hypotension, altered level of consciousness, and pain. The client must be assessed before, during, and after ambulation to maintain client safety. Ambulation may be delayed or terminated based on the registered nurse's assessments of the client.**
	4. **Client teaching is the responsibility of a nurse, who has the knowledge and judgment to select various teaching strategies and the ability to evaluate the client's understanding of the content taught.**
	5. Measuring the urinary output of a client who has an indwelling urinary catheter is not a complex task, has little potential for harm, requires simple problem-solving skills, employs a simple level of interaction with the client, and is within the scope of practice of a nursing assistant.
Eliminate incorrect options.	Options 2 and 5 can be eliminated because these actions do not require the education and skills of a registered nurse.

53.

CRITICAL-THINKING STRATEGY

Recognize keywords.	A nurse is providing dietary teaching for a client who follows a plant-based **(pure) vegan diet**. **Which food combination** that **is a** substitute for a **complete protein** should the nurse include in the dietary teaching?
Ask what the question is asking.	Which combination of food provides essential amino acids for a person who follows a pure vegan diet?
Critically analyze each option in relation to the question and the other options.	Recall what a person who follows a pure vegan diet does or does not eat. Identify the type of protein presented in each food combination. Analyze the food combinations presented, and conclude whether they provide essential amino acids and are included in a pure vegan diet. Rationales: 1. **Pasta is made from grains, and peas are legumes, which together provide amino acids that make a complete protein. Complete proteins supply all eight essential amino acids. Essential amino acids are those that cannot be manufactured by the human body and must be obtained from food.**

Continued

	2. Yogurt and fruit together do not provide a complete protein. In addition, a client who follows a pure vegan diet eats only plant-based food. 3. Bread and cheese together provide a complete protein. However, a client who follows a pure vegan diet eats only plant-based food, which includes grains, not dairy products. **4. Grains and legumes contain different amino acids. When these foods are combined, they substitute for a complete protein. Complete proteins supply all eight essential amino acids. Essential amino acids are those that cannot be manufactured by the human body and must be obtained from food.** 5. Peanut butter combined with a grain, not jelly, is a substitute for a complete protein.
Eliminate incorrect options.	Eliminate options 2, 3, and 5. A person who follows a pure vegan diet eats only plants, and the food combinations in the options do not provide essential amino acids.

54.

CRITICAL-THINKING STRATEGY

Recognize keywords.	A construction worker comes to the emergency department with an injury that occurred 3 days ago. The client has an open **wound** of the right calf that has **purulent drainage**. The medical professional decides to admit the client to the hospital for IV antibiotic therapy and prescribes **contact precautions**. Which should the nurse in the emergency department do before transporting the client to a room?
Ask what the question is asking.	What should the nurse do first to minimize the risk of contaminating others or objects with purulent drainage?
Critically analyze each option in relation to the question and the other options.	Compare and contrast nursing actions associated with contact precautions versus other types of transmission-based precautions. Recall nursing actions associated with the steps in the chain of infection. Determine which action prevents transmission of purulent drainage from others and objects in the environment. **Rationales:** 1. An airborne infection isolation room (AIIR) is associated with airborne precautions, not contact precautions. This type of room has negative pressure airflow of 6 to 12 air exchanges per hour via high-efficiency particulate air (HIPA) filtration or discharged to outside air. Airborne precautions are used for clients with an infectious agent that has droplet nuclei smaller than 5 mcg that can remain suspended in the air and travel by air currents. **2. Draining secretions that contain pathogens are capable of transmitting the infection to others by direct or indirect contact. With contact precautions, the wound should be covered to interrupt the potential for contamination of others or objects.** 3. It is not necessary to administer the prescribed antibiotic before transporting the client to a room. The antibiotic should be administered when it is received from the pharmacy and at the time it is prescribed.

Continued

Continued

	4. Wearing a gown, gloves, and goggles is unnecessary when transporting this client. With contact precautions, a gown and gloves are necessary only when anticipating direct contact with this client or the client's environment. The nurse should wear additional personal protective equipment (PPE), such as goggles or a face shield, when splashing of body fluids is anticipated.
Eliminate incorrect options.	Eliminate option 1 because it is associated with airborne precautions, not contact precautions. The actions in option 4 are unnecessary. Eliminate option 4. The prescribed antibiotic (option 3) can be administered when received and at the prescribed time. In addition, this action does not protect others or the environment from becoming contaminated with purulent drainage when transporting the client. Eliminate option 3.

55.

CRITICAL-THINKING STRATEGY

Recognize keywords.	A nurse is going to instill medicated **drops into the ear** of an **adult**. Which should the nurse do to **ensure** that the **medication flows toward the eardrum**?
Ask what the question is asking.	Which action disperses medication in the ear canal of an adult?
Critically analyze each option in relation to the question and the other options.	List the steps of administering medicated drops into a client's ear. Recall the difference in the procedure for an adult versus an infant/young child. Compare the list and the options presented. **Rationales:** 1. Pulling the pinna of the ear backward and downward is done to straighten the ear canal of an infant or a young child, not an adult. 2. Inserting the drops into the center of the auditory canal can injure the eardrum. Drops should be directed along the wall of the ear canal. 3. **Pressing gently on the tragus facilitates the flow of medication toward the eardrum.** 4. Rolling the client from the side-lying position to the supine position can result in medication flowing out of the ear. The side-lying position with the involved ear on the uppermost side should be maintained for 2 to 3 minutes after the medication is instilled.
Eliminate incorrect options.	Option 1 is a technique used with infants and young children. Option 2 can harm the eardrum and is unsafe. Option 4 will result in fluid draining away from the eardrum. Eliminate options 1, 2, and 4.

56.

CRITICAL-THINKING STRATEGY

Recognize keywords.	A nurse is caring for a client on bedrest. **Which client statement should alert the nurse to assess for** indications of **immobility-induced thrombophlebitis?**
Ask what the question is asking.	Which statement reflects clinical manifestations of thrombophlebitis?
Critically analyze each option in relation to the question and the other options.	Recall the pathophysiology and list the signs and symptoms associated with thrombophlebitis. Compare each option with the information you recalled. **Rationales:** 1. The skin will appear taut and shiny, not dry, with thrombophlebitis. **2. A slowed blood flow and increased viscosity of the blood allow platelets and calcium to settle out against the intimal lining of a vein, which can result in thrombus formation. The inflammatory process causes calf edema, pain, heat, and erythema.** 3. The client will feel discomfort or pain, not tingling sensations, with thrombophlebitis. 4. The area will feel warm, not cool, to the touch with thrombophlebitis. Cool toes may indicate lower extremity arterial disease.
Eliminate incorrect options.	Eliminate options 1, 3, and 4 because dry skin, tingling in the feet, and cool toes are not clinical manifestations of thrombophlebitis.

57.

CRITICAL-THINKING STRATEGY

Recognize keywords.	A nurse is obtaining a client's blood pressure. **Which** of the following **will result in an accurate blood pressure measurement?**
Ask what the question is asking.	Which is a step in obtaining a blood pressure measurement?
Critically analyze each option in relation to the question and the other options.	List the steps of the procedure for performing a blood pressure measurement. Compare and contrast the list with the options presented. **Rationales:** **1. Positioning the arm at the level of the heart will result in an accurate blood pressure measurement. The blood pressure will be inaccurately low if the arm is positioned higher than the level of the heart. The blood pressure will be inaccurately high if the arm is positioned lower than the level of the heart.** 2. Wrapping the lower edge of the cuff over the antecubital space will cover the brachial artery and interfere with the accurate assessment of blood pressure. The lower edge of the cuff should be approximately 1 inch (2.5 cm) above the antecubital space. **3. The sphygmomanometer should be pumped up 20 to 30 mm Hg above the palpatory blood pressure reading. This ensures an accurate systolic reading without exerting undue pressure on the tissues of the arm.**

Continued

Continued

	4. **Releasing the valve slowly ensures that all five Korotkoff's sounds are heard accurately. Deflating the cuff too rapidly can result in a falsely low systolic reading. Deflating the cuff too slowly can result in a falsely high diastolic reading.** 5. **When repeating a blood pressure measurement, the cuff should be completely deflated and the caregiver should wait 2 minutes before reinflating the blood pressure cuff. This action prevents congestion of the veins and an inaccurately high blood pressure reading.**
Eliminate incorrect options.	Inappropriate placement of the sphygmomanometer cuff will result in an inaccurate measurement. Eliminate option 2.

58.

CRITICAL-THINKING STRATEGY

Recognize keywords.	A nurse is caring for a client who is **unconscious**. Which should the nurse use to **best clean** this client's **oral cavity?**
Ask what the question is asking.	What should be used to clean the oral cavity of an unconscious client?
Critically analyze each option in relation to the question and the other options.	Consider the unique needs of a client who is unconscious, particularly in relation to the ABCs (airway, breathing, and circulation). Analyze each option in relation to how it will have an impact on the client's physical status. **Rationales:** 1. **Unconscious clients often bite down when something is placed in the mouth. Therefore, a padded tongue blade should be placed between the upper and lower teeth to help keep the mouth open during oral care. This prevents injury to the client and the nurse. Other padded tongue blades, wetted with a small amount of saline, should be used to clean the oral cavity. This technique does not require flushing the oral cavity with fluid, which may compromise the airway.** 2. Although half-strength mouthwash and saline may be used, it is not the best intervention because mouthwash contains ingredients that can be irritating to the mucous membranes. Also, fluid in the mouth may be aspirated, compromising the airway and respiratory functioning. 3. Glycerin is not a cleansing agent and is not effective in cleaning the oral cavity. 4. Toothpaste should be avoided because it requires flushing the mouth with adequate amounts of water to prevent leaving an irritating residue on the mucous membranes. An unconscious client usually has a diminished gag reflex and is at risk for aspiration.
Eliminate incorrect options.	Airway patency always is the priority. Options 2 and 4 require flushing the oral cavity with fluid, which may compromise the airway. Glycerin coats, rather than cleans, the oral mucosa. Eliminate options 2, 3, and 4.

59.

CRITICAL-THINKING STRATEGY

Recognize keywords.	A client is admitted to the hospital with the diagnosis of **diverticulitis**. Which is the **best question** the nurse should ask when obtaining an **admission history** from this client?
Ask what the question is asking.	Which initial question will obtain the client's perspective of the situation?
Critically analyze each option in relation to the question and the other options.	Review the purpose of obtaining an admission history from a client. Analyze each question to determine what information will be collected by the client's response. Identify the most significant information the nurse should collect. **Rationales:** 1. This question is too focused. 2. Although determining how long the client has had diverticulitis is information that eventually may be obtained, it is not the immediate priority. **3. This question invites the client to expand on and develop a topic of importance that relates to the current problem.** 4. Although identifying previous episodes of diverticulitis is information that eventually may be obtained, it is not the immediate priority.
Eliminate incorrect options.	Options 1, 2, and 4 are direct questions that obtain limited information. Eliminate these options.

60.

CRITICAL-THINKING STRATEGY

Recognize keywords.	A primary health-care provider prescribes peak and trough levels for a client receiving an intravenous antibiotic. **What time** should the nurse obtain a blood sample to determine a **trough level** when the **antibiotic was administered at 12 noon**?
Ask what the question is asking.	When should a blood specimen for a trough level of a drug be obtained?
Critically analyze each option in relation to the question and the other options.	Recall the parameters for obtaining a specimen for a trough level of a drug. Identify the interrelationship of when the drug was administered and the times offered in each of the options. **Rationales:** 1. 11 a.m. is too soon. The drug will not be at its lowest concentration in the blood. **2. Thirty minutes before or closer to the next scheduled dose is the most appropriate time for a trough blood level to be obtained. The serum level of the drug will be at its lowest.** 3. Peak, not trough, levels are obtained 30 minutes after completion of drug administration. 4. The blood level of the drug increases after the drug is administered. A value taken at this time will not reflect the lowest serum level, which is the purpose of identifying a trough level.
Eliminate incorrect options.	A specimen of blood for a trough level should be obtained when the drug is at its lowest level (about 30 minutes before the next dose). Option 1 is too early compared with option 2. Eliminate option 1. Options 3 and 4 are too soon after the drug was administered. Eliminate options 3 and 4.

61.

CRITICAL-THINKING STRATEGY

Recognize keywords.	A nurse is monitoring a client who is receiving an IV infusion because of dehydration. Which client **response most specifically indicates** that the **IV fluid replacement is adequate**?
Ask what the question is asking.	Which assessment most indicates that the expected outcome of IV fluid replacement therapy is achieved?
Critically analyze each option in relation to the question and the other options.	List clinical manifestations of adequate fluid volume, excess fluid volume, and deficient fluid volume. Compare and contrast your lists with the options in the question. Identify whether any of the clinical manifestations of adequate fluid volume you identified are one of the options. If it appears that there is more than one correct answer, as is the case in this question, examine the two options and identify the option that **most specifically** indicates that IV fluid replacement is adequate. **Rationales:** 1. Moist lips is a nonspecific and too-subjective assessment to determine the adequacy of IV fluid replacement. 2. A bounding pulse indicates excessive fluid in the intravascular compartment. 3. **The circulating blood volume perfuses the kidneys and produces a glomerular filtrate, of which varying amounts are either reabsorbed or excreted to maintain fluid balance. When a person without kidney disease is adequately hydrated, the minimally acceptable urinary output is 30 mL/hr.** 4. A blood pressure of 96/60 mm Hg reflects a decreased circulating blood volume (hypovolemia). The average blood pressure of a healthy adult is a systolic less than 120 and a diastolic less than 80 mm Hg.
Eliminate incorrect options.	Eliminate option 2 because a bounding pulse indicates excess fluid volume. Eliminate option 4 because this blood pressure indicates deficient fluid volume. Eliminate option 1 because moist lips is nonspecific and too-subjective an assessment to determine the adequacy of IV fluid replacement when compared with option 3.

62.

CRITICAL-THINKING STRATEGY

Recognize keywords.	A nurse is teaching a group of clients about correct body mechanics. Which **action reflects** teaching about the principle, *the greater the base of support, the more stable the body?*
Ask what the question is asking.	Which action provides a wide base of support?
Critically analyze each option in relation to the question and the other options.	Identify the projected outcome for the behavior in each option. Then consider the principle that underlines the behavior and its outcome. **Rationales:** 1. **A cane provides three points of contact with the floor. This wide base provides support for ambulation.**

Continued

	2. Locking the wheels of a wheelchair follows the principle, *an object with wheels that are locked will remain stationary.* **3. Assistance when getting out of bed widens the client's base of support because the base extends from the client's feet on the floor to the caregiver's feet on the floor.** 4. Holding objects close to the body when walking follows the principle, *the closer an object is held to the center of gravity, the greater the stability and the easier the object is to move.* 5. Keeping the back straight when lifting an object follows the principle, *balance is maintained and muscle strain is limited as long as the line of gravity passes through the base of support.*
Eliminate incorrect options.	Option 2 relates to safety, not to a wide base of support. Options 4 and 5 relate to principles associated with body mechanics other than a wide base of support. Eliminate options 2, 4, and 5.

63.

CRITICAL-THINKING STRATEGY

Recognize keywords.	A nurse is caring for a client who has been having difficulty sleeping. Which should the nurse do because it is the **most effective** nursing **intervention** to **promote sleep** that is appropriate for a client **in any situation**?
Ask what the question is asking.	Which is the best method to promote sleep for most clients?
Critically analyze each option in relation to the question and the other options.	Identify the commonalities and differences of nursing interventions that relate to promoting sleep. A commonality is an intervention that may work regardless of the client situation. A difference is an intervention that may work for a client in a specific situation. **Rationales:** 1. A back rub is the therapeutic manipulation of muscles and tissues that relaxes tense muscles, relieves muscle spasms, and induces rest or sleep. However, it may be contraindicated, and some people do not like a back rub or consider it an invasion of their personal space. 2. Music can be relaxing or stimulating, depending on the individual's perception of the music. 3. Although milk contains the amino acid L-tryptophan, which promotes sleep, many people have issues (e.g., lactose intolerance, gastroesophageal reflux disease) that contraindicate the intake of milk. **4. Following routines provides consistency and comfort in an unfamiliar environment. Bedtime rituals meet basic physiological needs and usually include physically and emotionally relaxing behaviors.**
Eliminate incorrect options.	Options 1, 2, and 3 may work for certain clients in specific situations. The nursing interventions in these options cannot be implemented for all clients. Eliminate options 1, 2, and 3.

64.

CRITICAL-THINKING STRATEGY

Recognize keywords.	A nurse is performing an assessment of a client. Place an X on the figure of the body where the nurse should **place the stethoscope** to assess for the **presence of borborygmi.**
Ask what the question is asking.	Where on the body are borborygmi heard?
Critically analyze each option in relation to the question and the other options.	Define borborygmi. Consider where these sounds are produced within the body. Place an X where a stethoscope should be placed to auscultate these sounds. **Rationale:** **An X in any part of the shaded area across the abdomen is a correct answer. A nurse should auscultate all four quadrants of the abdomen to determine the presence of borborygmi. Borborygmi are audible, high-pitched, loud, gurgling sounds caused by the propulsion of gas through the intestine.**
Eliminate incorrect options.	Other areas of the body will be eliminated when an X is placed over the shaded area indicated in the answer.

65.

CRITICAL-THINKING STRATEGY

Recognize keywords.	A nurse is caring for clients who are on a medical/surgical unit in a hospital. Which should the nurse do to **best prevent** clients from **falling due to physical hazards**?
Ask what the question is asking.	How can the nurse best prevent falls in a hospital?
Critically analyze each option in relation to the question and the other options.	Analyze the outcome of each intervention in relation to safety. Compare and contrast options to eventually identify the best intervention. **Rationales:** 1. Although positioning the telephone within easy reach should be done because it avoids having the client possibly lose balance and fall while reaching for a phone, it is not the most important intervention to prevent injury in a hospital. 2. Although storing belongings in a safe place should be done, this is not a physical hazard. **3. Adequate lighting provides for the safety of clients, staff, and visitors within a hospital. Inadequate lighting causes shadows, a dark environment, and the potential for misinterpreting stimuli (illusions). Inadequate lighting is a major cause of accidents in the hospital setting.** 4. An over-bed table has wheels and therefore cannot provide a firm base of support. Over-bed tables are physical hazards that may contribute to falls if used inappropriately.
Eliminate incorrect options.	Option 2 is unrelated to physical safety, and option 4 is unsafe because an over-bed table has wheels. Eliminate options 2 and 4. Options 1 and 3 both relate to safety. Option 1 relates to just one limited aspect of a safe environment. Option 2 relates to a more global issue—inadequate lighting. Therefore, eliminate option 1.

66.

CRITICAL-THINKING STRATEGY

Recognize keywords.	A client prefers and excessively maintains the **supine position**. For which **potential problem** associated with this position should the nurse assess the client?
Ask what the question is asking.	Which problem is associated with the supine position?
Critically analyze each option in relation to the question and the other options.	Visualize a client in the supine position. Examine each option in relation to the visualization. Identify the option that may place the client at risk for a negative outcome. **Rationales:** **1. The supine position is a back-lying position that results in pressure on the heels (calcanei), which have minimal tissue between the bone and skin, making them vulnerable to the development of pressure ulcers.** 2. External, not internal, rotation of the hips tends to occur when a client is in the supine position. 3. The knees are extended, not flexed, when in the supine position. 4. There is no pressure on either greater trochanter when a client is in the supine position. Pressure on a greater trochanter occurs when the client is in a lateral (side-lying) position.

Continued

Continued

| Eliminate incorrect options. | Eliminate option 2 because external, not internal, rotation of the hips occurs with the supine position if trochanter rolls are not used to maintain functional alignment. Eliminate option 3 because hyperextension of the knees, not flexion contractures of the knees, can occur in the supine position. Eliminate option 4 because pressure on the trochanters does not occur in the supine position. |

67.

CRITICAL-THINKING STRATEGY

Recognize keywords.	A client is using the call bell **numerous times** an hour and **requesting assistance** with activities that the client is **capable of achieving independently. Which should the nurse do** to help this client?
Ask what the question is asking.	Which should the nurse do when a client calls the nurse excessively?
Critically analyze each option in relation to the question and the other options.	Review concepts related to psychological responses to stress. Identify that the client's behavior reflects anxiety. Explore nursing actions that support emotional needs and reduce anxiety. Then examine each option in light of whether the action will increase or decrease anxiety. **Rationales:** 1. Demanding behavior is the client's coping mechanism. Setting limits will make the client more anxious and demanding. 2. Alternating care with another nurse can be confusing to the client and increase anxiety. Maintaining continuity in the nurse assignment will support the development of a trusting relationship and enable the nurse to explore the client's feelings, as well as plan and implement interventions that encourage choices, all of which support feeling in control. 3. Pointing out demanding behavior is too confrontational at this time. Confronting the behavior and taking away the client's coping mechanism will cause the client to become more anxious. **4. Attempting to see the situation from the client's perspective is an example of empathy, which is understanding a client's emotional point of view. An empathic response communicates that the nurse is listening and cares. Demanding behavior generally is a defense mechanism that reduces anxiety generated by powerlessness.**
Eliminate incorrect options.	Options 1, 2, and 3 will increase, not decrease, anxiety and can be eliminated.

68.

CRITICAL-THINKING STRATEGY

Recognize keywords.	A nurse going off duty is making rounds with the nurse coming on duty and provides a report about each client in the district. **Which information** reported by the nurse **is the most complete**?
Ask what the question is asking.	Which information is the most thorough?
Critically analyze each option in relation to the question and the other options.	Examine each option to determine if the information included is objective and comprehensive. **Rationales:** 1. **This information includes a nursing intervention and an evaluation of the outcome, which is the most specific and complete of all the options.** 2. No data are given to support the assumption that the client is happy. 3. The words "less anxious" are relative and do not clearly evaluate the client's status. 4. Every client has his or her own baseline. Indicating that a blood pressure is stable is incomplete and unclear.
Eliminate incorrect options.	Options 2 and 3 use the terms "happy" and "less anxious," which are subjective and not measurable. Option 4 fails to provide the blood pressure measurements before and after the current blood pressure measurement, making the information about the stability of the current blood pressure meaningless. Options 2, 3, and 4 can be eliminated.

69.

CRITICAL-THINKING STRATEGY

Recognize keywords.	A nurse is bathing a client. Which **action** is **associated with medical asepsis**?
Ask what the question is asking.	Which action is related to medical asepsis?
Critically analyze each option in relation to the question and the other options.	Visualize the steps of the procedure for bathing a client. Recall principles associated with maintaining medical asepsis. Integrate the principles of medical asepsis with the visualized steps of the procedure. Analyze the options in relation to this information. **Rationales:** 1. **The eye should always be washed from the inner to the outer canthus to prevent secretions from entering the lacrimal ducts, which may result in an infection.** 2. A bath blanket promotes privacy and prevents heat loss during a bath and is unrelated to asepsis. If not soiled, a client's bath blanket can be reused. 3. **Changing the bathwater after cleaning the perineum prevents transferring microorganisms from the genitals, perianal area, and urinary meatus to subsequent areas of the body that are being washed. This action promotes medical asepsis.** 4. Having a client void before beginning the bed bath is related to a client's comfort and elimination needs rather than asepsis. 5. **Clean gloves are required during this procedure to protect the nurse from being exposed to the client's body fluids.**
Eliminate incorrect options.	Although options 2 and 4 are part of the procedure of bathing, they are unrelated to principles of medical asepsis. Eliminate options 2 and 4.

70.

CRITICAL-THINKING STRATEGY

Recognize keywords.	A nurse is assessing the **oxygen status of a dark-skinned client**. Where should the nurse **assess for cyanosis** in this client?
Ask what the question is asking.	Which part of the body should the nurse assess for cyanosis in a client with dark skin?
Critically analyze each option in relation to the question and the other options.	Recall that cyanosis is the result of excessive concentrations of deoxyhemoglobin in capillary blood. Recall common body sites that contain minimal melanotic pigment because they are the best sites to assess for cyanosis. Recognize that a client with dark skin has higher amounts of melanin in the skin, which will eliminate common sites when assessing cyanosis in a person with light skin. Examine the options and identify which site has the least melanin. **Rationales:** 1. The lower legs are not as reliable a site to assess for cyanosis as are areas listed in another option. The legs are distal sites that already may be discolored because of diseases of peripheral arteries and veins. 2. The sclera of the eyes is an excellent location to assess for the presence of jaundice, not cyanosis. Jaundice is a yellow discoloration of skin and mucous membranes resulting from an increase in bilirubin in tissues. Blue coloration of the whites of the eyes can occur with several connective tissue disorders, not cyanosis. 3. Although the nailbeds are areas of lighter pigmentation in darker-skinned people, the feet are not a reliable body part to assess central cyanosis because they are distal sites that already may be discolored because of diseases of peripheral arteries and veins. **4. Cyanosis, a bluish discoloration of the tissues caused by a decreased amount of oxygen in the blood, is best identified in the mucous membranes of the oral cavity and the conjunctivae of the eyes. The mucous membranes usually are pink regardless of the person's skin color, which facilitates an accurate assessment for cyanosis.**
Eliminate incorrect options.	Eliminate option 1 and 3 because the lower legs and nailbeds of the toes are distal sites that may be discolored due to lower-extremity peripheral disease. Eliminate option 2, sclera of the eyes, because this site is not used for assessing cyanosis.

71.

CRITICAL-THINKING STRATEGY

Recognize keywords.	A client who self-administers an aerosol medication by a **metered-dose inhaler** reports a "**nasty taste** to the medication." **Which should the nurse** encourage the client to **do**?
Ask what the question is asking.	Which action will reduce the "nasty taste" to the medication delivered via a metered-dose inhaler?
Critically analyze each option in relation to the question and the other options.	Review the rationale for each step of the procedure when using a metered-dose inhaler. Identify the equipment that may be used when administering medication via a metered-dose inhaler. Compare and contrast this information in relation to resolution of the client's problem.

Continued

	Rationales:
	1. Sucking on a hard candy after the procedure addresses the nasty taste after, rather than before, it occurs.
	2. Shaking the cartridge longer before using it will ensure that the medication is dispersed throughout solution in the cartridge. It will not change the taste of the medication.
	3. Oral hygiene should be performed after, not before, the procedure.
	4. **The aerosolized medication enters the aerosol chamber, where the larger droplets fall to the bottom of the chamber. The smaller droplets are inhaled deep into the lungs rather than falling on the client's tongue.**
Eliminate incorrect options.	The action in option 1 will not prevent the problem. The action in option 2 will not change the taste of the medication. The action in option 3 is done after, not before, the procedure. Options 1, 2, and 3 can be eliminated.

72.

CRITICAL-THINKING STRATEGY

Recognize keywords.	A nurse is meeting a client for the first time. **Which should the nurse do** during the **orientation phase** of this **therapeutic relationship**?
Ask what the question is asking.	Which is the main function of the orientation phase of a therapeutic relationship?
Critically analyze each option in relation to the question and the other options.	Recall the phases of a therapeutic relationship. Determine what is significant about the orientation phase versus the other phases of the therapeutic relationship. Examine the options and identify which one accurately reflects the purposes of the orientation phase that you have identified.
	Rationales:
	1. Collecting data is not the most important purpose of the orientation phase of a therapeutic relationship.
	2. **The orientation phase (also called the introductory or pre-helping phase) of a therapeutic relationship sets the tone for the rest of the relationship. A rapport develops when the client recognizes that the nurse is willing and able to help and can be trusted.**
	3. Problems are identified, explored, and dealt with during the working, not the orientation, phase of a therapeutic relationship.
	4. Priority needs are identified and interventions planned and implemented during the working, not the orientation, phase of a therapeutic relationship.
Eliminate incorrect options.	Although data are collected during the orientation phase of the therapeutic relationship, this is not the most important purpose; therefore, option 1 can be eliminated. Options 3 and 4 relate to the working phase of a therapeutic relationship and can be eliminated.

73.

CRITICAL-THINKING STRATEGY

Recognize keywords.	A client has a temperature of 102°F and reports feeling cold. For which **additional response** should the nurse assess the client during this **onset phase (cold or chill phase) of a fever**?
Ask what the question is asking.	Which is a sign associated with the onset phase (cold or chill phase) of a fever?
Critically analyze each option in relation to the question and the other options.	Recall the different phases of a fever. List the physiological responses associated with each phase of a fever. Compare the list with the options provided. **Rationales:** 1. Lethargy, weakness, and aching muscles occur during the course phase (plateau phase), not onset phase (cold or chill phase), of a fever. **2. Pale skin occurs as the peripheral blood vessels constrict in an attempt to increase the core body temperature during the onset phase (cold or chill phase) of a fever.** **3. Feeling cold, having chills, and shivering are adaptations associated with the onset phase (cold or chill phase) of a fever. During this phase, the body responds to pyrogens by conserving heat to raise body temperature.** 4. Profuse diaphoresis (sweating) occurs during the defervescence phase (fever abatement, flush phase) of a fever. During this phase, the fever abates and body temperature returns to the expected range. 5. Dehydration can occur during both the course phase (plateau phase) and defervescence phase (fever abatement, flush phase) of a fever.
Eliminate incorrect options.	The response in option 1 is associated with the course phase (plateau phase) of a fever and can be eliminated. The responses in options 4 and 5 are associated with the defervescence phase (fever abatement, flush phase) of a fever and can be eliminated.

74.

CRITICAL-THINKING STRATEGY

Recognize keywords.	A nurse is delegating an assignment to a nursing assistant. **Which client** who will **benefit the most** from **soaking the feet** for several minutes as part of a bath should the nurse assign to the nursing assistant?
Ask what the question is asking.	Which client will gain the most from soaking the feet?
Critically analyze each option in relation to the question and the other options.	Identify whether soaking the feet is beneficial for the client in each option. Then compare and contrast each client situation and establish which client will benefit the most from soaking the feet. **Rationales:** 1. The feet can be washed thoroughly when taking a shower. 2. Although warm water used to soak the feet promotes vasodilation, it is contraindicated in a client who has lower-extremity arterial disease. Foot soaks can cause maceration of already delicate skin and remove natural skin oils that make the skin vulnerable to cracking.

Continued

	3. **A homeless person will benefit from a foot soak. Homeless people do not have regular access to bathing facilities and generally are in need of skin care. Soaking the feet loosens dirt and limits scrubbing, which prevents trauma to the skin. Soaking the feet should be done for just several minutes because prolonged soaking removes natural skin oils, which dries the skin and makes it prone to cracking.** 4. When a client is on bedrest, the feet do not get soiled with dirt. Bedrest does not necessitate soaking the feet during a bed bath.
Eliminate incorrect options.	The clients in options 1 and 4 do not require soaking the feet. Soaking the feet is contraindicated for the client in option 2. Options 1, 2, and 4 can be eliminated.

75.

CRITICAL-THINKING STRATEGY

Recognize keywords.	A nurse is assessing the **skin** of an **older adult**. Which **condition** is of **most concern** to the nurse?
Ask what the question is asking.	Which skin condition in an older adult is the most serious?
Critically analyze each option in relation to the question and the other options.	Explore the causes and consequences of the clinical finding presented in each option. Review the expected skin changes associated with aging. Compare and contrast the options in relation to this information to identify the most serious clinical finding. **Rationales:** 1. Flat, brown spots on the skin are an expected integumentary change in older adults. Brown spots *(lentigo senilis)* on the skin are caused by a clustering of melanocytes, which are pigment-producing cells. 2. A loss of subcutaneous fat and a reduced thickness and vascularity of the dermis that occur with aging result in thin, translucent skin in older adults. 3. **Tenting occurs when the skin of a dehydrated person remains in a peak or tent position after the skin is pinched together. This is a sign of a deficient fluid volume. Care must be taken when assessing an older person because some degree of tenting may occur, even when hydrated, because of the decrease in skin elasticity and decrease in tissue fluid associated with aging; however, in a hydrated older adult tenting will resolve, but slowly.** 4. A decrease in tissue fluid and sebaceous gland activity associated with aging commonly results in dry, flaky skin.
Eliminate incorrect options.	The signs in options in 1, 2, and 4 are expected changes associated with aging and are not as serious as tenting of the skin, which indicates dehydration. Options 1, 2, and 4 can be eliminated.

76.

CRITICAL-THINKING STRATEGY

Recognize keywords.	A nurse is caring for a client who is using an **incentive spiromete**r. Which client **behavior** observed by the nurse **indicates** that **the teaching was effective**?
Ask what the question is asking.	Which action demonstrates correct use of an incentive spirometer?
Critically analyze each option in relation to the question and the other options.	List the steps of the procedure—use of an incentive spirometer. The behavior in each option must be compared with the steps in the procedure. This question expects you to identify the action that demonstrates the correct use of an incentive spirometer. **Rationales:** 1. **Inhaling slowly and deeply using the spirometer is the correct way to inhale when using an incentive spirometer; this technique helps to keep the airways open.** 2. The client is using the incentive spirometer incorrectly and requires further teaching. An incentive spirometer must be held in an upright position. A flow-oriented device that is tilted requires less effort to reach the desired inspiratory volume. A volume-oriented device that is tilted will not function correctly. 3. **Inspiratory goals progressively should be increased daily or more frequently, depending on the client's ability to maintain the improved volume at the set goal, which promotes alveoli ventilation.** 4. **Taking several breaths using the spirometer, then breathing without using the spirometer and using the spirometer again, are desirable practices because they prevent hyperventilation and respiratory alkalosis.** 5. The client should be taught to remove the mouthpiece from the mouth before exhalation. An incentive spirometer is designed to encourage inhalation, not exhalation.
Eliminate incorrect options.	Options 2 and 5 are incorrect actions when using an incentive spirometer and can be eliminated.

77.

CRITICAL-THINKING STRATEGY

Recognize keywords.	A nurse on a postpartum unit is teaching a class for new mothers about umbilical cord care. The nurse identifies that **one mother does not become involved** with the discussion and **is withdrawn**. Which is the **best action** by the nurse **to help this new mother learn** about umbilical cord care?
Ask what the question is asking.	Which teaching intervention is the most helpful for a client who is withdrawn?
Critically analyze each option in relation to the question and the other options.	This question requires the integration of several concepts: teaching-learning principles, strengths and weaknesses of various teaching strategies, and how best to teach a client who is withdrawn. Examine the action presented in each option and determine if it will be effective for this client, considering what you explored about teaching-learning.

Continued

	Rationales: 1. Giving the mother written material about cord care assumes that the client can read at the reading level of the presented material. Also, it does not provide an opportunity for the nurse to communicate with the client. 2. If the client was not participating in the present formal class, it is unlikely that the client will participate in the next class. 3. Although an audiovisual cassette is an excellent strategy to provide instruction, it does not provide the nurse with an opportunity to individualize one-on-one instruction. **4. The nurse identified that the client was quiet and withdrawn in the group class. Individual instruction provides the nurse the opportunity to explore the client's concerns and address the client's individual needs in privacy.**
Eliminate incorrect options.	Options 1 and 3 support withdrawn behavior. Option 2 was not effective in the past, and the teaching plan should be revised. Eliminate options 1, 2, and 3.

78.

CRITICAL-THINKING STRATEGY

Recognize keywords.	A nurse is teaching a client with **dysphagia how to eat safely**. Which should the nurse **encourage the client to do**?
Ask what the question is asking.	Which should a client with dysphagia do when eating?
Critically analyze each option in relation to the question and the other options.	Identify the major problem associated with dysphagia—risk for aspiration. Identify a client's response to each of the actions presented in the options. Determine if the action in each option is safe or unsafe. Identify the option that will have a safe outcome. **Rationales:** 1. Tilting the head backward when swallowing increases the risk of aspiration because it straightens the trachea and anatomically makes it easier for food and fluid to enter the trachea rather than the esophagus. 2. Food and fluid should be consumed separately in the presence of dysphagia. Fluid is more difficult to control with dysphagia, and it may flush the solid food toward the trachea, where it can cause choking or a partial or total airway obstruction. **3. A client with dysphagia should concentrate on the acts of chewing and swallowing. Environmental stimuli can be distracting and can result in inadequate chewing or premature swallowing, which in turn can result in choking and aspiration.** **4. Ensuring that the mouth is empty after eating reduces the risk of aspiration of retained food.** 5. Chewing food in the front of the mouth will increase the risk for aspiration. Food should be placed in the posterior, not anterior, part of the mouth toward the side. The molars in the back of the mouth are designed for chewing. Placing food to the side keeps it close to the molars for chewing and out of direct line with the trachea. Placing food in the posterior of the mouth limits the need for the tongue to manipulate the bolus of food toward the back of the mouth in preparation for swallowing (deglutition).
Eliminate incorrect options.	Eliminate the options that increase the risk of aspiration. Options 1, 2, and 5 can be eliminated.

79.

CRITICAL-THINKING STRATEGY

Recognize keywords.	A nurse is assessing a client for clinical manifestations of an altered serum potassium level. **Which clinical manifestation is common to both hypokalemia and hyperkalemia?**
Ask what the question is asking.	Identify the clinical indicator that is associated with both hypokalemia and hyperkalemia.
Critically analyze each option in relation to the question and the other options.	Make a list of all the clinical manifestations associated with hypokalemia. Make a list of all the clinical manifestations associated with hyperkalemia. Identify the signs and symptoms that appear on both your lists. **Rationale:** 1. Increased bowel sounds are caused by intestinal hypermotility, which is associated with just hyperkalemia, not hypokalemia. 2. **A deficiency or excess of potassium can cause muscle weakness because of potassium's role in the sodium–potassium pump, cellular metabolism, and muscle contraction. Muscle weakness is associated with both hyperkalemia and hypokalemia.** 3. **A deficiency or excess of potassium can cause dysrhythmias because of potassium's role in the sodium–potassium pump, cellular metabolism, and muscle contraction. The heart is a muscle. Dysrhythmias are associated with both hyperkalemia and hypokalemia.** 4. Confusion is associated with just hyperkalemia, not hypokalemia. 5. **Hypokalemia causes slowed gastrointestinal motility. Hyperkalemia causes hyperactivity of the gastrointestinal smooth muscle. Both of these manifestations can result in nausea.**
Eliminate incorrect options.	Eliminate options 1 and 4 because increased bowel sounds and confusion are related only to hyperkalemia.

80.

CRITICAL-THINKING STRATEGY

Recognize keywords.	A nurse in charge is delegating assignments to a registered nurse and a nursing assistant on the nursing team. Which **assignment** should be **delegated to only the registered nurse?**
Ask what the question is asking.	Which action is within the legal scope of practice for a registered nurse?
Critically analyze each option in relation to the question and the other options.	In general terms, contrast the responsibilities of a registered nurse and a nursing assistant. Assess each option and designate which member of the team can perform the assignment. **Rationales:** 1. **Evaluating a client's response to activity requires the knowledge and judgment of a registered nurse. This evaluation requires multiple assessments (e.g., breathing, heart rate, and fatigue) and may require immediate nursing intervention if an activity intolerance is identified.**

Continued

	2. A task of this complexity requires the knowledge and judgment of a registered nurse. This assessment requires more than just obtaining a pulse rate. It requires an additional assessment of rhythm and volume. Nursing assistants can take routine vital signs of clients who are stable.
	3. Client teaching is a complex task and requires the expertise of a registered nurse. It requires knowledge of principles such as identifying readiness to learn, progressing from simple to complex information, using motivational theory, and evaluating outcomes. Also, it requires knowledge of principles related to colostomy care (e.g., the bag opening must be at least ⅛ inch larger than the stoma, a pale stoma may indicate ischemia, and what to include in an assessment of the characteristics of intestinal output).
	4. Applying a condom catheter is not a complex task. It requires simple problem-solving skills, involves a predictable outcome, and employs a simple level of interaction with the client. This task is within the scope of practice of a nursing assistant and does not require the more advanced competencies of a registered nurse.
	5. Making an occupied bed is not a complex task. It requires simple problem-solving skills, involves a predictable outcome, and employs a simple level of interaction with the client. This task is within the scope of practice of a nursing assistant and does not require the more advanced competencies of a registered nurse.
Eliminate incorrect options.	Doing health teaching and assessing clients who are experiencing complex problems or are in high-risk situations are responsibilities of a registered nurse. Assignments that include the activities of daily living can be assigned to a nursing assistant. Eliminate options 4 and 5.

81.

CRITICAL-THINKING STRATEGY

Recognize keywords.	A nurse is caring for a client who recently received a diagnosis of diabetes. The nurse institutes all of the following interventions. **Which** nursing **action reflects** teaching self-management in the **affective domain**?
Ask what the question is asking.	Which nursing intervention is an example of teaching in the affective domain?
Critically analyze each option in relation to the question and the other options.	Explore what you know about the three domains of learning—affective, cognitive, and psychomotor. Identify examples of learning that occur in each domain. Determine the domain in which beliefs, attitudes, feelings, emotions, and values are addressed. **Rationales:** 1. Providing a list of signs and symptoms of a high glucose level is an example of teaching/learning in the cognitive domain. In the cognitive domain, teaching/learning is concerned with intellectual understanding. 2. **Encouraging the client to express feelings is an example of teaching/learning in the affective domain. In the affective domain, teaching/learning is concerned with feelings, emotions, values, beliefs, and attitudes.**

Continued

Continued

	3. Instructing the client about which foods are high in glucose is an example of teaching/learning in the cognitive domain. In the cognitive domain, teaching/learning is concerned with intellectual understanding. 4. Coaching the client on how to self-administer insulin is an example of teaching/learning in the psychomotor domain. Teaching/learning in the psychomotor domain includes using motor and physical abilities to master a skill. It requires a demonstration by the nurse, supervised practice, and a return demonstration by the client.
Eliminate incorrect options.	Options 1 and 3 reflect the cognitive domain. Option 4 reflects the psychomotor domain. Eliminate options 1, 3, and 4.

82.

CRITICAL-THINKING STRATEGY

Recognize keywords.	A nurse is caring for a client with an infected leg ulcer. Which **common systemic response to an infection** should the nurse **assess for** when monitoring this client?
Ask what the question is asking.	Which is a systemic response to an infection?
Critically analyze each option in relation to the question and the other options.	Make a list of local responses to an infection. Examine the options and eliminate those that are local responses to infection that you identified. Make a list of systemic responses and ensure that the remaining options in the question are on your list of systemic responses to infection. **Rationales:** 1. Pain is a local, not a systemic, response to infection because swelling of inflamed tissue exerts pressure on nerve endings. 2. Edema is a local, not a systemic, response to infection. Chemical mediators (e.g., kinins) increase the permeability of small blood vessels, thereby causing fluid to enter the interstitial compartment, resulting in local edema. **3. An increased body temperature is a common systemic response to infection. With hyperthermia, microorganisms or endotoxins stimulate phagocytic cells that release pyrogens, which stimulate the hypothalamic thermoregulatory center, causing fever.** **4. Infection causes the hormonal response of an increase in the secretion of epinephrine and norepinephrine, which then causes an increase in the heart rate of more than 100 beats per minute (tachycardia).** **5. An increased white blood cell count is a systemic response to infection. Neutrophils, a type of white blood cell, are the body's main defense against invading pathogens. Neutrophils kill bacteria by ingesting them.**
Eliminate incorrect options.	Eliminate options 1 and 2 because pain and edema are local, not systemic, responses to infection.

83.

CRITICAL-THINKING STRATEGY

Recognize keywords.	A client with terminal cancer says to the nurse, "I've been fairly religious, but sometimes **I wonder if the things I did were acceptable to God.**" **How should the nurse respond**?
Ask what the question is asking.	Identify the therapeutic response by the nurse in this situation.
Critically analyze each option in relation to the question and the other options.	Review therapeutic communication techniques and barriers to communication. Examine the options and identify the response that promotes communication and the responses that are barriers to communication. **Rationales:** 1. **This response recognizes the client's feelings.** 2. This response denies the client's feelings and gives false reassurance. The client's statement does not include information about attending religious services. 3. This response denies the client's feelings and gives false reassurance. 4. This response denies the client's feelings and gives false reassurance.
Eliminate incorrect options.	Options 2, 3, and 4 deny the client's feelings and give false reassurance. Options 2, 3, and 4 can be eliminated.

84.

CRITICAL-THINKING STRATEGY

Recognize keywords.	A nurse is administering a **lozenge** to a client's **buccal area** of the mouth. **Which should the nurse do**?
Ask what the question is asking.	Which intervention is essential when administering a lozenge?
Critically analyze each option in relation to the question and the other options.	List the steps of the procedure—administering a lozenge to a client's buccal cavity. Examine the behavior in each option and compare it with the list. **Rationales:** 1. **If the client falls asleep, the client may aspirate the lozenge, which can cause an airway obstruction.** 2. Fluid will interfere with the action and absorption of the lozenge. This action is unsafe because it can cause the client to aspirate or swallow the lozenge. 3. Medication that dissolves under the tongue is administered via the sublingual, not buccal, route. 4. The cheeks should be alternated when placing a lozenge to limit irritation to the mucous membranes in the buccal area. 5. A lozenge should be administered after, or between, meals. Food will interfere with the action and absorption of the medication.
Eliminate incorrect options.	Eliminate the options that have actions that are not on your identified list, are associated with another route of administration, or are contraindicated. Options 2, 4, and 5 are incorrect actions. Option 3 addresses the sublingual route. Eliminate options 2, 3, 4, and 5.

85.

CRITICAL-THINKING STRATEGY

Recognize keywords.	The nurse is assessing a client who is in pain. **Which question should** the nurse ask to **assess** the client's **pain tolerance**?
Ask what the question is asking.	Which question assesses pain tolerance?
Critically analyze each option in relation to the question and the other options.	Several concepts must be explored: characteristics of pain, pain threshold, and pain tolerance. Characteristics of pain include intensity, location, quality, pattern (onset, duration, exacerbation, and remission), and factors that increase or decrease the intensity of pain. **Rationales:** 1. **Pain tolerance is the maximum amount and duration of pain that a person is willing to tolerate. Pain tolerance is influenced by psychosociocultural factors and usually increases with age.** 2. This question focuses on an alleviating factor, distraction, rather than on the concept of pain tolerance. 3. This question determines the client's perception of the intensity of pain, not pain tolerance. 4. This question focuses on an alleviating factor, medication, rather than on the concept of pain tolerance.
Eliminate incorrect options.	Options 2 and 4 focus on alleviating factors. Option 3 focuses on intensity. Options 2, 3, and 4 can be eliminated.

86.

CRITICAL-THINKING STRATEGY

Recognize keywords.	An obese client asks the nurse, "What should I do to help myself lose weight?" How should the nurse respond while considering the **best behavior modification strategy for controlling food intake**?
Ask what the question is asking.	Which is the best intervention to control food intake?
Critically analyze each option in relation to the question and the other options.	Examine each option while considering certain concepts: promoting independence, physiological responses to dieting, and strategies to achieve dietary success. **Rationales:** 1. Asking family members not to bring tempting food into the house imposes on family members. A person must learn to cope with temptation regardless of where they are being exposed to desirable foods. 2. Although pictures that reflect a positive outcome may be motivating to some people, they are not personalized to the individual. An intervention in another option is more effective in controlling personal food intake. 3. The rigidity and limitation of avoiding between-meal snacks may cause periods of hypoglycemia, overeating, and noncompliance. Between-meal snacks should be calculated into the weight-reduction program to meet both physical and emotional needs. 4. **Behavior modification strategies are most successful when the person has an internal locus of control and is actively involved in self-care. Research demonstrates that self-monitoring of food intake is the single most helpful strategy in weight reduction.**

Continued

Eliminate incorrect options.	Involving other people communicates to clients that they are unable to develop an internal locus of control. Pictures of others may not motivate this client. Avoiding snacks may not meet the client's psychological or physical needs. Options 1, 2, and 3 can be eliminated.

87.

CRITICAL-THINKING STRATEGY

Recognize keywords.	A primary health-care provider prescribes diltiazem (Cardizem) **75 mg** by mouth three times a day. The scored diltiazem **tablets are labeled 30 mg/tablet. How many tablets** should the nurse **administer**? Record your answer **using one decimal place.**
Ask what the question is asking.	How many tablets of a drug should the nurse administer when 75 mg by mouth is prescribed and 30 mg/tablets are available?

Critically analyze each option in relation to the question and the other options.	Analyze the situation to extract the information needed to calculate the number of tablets to be administered. Recall the formula to perform the calculation. Insert the information in the question into the formula. Perform the calculation.
	Rationale:
	Answer: 2.5 tablets.
	   Solve the problem by using ratio and proportion.
	$$\frac{\text{Desired}}{\text{Have}} \quad \frac{75 \text{ mg}}{30 \text{ mg}} \times \frac{x \text{ tablet}}{1 \text{ tablet}}$$
	   Cross-multiply and reduce.
	$$30 \, x = 75$$
	$$x = 75 \div 30$$
	$$x = 2.5 \text{ tablets}$$

Eliminate incorrect options.	There are no incorrect options to eliminate.

88.

CRITICAL-THINKING STRATEGY

Recognize keywords.	A primary health-care provider prescribes the insertion of an **indwelling urinary catheter** (retention, Foley) as part of the client's preoperative prescriptions. Place the following **steps of the procedure in the order** in which they should be **performed** by the nurse.
Ask what the question is asking.	What is the progression of steps for inserting an indwelling urinary catheter?
Critically analyze each option in relation to the question and the other options.	List the sequential steps of inserting an indwelling urinary catheter. Refer to your list as you examine the options presented. Order the steps presented according to the sequence you identified. **Rationales:** **2. The outside of the catheterization package is not sterile and can be opened with hands that have been washed with soap and water.**

Continued

Continued

	1. The inside of the catheterization package is sterile. Sterile gloves are on the top of the supplies included because all subsequent equipment in the package must remain sterile. 3. The nurse's sterile, gloved hands then place the fenestrated drape over the client's perineal area to continue with the establishment of a sterile field. 5. Cleansing the labia moves from areas that are less likely to be contaminated than the urinary meatus as well as reduces the spread of microorganisms toward the urinary meatus. 4. Cleansing the urinary meatus last reduces the possibility of introducing microorganisms into the urinary meatus and the bladder.
Eliminate incorrect options.	There are no incorrect options.

89.

CRITICAL-THINKING STRATEGY

Recognize keywords.	A client's vital signs are apical heart rate—100 beats per minute, radial heart rate—84 beats per minute, respirations—20 breaths per minute, blood pressure—140/84 mm Hg. **What is the client's pulse deficit?** Record your answer **using a whole number**.
Ask what the question is asking.	Calculate a pulse deficit from the information provided.
Critically analyze each option in relation to the question and the other options.	Define a pulse deficit. Analyze the situation to extract the information needed to calculate the pulse deficit. Perform the calculation. **Rationale:** **Answer: 16.** **The pulse deficit is the difference between the apical and radial pulse rates. Therefore, 100 (apical rate) minus 84 (radial rate) equals 16. The client's pulse deficit is 16.**
Eliminate incorrect options.	There are no incorrect options to eliminate.

90.

CRITICAL-THINKING STRATEGY

Recognize keywords.	A client is admitted to the emergency department after sustaining a crushing injury at work. For which **characteristic of blood pressure** should the nurse assess the client to identify **impending shock**?
Ask what the question is asking.	Which abnormality in blood pressure is an early sign of shock?
Critically analyze each option in relation to the question and the other options.	Explore each option in relation to the physiological response to impending shock (reduced oxygenation). Compare and contrast the options and determine which option is a response to impending shock relative to the information you explored. **Rationales:** 1. The diastolic blood pressure decreases, not increases, during shock.

Continued

	2. **The initial stage of shock begins when baroreceptors in the aortic arch and the carotid sinus detect a drop in the mean arterial pressure, resulting in a decrease in the systolic blood pressure. The systolic pressure is the pressure in the arteries during ventricular contraction.** 3. During shock, there will be a narrowing, not a widening, of pulse pressure. Pulse pressure is the difference between the systolic and diastolic pressures. 4. Weak or absent, not robust, Korotkoff's sounds are associated with shock. Korotkoff's sounds are the five distinct sounds that are heard when auscultating a blood pressure (I—faint, clear tapping; II—swishing sound; III—intense, clear tapping; IV—muffled, blowing sounds; V—absence of sounds).
Eliminate incorrect options.	Options 1, 3, and 4 are the opposite of what will happen with impending shock. Options 1, 3, and 4 can be eliminated.

91.

CRITICAL-THINKING STRATEGY

Recognize keywords.	A client's primary health-care provider prescribes **antiembolism stockings** to be worn when out of bed. Which is an **important action** about antiembolism stockings that the nurse should teach the client?
Ask what the question is asking.	Which action is essential when caring for a client with antiembolism hose?
Critically analyze each option in relation to the question and the other options.	Recall the steps and the rationale for each step in the procedure for applying and wearing antiembolism stockings. Identify the benefits and consequences of the action presented in each option. Compare and contrast the options relative to the recalled information. **Rationales:** 1. Massaging the legs is contraindicated because it can cause a blood clot to migrate to the lungs, resulting in a pulmonary embolus. Lotion should not be used because it increases resistance between the fabric of the stocking and the skin. The resulting combination of friction and pressure will cause a shearing force that can injure the skin. 2. **Elastic stockings provide external pressure on the legs and feet to prevent pooling of blood in the veins while not interfering with arterial circulation. Putting antiembolism stockings on before the legs are dependent is appropriate because there will be less fluid in the tissues. Putting the stockings on after the legs are dependent is unsafe because the pressure of the stockings can injure fluid-filled tissue.** 3. The top cuff of antiembolism stockings should not be rolled because this can create a tight band that acts as a tourniquet, which can compromise impaired circulation further. The entire stocking should be applied so that the fabric is smooth and free of folds, creases, bunches, and wrinkles, which can impair circulation further.

Continued

Continued

	4. Removing and reapplying the stockings every 4 hours is unnecessary. Most antiembolism stockings have openings in the area of the feet to allow for assessment of capillary refill and skin color. Elastic stockings that are prescribed for 24 hours a day should be removed for 30 minutes three times a day.
Eliminate incorrect options.	Eliminate options 1, 3, and 4 because these actions can injure tissue.

92.

CRITICAL-THINKING STRATEGY

Recognize keywords.	A nurse must perform a straight catheterization of a client to obtain a urine specimen. The nurse opens the prepackaged straight catheter kit. **Place an X on the item in the kit that the nurse should touch first.**
Ask what the question is asking.	Which item in a sterile catherization kit should the nurse touch first in order to maintain sterile technique?
Critically analyze each option in relation to the question and the other options.	Recall the steps in obtaining a sterile urine specimen when using a sterile straight catheter. Then identify what the nurse must do first before touching any other piece of equipment in a sterile catherization kit. **Rationale:** **The nurse opens the outer package of the straight catheter kit with ungloved hands and then must don sterile gloves before touching any other item in the kit. Touching an item in the kit other than the packet of sterile gloves will result in contaminating the contents of the kit. The insertion of a straight catheter to obtain a urine specimen is a sterile procedure.**
Eliminate incorrect options.	Eliminate all items in the catherization kit except the sterile gloves. The nurse must apply sterile gloves before touching anything else in a catheterization kit.

93.

CRITICAL-THINKING STRATEGY

Recognize keywords.	A primary health-care provider prescribes 1 g of an antibiotic to be administered via the intramuscular route twice a day. The nurse implements all of the following actions. **Which** nursing **action reflects** the **planning step** of the **nursing process**?
Ask what the question is asking.	Identify the action that is part of the planning step of the nursing process.
Critically analyze each option in relation to the question and the other options.	Recall the steps in the nursing process—assessment, analysis, planning, implementation, and evaluation. Examine each option and identify which step of the nursing process is reflected by the action presented. **Rationales:** 1. Collecting data about a client involves assessment. Therefore, this action is an example of the assessment step of the nursing process. 2. Eventually obtaining the medication is part of the procedure associated with giving a medication. Therefore, this action is an example of the implementation step of the nursing process. 3. Identifying body landmarks before giving an injection is part of the procedure for administering an injection. Therefore, this action is an example of the implementation step of the nursing process. **4. Determining when medications should be administered requires planning. Therefore, this action is part of the planning step of the nursing process. The prescription states that the medication should be given twice a day. The nurse has the responsibility to determine when the medication should be given. This decision is based on a variety of factors, such as hospital policy, physiological action of the medication, and whether it should be administered on an empty stomach or with food.**
Eliminate incorrect options.	Collecting data in option 1 is related to the assessment phase of the nursing process. Options 2 and 3 are examples of actions in the implementation phase of the nursing process. Options 1, 2, and 3 can be eliminated.

94.

CRITICAL-THINKING STRATEGY

Recognize keywords.	A nurse working in a nursing home routinely administers **digoxin** 0.125 mg by mouth to a client every morning. **Which** of the following **should alert** the nurse to **withhold the medication**?
Ask what the question is asking.	Which client response indicates digoxin toxicity?
Critically analyze each option in relation to the question and the other options.	Review the physiological action of digoxin. Analyze each option to determine if the content is unrelated to digoxin or is a toxic effect of digoxin requiring its discontinuation.

Continued

Continued

	Rationales:
	1. Digoxin can cause sensory changes, such as diplopia (double vision), halos, colored vision, blind spots, and flashing lights. If any of these symptoms of toxicity occur, the medication should be withheld and a serum digoxin level assessed to determine if the drug is exceeding its therapeutic range of 0.5 to 2 ng/mL. Toxicity occurs when the plasma concentration of the drug exceeds its therapeutic range, resulting in life-threatening responses.
	2. Nausea and vomiting are common clinical indicators of digoxin toxicity that result from irritation of the gastrointestinal system caused by an excessive dose.
	3. A respiratory rate of more than 20 breaths per minute (tachypnea) is not a sign of digoxin toxicity.
	4. Digoxin prolongs conduction through the sinoatrial and atrioventricular nodes, which slows the heart rate (negative chronotropic effect). When the heart rate is less than 60 beats per minute (bradycardia), the medication should be held to prevent a further decrease in the heart rate. Some primary health-care providers will stipulate the low and high levels of pulse rates at which the drug should be held.
	5. Dysrhythmias are a common sign of digoxin toxicity because of the negative chronotropic effect of digoxin on cardiac tissue.
Eliminate incorrect options.	As indicated in the rationales, option 3 is unrelated to digoxin toxicity and can be eliminated.

95.

CRITICAL-THINKING STRATEGY

Recognize keywords.	A nurse is giving a client a **bed bath**. Which should the nurse **do to increase circulation**?
Ask what the question is asking.	Which action will increase circulation during a bed bath?
Critically analyze each option in relation to the question and the other options.	Identify the consequences of the action in each option. Then identify whether the action will or will not increase circulation. Identify whether an option is unsafe. Rationales: 1. The pressure of firm strokes on the skin moving from distal to proximal areas increases venous return. When venous return increases, cardiac output increases. 2. Although warm water will increase circulation, 20 minutes is an excessive period of time to soak the feet. Prolonged soaking removes the protective oils on the skin, and the result is dry, cracked skin that is prone to further injury. 3. Exposing just the areas that are being washed prevents chilling rather than increasing circulation. 4. A temperature of 120°F to 125°F is too hot for bathwater because it may cause tissue injury. Bathwater should be 110°F to 115°F.
Eliminate incorrect options.	Options 2 and 4 are unsafe because they may cause tissue injury. Option 3 does not increase circulation. Options 2, 3, and 4 can be eliminated.

96.

CRITICAL-THINKING STRATEGY

Recognize keywords.	A nurse is planning a teaching program for a client regarding the learning of a new skill. The nurse assesses each of the following. Which **factor** does the nurse conclude is **most relevant** when **predicting success of the teaching program**?
Ask what the question is asking.	Which factor is essential to the success of a teaching program?
Critically analyze each option in relation to the question and the other options.	Examine each option relative to its importance in facilitating learning. Compare and contrast the options. **Rationales:** 1. Although the level of the client's education must be considered when designing a teaching program, of the options presented, it is not the most relevant factor when predicting success of the teaching program. 2. **The motivation of the learner to acquire new attitudes, information, or skills is the most important component for successful learning; motivation exists when the learner recognizes the future benefits of learning.** 3. Although family support is important, of the options presented, it is not the most relevant factor when predicting success of the teaching program. Not all clients have a family support system. 4. Although a teaching program must be designed within the client's cognitive and developmental abilities, of the options presented, they are not the most relevant factors when predicting success.
Eliminate incorrect options.	Progressively eliminate the least important action until you arrive at a single option. Options 1, 3, and 4 can be eliminated because the factors in these options are not as important as motivation of the learner.

97.

CRITICAL-THINKING STRATEGY

Recognize keywords.	A client who immigrated with her family to the United States 15 years ago is residing in a long-term care facility. The nurse sits down next to the client, who is crying. Eventually, the client states, "**Our son is** 30 years old and still is **not married. My husband and I want to arrange a marriage for him, but he refuses.** My husband and I have a wonderful marriage, and we had an arranged marriage 35 years ago. **Arranged marriages are accepted in our culture.**" What is the nurse's best response?
Ask what the question is asking.	Which is a therapeutic response by the nurse to a client's statements indicating a cultural divide among family members?
Critically analyze each option in relation to the question and the other options.	Examine each statement in the options and identify those that reflect a barrier to communication. Identify the option that demonstrates a therapeutic communication technique. Explore each option and identify whether the nurse's response focuses on the client's feelings and concerns.

Continued

Continued

	Rationales:
	1. This response is too blunt and may be an assumption.
	2. Although this response addresses arranged marriages, it does not focus on the central issue in the discussion—the son does not want an arranged marriage.
	3. This response focuses on the client's feelings. It provides an opportunity for the client to discuss personal concerns further.
	4. Although this may be a true statement, it is too brusque (direct, frank) and challenging. The client is coping with the issue in the present and is not ready to move forward with a resolution.
Eliminate incorrect options.	Options 1 and 4 are abrupt, challenging, and not therapeutic. Option 2 is a supportive statement, but it does not address the client's concern. Eliminate options 1, 2, and 4.

98.

CRITICAL-THINKING STRATEGY

Recognize keywords.	A client who is secretly smoking in bed falls asleep, and the **cigarette ignites** the client's **gown**. Which should the nurse **do first** after discovering the fire?
Ask what the question is asking.	What is the nurse's first action when a client's gown is on fire?
Critically analyze each option in relation to the question and the other options.	Identify the steps to follow when confronted with a fire and integrate the concept "oxygen supports combustion." Refer to the mnemonic RACE (**R**escue clients in immediate danger, **A**ctivate the alarm, **C**onfine the fire, **E**xtinguish the fire). Identify that to rescue the client, the nurse has to extinguish the fire. Identify ways in which the nurse can cut off oxygen that supports a fire. Examine options in light of the information you have explored. Rationales: **1. Smothering the flames with a blanket deprives the fire of oxygen. Without oxygen to support combustion, the fire will go out. This action protects the client. Rescuing the client is the first step of fire safety.** 2. Rolling the client from side to side will fan the flames, which will increase the intensity of the fire. 3. Activating the alarm is premature at this time, but it will be done eventually. 4. Closing the door will impede the evacuation of the client from the room if it becomes necessary.
Eliminate incorrect options.	Option 2 is unsafe. Option 3 is premature. Option 4 will impede departure from the room if it becomes necessary. Options 2, 3, and 4 can be eliminated.

99.

CRITICAL-THINKING STRATEGY

Recognize keywords.	A nurse **discovers** that a **client is taking natural herbal remedies. Which intervention is most important** for the nurse to do?
Ask what the question is asking.	Which action is most important when the nurse identifies that the client is taking natural herbal remedies?
Critically analyze each option in relation to the question and the other options.	Consider the significance of the word *discover* as it relates to the scenario—what is most important after discovering new information. Identify the action that will protect the client immediately. Analyze the options and determine which action is most critical to ensure the client's safety. **Rationales:** 1. It is essential for the nurse to be an informed provider of care, but it is not the priority of care for this client. 2. Although thinking of supplements as drugs should be done, it is not the priority of care for this client. **3. The primary health-care provider should be notified immediately because the herb may interact with prescribed medications or therapies.** 4. Although including the details about supplement use in the client's health history should be done, it is not the priority. Medications or therapies may interact with the herb before the primary health-care provider reads the information in the health history.
Eliminate incorrect options.	The actions in options 1 and 2 will not immediately provide for client safety. Although documentation is important, it is not the priority. Eliminate options 1, 2, and 4.

100.

CRITICAL-THINKING STRATEGY

Recognize keywords.	A client sustained a traumatic brain injury resulting in neurological deficits after falling off a ladder at work. Which **setting** is **most appropriate** for the nurse to explore with the client and the family to assist this client **to learn how to live with neurological limitations**?
Ask what the question is asking.	Which health-care setting is best for learning how to live with neurological deficits?
Critically analyze each option in relation to the question and the other options.	Identify the types of services provided by each of the health-care settings presented in the options. Examine the situation in the question and determine which of the settings best provides services that meet the needs of a client with neurological deficits. **Rationales:** 1. An assisted-living residence provides limited assistance with activities of daily living, meal preparation, laundry services, transportation, and opportunities for socialization. Residents are relatively independent.

Continued

Continued

	2. **Once stabilized and out of danger, the individual in this scenario needs intensive rehabilitation services that can be received in an extended care facility. An extended care facility is a setting where people live while receiving suba-cute medical, nursing, and rehabilitative care. Examples of extended care facilities include intermediate care facili-ties, rehabilitation centers, and nursing homes that provide subacute care/skilled nursing care.**
	3. An acute care setting generally is not the best setting to provide extensive rehabilitation services. The acute care setting provides services that medically and emotionally support the client during the critical and acute phases right after the traumatic event and until the client is stable and out of danger.
	4. Hospice care is inappropriate for this client because the client is not dying. Hospice programs provide supportive care to dying clients and their family members to pro-mote dying with dignity.
Eliminate incorrect options.	Assisted-living residences, hospitals, and hospice services are not designed to meet the intense rehabilitation needs of a client learning to live with neurological limitations. Options 1, 3, and 4 can be eliminated.

Glossary of English Words Commonly Encountered on Nursing Examinations

Abnormality — defect, irregularity, anomaly, oddity

Absence — nonappearance, lack, nonattendance

Abundant — plentiful, rich, profuse

Accelerate — go faster, speed up, increase, hasten

Accumulate — build up, collect, gather

Accurate — precise, correct, exact

Achievement — accomplishment, success, reaching, attainment

Acknowledge — admit, recognize, accept, reply

Activate — start, turn on, stimulate

Adequate — sufficient, ample, plenty, enough

Angle — slant, approach, direction, point of view

Application — use, treatment, request, claim

Approximately — about, around, in the region of, more or less, roughly speaking

Arrange — position, place, organize, display

Associated — linked, related

Attention — notice, concentration, awareness, thought

Authority — power, right, influence, clout, expert

Avoid — keep away from, evade, let alone

Balanced — stable, neutral, steady, fair, impartial

Barrier — barricade, blockage, obstruction, obstacle

Best — most excellent, most important, greatest

Capable — able, competent, accomplished

Capacity — ability, capability, aptitude, role, power, size

Central — middle, mid, innermost, vital

Challenge — confront, dare, dispute, test, defy, face up to

Characteristic — trait, feature, attribute, quality, typical

Circular — round, spherical, globular

Collect — gather, assemble, amass, accumulate, bring together

Commitment — promise, vow, dedication, obligation, pledge, assurance

Commonly — usually, normally, frequently, generally, universally

Compare — contrast, evaluate, match up to, weigh or judge against

Compartment — section, part, cubicle, booth, stall

Complex — difficult, multifaceted, compound, multipart, intricate

Complexity — difficulty, intricacy, complication

Component — part, element, factor, section, constituent

Comprehensive — complete, inclusive, broad, thorough

Conceal — hide, cover up, obscure, mask, suppress, secrete

Conceptualize — to form an idea

Concern — worry, anxiety, fear, alarm, distress, unease, trepidation

Concisely — briefly, in a few words, succinctly

Conclude — make a judgment, determine

Confidence — self-assurance, certainty, poise, self-reliance

Congruent — matching, fitting, going together well

Consequence — result, effect, outcome, end result

Constituents — elements, components, parts that make up a whole

Contain — hold, enclose, surround, include, control, limit

Continual — repeated, constant, persistent, recurrent, frequent

Continuous — constant, incessant, nonstop, unremitting, permanent

Contribute — be a factor, add, give

Convene — assemble, call together, summon, organize, arrange

Convenience — expediency, handiness, ease

Coordinate — organize, direct, manage, bring together

Create — make, invent, establish, generate, produce, fashion, build, construct

Creative — imaginative, original, inspired, inventive, resourceful, innovative

Critical — serious, grave, significant, dangerous, life-threatening

Cue — signal, reminder, prompt, sign, indication

Curiosity — inquisitiveness, interest, nosiness, snooping

Damage — injure, harm, hurt, break, wound

Deduct — subtract, take away, remove, withhold

Deficient — lacking, wanting, underprovided, scarce, faulty

Defining — important, crucial, major, essential, significant, central

Defuse — resolve, calm, soothe, neutralize, rescue, mollify

Delay — hold up, wait, hinder, postpone, slow down, hesitate, linger

577

Demand — insist, claim, require, command, stipulate, ask

Describe — explain, tell, express, illustrate, depict, portray

Design — plan, invent, intend, aim, propose, devise

Desirable — wanted, pleasing, enviable, popular, sought after, attractive, advantageous

Detail — feature, aspect, element, factor, facet

Deteriorate — worsen, decline, weaken

Determine — decide, conclude, resolve, agree on

Dexterity — skillfulness, handiness, agility, deftness

Dignity — self-respect, self-esteem, decorum, formality, poise

Dimension — aspect, measurement

Diminish — reduce, lessen, weaken, detract, moderate

Discharge — release, dismiss, set free

Discontinue — stop, cease, halt, suspend, terminate, withdraw

Disorder — complaint, problem, confusion, chaos

Display — show, exhibit, demonstrate, present, put on view

Dispose — get rid of, arrange, order, set out

Dissatisfaction — displeasure, discontent, unhappiness, disappointment

Distinguish — separate, classify, recognize differences

Distract — divert, sidetrack, entertain

Distress — suffering, trouble, anguish, misery, agony, concern, sorrow

Distribute — deliver, spread out, hand out, issue, dispense

Disturbed — troubled, unstable, concerned, worried, distressed, anxious, uneasy

Diversional — serving to distract

Don — put on, dress oneself in

Dramatic — spectacular

Drape — cover, wrap, dress, swathe

Dysfunction — abnormal, impaired

Edge — perimeter, boundary, periphery, brink, border, rim

Effective — successful, useful, helpful, valuable

Efficient — not wasteful, effective, competent, resourceful, capable

Elasticity — stretch, spring, suppleness, flexibility

Eliminate — get rid of, eradicate, abolish, remove, purge

Embarrass — make uncomfortable, make self-conscious, humiliate, mortify

Emerge — appear, come, materialize, become known

Emphasize — call attention to, accentuate, stress, highlight

Ensure — make certain, guarantee

Environment — setting, surroundings, location, atmosphere, milieu, situation

Episode — event, incident, occurrence, experience

Essential — necessary, fundamental, vital, important, crucial, critical, indispensable

Etiology — assigned cause, origin

Exaggerate — overstate, inflate

Excel — stand out, shine, surpass, outclass

Excessive — extreme, too much, unwarranted

Exertion — intense or prolonged physical effort

Exhibit — show signs of, reveal, display

Expand — get bigger, enlarge, spread out, increase, swell, inflate

Expect — wait for, anticipate, imagine

Expectation — hope, anticipation, belief, prospect, probability

Experience — knowledge, skill, occurrence, know-how

Expose — lay open, leave unprotected, allow to be seen, reveal, disclose, exhibit

External — outside, exterior, outer

Facilitate — make easy, make possible, help, assist

Factor — part, feature, reason, cause, think, issue

Focus — center, focal point, hub

Fragment — piece, portion, section, part, splinter, chip

Function — purpose, role, job, task

Furnish — supply, provide, give, deliver, equip

Further — additional, more, extra, added, supplementary

Generalize — take a broad view, simplify, make inferences from particulars

Generate — make, produce, create

Gentle — mild, calm, tender

Girth — circumference, bulk, weight

Highest — uppermost, maximum, peak, main

Hinder — hold back, delay, hamper, obstruct, impede

Humane — caring, kind, gentle, compassionate, benevolent, civilized

Ignore — pay no attention to, disregard, overlook, discount

Imbalance — unevenness, inequality, disparity

Immediate — insistent, urgent, direct

Impair — damage, harm, weaken

Implantation — insertion

Implement — employ, execute, carry out

Impotent — powerless, weak, incapable, ineffective, unable

Inadvertent — unintentional, chance, unplanned, accidental

Include — comprise, take in, contain

Indicate — point out, sign of, designate, specify, show

Ineffective — unproductive, unsuccessful, useless, vain, futile

Inevitable — predictable, expected, unavoidable, foreseeable

Influence — power, pressure, sway, manipulate, affect, effect

Initiate — start, begin, open, commence, instigate

Insert — put in, add, supplement, introduce

Inspect — look over, check, examine

Inspire — motivate, energize, encourage, enthuse

Institutionalize — place in a facility for treatment

Integrate — put together, mix, add, combine, assimilate

Integrity — honesty

Interfere — get in the way, hinder, obstruct, impede, hamper

Interpret — explain the meaning of, make understandable

Intervention — action, activity

Intolerance — bigotry, prejudice, narrow-mindedness

Involuntary — instinctive, reflex, unintentional, automatic, uncontrolled

Irreversible — permanent, irrevocable, irreparable, unalterable

Irritability — sensitivity to stimuli, fretful, quick excitability

Justify — explain in accordance with reason

Likely — probably, possible, expected

Liquefy — change into or make more fluid

Logical — using reason

Longevity — long life

Lowest — inferior in rank

Maintain — continue, uphold, preserve, sustain, retain

Majority — the greater part of

Mention — talk about, refer to, state, cite, declare, point out

Minimal — least, smallest, nominal, negligible, token

Minimize — reduce, diminish, lessen, curtail, decrease to smallest possible

Mobilize — activate, organize, assemble, gather together, rally

Modify — change, adapt, adjust, revise, alter

Moist — slightly wet, damp

Multiple — many, numerous, several, various

Natural — normal, ordinary, unaffected

Negative — no, harmful, downbeat, pessimistic

Negotiate — bargain, talk, discuss, consult, cooperate, settle

Notice — become aware of, see, observe, discern, detect

Notify — inform, tell, alert, advise, warn, report

Nurture — care for, raise, rear, foster

Obsess — preoccupy, consume

Occupy — live in, inhabit, reside in, engage in

Occurrence — event, incident, happening

Odorous — scented, stinking, aromatic

Offensive — unpleasant, distasteful, nasty, disgusting

Opportunity — chance, prospect, break

Organize — put in order, arrange, sort, categorize, classify

Origin — source, starting point, cause, beginning, derivation, etiology

Pace — speed

Parameter — limit, factor, limitation, issue

Participant — member, contributor, partaker, applicant

Perspective — viewpoint, view, perception

Position — place, location, point, spot, situation

Practice — do, carry out, perform, apply, follow

Precipitate — cause to happen, bring on, hasten, abrupt, sudden

Predetermine — fix or set beforehand

Predictable — expected, knowable

Preference — favorite, liking, first choice

Prepare — get ready, plan, make, train, arrange, organize

Prescribe — set down, stipulate, order, recommend, impose

Previous — earlier, prior, before, preceding

Primarily — first, above all, mainly, mostly, largely, principally, predominantly

Primary — first, main, basic, chief, most important, key, prime, major, crucial

Priority — main concern, giving first attention to, order of importance

Production — making, creation, construction, assembly

Profuse — a lot of, plentiful, copious, abundant, generous, prolific, bountiful

Prolong — extend, delay, put off, lengthen, draw out

Promote — encourage, support, endorse, sponsor

Proportion — ratio, amount, quantity, part of, percentage, section of

Provide — give, offer, supply, make available

Rationalize — explain, reason

Realistic — practical, sensible, reasonable

Receive — get, accept, take delivery of, obtain

Recognize — acknowledge, appreciate, identify, aware of

Recovery — healing, mending, improvement, recuperation, renewal

Reduce — decrease, lessen, ease, moderate, diminish

Reestablish — reinstate, restore, return, bring back

Regard — consider, look upon, relate to, respect

Regular — usual, normal, ordinary, standard, expected, conventional

Relative — comparative, family member

Relevance — importance of

Reluctant — unwilling, hesitant, disinclined, indisposed, adverse

Reminisce — recall and review remembered experiences

Remove — take away, get rid of, eliminate, eradicate

Reposition — move, relocate, change position

Require — need, want, necessitate

Resist — oppose, defend against, keep from, refuse to go along with, defy

Resolution — decree, solution, decision, ruling, promise

Resolve — make up your mind, solve, determine, decide

Response — reply, answer, reaction, retort

Restore — reinstate, reestablish, bring back, return to, refurbish

Restrict — limit, confine, curb, control, contain, hold back, hamper

Retract — take back, draw in, withdraw, apologize

Reveal — make known, disclose, divulge, expose, tell, make public

Review — appraisal, reconsider, evaluation, assessment, examination, analysis

Ritual — custom, ceremony, formal procedure

Robust — sturdy, vigorous

Rotate — turn, go around, spin, swivel

Routine — usual, habit, custom, practice

Satisfaction — approval, fulfillment, pleasure, happiness

Satisfy — please, convince, fulfill, make happy, gratify

Secure — safe, protected, fixed firmly, sheltered, confident, obtain

Sequential — chronological, in order of occurrence

Significant — important, major, considerable, noteworthy, momentous

Slight — small, slim, minor, unimportant, insignificant, insult, snub

Source — basis, foundation, starting place, cause

Specific — exact, particular, detail, explicit, definite

Stable — steady, even, constant

Statistics — figures, data, information

Subtract — take away, deduct

Success — achievement, victory, accomplishment

Surround — enclose, encircle, contain

Suspect — think, believe, suppose, guess, deduce, infer, distrust, doubtful

Sustain — maintain, carry on, prolong, continue, nourish, suffer

Synonymous — same as, identical, equal, tantamount

Systemic — affecting the entire organism

Thorough — careful, detailed, methodical, systematic, meticulous, comprehensive, exhaustive

Tilt — tip, slant, slope, lean, angle, incline

Translucent — see-through, transparent, clear

Unique — one and only, sole, exclusive, distinctive

Universal — general, widespread, common, worldwide

Unoccupied — vacant, not busy, empty

Unrelated — unconnected, unlinked, distinct, dissimilar, irrelevant

Unresolved — unsettled, uncertain, unsolved, unclear, in doubt

Utilize — make use of, employ

Various — numerous, variety, range of, mixture of, assortment of

Verbalize — express, voice, speak, articulate

Verify — confirm, make sure, prove, attest to, validate, substantiate, corroborate, authenticate

Vigorous — forceful, strong, brisk, energetic

Volume — quantity, amount, size

Withdraw — remove, pull out, take out, extract

Bibliography

Ackley BJ, Ladwig GB, Makic MBF. *Nursing Diagnosis Handbook: An Evidence-Based Guide to Planning Care.* 11th ed. St. Louis, MO: Mosby Elsevier; 2017.

Alfaro-LeFevre R. *Critical Thinking and Clinical Judgment: A Practical Approach to Outcome-Focused Thinking.* 4th ed. Philadelphia, PA: W.B. Saunders; 2009.

American Association of Colleges of Nursing. *2016-2017 Enrollment and Graduations in Baccalaureate and Graduate Programs in Nursing.* Washington, DC: American Association of Colleges of Nursing; 2017.

American Hospital Association. The patient care partnership: Understanding expectations, rights and responsibilities [patient brochure]. Chicago, IL; 2003. https://www.aha.org/system/files/2018-01/aha-patient-care-partnership.pdf. Accessed March 28, 2018.

Baranoski S, Ayello EA. *Wound Care Essentials: Practice Principles.* 4th ed. Philadelphia, PA: Wolters Kluwer; 2016.

Bastable SB. *Essentials of Patient Education.* 2nd ed. Burlington, MA: Jones & Bartlett Learning; 2017.

Bauer C, Arnold-Long M, Kent DJ. Colostomy irrigation to maintain continence: an old method revived. *Nurs.* 2016;46(8):59-62.

Betts VT. Nursing's agenda for health care reform: policy, politics, and power through professional leadership. *Nurs Adm Q.* Spring 1996;20(3):1-8.

Black BP. *Professional Nursing: Concepts and Challenges,* 8th ed. St. Louis, MO: Elsevier; 2016.

Bradshaw MJ, Hultquist BL, eds. *Innovative Teaching Strategies in Nursing and Related Health Professions.* 7th ed. Burlington, MA: Jones & Bartlett Learning; 2017.

Brous E. Lessons learned from litigation: maintaining professional boundaries. *Am J Nurs.* 2014;114(7):60-63.

Bryant RA, Nix DP. *Acute and Chronic Wounds: Current Management Concepts.* 5th ed. St. Louis, MO: Elsevier; 2015.

Bulechek GM, Butcher HK, Dochterman JM, Wagner C, eds. *Nursing Interventions Classification (NIC).* 6th ed. St. Louis, MO: Elsevier/Mosby; 2013.

Burton MA, Ludwig LJM. *Fundamentals of Nursing Care: Concepts, Connections & Skills.* 2nd ed. Philadelphia, PA: FA Davis Co; 2015.

Catalano J. *Nursing Now! Today's Issues, Tomorrow's Trends.* 7th ed. Philadelphia, PA: FA Davis Co; 2015.

Center for Nursing Classification and Clinical Effectiveness (CNC). www.nursing.uiowa.edu/center-for-nursing-classification-and-clinical-effectiveness. Accessed March 26, 2018.

Chaffee J. *Thinking Critically.* 11th ed. Stamford, CT: Cengage Learning; 2015.

Cherry B, Jacob SR. *Contemporary Nursing: Issues, Trends, and Management.* 7th ed. St. Louis, MO: Elsevier; 2017.

Clean hands count for safe healthcare. Centers for Disease Control and Prevention. https://www.cdc.gov/features/handhygiene/index.html. Accessed March 26, 2018.

Colbert A. Putting ethics into action. *Nurs.* 2017;47(8):13-14.

Costedio E, Powers J, Stuart TL. Change-of-shift report: from hallways to the bedside [Student voices]. *Nurs.* 2013;43(8):18-19.

Coyle R, Mazaleski A. Initiating and sustaining a fall prevention program. *Nurs.* 2016;46(5):16-21.

de Castillo SLM, Werner-McCullough M. *Calculating Drug Dosages: A Patient-Safe Approach to Nursing and Math.* Philadelphia, PA: FA Davis Co; 2017.

Dahlkemper TR. *Anderson's Caring for Older Adults Holistically.* 6th ed. Philadelphia, PA: FA Davis Co; 2016.

Dillon PM. *Nursing Health Assessment: The Foundation of Clinical Practice.* 3rd ed. Philadelphia, PA: FA Davis Co; 2016.

Doenges ME, Moorhouse MF, Murr AC. *Nursing Diagnosis Manual: Planning, Individualizing, and Documenting Client Care.* 5th ed. Philadelphia, PA: FA Davis Co; 2016.

Facts about the official "Do Not Use" List of Abbreviations. The Joint Commission. https://www.jointcommission.org/facts_about_do_not_use_list/. Accessed March 28, 2018.

Fahlberg B. Promoting patient dignity in nursing care. *Nurs.* 2014;44(7):14.

Finkelman A. *Leadership and Management for Nurses: Core Competencies for Quality Care.* 3rd ed. Upper Saddle River, NJ: Pearson Education; 2016.

Gibson M, Keeling A. Shaping family and community health: a historical perspective. *Family and Community Health.* 2014;37(3):168-169.

Gorski L. *Phillips's Manual of I.V. Therapeutics: Evidence-Based Practice for Infusion Therapy.* 7th ed. Philadelphia, PA: FA Davis Co; 2018.

Grant B, Chou SP, Saha TD, Pickering RP, Kerridge BT, Ruan WJ, et al: Prevalence of 12-month alcohol use, high-risk drinking, and DSM-IV alcohol use disorder in the United States 2001-2002 to 2012-2013. Results from the National Epidemiologic Survey on Alcohol and Related Conditions. *JAMA Psychiatry* 2017;74(9):911-923.

Grey J, Enoch S, Harding KG. Wound assessment. *BMJ.* 2006;332(7536):285-288. https://www.ncbi.nlm.nih.gov/pmc/articles/PMC1360405/. Accessed March 28, 2018.

Hargrove-Huttel RA, Colgrove KC. *Pharmacology Success: Applying Critical Thinking to Test Taking.* 2nd ed. Philadelphia, PA: FA Davis Co; 2014.

Hargrove-Huttel RA, Colgrove KC. *Prioritization, Delegation, and Management of Care for the NCLEX-RN® Exam.* Philadelphia, PA: FA Davis Co; 2014.

Healthcare-associated infections. Centers for Disease Control and Prevention. http://www.cdc.gov/hai/. Accessed March 24, 2018.

Hopp L. *Introduction to Evidence-Based Practice.* Philadelphia, PA: FA Davis Co; 2012.

Huston CJ. *Professional Issues in Nursing: Challenges and Opportunities.* 4th ed. Philadelphia, PA: Wolters Kluwer; 2017.

Important facts about falls. Centers for Disease Control and Prevention. https://www.cdc.gov/homeandrecreationalsafety/falls/adultfalls.html. Accessed March 26, 2018.

Jackson SA. Rapid response teams: what's the latest? *Nurs.* 2017;47(12):34-41.

Jones V, Grey JE, Harding KG. Wound dressings. *BMJ.* 2006;332(7544):777-780.

Kee JF, Marshall SM. *Clinical Calculations: With Applications to General and Specialty Areas.* 8th ed. St. Louis, MO: Elsevier Health Sciences; 2016.

Kelly P, Marthaler MT. *Nursing Delegation, Setting Priorities, and Making Patient Care Assignments.* 2nd ed. Clifton Park, NY: Delmar Cengage Learning; 2011.

Kirkland-Kyhn H, Zaratkiewicz S, Teleten O, Young HM. Caring for aging skin. *Am J Nurs.* 2018;118(2):60-63.

Kowalski SL, Anthony M. Nursing's evolving role in patient safety [CE]. *Am J Nurs.* 2017;117(2):34-48.

Kübler-Ross E. *On Death and Dying.* New York, NY: Macmillan; 1969.

Lange JW. *The Nurse's Role in Promoting Optimal Health of Older Adults: Thriving in the Wisdom Years.* Philadelphia, PA: FA Davis Co; 2011.

Laskowski-Jones L. The art of harmonious delegation. *Nurs.* 2014;44(5):6.

Leapfrog Group. Safe practices. http://www.leapfroggroup.org/ratings-reports/safe-practices. Accessed March 27, 2018.

Lindauer A, Sexson K, Harvath TA. Medication management for people with dementia. *Am J Nurs.* 2017;117(5 Suppl 1):S17-S21.

Lutz CA, Mazur EE, Litch NA. *Nutrition and Diet Therapy.* 7th ed. Philadelphia, PA: FA Davis Co; 2018.

Makic MBF, Bridges E. Managing sepsis and septic shock: current guidelines and definitions [CE]. *Am J Nurs.* 2018;118(2):34-39.

Maslow AH. *A Theory of Human Motivation.* Eastford, CT: Martino Fine Books Publishers; 2013.

McCarron K. Med check: routine labs for common meds. *Nursing Made Incredibly Easy!* 2013;11(2):50-53.

McFarland MR, Wehbe-Alamah H. *Leininger's Culture Care Diversity and Universality: A Worldwide Nursing Theory.* 3rd ed. Burlington, MA: Jones & Bartlett Learning; 2015.

Mick J. Call to action: how to implement evidence-based nursing practice. *Nurs.* 2017; 47(4):36-43.

Miller J, Hayes DD, Carey KW. 20 questions: evidence-based practice or sacred cow? *Nurs.* 2015;45(8):46-55.

Moorhead S, Swanson E, Johnson M, Maas M. *Nursing Outcomes Classification (NOC)— E-Book: Measurement of Health Outcomes.* 6th ed. St. Louis, MO: Elsevier; 2018.

Murdock A, Griffin B. How is patient education linked to patient satisfaction? *Nurs.* 2013; 43(6):43-45.

Multiple chronic conditions. Centers for Disease Control and Prevention. www.cdc.gov/chronicdisease/about/multiple-chronic.htm. Accessed August 7, 2018.

Nix, S. *Williams' Basic Nutrition and Diet Therapy.* 15th ed. St. Louis, MO: Elsevier Health Sciences; 2017.

Nugent PM, Vitale BA. *Davis Essential Nursing Content + Practice Questions, Fundamentals.* 2nd ed. Philadelphia, PA: FA Davis Co; 2017.

Nugent PM, Vitale BA. *Fundamentals of Nursing: Content Review PLUS Practice Questions.* Philadelphia, PA: FA Davis Co; 2014.

Nugent PM, Vitale BA. *Test Success: Test-Taking Techniques for Beginning Nursing Students.* 8th ed. Philadelphia, PA: FA Davis Co; 2018.

O'Keeffe M, Saver C (contributors). *Communication, Collaboration, and You: Tools, Tips, and Techniques for Nursing Practice.* Silver Spring, MD: American Nurses Association; 2014.

Ortega L, Parsh B. Improving change-of-shift report. *Nurs.* 2013;43(2):68.

Palmer JE. Reducing distress and medication use in patients with dementia. *Nurs.* 2017;47(5):18-21.

Phillips J, Stinson K, Strickler J. Avoiding eruptions: de-escalating agitated patients. *Nurs.* 2014;44(4):60-63.

Pozgar GD. *Legal and Ethical Issues for Health Professionals.* 4th ed. Burlington, MA: Jones & Bartlett Learning; 2016.

Pressure ulcers get new terminology and staging definitions. *Nurs.* 2017;47(3):68-69.

Primeau MS, Frith KH. Teaching patients with an intellectual disability. *Nurs.* 2013; 43(6):68-69.

Quinlan-Colwell A. Making an ethical plan for treating patients in pain. *Nurs.* 2013; 43(10):64-68.

Raines V. *Davis's Basic Math Review for Nursing and Health Professionals: With Step-by-Step Solutions.* 2nd ed. Philadelphia, PA: FA Davis Co; 2016.

Rank W. Performing a focused neurologic assessment. *Nurs.* 2013;43(12):37-40.

Riley JB. *Communication in Nursing*. 8th ed. St. Louis, MO: Elsevier; 2017.

Roe E, Williams DL. Using evidence-based practice to prevent hospital-acquired pressure ulcers and promote wound healing. *Am J Nurs*. 2014;114(8):61-65.

Rogers TL, Darden CR. How clinical nurse leaders can improve rural healthcare? *Nurs*. 2014;44(9):52-55.

Said AA, Kautz DD. Reducing restraint use for older adults in acute care. *Nurs*. 2013; 43(12):59-61.

Salladay SA. Ethical problems [Intimate Partner Violence]. *Nurs*. 2016;46(8):12-13.

Satorre J. Managing medication errors. *Am J Nurs*. 2017;117(4):13.

Scanlon VC, Sanders T. *Essentials of Anatomy and Physiology*. 8th ed. Philadelphia, PA: FA Davis Co; 2017.

Slachta PA, ed. *Wound Care Made Incredibly Easy!* 3rd ed. Philadelphia, PA: Wolters Kluwer; 2019.

Squires A. Evidence-based approaches to breaking down language barriers. *Nurs*. 2017; 47(9):34-40.

Stanhope M, Lancaster J. *Public Health Nursing: Population-Centered Health Care in the Community*. 9th ed. St. Louis, MO: Elsevier Health Sciences; 2014.

Ten leading causes of death and injury. Centers for Disease Control and Prevention. https://www.cdc.gov/injury/wisqars/LeadingCauses.html. Accessed March 26, 2018.

National Self-Help Clearinghouse. www.selfhelpweb.org. Accessed August 7, 2018.

Thompson GS. *Understanding Anatomy & Physiology: A Visual, Auditory, Interactive Approach*. 2nd ed. Philadelphia, PA: FA Davis Co; 2015.

Todd B. New CDC guidelines for the prevention of surgical site infection. *Am J Nurs*. 2017;117(8):17.

Townsend MC. *Psychiatric Nursing*. 9th ed. Philadelphia, PA: FA Davis Co; 2014.

Treas LS, Wilkinson JM. *Basic Nursing: Concepts, Skills & Reasoning*. Philadelphia, PA: FA Davis Co; 2014.

Ulbricht C. *Davis's Pocket Guide to Herbs and Supplements*. Philadelphia, PA: FA Davis Co; 2010.

US Food and Drug Administration. Changes to the Nutrition Facts Label. https://www.fda.gov/Food/GuidanceRegulation/GuidanceDocumentsRegulatoryInformation/LabelingNutrition/ucm385663.htm. Accessed March 27, 2018.

US Department of Health and Human Services. Healthy People 2020 Leading Health Indicators. https://www.healthypeople.gov/2020/leading-health-indicators/2020-LHI-Topics. Accessed March 28, 2018.

US Food and Drug Administration. How to Understand and Use the Nutrition Facts Label. https://www.fda.gov/Food/LabelingNutrition/ucm274593.htm. Accessed March 27, 2018.

Vallerand AH, Sanoski CA. *Davis's Drug Guide for Nurses®*, 15th ed. Philadelphia, PA: FA Davis Co; 2017.

Van Leeuwen AM, Bladh ML. *Davis's Comprehensive Handbook of Laboratory & Diagnostic Tests With Nursing Implications*. 7th ed. Philadelphia, PA: FA Davis Co; 2017.

Venes D, ed. *Taber's Cyclopedic Medical Dictionary*. 23rd ed. Philadelphia, PA: FA Davis Co; 2017.

Vitale BA. *NCLEX-RN Notes: Core Review & Exam Prep*. Philadelphia, PA: FA Davis Co; 2015.

Vitale BA. *NCLEX-RN Notes: Core Review & Exam Prep*. 3rd ed. Philadelphia, PA: FA Davis Co; 2017.

Weston D, Burgess A, Roberts S. *Infection Prevention and Control at a Glance*. Hoboken, NJ: Wiley Blackwell; 2017.

Williams LS, Hopper PD. *Understanding Medical-Surgical Nursing*. 5th ed. Philadelphia, PA: FA Davis Co; 2015.

Figure Credits

Chapter 1

Comprehensive-Level Question 4: Vitale BA. *NCLEX-RN® Notes*. 3rd ed. Philadelphia, PA: FA Davis Co; 2018, with permission.

Chapter 2

Question 28: Dunn HL. High-level wellness for man and society. *Am J Public Health Nations Health*. 1959;49(6):786-788, with permission.

Chapter 3

COMMUNICATION

Question 34: Burton M, Ludwig LJM. *Fundamentals of Nursing Care: Concepts, Connections, & Skills*. Philadelphia, PA: FA Davis Co; 2011, with permission.

PSYCHOLOGICAL SUPPORT

Question 27: Burton M, Ludwig LJM. *Fundamentals of Nursing Care: Concepts, Connections, & Skills*. Philadelphia, PA: FA Davis Co; 2011, with permission.

TEACHING AND LEARNING

Question 35: Wilkinson JM, Treas LS. *Fundamentals of Nursing*. Vol 1. 2nd ed. Philadelphia, PA: FA Davis Co; 2011, with permission.

Chapter 4

PHYSICAL ASSESSMENT

Question 40: Dillon PM. *Nursing Health Assessment*. 2nd ed. Philadelphia, PA: FA Davis Co; 2007, with permission.
Question 42: Courtesy of Kingfisher Regional Hospital. Kingfisher, OK.

INFECTION CONTROL

Question 21: Wilkinson JM, Treas LS. *Fundamentals of Nursing*. Vol 1. 2nd ed. Philadelphia, PA: FA Davis Co; 2011, with permission.
Question 24: Wilkinson JM, Van Leuven K. *Fundamentals of Nursing: Theory, Concepts, & Applications*. Philadelphia, PA: FA Davis Co; 2007, with permission.

SAFETY

Questions 29, 40: Wilkinson JM, Treas LS. *Fundamentals of Nursing*. Vol 1. 2nd ed. Philadelphia, PA: FA Davis Co; 2011, with permission.

MEDICATION ADMINISTRATION

Questions 38, 51, 56: Nugent PM, Vitale BA. *Fundamentals of Nursing: Content Review PLUS Practice Questions*. Philadelphia, PA: FA Davis Co; 2014, with permission.

Question 60: Wilkinson JM, Treas LS. *Fundamentals of Nursing*. Vol 1. 2nd ed. Philadelphia, PA: FA Davis Co; 2011, with permission.

Chapter 5

NUTRITION

Questions 34, 37: Nugent PM, Vitale BA. *Fundamentals of Nursing: Content Review PLUS Practice Questions*. Philadelphia, PA: FA Davis Co; 2014, with permission.

Question 42: Burton MA, Ludwig LJM. *Fundamentals of Nursing Care: Concepts, Connections, & Skills*. Philadelphia, PA: FA Davis Co; 2011, with permission.

OXYGENATION

Question 37: Wilkinson JM, Treas LS. *Fundamentals of Nursing*. Vol 2. 2nd ed. Philadelphia, PA: FA Davis Co; 2011, with permission.

Question 40: Burton M, Ludwig LJM. *Fundamentals of Nursing Care: Concepts Connections, & Skills*. Philadelphia: F.A. Davis Company; 2011, with permission.

FLUID & ELECTROLYTES

Question 29: Wilkinson JM, Treas LS. *Fundamentals of Nursing*. Vol 2. 2nd ed. Philadelphia, PA: FA Davis Co; 2011, with permission.

GASTROINTESTINAL SYSTEM

Question 38: Phillips LD. *Manual of I.V. Therapeutics: Evidence-Based Practice for Infusion Therapy*. 5th ed. Philadelphia, PA: FA Davis Co; 2010, with permission.

PERIOPERATIVE NURSING

Question 39: Nugent PM, Vitale BA. *Fundamentals of Nursing: Content Review PLUS Practice Questions*. Philadelphia, PA: FA Davis Co; 2014, with permission.

Question 43: Aldrete JA. The post-anesthesia recovery score revisited. *J Clin Anesth*. 1995;7(1):89-91, with permission from Elsevier.

Question 47: Wilkinson JM, Treas LS. *Fundamentals of Nursing*. Vol 2. 2nd ed. Philadelphia, PA: FA Davis Co; 2011, with permission.

Chapter 6

HOT-SPOT ITEMS

Question 2: Burton MA, Ludwig LJM. *Fundamentals of Nursing Care: Concepts, Connections, & Skills*. Philadelphia, PA: FA Davis Co; 2011, with permission.

Question 3: Dillon P. *Nursing Health Assessment*. 2nd ed. Philadelphia, PA: FA Davis Co; 2007, with permission.

Question 8: Wilkinson JM, Treas LS. *Fundamentals of Nursing*. Vol 2. 2nd ed. Philadelphia, PA: FA Davis Co; 2011, with permission.

GRAPHIC ITEMS

Questions 4, 7: Burton MA, Ludwig LJM. *Fundamentals of Nursing Care: Concepts, Connections, & Skills*. Philadelphia, PA: FA Davis Co; 2011, with permission.

Question 8: Wilkinson JM, Treas LS. *Fundamentals of Nursing*. Vol 2. 2nd ed. Philadelphia, PA: FA Davis Co; 2011, with permission.

Chapter 7

Question 37: Wilkinson JM, Treas LS. *Fundamentals of Nursing*. Vol 2. 2nd ed. Philadelphia, PA: FA Davis Co; 2011, with permission.

Questions 45, 64, 92: Burton MA, Ludwig LJM. *Fundamentals of Nursing Care: Concepts, Connections, & Skills*. Philadelphia, PA: FA Davis Co; 2011, with permission.

Index